Rhinologic Diagnosis and Treatment

RHINOLOGY AND SINUSOLOGY
Diagnosis • Medical Management • Surgical Approaches

Series Editor

Howard L. Levine, M.D., F.A.C.S.
Director, The Mt. Sinai Nasal-Sinus Center
Chief, Section of Nasal-Sinus Surgery
The Mt. Sinai Medical Center
Cleveland, Ohio

Rhinologic Diagnosis and Treatment

Thomas V. McCaffrey, M.D., Ph.D.
Department of Otorhinolaryngology—Head and Neck Surgery
Mayo Clinic

Professor of Otolaryngology
Mayo Medical School
Rochester, Minnesota

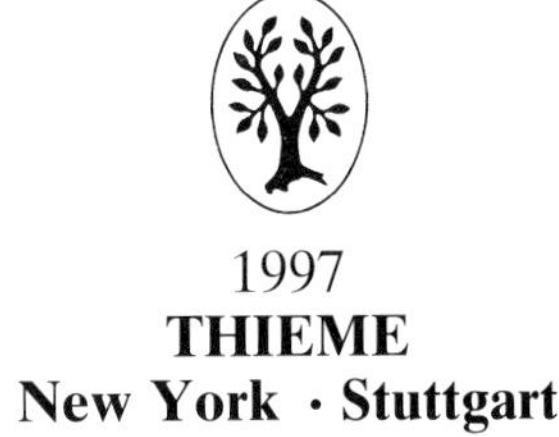

1997
THIEME
New York · Stuttgart

Thieme
381 Park Avenue South
New York, New York 10016

RHINOLOGIC DIAGNOSIS
Thomas V. McCaffrey

Library of Congress Cataloging-in-Publication Data
Rhinologic diagnosis and treatment / [edited by] Thomas V. McCaffrey.
       p.   cm.—(Rhinology and sinusology)
    Includes bibliographical references and index.
    ISBN 0-86577-619-9.—ISBN 3-13-103661-3
    1. Nose—Diseases—Diagnosis. 2. Paranasal sinuses—Diseases—Diagnosis.
    I. McCaffrey, Thomas Vincent. II. Series.
    [DNLM: 1. Nose Diseases—diagnosis. 2. Nose—physiology. WV 300
    R473   1996]
    RF345.R48   1996
    616.2'12075—dc20
    DNLM/DLC
    for Library of Congress   96-14922
                                                             CIP

Important note: Medical knowledge is ever-changing. As new research and clinical experience broaden our knowledge, changes in treatment and drug therapy may be required. The editors of the material herein have consulted sources believed to be reliable in their efforts to provide information that is complete and in accord with the standards accepted at the time of publication. However, in view of the possibility of human error by the authors, editors, or publisher of the work herein, or changes in medical knowledge, neither the editors or the publisher, nor any other party who has been involved in the preparation of this work, warrants that the information contained herein is in every respect accurate or complete, and they are not responsible for any errors or omissions or for the results obtained from use of such information. Readers are encouraged to confirm the information contained herein with other sources. For example, readers are advised to check the product information sheet included in the package of each drug they plan to administer to be certain that the information contained in this publication is accurate and that changes have not been made in the recommended dose or in the contraindications for administration. This recommendation is of particular importance in connection with new or infrequently used drugs.

Some of the product names, patents, and registered designs referred to in this book are in fact registered trademarks or proprietary names even though specific reference to this fact is not always made in the text. Therefore, the appearance of a name without designation as proprietary is not to be construed as a representation by the publisher that it is in the public domain.

Printed in the United States of America.

5   4   3   2   1

TMP ISBN 0-86577-619-9
GTV ISBN 3-13-103661-3

Contents

Contributors

Morgan Andersson, M.D., Ph.D.
University Hospital
Lund, Sweden

Fuad M. Baroody, M.D.
Departments of Otolaryngology
  and Pediatrics
University of Chicago
Pritzker School of Medicine
Chicago, Illinois

Holly H. Birdsall, M.D., Ph.D.
Department of Otolaryngology
Baylor University
Houston, Texas

T. Buisseret, M.D.
ENT Department
A.Z.-V.U.B.
Brussels, Belgium

P.A.R. Clement, M.D., Ph.D.
ENT Department
A.Z.-V.U.B.
Brussels, Belgium

D. Thane Cody II, M.D.
Department of Otorhinolaryngology
Mayo Clinic
Rochester, Minnesota

Jacquelynne P. Corey, M.D., F.A.C.S.
Department of Otolaryngology
University of Chicago
Chicago, Illinois

Kathelyne G. Delsupehe, M.D.
Department of Otolaryngology
Loyola University
Maywood, Illinois

Pamela M. Eller, M.A.
Department of Otolaryngology
University of Colorado
Denver, Colorado

Lennart Greiff, M.D., Ph.D.
University Hospital
Lund, Sweden

Anil Gungor, M.D.
Department of Otolaryngology
University of Chicago
Chicago, Illinois

A.R. Halama, M.D., Ph.D.
ENT Department
A.Z.-V.U.B.
Brussels, Belgium

Seok-Chan Hong, M.D.
Department of Otolaryngology
Kon-nuk University
College of Medicine
Chungbuk-do, Korea

Bruce W. Jafek, M.D.
Department of Otolaryngology
University of Colorado
Denver, Colorado

Edward W. Johnson, Ph.D.
Department of Otolaryngology
University of Colorado
Denver, Colorado

Jan L. Kasperbauer, M.D.
Department of Otorhinolaryngology
Mayo Clinic
Rochester, Minnesota

Eugene B. Kern, M.D.
Department of Otorhinolaryngology
Mayo Clinic
Rochester, Minnesota

David A. Khan, M.D.
Department of Otorhinolaryngology
Mayo Clinic
Rochester, Minnesota

Heinrich G. Lenders, Ph.D.
Ulm/Donau, Germany

Donald A. Leopold, M.D.
Department of Otolaryngology
Johns Hopkins University
Baltimore, Maryland

Sven Lindberg, M.D., Ph.D.
University Hospital
Lund, Sweden

Miriam R. Linschoten, Ph.D.
Department of Otolaryngology
University of Colorado
Denver, Colorado

Thomas V. McCaffrey, M.D., Ph.D.
Department of Otorhinolaryngology
Mayo Clinic
Rochester, Minnesota

Thomas J. McDonald, M.D.
Chair, Department of
  Otorhinolaryngology
Mayo Clinic
Rochester, Minnesota

Kerry D. Olsen, M.D.
Department of Otorhinolaryngology
Mayo Clinic
Rochester, Minnesota

John F. Pallanch, M.D.
Surgical Consultants, P.C.
Sioux City, Iowa

Carl Persson, Ph.D.
University Hospital
Lund, Sweden

Wolfgang Pirsig, M.D.
ENT Clinic
University of Ulm
Ulm, Germany

Saeed Sheikhali, M.D.
Department of Otolaryngology
University of Colorado
Denver, Colorado

David H. Slavit, M.D.
Veterans Affairs Medical Center
Brooklyn, New York

James A. Stankiewicz, M.D.
Department of Otolaryngology
Loyola University
Maywood, Illinois

Christer Svensson, M.D., Ph.D.
University Hospital
Lund, Sweden

Foreword

Rhinology and sinusology continue to generate interest for the general otolaryngologist and subspecialist. Numerous conferences, courses, workshops, journals, and textbooks provide ongoing updated information for the practitioner. This series, *Rhinology and Sinusology*, attempts to provide an ongoing method through which information may be gathered, summarized, and collated into a usable format for the health provider. The series attempts to include new topics, and at other times, material which merely has never been brought together within one volume.

Rhinologic Diagnosis and Treatment is one of the latest in this series. Thomas V. McCaffrey, M.D., Ph.D., has edited a volume which encompasses many well known methods of nasal diagnosis with some newer and less well known techniques. Topics such as olfaction, nasal imaging, nasal endoscopy, and objective testing of nasal function are included. Many less common nasal and sinus problems are discussed in several chapters. Some more complex nasal and sinus problems are also included, such as nose and sleep apnea, cerebrospinal fluid rhinorrhea, diagnosis and management of the difficult and unusual infection, trauma, neoplasia, vasculitis, granulomatous disease, and the pediatric patient.

This textbook should serve as aboth a volume which may be read and studied in its entirety, or which may be used as a quick and specific reference guide. It should be valuable for students and health practitioners with all levels of interest in rhinology and sinusology.

Howard L. Levine, M.D., F.A.C.S.

Preface

Largely due to recent developments in endoscopic sinus surgery and aesthetic nasal surgery, there has been a general renaissance in rhinology that has led to the reestablishment of its status as an equal in the triumvirate of otology, rhinology, and laryngology. With advances in the basic understanding of rhinologic disease have come improvements and innovation in all areas of rhinologic diagnosis and treatment. Diagnostic techniques which were not available just a few years ago are now regularly applied to the diagnosis of nasal disease. Detailed descriptions of these methods have only been available in widely scattered specialty journals because of the rapid innovation and development of new techniques. Now appears to be a good time to bring together in a comprehensive volume the latest techniques and methods used to diagnose nasal disease and quantify nasal function. This book has been produced to be a comprehensive collection of the most current applications of diagnostic methodology to rhinologic disease.

The book's nineteen chapters have been divided into two major sections. The first section of the book deals with the technical aspects of specific diagnostic methodologies. These include the diagnosis of olfactory disorders both using histopathologic techniques and sensory assessment covered in the first two chapters. The next few chapters deal with the anatomical and functional assessment of the nasal airway using rhinomanometry, acoustic rhinometry, imaging, and endoscopic techniques. The epithelium of the nasal airway is the interface between the environment and the organism, and its assessment is treated in the two chapters that follow. These present the diagnostic techniques for mucociliary function and mucosal cytology. Finally, the diagnosis of nasal allergy by skin testing, in vitro testing, and nasal challenge is covered in the final chapters of the first section of the book.

The second section of the book approaches nasal diagnosis from a disease oriented perspective. The chapters in this part of the book emphasize the clinical use of the diagnostic techniques described in the first part. Chapters are devoted to difficult clinical areas were nasal diagnostic testing is essential in treatment planning. These chapters cover obstructive sleep apnea, cerebrospinal fluid rhinorrhea, bacterial infections, fungal infections, allergic fungal sinusitis, neoplasms, trauma, and the vasculidites affecting the upper airway.

To achieve a balanced international perspective, authors from both North America and Europe have been included. It is hoped that this book, by providing a compendium of diagnostic methodologies, will demonstrate the depth and extent of modern rhinology. It should be useful to clinicians wishing to implement these diagnostic techniques, as well as provide a starting point for those advancing the art and science of rhinology in the future.

Thomas V. McCaffrey, M.D., Ph.D.

Histopathology of Olfactory Mucosa

BRUCE W. JAFEK, M.D.
PAMELA M. ELLER, M.A.
EDWARD W. JOHNSON, Ph.D.
MIRIAM R. LINSCHOTEN, Ph.D.
SAEED SHEIKHALI, M.D.

More than 2 million adult Americans have a chemosensory disorder, primarily a smell deficit. As a means to better understand the nature of the dysfunction, as a guide to both cause and therapy, biopsy of the olfactory epithelium was developed in 1982 as a research tool.[1] The original hypothesis was that olfactory dysfunction is due to histopathologic change, a logical extension of Virchow's postulate that dysfunction is due to structural abnormality.[2] Electron microscopic study of specimens confirmed that, indeed, dysfunction was associated with histopathologic change and that the specific type of change correlated with the cause of the dysfunction. This observation served as a guide to pathogenesis and therapy, allowing improvement in the care of patients. This chapter discusses the histopathologic changes in several of these disorders and their implications for management. Additional evaluation and understanding of olfactory dysfunction require subsequent immunohistochemical and genetic analyses of the dysfunctional receptors or central processing mechanism, studies that are ongoing.

PRELIMINARY EVALUATION

Before a biopsy specimen is obtained, the patient with a chemosensory complaint completes a detailed history and undergoes a focused and pertinent general physical examination.

At the Rocky Mountain Taste and Smell Center (RMTSC), the evaluation is initiated by completion of the AChemS Multicenter history. Because this is a "standardized" historical review, the data can be entered into a computer database, allowing interinstitutional comparisons and subsequent statistical analyses in reference to the findings. The physical examination includes a complete otolaryngologic examination of the head and neck region, followed by whatever neurologic and general examinations are indicated by the results of the first two portions of the evaluation.

Evaluation of chemosensory function includes a butyl alcohol threshold test, a seven-item smell identification test, the University of Pennsylvania Smell Identification Test (UPSIT), the Q-Tip spatial taste test, a sucrose threshold determination, a citric acid magnitude estimation test, and electrogustometry. The details of these testing procedures are not pertinent to this chapter and have been published previously.[3]

Radiologic evaluation of the olfactory system often consists of limited (5-mm cuts without contrast) coronal ethmoid computed tomography (CT), but with recent improvements in magnetic resonance imaging (MRI) technology, the central olfactory pathway area may be successfully imaged.[4,5] Truwit and Kelly[5] reviewed the pertinent neuroembryology and normal anatomy, followed by a detailed consideration of the MRI findings, in a wide variety of olfactory disorders. They concluded that "high-resolution coronal MRI images, both before and after contrast material, with and without fat suppression techniques, offer the best opportunity to study the olfactory bulbs and tracts." Sites of pathology (e.g., olfactory groove meningioma, olfactory bulb agenesis) are clearly apparent on these studies.

Other routine tests (e.g., complete blood cell count, chemistries) rarely produce diagnostic results in olfactory dysfunction and are not administered routinely.[3]

OLFACTORY BIOPSY

The olfactory epithelium occupies the anterior superior portion of the nasal vault: the superior $2\,cm^2$ of the nasal septum, the cribriform plate, and the superior aspect of the superior turbinate, or $1\frac{1}{4}\%$ of the nasal mucosa. This area contains an estimated total of approximately 6×10^6 total receptors; thus, humans are "microsmatic" relative to other vertebrates.[6] The olfactory epithelium is interspersed with respiratory epithelium, in a checkerboard fashion, and appears to decrease in total area with certain pathologic conditions (e.g., postviral olfactory dysfunction).

Obtaining a Specimen

The biopsy specimen is obtained while the patient is under local, topical anesthesia (usually 4% cocaine, although a mixture of xylocaine and ephedrine or other vasoconstrictor may be an acceptable alternative) from the uppermost epithelium of the nasal septum. Patients are told not to blow their nose for 24 hours and to avoid heavy lifting or straining (Valsalva maneuver) for the same period. Occasionally, minimal blood-tinged mucus is seen, but patients are cautioned to return if there is major bleeding (this has not occurred, to date). Subsequent follow-up evaluations have shown that biopsy is accomplished without loss of olfactory acuity.[7]

Processing of Specimen

The specimen, contained in the trough of the instrument, is immediately placed in fixative. Electron microscopy specimens are fixed in a solution of 2% glutaraldehyde and 0.6% paraformaldehyde buffered to a pH of 7.2 with 0.06 M sodium cacodylate. Preservation is improved by the addition of 0.05 M $CaCl_2$ to the fixative. Tissues are fixed overnight at room temperature, rinsed in buffer, and postfixed in Spurr's low-viscosity resin. Thin sections are cut on a Reichert UltraCutE ultramicrotome, mounted on Formvar-coated slot grids by the method of Rowley and Moran, double-stained with uranyl acetate and lead citrate, and examined and photographed with a CM 10 operated at 80 kV.[8]

Microscopic Structure

Five types of epithelium line the nasal (upper respiratory) passages in humans. Anteriorly, in direct contact with the environment, the epithelium is a keratinized, stratified, squamous epithelium. The subepithelial region contains sebaceous and sweat glands and the basal follicles of coarse hairs that aid in the initial filtration. Anterolaterally, the sinus cavities are lined by low pseudostratified respiratory epithelium, which is flattened and modified to a simple cuboidal type in some areas and contains a few goblet cells and a very few seromucinous glands. The lamina propria is thin here and blends in with the underlying periosteum. Posterolaterally, where the nose has less filtration/monitoring function, there is an abrupt transition to a moist, nonkeratinized, stratified, squamous eptithelium (mucous membrane). This epithelium is similar to that found throughout the oral cavity.

Superiorly, respiratory epithelium lines the nasal cavity from the posterior nasal vestibule (entrance of the nose) to the nasopharynx, superiorly up to the olfactory region. In the most superior aspect of the nasal vestibule, the respiratory epithelium and olfactory epithelium interdigitate irregularly, with "islands" of each surrounded by the other.[9] In the most superior area of the nasal vestibule, there is little respiratory epithelium. The respiratory epithelium is a pseudostratified columnar epithelium made up of ciliated respiratory cells, goblet cells, and intermediate cells with basal cells resting on a basement membrane. It is supported by a deeper, loose lamina propria. The lamina propria contains small blood vessels with a unique concentration of venous plexi and wandering blood cells. The function of the respiratory portion of the nasal mucosa, as opposed to the olfactory mucosa, is to initially condition the air before its entry into the lower respiratory passages through the action of filtration, warming, and humidification.

The human *olfactory epithelium* is a pseudostratified columnar epithelium resting on a highly cellular lamina propria, which extends down more than 150 μm to the underlying bone or cartilage and contains Bowman's glands (Fig. 1–1). It has no submucosa and consists of four major cell types: ciliated bipolar olfactory receptors, microvillar cells, support (sustentacular) cells, and basal cells. All except the basal cells project to the epithelial surface. In addition, occasional degenerating cells and wandering inflammatory cells, primarily lymphocytes, are present.

More detailed descriptions of the ultrastructure of the olfactory epithelium, and a comparison with that of the respiratory epithelium, and an analysis of the functional significance are available, but they are beyond the scope of this chapter.[9–11]

Pathology

The histopathology of the olfactory epithelium of dysfunctional patients confirms the hypothesis that olfactory dysfunction is accompanied by ultrastructural change that can be correlated with the nature and degree of dysfunction.

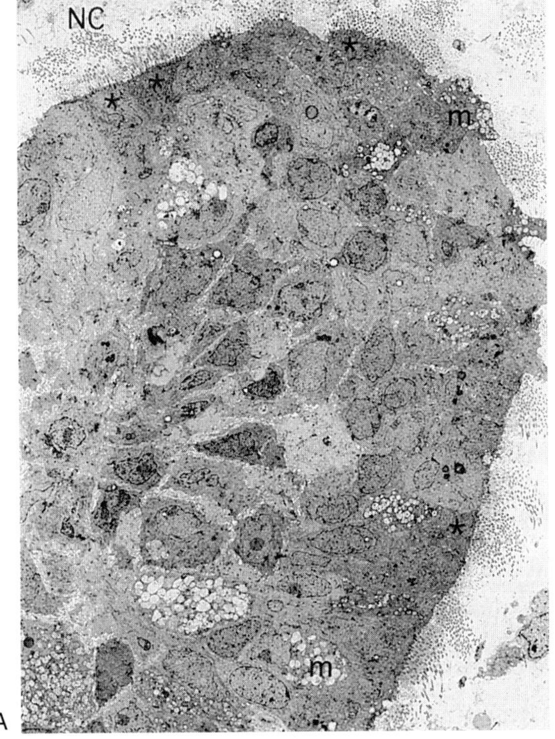

Figure 1–1.   Normal respiratory and olfactory epithelium. *A*, Low-power electron micrograph of longitudinal section through a biopsy specimen of *respiratory* mucosa. Note the mucous cells (*m*) and ciliated respiratory cells (*). The nasal cavity (*NC*) is identified. *B*, Low-power electron micrography of longitudinal section through a biopsy specimen of *olfactory* mucosa. Note the olfactory receptor cells (*r*) with their vesicles (*arrows*) projecting into the nasal cavity (*NC*) and support cells (*s*). Basal cells rest on the lamina propria (*lp*), below which a Bowman's gland acini is seen. *C*, High-power view of olfactory vesicle/dendrite (*OV*) projecting into nasal cavity (*NC*). The adjacent support cells (*s*) contain electron-dense vesicles and have branched microvilli projecting from their surfaces. The olfactory cilia (*arrowheads*) have basal bodies, and the axoneme has the usual "9 + 2" pattern of microtubular arrangement, centrally, except that the tubules lack dynein arms, indicating that they are immotile.

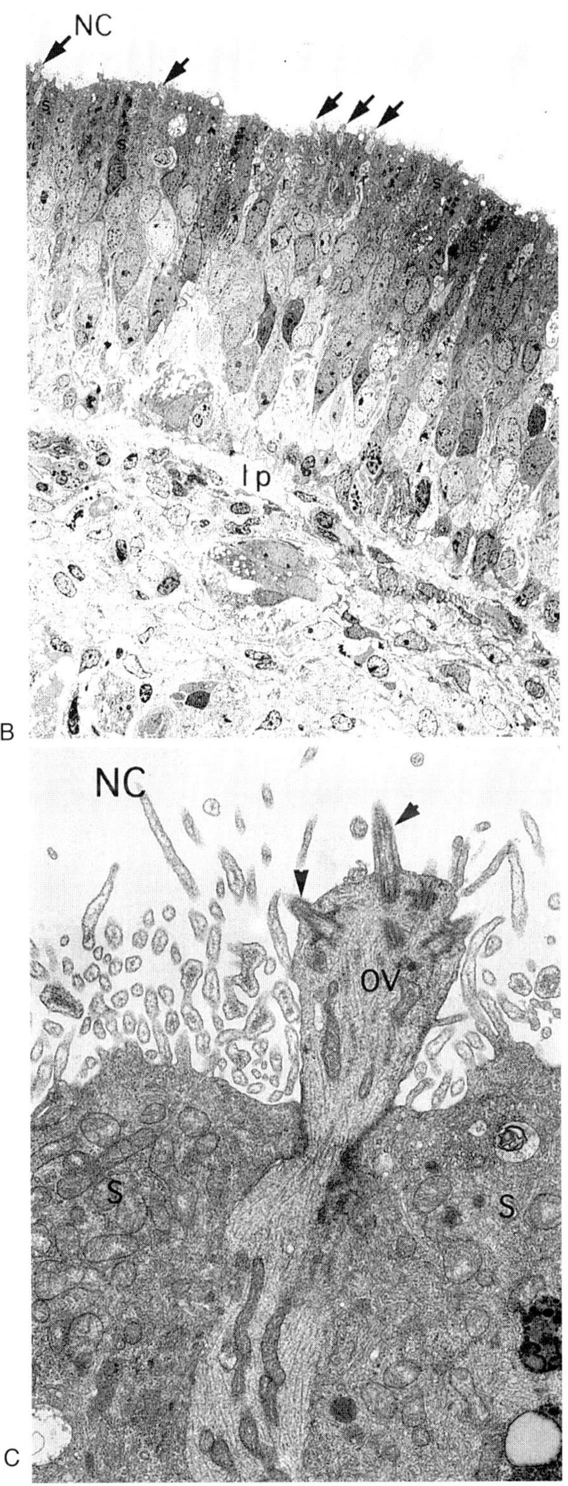

Figure 1–1 (*Continued*).

SINONASAL INFLAMMATORY DISEASE

The most common cause of prolonged olfactory loss is sinonasal inflammatory disease (SNID).[12] This category includes sinusitis with rhinitis, postviral olfactory disorder (PVOD), nasal polyposis, and allergic rhinitis, along with combinations of each. These processes usually affect olfaction because of the obstruction of the passage of odorants through the air to reach the olfactory epithelium (*obstructive* or *transport* losses), although a local increase in mucous viscosity (rheological index increase) or similar alteration of mucous, producing delayed odorant transit, may be present.[13] Physiologically, airborne odorants diffuse through the mucous layer of the olfactory epithelium to reach the cilia and terminal process of the olfactory receptor cells and reversibly bind to the receptor sites located on these structures. The binding of the odorant ligand to olfactory receptor proteins of the cilium is thought to induce a conformational change in receptor proteins that sets off a chain of intracellular events, resulting in production of an action potential that is conducted centrally, completing olfactory signal transduction.[14] When the odorant molecules fail to reach the olfactory epithelium because of mechanical obstruction, medical or surgical therapy is most promising. Alternatively, in PVOD, the defect is in the olfactory epithelium (*sensory* loss) or nerve (*neural* loss) or a combination of these (*sensorineural* loss), and the prognosis is not nearly so promising.

The most common historical complaint in SNID is that of fluctuant loss, suggesting intact olfactory epithelium, although with nasal polyps, the anosmia or hyposmia may be of long-standing, constant duration. Many cases are, however, fully reversible. Other specific types of loss, as mentioned previously, are not so reversible.

Chronic or Recurrent Sinusitis

Patients with chronic sinusitis usually present with recurrent postnasal discharge. Pain and fever, which occur with acute sinusitis, are usually absent during the chronic condition, but there may be a chronic "discomfort" in the area of the involved sinus (e.g., forehead in frontal sinusitis, teeth in maxillary involvement). There may be a history of recurrent sore throat, halitosis, or nocturnal cough. Systemic or predisposing factors for the sinusitis include recurrent acute sinusitis; cystic fibrosis; primary or secondary ciliary dyskinesia; Young's syndrome (thickened mucus); immune deficiencies; acquired immunodeficiency syndrome (AIDS); anatomic abnormalities; environmental and genetic factors; and hyperreactive respiratory lining, especially in patients with asthma (Samter's syndrome or triad asthma: asthma, nasal polyps, aspirin sensitivity).[15]

The cause of the sinusitis is obstruction, producing a recurrent cycle of secretion stagnation, ciliary and epithelial damage, and mucosal change. Physical examination often shows mucopus in the nose, although this may not be seen if obstruction is severe; this examination is greatly facilitated by the use of the nasal endoscope. Transillumination is inexpensive, but it is of limited value. Ultrasonography is similarly cheaper than radiography, but it is of dubious value, especially if the operator is inexperienced. Coronal CT of the ethmoid region is usually confirmatory of mucosal disease and extremely useful in planning the proper surgical correction of the obstruction. Even slight ostiomeatal complex disease (mucosal changes in the area of the ostiomeatal complex: infundibulum, uncinate process, bulla ethmoidalis, nasofrontal recess, middle turbinate) can produce significant olfactory impairment.[15]

Histopathologically, the olfactory epithelium is normal in chronic sinusitis, although the recurrent epithelial damage, or coexistent postviral olfactory disorder, may irreversibly damage the olfactory receptors, making the olfactory dysfunction permanent (sensory loss) even though the inciting factor, infection, is relieved. There is no way to determine whether the dysfunction is obstructive, sensory, or sensorineural without relieving the obstruction.

Surgery is usually indicated for relief of obstruction, relieving the sinusitis, with relief of anosmia, hyposmia, or dysosmia as a secondary benefit.

Steroid-Dependent Anosmia

One type of specific sinonasal inflammatory disease is steroid-dependent anosmia (SDA). This is a syndrome consisting of inhalant allergy, nasal polyps, and anosmia.[16] The anosmia is temporarily reversible by high doses of oral corticosteroids. In the past, SDA has been attributed simply to obstruction of the nasal airways by polyps, preventing odorant molecules from reaching the olfactory epithelium. Restoration of the sense of smell with steroids was "proportional to the amount of (polyp) shrinkage produced."[17] However, it has now been found that some patients do not have gross obstruction to neuroepithelium, as evidenced by fiberoptic examination.[16]

The workup of a patient with suspected SDA consists of a complete otolaryngologic examination (which usually shows nasal polyposis), detailed chemosensory testing (which usually shows anosmia or severe hyposmia on UPSIT testing), ethmoid CT (which usually shows extensive sinus mucosal disease), and a "trial of steroids." The authors' trial of steroids consists of a burst of steroids (prednisone, 60 mg tapered by 5 mg/day for a 12-day course), covered by a course of a broad-spectrum antibiotic (e.g., amoxicillin 250 mg three times daily for 10 days). In patients with SDA, restoration of the sense of smell is subjectively apparent on the third or fourth day of therapy, but the sense of smell is lost again after completion of medical therapy. In these patients, surgical clearance of a path for the odorant molecule to travel through the nose to reach the olfactory epithelium (e.g., polypectomy, ethmoidectomy) can be predicted to restore the sense of smell. Maintaining the sense of smell sometimes requires a small dose of topical (e.g., beclomethasone dipropionate) or systemic (e.g., prednisone, 2.5 to 7.5 mg/day) steroid. Alternatively, if the steroid trial is unsuccessful, restoration of the sense of smell surgically is unlikely to be successful, although the procedure might be indicated for other reasons (e.g., recurrent or chronic sinusitis), and the patient can be so advised.

A case report illustrates the typical patient with SDA. The patient is a 49-year-old man who noted that he became "slowly" anosmic 15 years previously. He had "always" had seasonal allergies and was sensitive to aspirin but did not have asthma.

He did not smoke. Nasal polypectomies had been performed 13 and 4 years previously and a septoplasty 3 years previously, improving his ability to breathe but not the anosmia. Allergic hyposensitization and topical steroids had not improved his anosmia. Chemosensory testing showed an UPSIT of 10/40 with a 7-item score of 0/0 [R/L]. Radiography showed pansinusitis. A preoperative burst of steroids, according to the regimen outlined above, subjectively restored his sense of smell, which then disappeared as the steroids were tapered. Intranasal sphenoethmoidectomy, followed by postoperative oral steroids (prednisone, 5 mg/day) maintained his sense of smell (UPSIT 31/40) at 1 year of follow-up, also greatly improving his nasal obstruction.

The histopathology of the olfactory epithelium in SDA is entirely normal (Fig. 1–2).[16] Specifically, the receptors are normal in number and fine structure. Thus, the pathogenesis of this olfactopathy is purely conductive in nature (obstructive or transport loss) but not specifically attributable to the bulk of the polypoid tissue. Simple polypectomy is unsuccessful in relieving the anosmia, despite the removal of most of the obstructive tissue mass. Oral steroids, however, temporarily relieve the anosmia but do not significantly or immediately decrease the obstructive mass, as does operation. The receptors are normal. Thus, it seems likely that the combined approach (operation plus medication) is successful because the steroids may produce a secondary effect in addition to their anti-inflammatory action, possibly on the olfactory epithelium directly, the surface of the olfactory receptors, the mucus in which the receptors are bathed, or a combination of sites.[16]

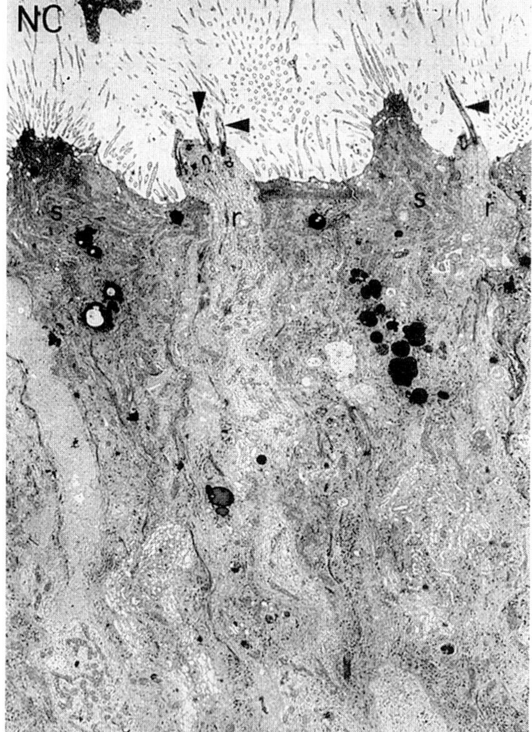

Figure 1–2. Steroid-dependent anosmia. Low-power electron micrograph of longitudinal section through a biopsy specimen of olfactory mucosa from a patient with steroid-dependent anosmia. The olfactory receptor cells (*r*) with their vesicles (*arrowheads*) projecting into the nasal cavity (*NC*) and support cells (*s*) appear entirely normal.

The therapy for SDA remains somewhat controversial in that postoperative steroids are required.[12] However, the important point, based on the histopathology, is that the receptors are intact despite the anosmia. In the patient with a positive trial of steroids, documented correction of the anosmia has been reported,[16] although the long-term success of this approach is unknown, and this can now be offered to select patients. The treatment consists of intranasal sphenoethmoidectomy, followed by long-term, low-dose topical or systemic steroids.[18–20] More recent observations suggest that the topical steroid is more effective if administered with the patient in a head-down-forward position.[21]

Postviral Olfactory Disorder

A second type of specific sinonasal inflammatory disease is PVOD. The olfactory loss in this condition is purely sensory (or sensorineural, if the nerves are primarily or secondarily involved) and is thought to result from viral infection and destruction of the olfactory epithelium.[13] This is in contrast to chronic or recurrent or allergic sinusitis, in which the loss is due to obstruction and is therefore potentially reversible. In PVOD, the olfactory loss acutely follows a viral-like upper respiratory tract infection. Surprisingly, often the patient knows the exact date of the loss and is able to remember and characterize the infection. The loss is most commonly partial, but it may be complete, occasionally with dysosmia, phantoms, or parosmias, usually unpleasant in nature. Women are more commonly affected than men, and all patients tend to be older in age.[15] The physical examination is usually unremarkable and directed at ruling out other causes of the loss, although Davidson believed that there might be some pallor of the olfactory mucosa.[22] Laboratory testing is not indicated in the presence of a characteristic history and absent positive physical findings.

Two brief case reports illustrate the findings characteristic of PVOD and are presented in detail. One patient was anosmic and the other was hyposmic.

A 75-year-old male nonsmoker presented 2 years after a bout of the "flu," following which he had noted persistent bilateral anosmia. He had otherwise been in good general health and was not taking medications. Nasal examination showed only a slight right septal deviation. No polyps were observed, and the nasal mucous membranes were moist without erythema. The results of detailed chemosensory testing (UPSIT: 11/40; butyl alcohol: no dilution [0/0] [L/R]; 7-item test: 1/0 [L/R]) showed that he was anosmic.

A 61-year-old female nonsmoker presented 18 months after having had a "bad cold," following which she experienced a partial loss of the sense of smell with some distortion (phantosmia). The decrease in olfactory function was immediate and stable after her illness. Detailed chemosensory testing (UPSIT: 32/40; butyl alcohol: 3/4 [L/R]; 7-item: 2.5/3 [L/R]) showed that she was hyposmic.

Olfactory biopsy specimens of patiens with PVOD show a very characteristic histopathology (Fig. 1–3).[13] In patients with *an*osmia, the olfactory epithelium is markedly disorganized. The primary structural abnormality is the greatly reduced number of olfactory receptors. Large areas of the epithelium are searched to find any receptors at all. Those that are present usually have dendrites that do not reach

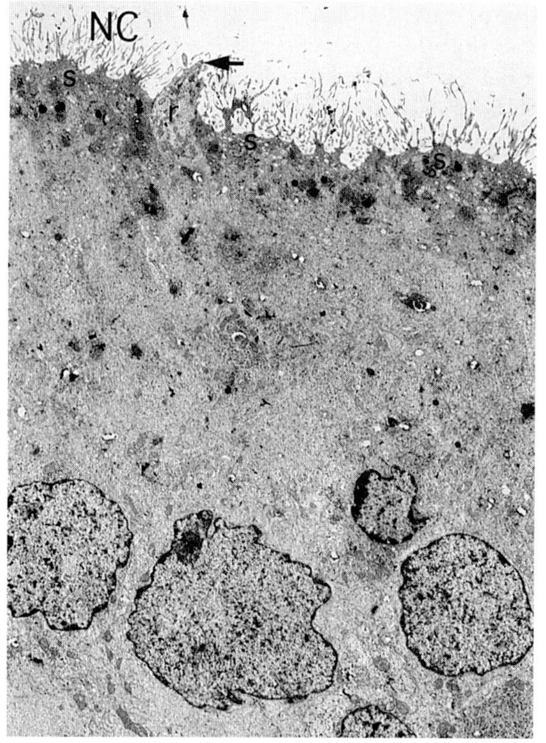

A

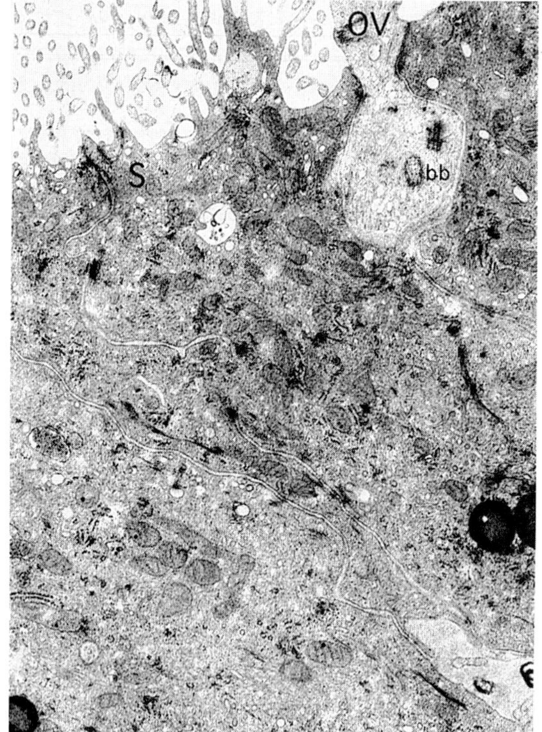

B

Figure 1–3.   Postviral olfactory disorder. *A*, Low-power electron micrograph of longitudinal section through a biopsy specimen of olfactory mucosa from *hyposmic* patient with postviral olfactory dysfunction (PVOD). The support cells (*s*) appear relatively unaffected, but the olfactory receptors (r) are diminished in number. The olfactory vesicle projecting into the nasal cavity (*NC*) has two relatively normal-appearing cilia (*arrow*). *B*, Low-power electron micrograph of longitudinal section through a biopsy specimen of olfactory mucosa from *anosmic* patient with PVOD. The support cells (*s*) appear relatively unaffected, and the olfactory receptors (r) are diminished in number. The single olfactory vesicle projecting into the nasal cavity (*NC*) lacks cilia, thought to be the site of olfactory transduction, although a single basal body (*bb*) is seen.

the epithelial surface. The occasional dendrites that are present at the free surface of the olfactory epithelium usually lack sensory cilia, the organelles believed responsible for bearing the macromolecular sites that function in sensory transduction of odorant molecules.[14] Our previous experience suggests that this finding is consistent with a receptor that has undergone regeneration but lacks central axonal contact with the central nervous system.[23] A single degenerating microvillar cell was found.[13] The support cells, while normal-appearing, are somewhat disorganized. The underlying connective tissue (lamina propria) appears normal.

In the olfactory biopsy specimens of PVOD patients with *hyp*osmia, the olfactory epithelium appears almost normal, with one major exception: the number of ciliated olfactory receptors and microvillar cells are greatly reduced, but not to the extent seen in patients with anosmia.[13] Where present, the olfactory receptors have the normal complement of basal bodies and intact sensory cilia on the olfactory vesicle. The dendrites of the receptor cells consistently contain large numbers of cytoplasmic inclusions reminiscent of myelin figures. Although the functional significance of the presence of these electron-dense bodies is unknown, their presence is remarkably consistent and limited only to the receptor cells themselves. Microvillar cells are observed. Their number, like that of the ciliated olfactory receptors, is reduced. Their structure appears normal. The support cells appear normal in structure and orientation, as do the basal cells and underlying connective tissues.

Hyposmic patients tend to have more olfactory receptors than anosmic patients; more of their dendrites reach the surface. Some of the dendrites possess sensory cilia, whereas others do not. The support and basal cells appear normal.[13]

These observations offer information on the pathogenesis of PVOD. The reasoning is as follows: PVOD clearly produces peripheral receptor/epithelial damage. The extent of this damage can be directly correlated with the degree of change in olfactory acuity. PVOD patients with *an*osmia have severely damaged or destroyed olfactory epithelium. PVOD patients with *hyp*osmia, however, have less severely damaged epithelium and receptors.

A possible mechanism for the observed histopathologic changes is as follows: respiratory viruses cause edema and hyperemia of the nasal membranes, necrosis of cilia, and cellular destruction.[24] This mechanism, followed by resolution of the infection and regeneration, probably explains the reversal of the occasional transient sensory loss occurring in the "usual" upper respiratory tract infection, in addition to the "conductive" loss caused by mucosal edema and increased mucous production. Recovery is generally complete in 3 weeks. In some cases, however, the destruction is more severe, and regeneration and resolution are incomplete.

A central destructive process (neural loss) might also be postulated. Although there is circumstantial evidence to suggest that in PVOD a virus or toxic products could ascend to the olfactory tracts or bulbs to cause subsequent degeneration and dysfunction, the clinical course of the disease does *not* support this. If the lesion were central, one would not expect some patients to slowly improve, which is often the course of the illness.[25] The clinical course of the illness is more suggestive of a peripheral insult that, over time, can improve as reinnervation and regeneration occur; this appears to be the case histologically. So, although it has been shown that viruses or their products can enter the central nervous system via the nasal epithelium, it has yet to be proved that a local viral infection could cause a central chemosensory dysfunction, either in humans or in animals.[26,27]

A combination of the two possibilities, peripheral and central pathologic change (sensorineural loss), offers an attractive correlation of the observed histopathologic changes and the clinical course of the disease. Graziadei[28] showed that interruption of the olfactory nerves is followed by regeneration of olfactory receptor bipolar neurons and central reattachment of their axons. Some of this axonal regeneration, however, may be displaced to the extent that "misguided" regenerating axons could reach abnormal locations in the brain.[28] This might be responsible for the distortion of olfactory sensation that occurs (e.g., phantosmia, parosmia).

Alternatively, destruction or regeneration of the olfactory receptors in a patchy, checkerboard fashion could produce distortion of the sense of smell by altering Mozelle's spatiotemporal, chromatographic orientation of the olfactory receptor sheet. Sorption of the odorant molecules could be changed, altering the central perception of the odorant.[29]

Thus, the data indicate that viral infection produces varying degrees of olfactory epithelial destruction. In the worst case, it may produce severe destruction of the olfactory epithelium, lack of regeneration, and anosmia. In milder cases, only patchy degeneration (or incomplete regeneration) occurs, resulting in hyposmia or pathologic changes that may be followed by complete regeneration with normosmia. Interestingly, the sensory neurons seem to be relatively selectively affected by the destructive process with preservation of the support cells. In some cases, faulty or patchy regeneration of the neurons may occur, possibly explaining the distortion of the sense of smell. Alternatively, the checkerboard distribution of the functional olfactory neurons may alter the sorptive characteristics of the receptor sheet, producing parosmia or phantosmia. Another explanation is that the virus or viral products may ascend via the olfactory neurons, possibly producing a central deficit or derangement, or abnormal axonal reconnections, resulting in distorted olfactory perception. Additional work with more specific neuronal tracers should offer additional information on the last situation. Specific viral "stains" or culture techniques may be helpful.[27]

The olfactory deficit can be correlated directly with the severity of the histopathologic change. The clinical correlation is that medical therapy is unlikely to alter the course of the disease. When severe destruction (anosmia) of the olfactory epithelium occurs, this appears to be permanent, and the patient should be so informed.

NASAL POLYPOSIS AND ALLERGIC RHINITIS

Considering only the olfactory deficit, an approach similar to that for steroid-dependent anosmia is used for extensive nasal polyposis and allergic rhinitis. A trial of steroids is used and, if positive, intact olfactory epithelium is probable. Intranasal polypectomy with sphenoethmoidectomy and follow-up topical or low-dose oral steroids should then maintain the normosmia. If inhalant allergies are diagnosed, elimination, medical management, or immunotherapy may be helpful. Management for other manifestations of these conditions (e.g., nasal obstruction, recurrent sinusitis) is dictated by the severity of symptoms. If, however, the steroid trial is negative (no subjective improvement in olfactory function), then the indications for operation are the standard ones, such as nasal obstruction and recurrent sinusitis.

CONGENITAL ANOSMIA

Congenital anosmia is defined as constant and lifelong.[30] Several forms of congenital olfactory dysfunction have been described, ranging from the inability to detect only one or a few compounds (specific anosmia) to complete anosmia. The best known form of congenital anosmia occurs in Kallmann's syndrome, in which it is associated with hypogonadotropic hypogonadism.[31] Genetically, this syndrome, reflects an autosomal dominant mode of inheritance with variable penetrance. The incidence has been put at 1:10,000 in men and 1:50,000 in women. Other developmental anomalies, primarily of the midline, include cryptorchidism, osteopenia, obesity, mild sensorineural hearing loss, cleft lip or palate (or both), metacarpal abnormalities, icthyosis, renal agenesis, and cardiac and intracranial abnormalities.[32,33]

Pathologic and surgical studies of patients with Kallmann's syndrome have shown absence of the olfactory bulbs.[34] More recent magnetic resonance studies have shown abnormalities of the central olfactory projections as well.[5] Laboratory findings include decreased levels of serum follicle-stimulating hormone and luteinizing hormone and decreased urinary gonadotropins.[32] Evidence from hormonal stimulation studies suggests that the defect exists in the hypothalamus with decreased production or release of gonadotropin-releasing hormone.[35] It was once hypothesized that the anosmia was the cause of the hypothalamic dysfunction, through lack of afferent innervation to the hypothalamus.[32] There is some evidence that odors activate hypothalamic factors, which then allow pituitary release of tropic hormones affecting gonadal and adrenal function.[36] Extending these observations, the olfactory bulb agenesis, which interrupts the afferent olfactory pathways to the hypothalamus, was thought to be indirectly responsible for the hypogonadal dysfunction.[37] Current theory, however, suggests that the anosmia and hypothalamic dysfunction are simply separate anomalies associated with the same syndrome.[32]

Two case reports are illustrative. In one case, a 16-year-old girl was not aware of ever having been able to smell. There was no history of any acquired cause for her anosmia. Subjectively, her sense of taste was unaffected. She enjoyed eating and did not avoid any particular foods. There were no associated congenital abnormalities nor delay in puberty. She was a nonsmoker. There was a possible history of anosmia in a maternal great-aunt, but this could not be confirmed. Composite chemosensory testing (UPSIT 14/40, 7-item test score 0/7 bilaterally, butanol 4/0 [R/L]) indicated anosmia, with some slight questionable function on the right side. Taste testing was within normal limits. Electron microscopic analysis of four biopsy specimens of the olfactory region showed only respiratory epithelium.

In the second case, a 19-year-old man had lifelong anosmia, associated with delayed puberty, and had been diagnosed as having Kallmann's syndrome. He was taking 200 mg of depotestosterone every 2 weeks and had finally achieved puberty. His sense of smell was subjectively absent; he thought that his sense of taste was slightly decreased from normal but was not absent. He had intermittent problems with nasal stuffiness and sneezing, consistent with rhinitis. He was a nonsmoker. Physical examination showed no polyps, and the nasal septum was in the midline. After olfactory testing (UPSIT 14/40, 7-item test 0 bilaterally, butanol 0/0 [R/L]), a diagnosis of anosmia due to Kallmann's syndrome was made. Four biopsy specimens of the olfactory region showed only respiratory epithelium.

Congenital anosmia may also be associated with other rare abnormalities, such as Refsum's syndrome. Specific familial anosmias for certain odors also have been reported.[38] Congenitally anosmic patients may, however, have no associated abnormalities, but only a few studies of such patients have been performed. In isolated cases of apparently "congenital" anosmia, the possibility always exists that some form of unrecognized or forgotten insult, such as a viral infection or trauma, occurred to the olfactory system at a very early age.

The evaluation of a patient with congenital anosmia consists of a general history and physical examination, followed by a detailed endocrinology examination, if suggested by the initial evaluation.

Biopsy specimens from seven patients with congenital anosmia showed only respiratory epithelium.[30] Leopold, however, identified olfactory epithelium in two patients with congenital anosmia, one with Kallmann's syndrome and the other with isolated congenital anosmia.[39] The mucosa was abnormal in both cases, consisting mainly of immature neurons (i.e., those lacking ciliated olfactory bulbs). The epithelium from the patient with Kallmann's syndrome showed disordered axonal growth and intraepithelial neuromas. There was widespread degeneration of olfactory axons, suggesting that neuronal turnover was rapid. These findings are consistent with the inability to make a synaptic connection with the olfactory bulb and suggest the diagnosis of posttraumatic anosmia, although there was no known history of trauma.[23]

In considering the pathogenesis of congenital anosmia, the usual absence of olfactory epithelium in association with normal respiratory epithelium raises the question of whether the olfactory placode is deficient, with no anlage for epithelium or whether this condition is produced by epithelial atrophy sometime early after normal embryonic development. The first possibility is very unlikely because the patients have normal nasal development. Because the nasal placode develops as a pit between the medial and lateral nasal processes, which subsequently enlarge and fuse to form the lower nose and upper lip, one can postulate that an embryologic malformation as early as 4 weeks, at the development of the placode, would produce a relatively serious congenital abnormality of the nose. The more likely pathogenesis is epithelial atrophy, possibly associated with an abnormal placode that invaginates normally. On the basis of the total lack of peripheral receptors or support cells, routine sampling of normal respiratory epithelium, and a review of the literature, the most likely explanation for congenital anosmia is a combination of the two previous explanations: the olfactory placode forms, possibly in a slightly abnormal state, and invaginates normally, and at some later date, the progenitor of the olfactory epithelium, or olfactory epithelium itself, degenerates partially or completely and is replaced by respiratory epithelium.

Therapy is focused on associated abnormalities, if present. The endocrinologic abnormality, if present, can be corrected by administration of exogenous testosterone, primarily to achieve puberty in the male with Kallmann's syndrome. Because no treatment is currently available for patients with lifelong anosmia, the main objective of studying these patients is to gain further information about possible causes, congenital or acquired, and to counsel such patients about the often unrecognized hazards of anosmia. Interestingly, most of these patients are not unduly distressed by their anosmia and enjoy eating. This finding is in distinct contrast to adults who lose their sense of smell, who often have an acute awareness of a loss of enjoyment in eating. Most of the patients studied lack any expectations that their anosmia can be cured. The intimate relationship of taste and olfaction is demonstrated by the fact that nearly all patients thought that their sense of taste was not as good that of other people, but gustatory testing showed normal taste function in all patients.[30]

POSTTRAUMATIC OLFACTORY DISORDER

The association of anosmia and head injury was first documented in 1864, but it was rarely reported until a major series of war injuries was analyzed in 1943.[40] Subsequent analysis indicates that as many as 5% to 60% of patients with concussion manifest some degree of anosmia, hyposmia, or dysosmia. The degree of dysfunction is often, but not always, proportional to the degree of trauma. The prognosis is variable, with rare cases of recovery reported as late as 5 or more years after the trauma. However, anosmia resulting from trauma is usually associated with a poor prognosis and is usually considered irreversible, particularly if it persists for more than 1 year.

The usual patient with posttraumatic olfactory disorder (PTOD) presents with olfactory loss and a history of "concussion" (period of unconsciousness after head trauma). Depending on how long the patient was unconscious and on associated injuries and length of hospitalization, the direct relationship of the observation of the loss and head trauma may be variable. No other cause for the loss is apparent from the history. Physical examination is normal, except for any sequelae of the trauma (e.g., facial trauma, cast). Radiographic studies have usually been completed coincident to the trauma and validate the degree of trauma (e.g., skull fracture, cerebral hematoma). Additional studies are rarely indicated.

A case history is illustrative. A 23-year-old man was evaluated 10 months after a fall from a roof, following which he was unconscious for several days. Skull radiographs at the time had shown a right temporoparietal skull fracture, and MRI had shown no evidence of intracranial bleeding or contusion. He had been hospitalized for 7 days and was recovering appropriately from a right humerus fracture, which was treated with casting. Approximately 3 weeks after the accident, he noted that he could no longer smell his morning coffee. Detailed otolaryngologic evaluation was normal, and there was no evidence of nasal trauma. UPSIT testing was 13/40, and Cain's 7-item testing and butanol threshold testing were confirmatory of anosmia. He was seen again 1 year after the trauma, and similar findings were observed. No specific therapy was instituted.

The ultrastructure of the olfactory epithelium from patients with PTOD is abnormal in three principal ways (Figs. 1–4 and 1–5). First, the general epithelial

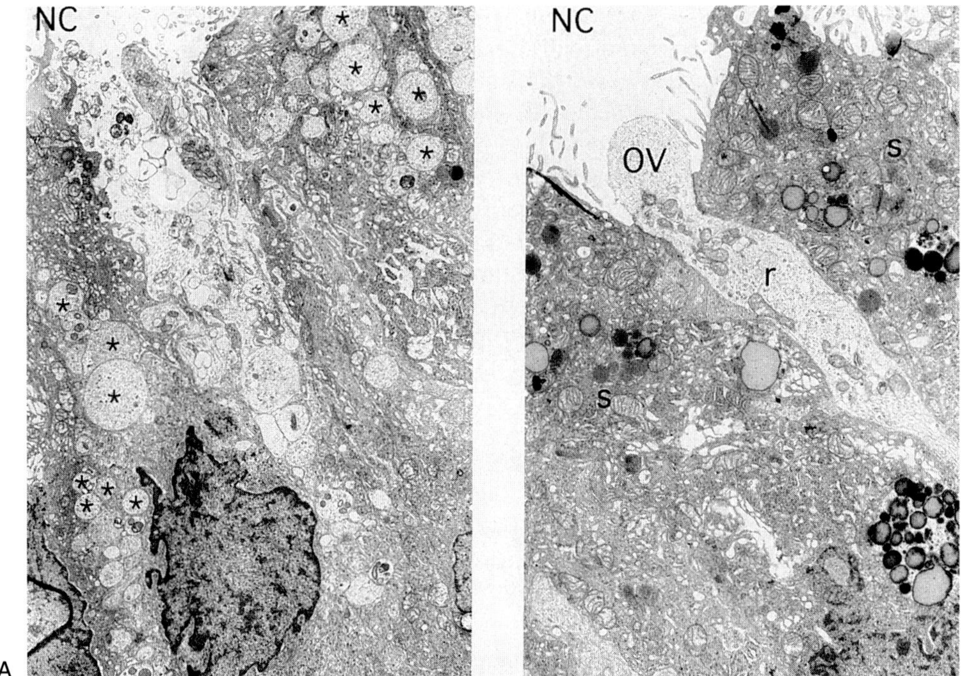

Figure 1–4. Posttraumatic olfactory disorder (PTOD). *A*, Low-power electron micrograph of longitudinal section through a biopsy specimen of olfactory mucosa from patient with PTOD. Axon profiles are seen throughout the epithelium (*). The support cells (s) appear somewhat disrupted, and the olfactory receptors are diminished in number (paler profile in center of photomicrograph) and often do not project to the surface (nasal cavity, *NC*). *B*, Low-power electron micrograph of longitudinal section through a biopsy specimen of olfactory mucosa from PTOD. The olfactory receptor (*r*) projects to the surface (*NC*) but is aciliate ("bald"). The adjacent support cells appear somewhat disrupted and contain increased amounts of electron-dense vesicles, the significance of which is unknown.

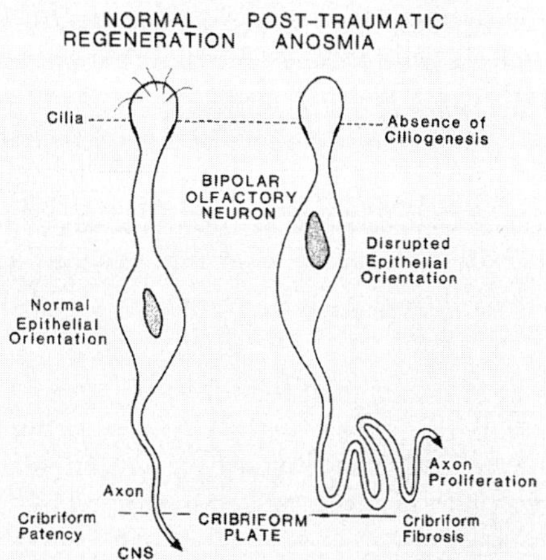

Figure 1–5. Posttraumatic olfactory disorder (PTOD). Changes that occur in the olfactory receptor cells of patients with PTOD. Three consistent changes are noted: disrupted epithelium, absence of ciliogenesis, and the presence of axon tangles, both below and within the epithelium. These are thought to result from disruption of the fila olfactoria at the cribriform plate, with subsequent fibrosis at the plate perforations and failure of axon regeneration centrally. CNS, central nervous system.

orientation is disorganized. The degree of abnormality varies from patient to patient and may, at times, be subtle. The epithelium appears thicker as individual cells are enlarged and bloated. The cellular nuclei, which are usually arranged in a band across the middle of the epithelium, are dispersed throughout the epithelium and may even lie close to the epithelial surface. Second, the PTOD epithelium contains many axon profiles, most of which are just below the basement membrane; there are some large nerve bundles in this region. A considerable additional number of axons can be seen throughout the epithelium, all the way to the surface. The axons are distinguished on the basis of their small diameter and the presence of microtubules and mitochondria. Third, olfactory receptors are diminished in number, but those that are seen are often "bald," lacking olfactory cilia projecting from their dendritic knobs (olfactory vesicles). Occasionally, basal bodies are seen within the vesicles, but cilia are almost nonexistent. In other patients, olfactory vesicles are absent and remaining receptors do not appear to reach the mucosal surface.

The three consistent observations in PTOD, epithelial disruption, axon proliferation, and absence of ciliogenesis, allow speculation on the pathogenesis of this disorder as well as the therapy of PTOD.

The epithelial disruption and disorder are significant and consistent with the appearance of regenerating epithelium. With rapid cell turnover and proliferation, the nuclear disorientation is characteristic of swollen, metabolically active epithelium. The increased number of axons suggests axon proliferation with failure to reach proximal synapses. Although we have not yet followed serial sections of these axons, their increased presence suggests that as the epithelium regenerates after head trauma, the receptor cells attempt to send axons centrally. Assuming that the cribriform plate has undergone fibrosis, after hemorrhage in the area, the axon is deflected back into the mucosa and submucosa, where it coils and possibly turns again toward the cribriform plate to attempt to achieve central synaptic contact with the olfactory bulb. The absence of ciliogenesis is possibly the most interesting finding. During embryonic development in mice, the sprouting of olfactory cilia (ciliogenesis) occurs approximately coincidentally with the receptor cell axon reaching synaptic contact with the central nervous system.[23] In fetal olfactory cell explants, ciliogenesis does not occur unless presynaptic central nervous tissue (olfactory bulb) is added to the culture, suggesting that ciliogenesis is dependent on axon contact with the central nervous system and initiated by some yet uncharacterized central ciliogenic factor. Conversely, the absence of ciliogenesis observed in the pathologic PTOD epithelium confirms the failure of the regenerating axons to reach the central nervous system, additionally supporting the observations of axon tangles previously described. All of these findings lend support to the hypothesis that PTOD epithelium is metabolically active, attempting regeneration, but that this regeneration is thwarted by fibrosis in the cribriform plate region.

Because of the above observations, it is suggested that patients with PTOD have traumatically severed their fila olfactoria in the cribriform plate region and that the olfactory epithelium is preserved and attempting central contact. Assuming that this is the case, it is unlikely that either medical therapy or additional observation would be curative. However, newer neurosurgical techniques might allow removal of the cribriform plate fibrosis with restoration of the sense of smell.[18] This theoretical approach would have to be considered carefully to prevent nasal contamination or infection from traveling the same pathway as the regenerating axons. Preventing this by using some sort of biologic seal might thwart the entire regenerative attempt, negating the operation. Additional evaluation of this proposal is warranted.

NEURODEGENERATIVE DISORDERS

In an additional group of patients, olfactory losses can be broadly grouped as due to neurodegenerative disorders. These include Alzheimer's disease, aging, Wernicke's encephalopathy/Korsakoff's psychosis, Parkinson's disease, stroke, and possibly epilepsy, multiple sclerosis, Down's syndrome, Huntington's disease, and AIDS dementia.[12,41,42]

Alzheimer's Disease

Alzheimer's disease is the most common degenerative disorder of the brain and the major cause of dementia. The disease is characterized neuropathologically by neurofibrillary tangles and neuritic plaques. Clinically, the disease is characterized by progressive deterioration of cognitive function. The diagnosis can only be confirmed at autopsy.[43]

The workup of a patient who potentially has Alzheimer's disease is usually conducted by an experienced neurologist and includes evaluation to exclude other cause of dementia, possibly including CT or MRI of the brain, electroencephalography, and appropriate blood studies. Olfactory studies may have to be altered to correct for cognitive identification deficits, with use of the Picture Identification Test to screen out patients too demented to allow interpretation of testing data.[43] Correcting for this problem in testing, patients with Alzheimer's disease are still shown to be anosmic or hyposmic, as compared with sex- and age-matched controls (necessary because patients with Alzheimer's disease are usually elderly).[44]

Histopathologically, olfactory biopsy specimens from patients with Alzheimer's disease exhibit three distinct changes (Figs. 1–6 and 1–7).[43] First, there is severe epithelial disruption. The normally organized appearance of pseudostratified epithelium is gone and cell types are often difficult to discern. Receptors are decreased in number, and those that remain often lack dendritic contact with the epithelial surface. Second, the support cells, although normal in number, often contain increased numbers of enlarged mitochondria and electron-dense particles. Finally, the most striking change is the presence of crystals overlying the surface of the epithelium at the light microscopic level; these stain metachromatically with toluidine blue. Radiographic microanalysis indicates a high concentration of silicon in the area of crystal deposit. Biopsy specimens of adjacent respiratory epithelium show no evidence of the crystals, and on radiographic microanalysis, no silicon is detected. More recently, olfactory epithelium from patients with Alzheimer's disease also has been shown to contain areas of increased activity to some neurofilament antibodies and abnormal neuronal structures, where-

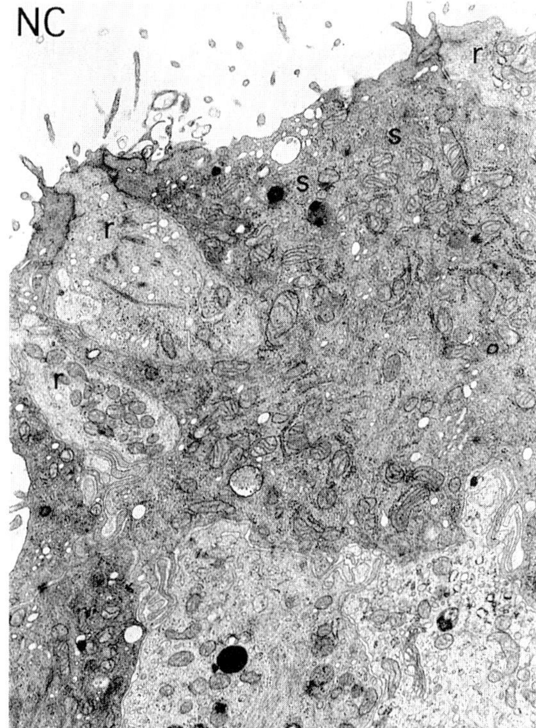

Figure 1–6. Alzheimer's disease. Medium-power electron micrograph of longitudinal section through a biopsy specimen of olfactory mucosa from a patient with Alzheimer's disease. The olfactory receptors are diminished in number (*r*) and often do not project to the surface (nasal cavity, *NC*). Cilia are often absent. The adjacent support cells (*s*) appear somewhat disrupted and are crowded with enlarged mitochondria.

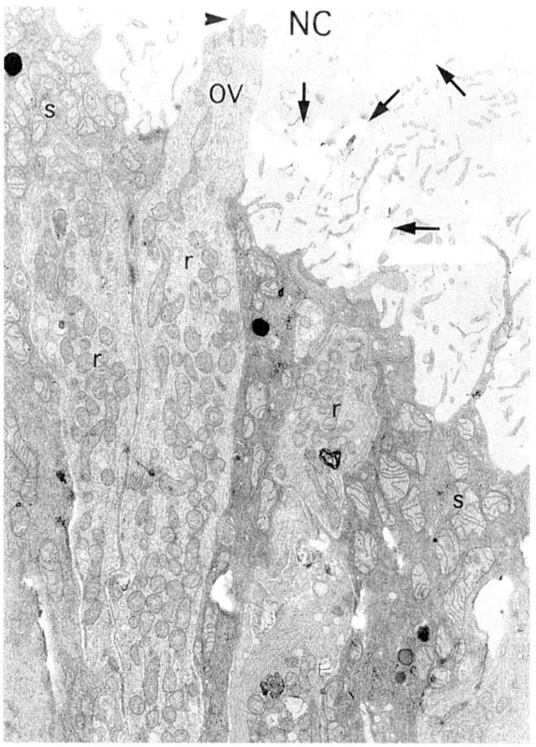

Figure 1–7. Alzheimer's disease. Medium-power electron micrograph of longitudinal section through a biopsy specimen of olfactory mucosa from a patient with Alzheimer's disease. One (*OV*) of three olfactory receptors projects to the surface (nasal cavity, *NC*) and has a single cilium (*arrow*). Cilia are often absent. The support cells (*s*) are disrupted and crowded with enlarged mitochondria. The most unusual (and consistent) finding is of crystals (lighter surface profiles because the crystalline material largely dissolves away in the processing) on the surface of the epithelium. Subsequent radiographic microanalysis indicated a high concentration of silicon in the area of crystal deposit.[43]

as normal olfactory epithelium lacks the neurofilament proteins.[45,46] Tabaton et al.[47] and Yamagishi et al.[48] have shown that the olfactory mucosa of patients with Alzheimer's disease contains tau- and ubiquitin-reactive neurites and concluded that the neuronal changes are morphologically similar to those in the brain.

More recent neuropathologic investigations indicate that the most extensive structural alterations associated with Alzheimer's disease may occur in the olfactory system.[49] Prominent changes (neurofibrillary tangles and neuritic plaques) are found in the periamygdaloid nucleus and entorhinal cortex major cortical relays for olfactory stimuli. Because the olfactory neurons are unique in that they extend from the environment (nasal mucosa) to the central nervous system, it is possible that they might conduct substances from the outside to the brain. Whether the crystals in patients with Alzheimer's disease are entering the brain, being released, or simply contaminants is unknown.

Therapy for olfactory loss due to Alzheimer's disease is not currently being contemplated. What remains interesting is the possibility of using olfactory biopsy for early diagnosis, possibly allowing the introduction of medical or behavioral intervention to ameliorate the effects of this devastating, extremely expensive public health problem. Brain biopsy to confirm the diagnosis is obviously possible only at autopsy, when the advantage is less apparent.

Aging

It is clear that olfactory acuity decreases with aging, as shown on UPSIT testing. In addition to absolute decreases in detection thresholds, the perception and identification of suprathreshold odors also appear to decline with advancing age. Women remain better at recognizing odorants than men, but UPSIT scores decline fairly markedly after age 69; this decline, however, appears to vary from individual to individual independent of age.[50] It is unclear, however, whether this decline is the result of a decreased number of receptors or of degenerative changes within the individual receptors. Morrison and Moran[51] suggested that the number of receptors decreases with age, and Trojanowski et al.[46] have shown dystrophic olfactory neurons in the epithelium of neurologically normal adults.

Other Neurodegenerative Disorders

Characterization of changes in other neurodegenerative disorders awaits further study. Trojanowski et al.[46] showed dystrophic olfactory receptors in Parkinson's disease, Down's syndrome, Shy-Drager syndrome, progressive supranuclear palsy without dementia, diffuse cortical Lewy body disease with dementia, schizophrenia, and idiopathic degeneration of the substantia nigra with Parkinson's disease. Patients with multiple sclerosis appear to have a preponderance of gustatory deficits, with smell impairment being less common.[15] Several other neurodegenerative disorders are variously reported to have associated olfactory losses.[38,42]

Patients with Parkinson's disease have been shown to have decreased olfactory acuity, independent of any age-related impairment.[52] Biopsy specimens from two patients in our laboratory showed only nonspecific changes in the olfactory mucosa, although there appeared to be some "siddness" of the changes related to the severity of symptoms (Fig. 1–8). Pharmacologic treatment of Parkinson's disease with dopaminergic or cholinergic agents did not appear to alter olfactory thresholds or acuity, a finding suggesting that the epithelial changes are not reversible.

TOXIC CAUSES

Patients with exposure to toxins and resultant anosmia or hyposmia usually remember the particular date and circumstances of the exposure. They characteristically describe the acute onset of pain and rhinitis, with immediate olfactory loss. Loss due to exposure to various liquids, mostly high concentrations of more volatile substances (e.g., formaldehyde, chlorine, industrial chemicals) and various powdery solids (e.g., cadmium, lead, potash, cement) is anecdotally described.[38,42] Few of the patients have undergone comprehensive chemosensory testing, and even fewer have undergone olfactory biopsy. The biopsy specimens that have been obtained have shown severe disorganization of the olfactory epithelium, metaplastic change, or replacement with respiratory epithelium.

Direct application of heavy metals, especially those with divalent ions, is known to produce olfactory dysfunction.[53] Both zinc and copper (interestingly, two of the

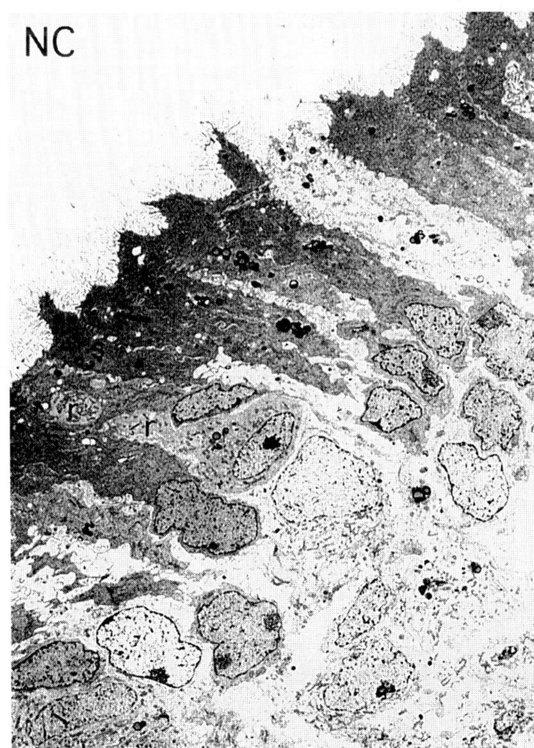

Figure 1–8. Parkinson's disease. Low-power electron micrograph of longitudinal section through a biopsy specimen of olfactory mucosa from a patient with Parkinson's disease. The olfactory receptors are diminished in number (*r*), and mild epithelial disruption is seen. These changes are nonspecific, but they are thought to be responsible for the olfactory dysfunction that occurs in these patients. *NC*, nasal cavity.

same trace substances in which deficiency is implicated in dysfunction) have been shown to be toxic when applied to the olfactory epithelium.

Cocaine abuse has been specifically studied. In the rat, cocaine exposure resulted in severe disorganization of the olfactory epithelium; in the human, however, this did not seem to be the case.[54] Eleven cocaine abusers were identified from a drug treatment clinic. Olfaction was assessed as described previously. Only one heavy user tested as being anosmic; this did not improve after 3 weeks off cocaine. One other patient had a normal butanol threshold but had reduced scores on the 7-item test and UPSIT. One heavy user had a large septal perforation, but was normosmic.

From this study, it appears that most cocaine abusers, even heavy users or those with intransasal damage, do not develop permanent olfactory dysfunction. It is not clear what factors may have resulted in complaints of olfactory loss in other studies. None of the patients had a taste dysfunction on gustatory testing.

OTHER CAUSES

Several conditions, which can be broadly grouped, have been described as causing olfactory dysfunction, although the histopathology of the olfactory epithelium, and therefore the pathogenesis, is poorly understood or unknown.

Endocrine causes of olfactory dysfunction include hypothyroidism, Addison's disease, and Cushing's syndrome, exclusive of Kallmann's syndrome, which was characterized previously.[42] Women with primary amenorrhea occasionally have coexistent anosmia.[38,55]

Hepatic dysfunction, such as cirrhosis, has also been associated with olfactory dysfunction. Whether this is the mechanism by which Korsakoff's psychosis and Wernicke's encephalopathy produce olfactory dysfunction is unknown. The olfactory dysfunction occurs with more severe cirrhosis, but it does not always occur. Some authors have suggested that the loss was associated with resultant zinc deficiency, and replacement therapy with zinc sulfate seems to help, but this was most useful for associated dysgeusia.[15]

Renal dysfunction, producing chronic renal failure and uremia, is sometimes associated with olfactory loss of varying degree. Some investigators have suggested that this loss was also associated (like hepatic dysfunction) with resultant zinc deficiency, and replacement therapy with zinc sulfate seems to help, but this was again most useful for associated dysgeusia.[15]

Metabolic and nutritional deficiencies have long been associated with olfactory loss (e.g., diabetes mellitus). Taste losses also have been described with pellegra and pernicious anemia. Henkin et al.[56] attributed the losses to zinc, copper, or magnesium deficiencies and recommended therapy with $ZnSO_4$ or $CuSO_4$. Zinc, vitamin, and trace metal therapy has since been widely used empirically. Double-blind, crossover clinical studies have been unable to validate the efficacy of this therapy, however, and it is not recommended except in the case of hepatic or renal dysfunction with serologic evidence of specific trace metal deficiency.[15]

Medication or medical iatrogenic causes of olfactory dysfunction are largely confined to single case reports and are generally poorly documented. Most classes of drugs have been implicated in losses (e.g., anesthetics, antimicrobials, opiates). The pathogenesis is poorly understood, and olfactory histopathology has not been described.[38,42]

Local or mechanical causes for olfactory loss include severe septal deviation, choanal atresia, local nasal inflammatory causes (e.g., syphilis, tuberculosis), and tumors. Unless the tumor specifically involves the olfactory epithelium or region (e.g., olfactory neuresthesioblastoma or olfactory groove meningioma), the olfactory epithelium is intact and normal, although developmental failure has been suggested, similar to optic atrophy, in early and persistent obstruction. In the murine animal model, closure of one nostril at an early age results in central atrophy of olfactory connections.[57,58] Whether this occurs in humans has not been extensively studied. Disuse atrophy apparently does not occur, based on preservation of olfactory function in laryngectomy patients.[59]

AIDS has been associated with olfactory loss, the severity of the loss being correlated with the severity of the AIDS.[60] Whether this is due to recurrent or chronic infection (peripheral destruction of the olfactory epithelium) or central involvement is unknown. Olfactory epithelial biopsy specimens have not been studied.

Psychogenic causes for olfactory dysfunction have been described.[38] The dysfunction is usually hyposmia or anosmia (e.g., due to depression), but *hyper*function also has been described. The structural basis for this dysfunction has not yet been elucidated, nor has the pathogenesis.

Other causes of olfactory loss, not clearly categorized, include cystic fibrosis (in which acuity may be increased), iatrogenic causes (e.g., radiotherapy, craniotomy), and sarcoidosis.[38,42] The mechanisms for these olfactory dysfunctions are unknown.

IDIOPATHIC CAUSES

Despite the lengthy list of categories, and even lengthier list of possible causes and associated conditions, there remains a group of "idiopathic" olfactory losses or distortions.[15,38,42]

COMBINED OR MULTIPLE CAUSES

In some cases of olfactory dysfunction, there appear to be two or several possible or actual causes. In these cases, the olfactory histopathology reflects multiple changes.

FUTURE

Olfactory marker protein (OMP) is a robust marker of olfactory receptor neurons. An antiserum was generated against OMP more than 2 decades ago.[61] Studies have established that OMP is expressed in olfactory receptor neurons early during development and in regenerated olfactory neurons in the adult. Although not done extensively,[62] OMP would undoubtedly be a valuable tool in studying olfactory neuron regeneration in humans; this would help in evaluating olfactory pathologies.

Complementing the light microscopic observations, immunoelectron microscopy has shown that OMP immunoreactivity extends into the cilia of the receptor neurons.[63,64] By obtaining biopsy specimens from patients with olfactory deficits and examining the tissue after exposure to OMP antisera, it may be possible to estimate the number of mature, and presumably functional, receptor neurons. Immunoelectron microscopy may be an aid in determining the morphology of OMP immunoreactive neurons in various conditions.

Immunocytochemical studies using antisera against nerve growth factor have demonstrated this growth and maintenance molecule in olfactory receptor neurons during development.[65,66] Nerve growth factor may be important in regeneration of olfactory receptor neurons.

Neural cell adhesion molecule and Thy-1, surface molecules that may be important in olfactory morphogenesis, have been identified on developing olfactory neurons through immunocytochemistry.[67] Immunocytochemistry has been a useful tool for identifying subsets of olfactory receptor neurons within the olfactory epithelium.[68–73]

We have recently observed subsets of calbindin-like immunoreactive olfactory receptor neurons in developing rats and humans.[74] These findings are consistent with reports on calbindin immunoreactivity in olfactory receptor cells in the rodent.[75] The role of calbindin in olfaction is not known. Nevertheless, these findings support the view that there are unique biochemical differences among olfactory receptor neurons early in development.

Some of the biochemical differences observed among olfactory receptor neurons may be involved in odor recognition and transduction of that information to the central nervous system.

Progress in identifying components of the olfactory receptor neuron transduction mechanism has included immunocytochemical localization of putative transduction molecules.[76–82] These types of studies will help define how olfactory transduction takes place.

Other proteins that are found in both neurons and neuroendocrine cells have been immunocytochemically localized to olfactory receptor neurons (e.g., neuron-specific enolase, protein gene product 9.5).

Immunocytochemistry has given us some insight into another cell type in the mammalian olfactory epithelium. This cell, named the microvillar cell, was identified originally in human adults by our laboratory.[10,11] The role of the microvillar cell is unknown. Future immunocytochemical studies, in conjunction with other tools, will identify the role of the enigmatic microvillar cell and thus contribute to our understanding of the olfactory system.

CONCLUSION

In conclusion, several important observations and clarifications are apparent from a review of the histopathology of human olfactory epithelium:

1. Nasal mucosa, both respiratory and olfactory, is unique. Although it possesses certain general and specific ultrastructural features similar to those of various vertebrate epithelia, a description of its features clearly indicates its uniqueness.

2. An exact understanding of the normal *human* olfactory epithelial ultrastructure is essential before embarking on an interpretation of the pathologic. We have described some previously unelucidated features of human olfactory epithelium: the existence of a fourth olfactory epithelial cell, the "microvillar cell," a putative second receptor; the absence of dynein arms on the olfactory cilia; the absence of olfactory pigment in olfactory bipolar neurons (and therefore its lack of functional significance in the olfactory transduction process); an ultrastructural basis for the "olfactomotor response"; and the presence of both branched and unbranched microvilli on both types of ciliated cells (human respiratory and olfactory).[10,11]

3. Human olfactory epithelial biopsy is an important, safe research tool.

4. Olfactory dysfunction is correlated with ultrastructural change; many histopathologic pictures are diagnostic and help to explain the pathogenesis and therefore provide a basis for therapy of the condition.

5. Studies of immunocytochemical, molecular, and genetic function will provide further insights into olfactory function and dysfunction.

Acknowledgments—Department of Otolaryngology-Head and Neck Surgery and Rocky Mountain Taste and Smell Center, University of Colorado School of Medicine, Denver, Colorado.

Supported in part by NIH/NIDCD #PO1-DC-00244 (Rocky Mountain Taste and Smell Center).

REFERENCES

1. Lovell MA, Jafek BW, Moran DT, Rowley JC III: Biopsy of human olfactory mucosa: an instrument and a technique. *Arch Otoloryngol* 1982; 108:247–249.
2. Goodman SR (ed.): *Medical Cell Biology.* Philadelphia, JB Lippincott Company, 1994, pp 1–23.
3. Hill DP, Jafek BW: Initial otolaryngologic assessment of patients with taste and smell disorders. *Ear Nose Throat J* 1989; 68:362, 365–366, 368.
4. Zinreich SJ, Kennedy DW, Rosenbaum AE, Gayler BW, Kumar AJ, Stammberger H: Paranasal sinuses: CT imaging requirements for endoscopic surgery. *Radiology* 1987; 163:769–775.
5. Truwit CL, Kelly WM: The olfactory system. *Neuroimaging Clin N Am* 1993; 3(1):47–70.
6. Douek E: *The Sense of Smell and Its Abnormalities.* Edinburgh, Churchill Livingstone, 1974, p 37.
7. Lanza DC, Deems DA, Doty RL, Moran D, Crawford D, Rowley JC III, et al: The effect of human olfactory biopsy upon olfaction: a preliminary report. *Laryngoscope* 1994; 104:837–840.
8. Rowley JC III, Moran DT: A simple procedure for mounting wrinkle-free sections on Formvar-coated slot grids. *Ultramicroscopy* 1975; 1:151–155.

9. Morrison EE, Costanzo RM: Morphology of the human olfactory epithelium. *J Comp Neurol* 1990; 297:1–13.

10. Moran DT, Rowley JC III, Jafek BW, Lovell MA: The fine structure of the olfactory mucosa in man. *J Neurocytol* 1982; 11:721–746.

11. Jafek BW: Ultrastructure of human nasal mucosa. *Laryngoscope* 1983; 93:1576–1599.

12. Seiden AM, Duncan HJ, Smith DV: Office management of taste and smell disorders. *Otolaryngol Clin North Am* 1992; 25:817–835.

13. Jafek BW, Hartman D, Eller PM, Johnson EW, Strahan RC, Moran DT: Postviral olfactory dysfunction. *Am J Rhinol* 1990; 4:91–100.

14. Lancet D: Vertebrate olfactory reception. *Annu Rev Neurosci* 1986; 9:329–355.

15. Duncan HJ, Smith DV: Clinical Disorders of Olfaction: A Review, in Doty RL (ed.): *Handbook of Olfaction and Gustation*. New York, Marcel Dekker, Inc., 1995, pp 345–365.

16. Jafek BW, Moran DT, Eller PM, Rowley JC III, Jafek TB: Steroid-dependent anosmia. *Arch Otolaryngol Head Neck Surg* 1987; 113:547–549.

17. Hotchkiss WT: Influence of prednisone on nasal polyposis with anosmia. *Arch Otolaryngol* 1956; 64:478–479.

18. Jafek BW, Hill DP: Surgical management of chemosensory disorders. *Ear Nose Throat J* 1989; 68:398, 400, 402–404.

19. Mauricio M, Davidson TM, Jalowayski AA, et al: Nasal disease and olfaction in chronic sinusitis patients. *Chem Senses* 1994; 19:515.

20. Seiden AM, Smith DV: Endoscopic intranasal surgery as an approach to restoring olfactory function. *Chem Senses* 1988; 13:736.

21. Mott A, Lafreniere D, Apter A, et al: Topical corticosteroid treatment of nasal/sinus disease olfactory loss. *Chem Senses* 1994; 19:525–526.

22. Davidson TM: Personal communication.

23. Farbman AI: Differentiation of olfactory receptor cells in organ culture. *Anat Rec* 1977; 189:187–199.

24. Snow JB Jr: The classification of respiratory viruses and their clinical manifestations. *Laryngoscope* 1969; 79:1485–1493.

25. Scott AE: Clinical characteristics of taste and smell disorders. *Ear Nose Throat J* 1989; 68:297–298, 301, 304–310.

26. Baker H, Spencer RF: Transneuronal transport of peroxidase conjugated wheat germ agglutinin from the olfactory epithelium to the brain of the adult rat. *Exp Brain Res* 1986; 63:461–473.

27. Monath TP, Cropp CB, Harrison AK: Mode of entry of neurotropic arbovirus into the central nervous system. Reinvestigation of an old controversy. *Lab Invest* 1983; 48:399–410.

28. Graziadei PPC, Levine RR, Monti Graziadei GA: Plasticity of connections of the olfactory sensory neurons: regeneration into the forebrain following bulbectomy in the neonatal mouse. *Neuroscience* 1979; 4:713–727.

29. Hornung DE, Mozell MM: Factors influencing the differential sorption of odorant molecules across the olfactory mucosa. *J Gen Physiol* 1977; 69:343–361.

30. Jafek BW, Gordon ASD, Moran DT, Eller PM: Congenital anosmia. *Ear Nose Throat J* 1990; 69:331–337.

31. Jones JR, Kemmann E: Olfacto-genital dysplasia in the female. *Obstet Gynecol Annu* 1976; 5:443–466.

32. Lieblich JM, Rogol AD, White BJ, Rosen SW: Syndrome of anosmia with hypogonadotropic hypogonadism (Kallmann syndrome): Clinical and laboratory studies in 23 cases. *Am J Med* 1982; 73:506–519.

33. Hermanussen M, Sippell WG: Heterogenity of Kallmann's syndrome. *Clin Genet* 1985; 28:106–111.

34. Males JL, Townsend JL, Schneider RA: Hypogonadotrophic hypogonadism with anosmia— Kallmann's syndrome. A disorder of olfactory and hypothalamic function. *Arch Intern Med* 1973; 131:501–507.

35. Soules MR, Hammond CB: Female Kallmann's syndrome: evidence for a hypothalamic luteinizing hormone-releasing hormone deficiency. *Fertil Steril* 1980; 33:82–85.

36. Schneider RA: Newer insights into the role and modifications of olfaction in man through clinical studies. *Ann NY Acad Sci* 1974; 237:217–223.

37. Rosen SW, Gann P, Rogol AD: Congenital anosmia: detection thresholds for seven odorant classes in hypogonadal in eugonadal patients. *Ann Otol Rhinol Laryngol* 1979; 88:288–292.

38. Schiffman SS: Taste and smell in disease. *N Engl J Med* 1983; 308:1275–1279.

39. Schwob JE, Szumowski KE, Leopold DA, Emko P: Histopathology of olfactory mucosa in Kallmann's syndrome. *Ann Otol Rhinol Laryngol* 1993; 102:117–122.

40. Jafek BW, Eller PM, Esses BA, Moran DT: Post-traumatic anosmia. Ultrastructural correlates. *Arch Neurol* 1989; 46:300–304.

41. Nordin S, Viazcan C, Ackerman K, et al: Sensory- and cognition-based olfactory functioning in Huntington's disease. *Chem Senses* 1994; 19:531–532.
42. Doty RL, Bartoshuk LM, Snow JB Jr: Causes of Olfactory and Gustatory Disorders, in Getchell TV, Doty RL, Bartoshuk LM, Snow JB Jr (eds.): *Smell and Taste in Health and Disease*. New York, Raven Press, 1991, pp 449–462.
43. Jafek BW, Eller PM, Johnson EW, Chapman MM, Filley CM: Ultrastructural changes of the olfactory epithelium in Alzheimer's disease. *Am J Rhinol* 1992; 6:219–225.
44. Doty RL: Olfactory Dysfunction in Neurodegenerative Disorders, in Getchell TV, Doty RL, Bartoshuk LM, Snow JB Jr (eds.): *Smell and Taste in Health and Disease*. New York, Raven Press, 1991, pp 735–751.
45. Talamo BR, Rudel R, Kosik KS, Lee VM, Neff S, Adelman L, et al: Pathological changes in olfactory neurons in patients with Alzheimer's disease. *Nature* 1989; 337:736–739.
46. Trojanowski JQ, Newman PD, Hill WD, Lee VM: Human olfactory epithelium in normal aging, Alzheimer's disease, and other neurodegenerative disorders. *J Comp Neurol* 1991; 310:365–376.
47. Tabaton M, Cammarata S, Mancardi GL, Cordone G, Perry G, Loeb C: Abnormal tau-reactive filaments in olfactory mucosa in biopsy specimens of patients with probable Alzheimer's disease. *Neurology* 1991; 4:391–394.
48. Yamagishi M, Ishizuka Y, Seki K: Pathology of olfactory mucosa in patients with Alzheimer's disease. *Ann Otol Rhinol Laryngol* 1994; 103:421–427.
49. Pearson RCA, Esiri MM, Hiorns RW, Wilcock GK, Powell TP: Anatomical correlates of the distribution of the pathological changes in the neocortex in Alzheimer disease. *Proc Natl Acad Sci USA* 1985; 82:4531–4534.
50. Doty RL, Shaman P, Dann M: Development of the University of Pennsylvania Smell Identification Test: a standardized microencapsulated test of olfactory function. *Physiol Behav* 1984; 32:489–502.
51. Morrison EE, Moran DT: Anatomy and Ultrastructure of the Human Olfactory Neuroepithelium, in Doty RL (ed.): *Handbook of Olfaction and Gustation*. New York, Marcel Dekker, Inc., 1995, pp 75–101.
52. Ward CD, Hess WA, Caine DB: Olfactory impairment in Parkinson's disease. *Neurology* 1983; 33:943–946.
53. Moran DT, Rowley JC III, Aiken GR, Jafek BW: Ultrastructural neurobiology of the olfactory mucosa of the brown trout, Salmo trutta. *Microsc Res Tech* 1992; 23:28–48.
54. Gordon ASD, Moran DT, Jafek BW, Eller PM, Strahan RC: The effect of chronic cocaine abuse on human olfaction. *Arch Otolaryngol Head Neck Surg* 1990; 116:1415–1418.
55. Marshall JR, Henkin RI: Olfactory acuity, menstrual abnormalities, and oocyte status. *Ann Intern Med* 1971; 75:207–211.
56. Henkin RI, Schechter PJ, Hoye R, Mattern CF: Idiopathic hypogeusia with dysgeusia, hyposmia, and dysosmia. A new syndrome. *JAMA* 1971; 217:434–440.
57. Webster DB, Webster M: Neonatal sound deprivation affects brain stem auditory nuclei. *Arch Otolaryngol* 1977; 103:392–396.
58. Maruniak JA: Deprivation and the Olfactory System, in Doty RL (ed.): *Handbook of Olfaction and Gustation*. New York, Marcel Dekker, Inc., 1995, pp 455–469.
59. Schwartz DN, Mozell MM, Youngentob SL, Leopold DL, Sheehe PR: Improvement of olfaction in laryngectomized patients with the larynx bypass. *Laryngoscope* 1987; 97:1280–1286.
60. Mattes RD, Wysocki CJ, Graziani, et al: Chemosensory assessment of HIV-infected adults. *Chem Senses* 1994; 19:514.
61. Margolis FL: A brain protein unique to the olfactory bulb. *Proc Nat Acad Sci USA* 1972; 69:1221–1224.
62. Nakashima T, Kimmelman CP, Snow JB Jr: Immunohistopathology of human olfactory epithelium, nerve and bulb. *Laryngoscope* 1985; 95:391–396.
63. Menco BPhM: Electron-microscopic demonstration of olfactory-marker protein with protein G-gold in freeze-substituted, Lowicryl K11M-embedded rat olfactory-receptor cells. *Cell Tissue Res* 1989; 256:275–281.
64. Johnson EW, Eller PM, Jafek BW: An immuno-electron microscopic comparison of olfactory marker protein localization in the supranuclear regions of the rat olfactory epithelium and vomeronasal organ neuroepithelium. *Acta Otolaryngol (Stockh)* 1993; 113:766–771.
65. Aiba T, Mori J, Nakai Y: Nerve growth factor (NGF) and its receptor in rat olfactory epithelium. *Acta Otolaryngol Suppl (Stockh)* 1993; 506:37–40.
66. Williams R, Rush RA: Electron microscopic immunocytochemical localization of nerve growth factor in developing mouse olfactory neurons. *Brain Res* 1988; 463:21–27.
67. Terkelsen OBF, Bock E, Møllgård K: NCAM and Thy-1 in special sense organs of the developing mouse. *Anat Embryol (Berl)* 1989; 179:311–318.

68. Fujita SC, Mori K, Imamura K, Obata K: Subclasses of olfactory receptor cells and their segregated central projections demonstrated by a monoclonal antibody. *Brain Res* 1985; 326:192–196.
69. Key B, Akeson RA: Distinct subsets of sensory olfactory neurons in mouse: possible role in the formation of the mosaic olfactory projection. *J Comp Neurol* 1993; 335:355–368.
70. Mori K, Fujita SC, Imamura K, Obata K: Immunohistochemical study of subclasses of olfactory nerve fibers and their projections to the olfactory bulb in the rabbit. *J Comp Neurol* 1985; 242:214–229.
71. Plank J, Mai JK: Developmental expression of the 3-fucosyl-N-acetyl-lactosamine/CD15 epitope by an olfactory receptor cell subpopulation and in the olfactory bulb of the rat. *Brain Res Dev Brain Res* 1992; 66:257–261.
72. Schwarting GA, Crandall JE: Subsets of olfactory and vomeronasal sensory epithelial cells and axons revealed by monoclonal antibodies to carbohydrate antigens. *Brain Res* 1991; 547:239–248.
73. Schwarting GA, Deutsch G, Gattey DM, Crandall JE: Glycoconjugates are stage- and position-specific cell surface molecules in the developing olfactory system, 1: The CC1 immunoreactive glycolipid defines a rostrocaudal gradient in the rat vomeronasal system. *J Neurobiol* 1992; 23:120–129.
74. Johnson EW, Eller PM, Jafek BW: Calbindin-like immunoreactivity in epithelial cells of the newborn and adult human vomeronasal organ. *Brain Res* 1994; 638:329–333.
75. Abe H, Watanabe M, Kondo H: Developmental changes in expression of a calcium-binding protein (spot 35-calbindin) in the Nervus terminalis and the vomeronasal and olfactory receptor cells. *Acta Otolaryngol (Stockh)* 1992; 112:862–871.
76. Anholt RRH, Mumby SM, Stoffers DA, Girard PR, Kuo JF, Snyder SH: Transduction proteins of olfactory receptor cells: identification of guanine nucleotide binding proteins and protein kinase C. *Biochemistry* 1987; 26:788–795.
77. Asanuma N, Nomura H: Cytochemical localization of adenylate cyclase activity in rat olfactory cells. *Histochem J* 1991; 23:83–90.
78. Asanuma N, Nomura H: Cytochemical localization of cyclic 3′,5′-nucleotide phosphodiesterase activity in the rat olfactory mucosa. *Histochem J* 1993; 25:348–356.
79. Jones DT, Reed RR: Golf: An olfactory neuron specific-G protein involved in odorant signal transduction. *Science* 1989; 244:790–795.
80. Mania-Farnell B, Farbman AI: Immunohistochemical localization of guanine nucleotide-binding proteins in rat olfactory epithelium during development. *Brain Res Dev Brain Res* 1990; 51:103–112.
81. Menco BPM, Bruch RC, Dau B, Danho W: Ultrastructural localiztion of olfactory transduction components: the G protein subunit $G_{olf\alpha}$ and type III adenylyl cyclase. *Neuron* 1992; 8:441–453.
82. Shinohara H, Kato K, Asano T: Differential localization of G proteins, G_i and G_o, in the olfactory epithelium and the main olfactory bulb of the rat. *Acat Anat (Basel)* 1992; 144:167–171.

2
Olfactory Evaluation

DONALD A. LEOPOLD, M.D.
SEOK-CHAN HONG, M.D.

Patients who have olfactory complaints require not only specialized testing of their chemosensory abilities but also a medical history and physical examination that assess necessary information related to this area. Because management and treatment of olfactory problems are dependent on an accurate diagnosis, it is important to gather and use all the information that is available. Figure 2–1 provides a flowchart summary of this process.

HISTORY TAKING FOR OLFACTORY CONCERNS

Patients with concerns about their perception of odors often have been shunned or have received an inaccurate diagnosis, perhaps because of a perception by clinicians that there is nothing that will help these patients or that the problems are psychiatric in nature. Patients are often reluctant to give reliable historical information about their odor concerns because it is a socially awkward area. If a considerate and empathetic attitude is maintained during the interview, much more useful information is obtained which will help in making the proper diagnosis.

Taste vs. Smell

Many patients initially complain of a loss of or problem with taste and smell. Both senses are likely mentioned because both taste and smell contribute in an additive way to the appreciation of flavor. In fact, the sense of smell is often responsible for 75% to 85% of the flavor of a meal. When a person licks a pink ice cream cone, for example, the trigeminal and taste receptors in the tongue determine that it is cold, smooth, and sweet. The sense of smell identifies the strawberry (olfactory) component of flavor. Early in the interview, it is helpful to determine whether the patient's complaint is related to gustation or olfaction. Rarely, testing is needed to assist in this determination. More often, testing is needed to document the degree of chemosensory dysfunction.

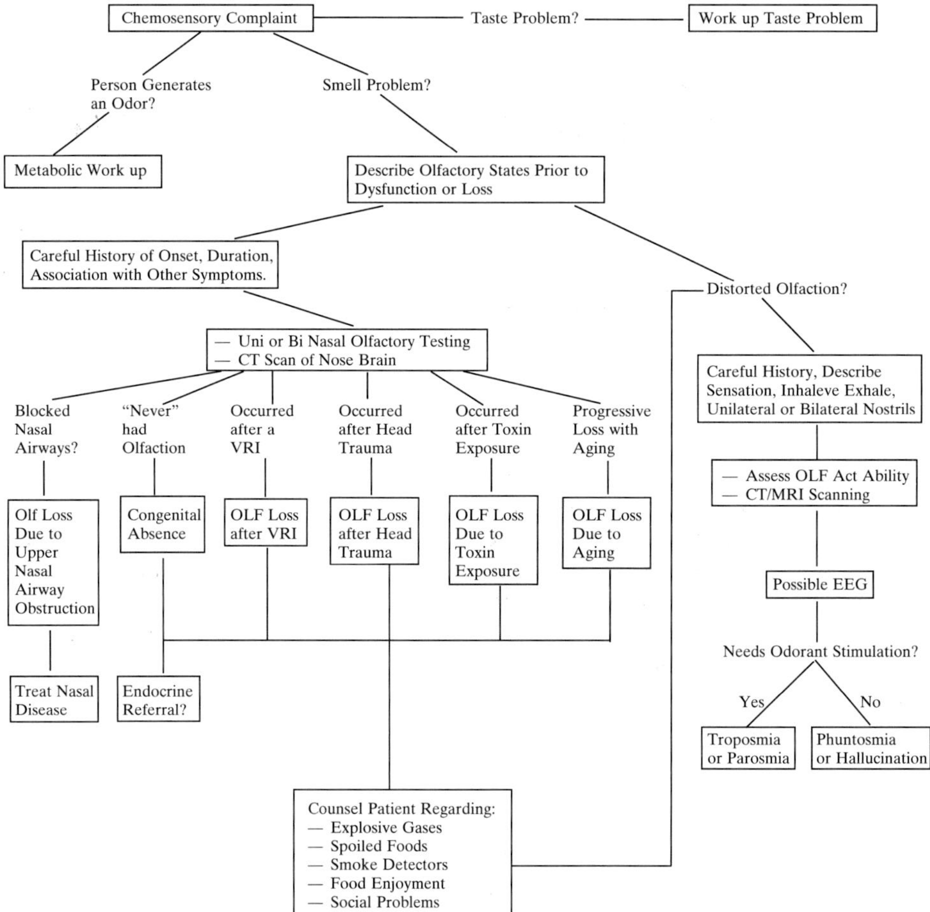

Figure 2–1.   Flowchart for management of a chemosensory (taste or smell) complaint.

Usually, even without testing, the status of the senses of taste and smell can be determined from the history. Questions about changes in food usage before and after the chemosensory problem began may reveal an increase in the use of salt or sweetener in someone who can still appreciate tastes but who has little olfactory ability. Similarly, asking the patient to describe the flavor of coffee (a warm, bitter liquid) and what amounts of sugar and cream, milk, or whitener the patient uses may help determine the problem. Additional questions about the flavor of salty foods like potato chips ("very flat" for someone without taste) or pizza ("like cardboard" without olfactory ability) can also help. It is rare for a patient to lose general taste (gustatory) ability; in most cases the problem is olfactory.[1]

Internally Generated Odorants

By carefully listening to the complaint of the patient, the clinician can differentiate patients who may complain of a bad smell or taste and those who **actually are** generally odorants. These rare persons usually have a metabolic problem, and the diagnosis can be established with special metabolic testing.[2]

Prior Olfactory Ability

After determining that the complaint is related to the sense of smell, the clinician should determine the status of the patient's olfactory ability before the problem began. Because patients rarely have had formal assessment of their olfactory ability, we ask them to list five odorants they remember smelling, like freshly cut grass, turpentine, manure, bath soap, or roasting turkey. Often they can even give information about the intensity, like "chocolate chip cookies two rooms away." An understanding of the patient's prior olfactory ability is useful for interpreting the results of olfactory tests, in legal cases, and for understanding the impact of the olfactory problem on the patient's life.

At this point in the interview, the clinician knows that the patient's complaint is related to the sense of smell and also the approximate level of olfactory function before the problem began. The goals are to identify what may have caused the patient's olfactory problem and, from this, make a diagnosis that will lead to a treatment plan.

Causes of Olfactory Dysfunction

Most olfactory dysfunctions result from six causes: (1) upper nasal airway obstruction due to inflammatory disease, (2) upper respiratory tract infection (due to viruses?), (3) head trauma, (4) toxins, (5) aging, and (6) congenital. Upper nasal airway obstruction generally causes only a decrease in the ability to perceive odorants (hyposmia or anosmia), which is potentially reversible. The damage to the olfactory system from the other causes can present as hyposmia or anosmia, a distortion in the perception of odorants (troposmia), a continuing perception of odor in the absence of an odorant (phantosmia), or any combination of these. From biopsy studies (see Chapter 1), we know that this damage often results in the loss of olfactory receptors and neurons. Without these neural elements, recognition of odorants at low concentrations is difficult, and coding for odorants may be affected. The following pages outline the historical characteristics that can help in determining the cause and the chemosensory symptoms of the patient.

Olfactory loss due to upper nasal airway obstruction

In patients who have a personal or family history of nasal disease or previous sinonasal operation, upper nasal airway obstruction is always suspected as a cause of their olfactory dysfunction, even if they have an otherwise convincing history for another type of loss. In the beginning of the dysfunction, the patients often have an on-again, off-again pattern to the loss, in which the decreased ability occurs during upper respiratory tract infections, when recumbent, or after allergen exposure or accompanies any other stimulus that causes nasal mucosal congestion or mucous production. A key factor is the quality of the olfactory ability when it is present. If even a tiny upper nasal airway develops, it usually allows enough odorant molecules into the olfactory cleft to allow essentially normal olfactory ability.

Another aspect of the history relates to the patient's response to medications. Sometimes patients have been given oral or parenteral steroids, like prednisone. This strong anti-inflammatory medication shrinks the thickened nasal mucosa and often allows olfaction to occur. Less often, nonsteroidal anti-inflammatory medications like ibuprofen have the same effect. If the upper nasal airway obstruction is related to an infection, especially an acute episode, antibiotics may also improve olfactory ability.

Neural olfactory damage

The remaining five types of olfactory damage are all due to damage or absence of the primary olfactory neurons in the nasal olfactory epithelium. When neurons are lost, patients can experience a decreased ability to perceive faint odorants. They may also lose the number or type of neurons needed to code odorants properly and thus have a distorted olfactory ability. Normal mammals have a constant turnover of olfactory neurons, with the entire epithelial sheet being replaced in approximately 60 to 90 days.[3] This replacement of neurons does not seem to occur after insults. Much current research is directed toward understanding this reparative process of nerve growth, in the hope that it may allow treatment for the insults.

Although damage can also occur in the central neural connections of the olfactory system, such as in Alzheimer's disease, it rarely occurs without accompanying peripheral damage.[4]

Olfactory loss after an upper respiratory tract infection. The most common type of neural olfactory damage occurs in conjunction with an upper respiratory tract infection (URTI).[5] Olfactory ability is frequently lost during a URTI. Although this "routine" loss may be due to damaged olfactory receptors, it is more likely due to obstruction of the upper nasal airways. Most people regain olfactory ability in 2 to 3 days as the inflammation resolves. Rarely, the sense of smell does not return, and the person is left with a permanent olfactory loss, which can be partial or near total. It usually occurs in adults, most often women (approximately 70%).[1,5]

Olfactory loss after head trauma. Major and minor head trauma can result in damage to the olfactory neural tissue. The most likely explanation for this is the tearing of the olfactory nerve, which occurs between the bony cribriform plate and the olfactory bulbs with sudden deceleration injuries. This results in decreased olfactory receptors due to degeneration. Although most people notice the loss of olfactory ability within hours or days, some do not notice the loss for weeks or months. This delay may be due to concomitant neural injury, like concussion. Sometimes olfactory ability returns spontaneously, but this is unusual.

Olfactory loss due to toxin exposure. Some chemicals can damage the olfactory tissues.[6] The diagnosis of a chemical cause requires a temporal connection between the exposure and the loss. The time course of the loss depends on the toxicity of the toxin, and can range from days to years.

Olfactory loss associated with aging. Measurement of olfactory ability in many persons of all ages has shown a major loss that begins around the sixth decade of life.[7] Although this loss could be due to an increased susceptibility to and incidence of the other types of olfactory loss, the gradual nature and prevalence of it suggest that it is a natural part of aging. The loss is generally gradual and occurs over months to years. Often the loss is so gradual that the person either does not notice it or notices it only when comparing over long time spans, with statements like "The lilacs do not smell this year."

Congenital loss of olfactory ability. In rare cases, a person has never had an olfactory ability.[8] Searching for a history of childhood head trauma or infections allows differentiation of these persons from the other groups discussed. Patients with congenital anosmia do not understand the concept of smell; instead, they relate better to taste or trigeminal sensations. One feature of the presentation is that the patient or the parents do not appreciate that the sense of smell is absent until the patient is about ages 8 to 12 years. Sometimes there is a family history of anosmia, and there can be associated medical problems, like Kallmann's syndrome (hypogonadotropic hypogonadism) with failure of secondary sexual characteristics to develop at puberty.

Olfactory Symptoms

As mentioned, patients can have a range of olfactory symptoms. Most commonly, the complaint is one of decreased ability to perceive odorants, but the odorants that are perceived are of normal quality. During times of active olfactory loss or gain, and at other times, patients can notice distortions. These distortions can be of odorants they are smelling (troposmia or parosmia), or they may be perceived spontaneously, without an odorant stimulus (phantosmias or olfactory hallucinations).[9] In our experience, they tend to occur with olfactory losses after a URTI, head trauma, or toxin exposure.

Rarely, a patient has phantosmia in only one nostril. Such patients are usually female, are in the second or third decade of life, and often have had spontaneous onset of a very foul odor perception. The odor can be eliminated simply by blocking the offending nostril.

Finally, some patients have olfactory hallucinations that accompany their psychiatric disease. This can occur with schizophrenia, alcoholic psychosis, depression, and seizures. Usually these hallucinations are relatively short, measured in seconds or minutes. These patients have no nasal symptoms, and the olfactory complaints go along with the psychiatric disease.

PHYSICAL EXAMINATION FOR CHEMOSENSORY CONCERNS

In general, the physical examination for chemosensory problems is a thorough general examination, with special emphasis on nasal endoscopy and oral examinations. When the tympanic membranes are examined, there should be no evidence of inflammation or masses near the chorda tympani nerve in the posterior tympanum. The anterior nasal examination should ensure that there is sufficient nostril patency for airflow, without scarring or stenosis. Signs of nasal mucosal inflammation may suggest an obstructive process higher in the nose.

When the oral cavity is examined, the tongue is particularly important to the sense of taste. Notice should be made of the quantity and distribution of taste papillae on both sides, in the front, and along the posterolateral aspect. As in the nose, mucosal inflammation can affect taste ability.

Nasal endoscopy is mandatory to evaluate the upper nasal airways. Rigid or flexible endoscopes smaller than 3 mm are useful for evaluating the space medial to the middle turbinate and, occasionally, the olfactory clefts. It is useful to estimate the potential airflow through the olfactory cleft. Note should be made of polyps or other inflammatory mucosal changes.

For patients who are suspected of having psychiatric problems, a mental status assessment is appropriate. This may be supplemented with psychometric tests. Finally, because general diseases like diabetes have been associated with taste and smell problems, a general examination is helpful.

IMAGING FOR OLFACTORY CONCERNS

Until relatively recently, the ability of a physician to image the olfactory pathway was limited. Even small endoscopes could reveal only the more peripheral portions of this pathway. Technologic development has revolutionized the ability to determine the integrity of chemosensory pathways and has permitted identification of treatable causes of chemosensory dysfunction.

Plain Radiography

In the past, plain radiographs were the standard images obtained when evaluating nasal and paranasal sinus disorders, but they have been completely usurped over the past 2 decades by computed tomography and magnetic resonance imaging. Subtle changes high in the nasal cavity may totally occlude the olfactory region, yet plain radiographs[10] may be interpreted as normal. Additionally, changes from trauma or small neoplasms may be difficult to detect with plain radiographs. For these reasons, they are not useful in the imaging evaluation of chemosensory dysfunction.

Computed Tomography (CT)

First introduced in the early 1970s, CT has evolved over several generations of instruments into a sensitive, accurate, and reliable means of imaging the head and neck. It is now the preferred technique for imaging the nose and paranasal sinuses, and it can be performed in both the coronal and the axial planes for the most complete assessment of the complex anatomy of the nasal cavity and paranasal sinuses.[10]

The nasal olfactory area is well imaged in coronal section CT. The images can reveal olfactory region encroachment or obstruction of airflow by mucosal edema, polyps, or neoplasms. Small obstructions or lesions of the ostiomeatal complex region secondarily affect the olfactory region because of the consequent alteration of airflow and extension of inflammation.[11] Injury to the olfactory pathway in the anterior cranial fossa, such as from intracerebral hemorrhage, contusion, or tumor, may be viewed on CT.

Magnetic Resonance Imaging (MRI)

Over the past decade, physicists have applied the technique of nuclear magnetic resonance combined with computerized analysis to form images of biologic structures. There are three kinds of images: the T1-weighted images, the T2-weighted images, and the proton density images.[12]

MRI is the only available technology that can image the olfactory bulbs and nerves.[13] These can be demonstrated to be absent in patients with congenital lack of olfactory ability. MRI is also superior for the detection of parenchymal brain lesions. For example, lesions due to multiple sclerosis are readily detected and are better seen than in CT images.[10]

MRI can also help differentiate between benign and malignant lesions, because of its superior soft tissue resolution.[14] For example, it can differentiate neoplasms from mucoceles because of differences in water content. MRI has a further advantage over CT in cases of suspected intracranial or intraorbital extension of tumor[15] because it shows this extension more clearly. Gadolinium-DTPA-enhanced MRI further improves the definition of a tumor. Esthesioneuroblastoma, for example, can be delineated from surrounding structures more accurately by this enhancement.

Because of its inability to image bone and vascular structures and its tendency to magnify mucosal thickness, MRI is not the preferred method for imaging the nasal and sinus cavities.

Functional MRI and PET Scanning

Koizuka et al.[16] applied functional MRI with odor stimulation to clarify the localization of olfactory cortices in the human. They obtained a significant increase in cerebral blood flow in the piriform cortex, orbitofrontal cortex, and inferior medial frontal lobe, corresponding to olfactory cortices. Positron emission tomography (PET) has also been used to evaluate the functional intracranial aspects of olfaction.[17,18] Both glucose utilization and blood flow can be assessed with this technique.

Other Imaging Techniques

Ultrasonography and radionuclide scanning produce images that do not provide enough information for careful delineation of the olfactory apparatus. The use of angiography is probably limited to the visualization of highly vascular neoplasms such as juvenile nasopharyngeal angiofibroma or chemodectoma.[10] Myelography is of some value in the chemosensory evaluation when a cerebrospinal fluid leak of the anterior cranial fossa is suspected.

PSYCHOPHYSICAL EVALUATION

Measurement of Odorant Detection

The lowest concentration of an odorant that can be perceived is commonly termed the odorant detection threshold. This concentration is not a fixed entity, but varies from one trial to another and is somewhat elusive to measure. Therefore, mathematical estimates of an average threshold are established. Three psychophysical methods are used for measuring the odorant detection threshold.

The method of constant stimuli

In this method, also called the method of right and wrong cases, the subject is presented with a series of concentrations of an odorant, from imperceptible to clearly perceptible. The order of presentation of concentrations is typically randomized, and hundreds of trials are usually made in an effort to obtain a reliable result. The proportion of correct responses is plotted as a function of odorant concentration. The threshold is defined as that concentration corresponding to the 75% correct performance level in two-choice task (odorant vs. blank) or the 66.67% correct performance level in three-choice task (two blanks and an odorant).

This method is less popular than the other methods, mainly because of the large number of trials and the attendant amount of time required to obtain a meaningful threshold estimate. In addition, there is potential for subject fatigue and boredom and for the introduction of adaptation, habituation, or facilitation.

The method of limits

In the classic method of limits (the method of minimal changes), alternating series of ascending and descending concentrations of a test odorant are presented. During an ascending trial series, an odorant is increased incrementally in concentration from an initially nondetectable level until it is reported as being detected by the subject. During a descending trial series, the stimulus is decreased incrementally from an initially detectable level until it is no longer discernible. The average concentration of the transition points where nondetection and detection occur is used as the threshold estimate.

A variation of this method described by Cain et al.[19] is the ascending method of limits, in which investigators present one or more ascending series only. Although this method is economical of time and has clinical utility, it provides a threshold estimate that is higher (indicative of less sensitivity) than that obtained from averaging data from multiple ascending series or from other procedures that more thoroughly sample the perithreshold region.

The staircase method

This method (the up-down method) is a common variant of the method of limits which requires a minimal number of trials. Its advantage is that it concentrates the stimulus presentations near the threshold region and eliminates most of the ascending or descending trials of the method of limits.[20]

In the laboratory of Deems and Doty,[21] the staircase is begun at the $-6.50\log_{10}$ odorant concentration (vol/vol) step and moved upward in full log steps.[1] Successive blank-odorant pairs are presented at each step until an incorrect response is made or five consecutive correct responses are made. When an incorrect response is made, the next higher log concentration is presented. When five consecutive correct responses are made, the staircase is reversed and the subsequent pair of trials is presented at a concentration 0.5 log step lower. From this point on, only one or two trials are presented at each step, that is, two correct trials are required for the staircase to descend and only one incorrect trial is required for the staircase to ascend. The geometric mean of the last four staircase reversal points of a total of seven is used as the threshold estimate. The threshold concentration determined by this method represents the value chosen correctly by the subject 71% of the time, not 50% of the time as in other methods.[22]

Measurement of Odorant Discrimination

Odorant discrimination is among the least demanding of olfactory tasks that a subject can be asked to perform, in that he or she merely needs to distinguish among odorants, not to recognize, identify, or remember them. Three procedures are used for odorant quality discrimination.

The most basic odorant discrimination test requires a decision as to whether two odorants are the same or different. Several same- and different-odorant pairs are presented, and the proportion of the pairing correctly identified as same or different can be used as the measure of discrimination. Alternatively, data from this type of paradigm can be quantified using measures derived from signal detection theory.[23]

A more commonly used odorant discrimination test requires the subject to choose an odd stimulus from a set of stimuli that, except for the odd stimulus, are identical to one another. Usually the stimuli are presented to the subject in counterbalanced order. The proportion of correct trials is a common measure of a subject's discrimination ability. Also, measures derived from signal detection theory can be used in data evaluation.[24]

A third odor discrimination test makes use of an odorant confusion matrix.[25] Each odorant of a set is presented in counterbalanced order to a subject. The subject's task is to determine which one of a set of codes previously assigned to each of the odorants best describes the odor sensation on a given trial. The percentages of responses given to each alternative for each odorant are displayed in a rectangular matrix (stimuli making up rows and response alternatives making up equivalently ordered columns) and subsequently converted to distance values and subjected to multidimensional scaling analysis.

Measurement of Odor Recognition

Suprathreshold odor quality recognition tests can be divided into two categories.

In the first category, a small set of odorants (often two or three) are presented in succession and the subject is asked to report in each case whether any odor is recognized. Identification of the stimuli is not required. This method is relatively unsophisticated, because it is very subjective.

In the second category, a subject is presented on a given trial with a target odorant and is subsequently provided with a set of several odorants that include the target stimulus. The subject's task is to report which odor of the set is the same as the previously presented target. The number correct in a series of such presentations provides the test score. This forced choice test eliminates the subjectivity of a simple yes or no response.

An odor matching test, a variant of this general theme, was presented by Abraham and Matha.[26] Four odorants are contained in eight vials (two vials per odorant). The subject is simply required to pair up the equivalent two-vial containers. Scoring consists of giving a single point to each pair correctly matched (0 to 4). The test is given twice.

If the first and second tests are discrepant, a third test is administered, and the average of the three tests is taken.

Measurement of Odor Identification

There are three basic methods for odor quality identification testing.

The odorant naming test requires a subject to provide a name for each of a set of odorants. Despite its use in clinical settings, many normal persons have difficulty in naming or identifying even familiar odorants without cues.

The yes/no odor identification test requires a subject to signify whether a stimulus smells like a particular odorant. It is relatively simple and less influenced by cognitive and memory demands. Because chance performance on this type of test is 50%, its range of discriminability is considerably lower, and therefore more trials are needed for good discriminability.

The multiple-choice odorant identification test requires a subject to identify the odorant from a list of odorant names. Several types of multiple-choice odor identification tests have been described,[19,27–29] and they are conceptually similar. The most widely used of these tests is the University of Pennsylvania Smell Identification Test (UPSIT), which is commercially available as the Smell Identification Test (Sensonics, Haddon Heights, NJ). This test focuses on the ability of a subject to identify each of 40 microencapsulated odorants.[27] The stimuli are released by scratching the strips with a pencil tip in a standardized manner. Above each odorant strip are four words representing possible odorant choices. The test is forced-choice, the subject having to mark one of the four alternatives, even if no smell is perceived. This test is scored as the number of items correct out of 40 and has the age- and gender-related norms that are based on thousands of subjects.[30]

ELECTROPHYSIOLOGIC EVALUATION

Electro-olfactogram

In 1956, Ottoson[31] demonstrated a slow, negative, monophasic potential from the olfactory region of the frog when it was stimulated by odorant-saturated air. It was also certain that the response was derived from the receptor cells proper, and not from the nerve fibers, because it remained unchanged after blocking with cocaine, which was known from other sense organs to affect nerve fibers and not the sensory cells. Moreover, a difference has been found between the responses to various substances. The composition of the mucous covering of the olfactory region is also different from respiratory mucus.

In 1969, Osterhammel et al.[32] discovered that the negative electrical potential recorded from the olfactory mucosa of two patients increased in relation to an incremental flow rate of coffee-saturated air. The response seemed to be proportional to the logarithm of the stimulus intensity.

In 1981, Kobal[33] utilized his stimulation method so that mechanical or thermal alterations of the stimulated mucosa due to different flow rates of the stimulant were eliminated. The odorants amyl acetate, hydrogen sulfide, and engenol were presented to four subjects. The responses were dependent on the concentration of the stimulus. When stimuli (hydrogen sulfide) of longer durations were applied, temporal integration over a period of 10 seconds was observed. During the past decade, further refinements have been made in the stimulating and recording systems for this technique, and the electro-olfactogram is being used for clinical evaluation in several centers worldwide. Its place as a research and clinical tool for objective olfactory testing is still being determined.

Olfactory Evoked Potential and Contingent Negative Variation

Finkenzeller,[34] in 1966, and Allison and Goff,[35] in 1967, first described cerebral evoked potentials in humans to chemical stimuli, which they assumed to be of olfactory origin. However, in 1971, Smith et al.[36] contested the olfactory nature of these responses on the grounds that they were not obtainable in patients who had lost trigeminal sensitivity.

In 1978, Kobal and Plattig[37] introduced a stimulator that delivered odorants in a constantly flowing airstream, thus avoiding the undesired stimulation of thermoreceptors and mechanoreceptors, while steep stimulus onsets were maintained. After introduction of a new stimulation technique, Kobal[38] tested anosmic patients who yielded no evoked potentials after stimulation with 2 phenylethyl alcohol or vanillin. These findings were concordant with the results of Doty et al.,[39] who reported that these substances were not perceived by anosmics. Thus, olfactory evoked potentials indeed exist and can be recorded if precise and well-controlled stimulation techniques are used.[40] So far, non-odorous carbon dioxide has been perceived by all anosmics investigated and has elicited chemosomatosensory evoked potentials that were mediated by the trigeminal nerve.

As an addition to earlier findings concerning the topographical distribution of evoked potentials,[41] recent investigations indicate that different stimulants effect different topographical patterns of chemosensory evoked potential.[42] Maximal amplitudes of potentials evoked by substances (high concentrations of carbon dioxide, menthol, acetaldehyde) that partly or exclusively excite the trigeminal nerve were found at the vertex and are defined as chemosomatosensory evoked potentials. Substances that exclusively, or to a great extent, excite the olfactory nerve (H_2S, vanillin) effected maximal responses in the parietal area and are defined as olfactory evoked potentials.

Another type of induced brain wave activity is the endogenous component, called the contingent negative variation.[43] These components are termed endogenous, because their presence depends on subjective response strategies rather than on stimulus characteristics. In 1993, Auffermann et al.[44] demonstrated the objective diagnosis of olfaction by simultaneous recording of olfactory evoked potentials and contingent negative variation. Anosmia can be determined by the lack of both olfactory evoked potentials and contingent negative variation, although the latter shows less variability. Patients with parosmia generally have only contingent negative variation. Hyposmia can also be detected; just above the discrimination threshold, the amplitude of contingent negative variation tends to be enhanced, whereas the amplitudes of olfactory evoked potentials may still be undetectable. Thus, olfactory evoked potentials and contingent negative variation can be used for olfactory testing.

CONCLUSION

Although many of the tests and evaluations described in this chapter can be time-consuming and involve expensive technology, most of the evaluation that is clinically relevant can be performed with routine clinical technologies. Of these, the most important is the history, which should allow the examiner to determine whether the olfactory concern is related to nasal disease and, if so, whether it seems to be lateralizing to one side of the nose. This information is important because, at this point, a blocked upper nasal airway or symptoms lateralizing to one side only relates to only the olfactory conditions that can reasonably be treated. Advances are being made in the treatment of primary neuron sensory loss and olfactory conditions related to central brain function. Currently, however, these are not well understood. By far the most important aspects of the evaluation of the patient with olfactory dysfunction are a thorough history, examination, imaging, and testing resulting in an accurate diagnosis. Empathy and understanding for the patient's situation will result in greater patient satisfaction and a safer adaptation to his or her own environment.

REFERENCES

1. Deems DA, Doty RL, Settle RG, et al: Smell and taste disorders, a study of 750 patients from the University of Pennsylvania Smell and Taste Center. *Arch Otolaryngol Head Neck Surg* 1991; 117:519–528.

2. Leopold DA, Preti G, Mozell MM, Youngentob SL, Wright HN: Fish-odor syndrome presenting as dysosmia. *Arch Otolaryngol Head Neck Surg* 1990; 116:354–355.
3. Monti Graziadei GA, Graziadei PPC: Neurogenesis and neuron regeneration in the olfactory system of mammals. II. Degeneration and reconstitution of the olfactory sensory neurons after axotomy. *J Neurocytol* 1979; 8:197–213.
4. Doty RL, Reyes PF, Gregor T: Presence of both odor identification and detection deficits in Alzheimer's disease. *Brain Res Bull* 1987; 18:597–600.
5. Mott AE, Leopold DA: Disorders in taste and smell. *Med Clin North Am* 1991; 75:1321–1353.
6. Leopold DA: Nasal toxicity: end points of concern in humans. *Inhalation Toxicol* 1994; 6 Supp:23–39.
7. Stevens JC, Cain WS: Old-age deficits in the sense of smell as gauged by thresholds, magnitude matching, and odor identification. *Psychol Aging* 1987; 2:36–42.
8. Leopold DA, Hornung DE, Schwob JE: Congenital lack of olfactory ability. *Ann Otol Rhinol Laryngol* 1992; 101:229–236.
9. Leopold D: Distorted Olfactory Perception, in Doty RL (ed.): *Handbook of Olfaction and Gustation*. New York, Marcel Dekker, 1995, pp 441–454.
10. Kimmelman CP: Medical imaging of smell and taste disorders, in Doty RL, Bartoshuk LM, Brow JB Jr, Setchell TV (eds.): *Smell and Taste in Health and Disease*. New York, Raven Press, 1991, pp 471–479.
11. Leopold DA: The relationship between nasal anatomy and human olfaction. *Laryngoscope* 1988; 98:1232–1238.
12. Shapiro MD, Som PM: MRI of the paranasal sinuses and nasal cavity. *Radiol Clin North Am* 1989; 27:447–475.
13. Yousem DM, Turner WJ, Li C, Snyder PJ, Doty RL: Kallmann syndrome: MR evaluation of olfactory system. *AJNR* 1993; 14:839–843.
14. Makow LS: Magnetic resonance imaging: a brief review of image contrast. *Radiol Clin North Am* 1989; 27:195–218.
15. Shankar L, Evans K, Hawke M, Stammberger H: *An Atlas of Imaging of the Paranasal Sinus*. Philadelphia, J.B. Lippincott, 1994, pp 148–171.
16. Koizuka I, Yano H, Nagahara M, et al: Functional imaging of the human olfactory cortex by magnetic resonance imaging. *ORL* 1994; 56:273–275.
17. Leopold DA, Meyerrose G: Diagnosis and Treatment of Distorted Olfactory Perception, in Kurihara K, Suzuki N, Ogawa H (eds.): *Olfaction and Taste XI*, Tokyo, Springer-Verlag, 1994, pp 618–622.
18. Jagust WJ, Eberling JL: MRI, CT, SPECT, PET: their use in diagnosing dementia. *Geriatrics* 1991; 46:28–35.
19. Cain WS, Gent JF, Goodspeed RB, Leonard G: Evaluation of olfactory dysfunction in the Connecticut Chemosensory Clinical Research Center. *Laryngoscope* 1988; 98:83–88.
20. Cornsweet TN: The staircase-method in psychophysics. *Am J Psychol* 1962; 75:485–491.
21. Deems DA, Doty RL: Age-related changes in the phenylethyl alcohol odor detection threshold. *Trans Pa Acad Ophthalmol Otolaryngol* 1987; 39:646–650.
22. Wetherill GB, Levitt H: Sequential estimation of points on a psychometric function. *Br J Math Statist Psychol* 1965;18:1–10.
23. O'Mahony MAPD: Short-cut signal detection measures for sensory analysis. *J Food Sci* 1979; 44:302–303.
24. Frijters JER: Three-stimulus procedures in olfactory psychophysics: an experimental comparison of Thurstone-Ura and three-alternative forced-choice models of signal detection theory. *Percept Psychophys* 1980; 28:390–397.
25. Koster EP: Human Psychophysics in Olfaction, in Moulton DG, Turk A, Johnston JW (eds.): *Methods in Olfactory Research*. New York, Academic Press, 1975 pp 345–374.
26. Abraham A, Matha KV: The effect of right temporal lobe lesions on matching of smells. *Neuropsychologia* 1983; 21:277–281.
27. Doty RL, Shaman P, Dann M: Development of the University of Pennsylvania Smell Identification Test: a standardized microencapsulated test of olfactory function. *Physiol Behav* 1984; 32:489–502.
28. Wood JB, Harkins SW: Effects of age, stimulus selection, and retrieval environment on odor identification. *J Gerontol* 1987; 42:584–588.
29. Wright HN: Characterization of olfactory dysfunction. *Arch Otolaryngol Head Neck Surg* 1987; 113:163–168.
30. Doty RL: Influence of age and age-related disease on olfactory function. *Ann NY Acad Sci* 1989; 561:76–86.
31. Ottoson D: Analysis of the electrical activity of the olfactory epithelium. *Acta Physiol Scand* 1956; 35 Suppl 122:1–83.

32. Osterhammel P, Terkildsen K, Zilstorff K: Electro-olfactograms in man. *J Laryngol Otol* 1969; 83:731–733.
33. Kobal G: *Elektrophysiologische Untersuchungen des Menschlichen Geruchssinns.* Stuttgart, Thieme, 1981.
34. Finkenzeller P: Gemittelte EEG-Potentiale bei olfaktorischer Reizung. *Pfluegers Arch* 1966; 292:76–80.
35. Allison T, Goff WR: Human cerebral evoked potentials to odorous stimuli. *Electroenceph Clin Neurophysiol* 1967; 23:558–560.
36. Smith DB, Allison T, Goff WR, Principato JJ: Human odorant evoked potentials: effects of trigeminal or olfactory deficit. *Elecroencephalogr Clin Neurophysiol* 1971; 30:313–317.
37. Kobal G, Plattig K-H: Methodische Anmerkungen zur Gewinnung olfaktorischer EEG- Antworten des wachen Menschen (objektive Olfaktometrie). *EEG EMG Z Elektroenzephalogr Elektromyogr Verwandte Geb* 1978; 9:135–145.
38. Kobal G: A New Method for Determination of the Olfactory and the Trigeminal Nerve's Dysfunction: Olfactory (OEP) and Chemical Somatosensory (CSSEP) Evoked Potentials, in Rothenberger A (ed.): *Event-related Potentials in Children: Basic Concepts and Clinical Application.* Amsterdam, Elsevier Biomedical Press, 1982, pp 455–461.
39. Doty RL, Brugger WE, Jurs PC, Orndorff MA, Snyder PJ, Lowry LD: Intranasal trigeminal stimulation from odorous volatiles: psychometric responses from anosmic and normal humans. *Physiol Behav* 1978; 20:175–185.
40. Kobal G, Hummel C: Cerebral chemosensory evoked potentials elicited by chemical stimulation of human olfactory and respiratory nasal mucosa. *Electroencephalogr Clin Neurophysiol* 1988; 71:241–250.
41. Plattig K-H, Kobal G: Spatial and Temporal Distribution of Olfactory Evoked Potentials and Techniques Involved in Their Measurement, in Lehmann D, Callaway E (eds.): *Human Evoked Potentials: Applications and Problems.* New York, Plenum Press, 1979, pp 285–301.
42. Kobal G, Hummel TH, Van Toller C: Olfactory and chemosomatosensory evoked potentials from stimuli presented to the left and right nostrils. *Chem Senses* 1987; 12:183.
43. Walter WG, Cooper R, Aldridge VJ, McCallum WC, Winter AL: Contingent negative variation: an electric sign of sensorimotor association and expectancy in the human brain. *Nature* 1964; 203:380–384.
44. Auffermann H, Gerull G, Mathe F, Mrowinski D: Olfactory evoked potentials and contingent negative variation simultaneously recorded for diagnosis of smell disorders. *Ann Otol Rhinol Laryngol* 1993; 102:6–10.

3

Imaging the Nasal Airway

P.A.R. CLEMENT, M.D., Ph.D.
A.R. HALAMA, M.D., Ph.D.
T. BUISSERET, M.D.

For decades, the standard routine radiographic examination of the paranasal sinuses was considered to be a standard x-ray series consisting of five views: Waters, Caldwell, Rhese, lateral, and openmouth Waters.[1-3] More sophisticated investigations of this region needed multidirectional tomography, a technique that was still advocated in the early 1980s,[4] although computed tomography (CT)[5] of the paranasal sinuses was also being discussed. At that time, CT had a rather low resolution capacity. CT had been introduced 9 years earlier by Ambrose[6] and Hounsfield.[7] In 1982, the vast potential of magnetic resonance imaging (MRI) also was mentioned by Mancuso and Hanafee,[8] and these authors anticipated that a combination of CT and MRI would assume all the roles that were formerly contributed by the latest generation of CT[9] and MRI[10] scanners, surpassing by far the diagnostic possibilities of the combination of standard radiographic and pluridirectional tomography and making these investigations almost completely obsolete.

In recent years, CT scanners of the latest generation have become much faster (1 second per scan) than those of the first generation, and they now have an increased degree of resolution (structures down to 0.6mm can be visualized). The only drawback of the scanners was their availability and the high costs involved. Because the number of CT and MRI scanners has increased in the Western world, these drawbacks have been reduced considerably. Actually, in Belgium, a series of CT scans of the paranasal sinuses in one plane costs only 43% (less than US $76) more than a standard x-ray series (US $53) and the radiation load is nearly similar.

Because standard radiography show well only the changes of the nasal mucosa that occur in voluminous paranasal sinuses such as the frontal, sphenoidal, and maxillary sinuses, its use is very limited. As long as some air remains in these sinuses, one can visualize only gross anomalies such as the presence of secretions, major mucosal swelling, polyps, and cysts. To be visible on standard radiography, the sinus mucosa requires thickening by a factor of 10 or more.[11] Mostly, the origin of these inflammatory changes must be looked for at the level of the ostiomeatal complex (infundibulum, frontal recess, anterior ethmoid), a region that is very poorly visualized by standard radiography. Therefore, in countries with easy access to CT scanners and in which the costs are low, and because of all the reasons mentioned before, CT can now fully obviate ordinary radiographic examination of the paranasal sinuses.

Echography in its most sophisticated way has even greater drawbacks than standard radiographic evaluation. It is far less accurate (in resolution as well as in differentiation) than any other investigation, except transillumination. Especially in children, in whom it was supposed to be a most desirable examination because it cuts down on the radiation load by avoiding repetitive radiographic examination, it has proved to be completely unreliable. This investigation was therefore not recommended by the International Conference on Sinus Disease[12] because (1) it is of dubious value, is difficult to perform, and provides variable results and (2) the information obtained is similar in reliability and quality to that of transillumination.

INFLAMMATORY DISEASES

The most common nasal disease in humans is the common cold. This disease is characterized during the early phase by sneezing, watery rhinorrea, blocked nose, and general malaise. Sinus involvement is present much earlier in colds and lasts longer after resolution of symptoms than was accepted before.[13] Among otherwise healthy adults with common colds of 48 to 96 hours in duration, CT showed that 77% of the patients had reduced ethmoidal infundibula, 87% had abnormalities of one or both maxillary cavities, 65% had ethmoid sinus abnormalities, 32% had frontal sinus abnormalities, and 39% had sphenoid sinus abnormalities. Although these are interesting data, they do not mean that a common cold is an indication for CT. This disease seems to induce a rhinosinusitis of short duration which in most cases is followed by a complete, spontaneous recovery. Therefore, CT has no therapeutic benefit and cannot be advocated for the common cold.

Chronic rhinosinusitis is by far the most common indication for CT of the paranasal sinuses. During the Princeton meeting (1993),[12] the old concept of "chronic sinusitis being a sinusitis that exists for longer than 3 weeks" was replaced by the new understanding of "chronic sinusitis being a sinusitis that does not resolve without significant mucosal damage." Sequential MRI studies have shown that although clinical resolution of acute maxillary symptoms occurs within 1 week after treatment, mucosal changes can persist for 8 weeks or more.[14] Therefore, duration does not seem to be an effective factor for differentation between acute and chronic sinusitis. Another old concept that has been changed is that chronic sinusitis is characterized by irreversible mucosal damage. In both acute and chronic sinusitis, the damaged mucosa may regenerate with removal of the ostial obstruction and adequate aeration of the affected sinuses. This new understanding highlights the importance of the ostiomeatal complex, and this can be visualized adequately only by high-resolution CT.

For the diagnosis in advanced care, the physician needs extensive information immediately, not only for staging and mapping the anatomy precisely when operation is a consideration but also for demonstrating why a patient has chronic or recurrent symptoms. According to Zinreich,[8] plain radiography is inadequate for evaluating the anterior ethmoid air cells, the upper two-thirds of the nasal cavity, infundibulum, middle meatus, and frontal recess air passages. During the consensus meeting (Princeton 1993),[12] all authorities agreed, however, that endoscopy should precede CT scanning. Many authors state[15-19] that *nasal endoscopic examination* can reveal or rule out indications for surgical intervention, provide objective information on the patient's response to antibiotic and decongestant therapy, and obviate repeated radiographic examination. Because endoscopy displays the surface mucosa of the ethmoid cells and CT shows the deep hidden air chambers, the two procedures are usually complementary. Finally, the consensus meeting[12] restricted CT to the following indications and requirements in chronic or recurrent sinusitis: (1) when nasal endoscopy is unrevealing and severe symptoms persist, CT is indicated to demonstrate disease in the anterior ethmoid sinuses; (2) when a patient is a candidate for operation, a full CT examination is necessary to define sinus anatomy (axial and coronal scans if possible); (3) when CT is done after medical therapy, it can reveal the extent of mucosal disease deep in the ostiomeatal complex and, once secondary inflammatory changes have resolved, serve as a guide to detailed mapping of surgical anatomy before an invasive procedure; and (4) in order to yield optimal information, the mucosa should be as free as possible from inflammation, so an appropriate course of medical therapy should precede CT examination.

From the preceding, it is obvious that anatomical variations are an important factor, if not the most important factor, in chronic and recurrent rhinosinusitis. From a CT scan study in 196 children,[20] it was clear that the prevalence of anatomical variations (such as septal deviation, concha bullosa, and "Haller" cells) increases with age (Table 3–1). Thus, anatomy seems subject to chronic changes in the growing child, changes that go on during adulthood. This finding does not mean that an anatomical anomaly is an indication for operation. Only when the anatomical variation is responsible for the sinusitis and medical treatment does not resolve the inflammation should an operation be considered.

In 350 adults with chronic nasal complaints,[29] CT showed a similar percentage of anatomical variations (concha bullosa, "Haller" cells, and processus uncinatus

Table 3–1 Anatomical Anomalies on Computed Tomography in 196 Children With Chronic Nasal Complaints

		ANATOMICAL ANOMALY, %			
			CONCHA BULLOSA		
AGE, YR	NO. OF PATIENTS	SEPTAL DEVIATION	MEDIA	SUPERIOR	"HALLER" CELL
3–4	38	16	0	0	0
5–6	46	37	8	0	3
7–8	42	55	4	2	2
9–10	21	48	2	0	2
11–12	20	65	15	0	10
13–14	29	72	20	3	3

bullosa) in a group that showed signs of mucosal disease and a group that did not show these signs (Table 3–2). This finding indicates that the existence of an anatomical variation of itself is not the cause of recurrent sinusitis, but an anatomical variation that is impeding the drainage or ventilation of any paranasal sinus will result in chronic inflammation of the mucosa with rhinosinusitis (Fig. 3–1). Zinreich et al.[21] and Bolger et al.[22] also were unable to show an overall increase in ostiomeatal disease when patients with concha bullosa were compared with 100 consecutive patients without concha bullosa. As in the previous study,[29] authors in both of these studies[21,22] counted every concha bullosa regardless of its size, and all patients in both studies were symptomatic. So, these studies did not necessarily reflect the "natural history" of the contribution of concha bullosa to the genesis of ostiomeatal disease.

The anatomical anomalies are not limited to concha bullosa and "Haller" cells but can also be a paradoxical middle turbinate (reversed or concave curvature),

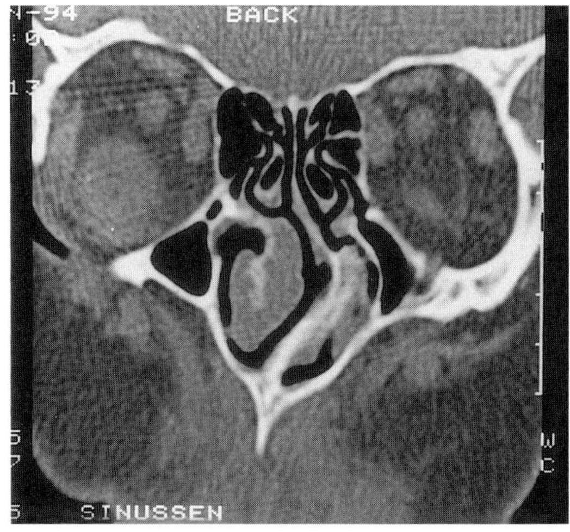

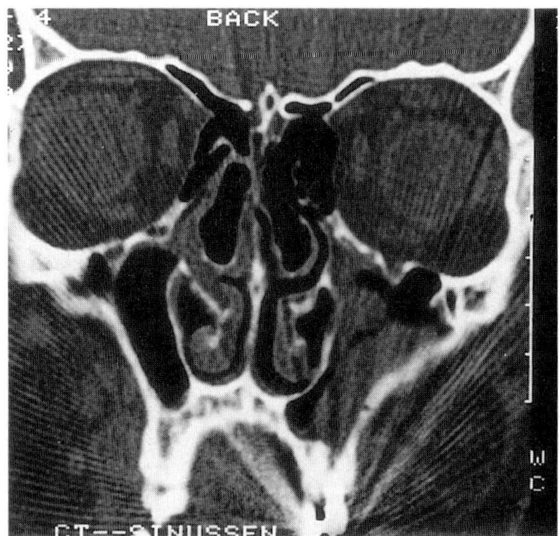

Figure 3–1. Coronal computed tomographic scans. *A*, Huge septal deviation and small bilateral bullous middle turbinate without sinusitis. *B*, Bilaterally huge bulla in middle turbinates with maxillary sinusitis on the right and mucosal swelling in the ostiomeatal complex on the left.

**Table 3–2 Anatomical Variations in 350 Adults With
Chronic Nasal Complaints**

ANATOMICAL VARIATION	CT SIGNS OF SINUS INFLAMMATION, %	
	YES	NO
Septal deviation	45	75
Concha bullosa	44	32
"Haller" cell	10	1
Processus uncinatus bullosa	2	1

enlarged or rotated uncinate process, enlarged ethmoidal bulla, agger nasi cell, and septal spurs.[18,23–26] As already stressed, CT is the method of choice to show the anatomical variations as well as the inflammation of the mucosa. One should remember, however, that thickening of the sinus mucosa due to nasal cycling up to 3 mm in the sinonasal mucosa is considered to be clinically insignificant[25,26] (Fig. 3–2).

There is some disagreement in the literature about which sinuses are most often involved in chronic recurrent rhinosinusitis (Table 3–3). Most authors found a higher percentage of involvement of the ethmoidal sinus and of the maxillary sinus. Clement et al.[29] found more cases of maxillary sinusitis. This observation was also noted during operation by Friedrich,[32] who, in patients operated on for chronic sinusitis of the anterior complex (maxillary, frontal, and ethmoidal sinuses), noted involvement of the maxillary sinus in 94%, 32% of which were isolated cases of maxillary sinusitis only. Clement et al. also found that the maxillary sinus was more often involved unilaterally than bilaterally. In 402 sinuses (in 201 patients), the percentage of involvement of the maxillary sinus was nearly equal to that of the ethmoidal sinuses 42% and 34% if each sinus is considered separately, and 73% and 34% if each patient is considered separately. Thus, the maxillary sinus is much more frequently involved unilaterally than the ethmoid sinus. Among the 42% with maxillary sinus involvement, 3% had minimal mucosal involvement (less than 2 mm) of the maxillary sinus, 4% had mucosal swelling occupying less than 50% of the volume, 12% had up to 75%, and 22% had a completely opaque maxillary sinus.

Polyps and cysts can be recognized easily (but not differentiated) in the maxillary sinus as rounded structures; in the adult population, 4% had a small polyp or cyst, 23% had one big polyp, and 4% had multiple polyps. All of these differences in percentages are of course highly influenced by the selection and assessment criteria. The series reported by Clement et al.[29] consisted of patients with chronic nasal complaints (including allergy, septal deviation, vasomotor rhinitis), and the other series included mainly patients selected for operation in whom infection of the sinuses was confirmed by nasal endoscopy.

In the authors' opinion,[20,33] *age* is a very important factor in the prevalence of rhinosinusitis as well as in which sinus is most frequently involved. During childhood, the number of children with chronic rhinosinusitis is higher in lower age

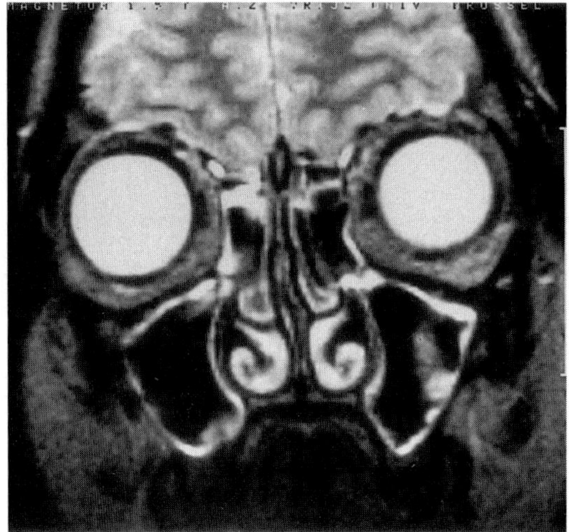

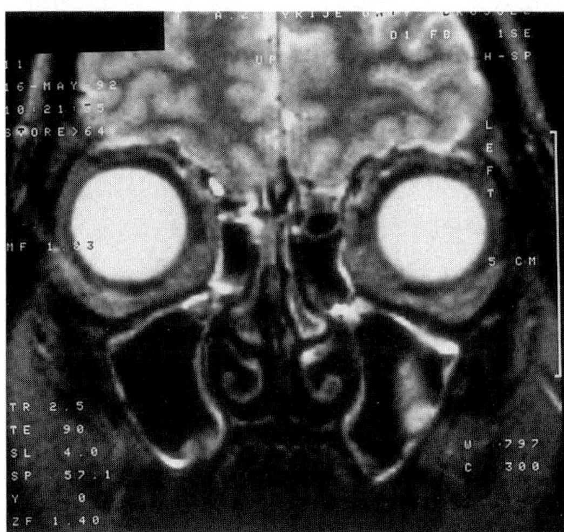

Figure 3–2. Magnetic resonance T_2-weighted images of the same test subject without decongestion (*A*) and after decongestion (xylometazoline spray 0.1%) (*B*). Note that there is marked decongestion of the mucosa of both inferior and middle turbinates and also of the mucosa of both ethmoids and maxillary sinuses.

groups, and it decreases between the ages of 8 and 9 years (Table 3–4). Younger children show a higher percentage of involvement of the anterior and posterior ethmoid and sphenoid sinuses (except of course the frontal sinus, which is not present before the age of 7 years). The maxillary sinus, however, shows a rather constant percentage of involvement in all age groups. The authors also found more extensive and bilateral sinusitis in children; the maxillary sinus is involved in 13% (5% in the age group younger than 9 years and 31% in the age group older than 9 years), the ethmoid sinus in 0.5%, the sphenoid sinus in 1.0%, and the frontal sinus in 0.5%. All these data point to the fact that chronic rhinosinusitis is more common in younger children, probably because of an immature immune system, whereas in older children, as in adults, the anatomical variations are more important in the pathogenesis of sinusitis.

Most authors agree that chronic maxillary and frontal sinusitis is linked to

Table 3–3   Involvement of Different Sinuses in Adults With Chronic or Recurrent Rhinosinusitis, According to Different Studies

	STUDY					
	ZINREICH ET AL. 1987[28]	CLEMENT ET AL. 1989[29]		BOLGER ET AL. 1991[22]	VLEMING 1991[25]	WEBER ET AL. 1992[30]	MAY ET AL. 1993[31]
No. of patients	100	201		202	103	123	184
No. of sinuses	NK		402	NK	NK	NK	NK
Sinus, %							
Maxillary	65	73	42	78	74	94	82
Anterior ethmoid	72	34	34	84	77	82	88
Posterior ethmoid	40	19		39	44	44	73
Frontal	34	13		37	26	24	31
Sphenoid	21	13		25	31	21	33

NK, not known.

Table 3–4   Mucosal Inflammation of the Sinuses in 196 Children and 284 Adults With Chronic Nasal Complaints

AGE, YR	NO.	SINUS AFFECTED, %				
		MAXILLARY	ANTERIOR ETHMOID	POSTERIOR ETHMOID	SPHENOID	FRONTAL
Children						
3–4	38	63	53	34	29	0
5–6	46	39	24	24	13	0
7–8	42	52	38	26	26	7
9–10	21	33	14	14	19	5
11–12	20	45	20	5	10	15
13–14	29	65	10	3	0	0
Adults						
20–30	64	56	36	12	8	8
30–40	82	54	36	12	12	12
40–50	48	56	38	14	16	6
50–60	36	90	42	30	22	24
60–70	34	86	44	22	18	18
>70	20	80	20	20	16	20

abnormality of the infundibulum ethmoidale. In 196 children (354 sinuses), there was a statistically significant relationship between infundibulum involvement and maxillary sinusitis on one hand ($P < 0.00$ and $\chi^2 = 149$) and anterior ethmoiditis ($P < 0.00$ and $\chi^2 = 94$) on the other hand. In adults, frontal sinusitis is always an extension of frontal recess abnormality (frontal recess abnormality always exceeds frontal sinus abnormality in all age groups) (Fig. 3–3), whereas for the maxillary sinus this is true to a lesser extent (infundibulum abnormality follows maxillary sinus abnormality, but maxillary sinusitis always exceeds the infundibulum abnormality), and this relationship applies to children and adults. Thus, isolated maxillary sinusitis can probably also be induced not only by an extension of infundibulum abnormality but also by other causes (dental, septal deviation). In adults with chronic nasal complaints, the absolute number of patients is more important during the third to the fifth decade of life, but in older age groups the percentage of rhinosinusitis in patients with chronic nasal complaints is higher (Fig. 3–4). Thus,

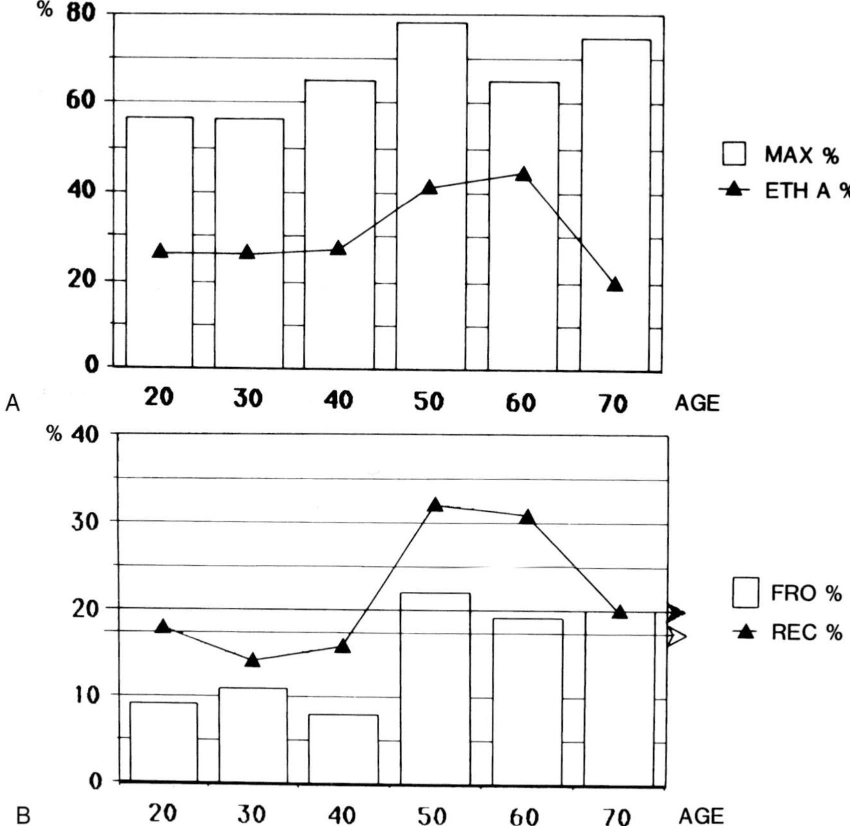

Figure 3–3.   Prevalence of inflammatory mucosal disease in 350 patients with chronic nasal complaints, according to age. *A*, Percentage of patients with maxillary and anterior ethmoidal disease. The ethmoidal disease follows the maxillary disease, but the maxillary sinus is more often involved for all age groups. So maxillary sinus disease is not always an extension of anterior ethmoidal disease. *B*, Percentage of patients with frontal recess and frontal sinus disease. Frontal sinus disease follows frontal recess disease, but frontal recess is involved more often. Frontal sinus disease seems to always be an extension of frontal recess disease.

during ages 20 to 50 years, other factors are also important for inducing nasal complaints, such as allergy, vasomotor rhinitis, and septal deviation.

Some authors claim that *allergy* plays an important role in the pathogenesis of sinusitis. In our group of 196 children with chronic nasal complaints, the prevalence of sinusitis decreased with age and the prevalence of allergy increased; therefore, allergy is certainly not a major cause of sinusitis. Study of populations with allergy,[34] however, shows that the percentage of mucosal inflammation in children and adults for the different sinuses is equally distributed (Table 3–5). Also the severity of the sinusitis is equally distributed for both groups (except for children 3 to 6 years old) (Table 3–6). Thus, allergy is not a major cause of chronic rhinosinusitis (Fig. 3–5). However, in an allergic population the distribution of the inflammation of the different sinuses and the severity are similar to those of an infection. Therefore, any condition that induces inflammation of the paranasal sinuses (except

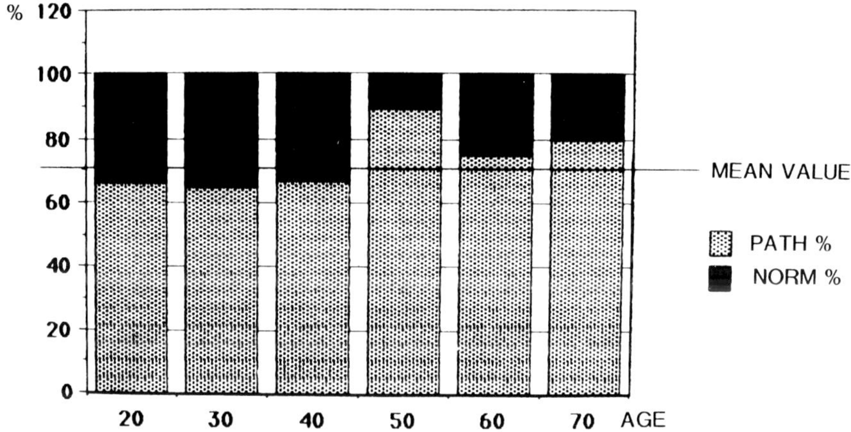

Figure 3–4. Computed tomography study (percentage) of patients (n = 350) with chronic nasal complaints who had signs of mucosal inflammation.

Table 3–5   Computed Tomography Signs of Mucosal Inflammation of the Paranasal Sinuses in Atopic Patients

	CHILDREN 3–14 YEARS (N = 59)	ADULTS 15–55 YEARS (N = 62)
% with sinus disease*	61	58
Maxillary	83	89
Anterior ethmoid	55	44
Posterior ethmoid	30	28
Sphenoid	40	11
Frontal	14	5

*Percentage of total population.

Table 3–6 Severity of Computed Tomography Signs of Mucosal Inflammation in Atopic Patients

AGE, YR	NO.	SINUSITIS, %	
		MILD (LESS THAN 50% OPAQUE)	SEVERE (MORE THAN 50% OPAQUE)
Children			
3–6	8	0	50
6–9	19	31	31
9–12	14	50	14
12–14	18	44	16
Adults			
15–55	62	45	13

some special conditions) will lead to a similar distribution and severity of the sinusitis.

Special conditions that also can induce chronic or recurrent rhinosinusitis are described below:

1. Any kind of *"immotile cilia syndrome,"* ranging from mild ciliary anomalies to its most extreme form, that is, Kartagener's syndrome (bronchiectasis, chronic sinusitis, and situs inversus, which can be seen on a standard chest radiograph).
2. *Massive nasal polyposis*: this is caused in 40% by aspirin intolerance,[35] and 36% to 60% of patients suffering from aspirin intolerance will develop massive nasal polyposis and 39% have the triad of aspirin intolerance, asthma, and nasal polyposis (Samter's syndrome).

The CT scan in massive polyposis can show two typical images:

    a. a complete "whiteout," which means that all paranasal cavities are completely filled with polyps or secretions and show a complete white shadow on the CT scan (Fig. 3–6) or

    b. a "halo" image, which means that the polyps are confined to the proximal part of the paranasal sinus and on CT scan show a black halo (air-containing spaces) surrounding the white image caused by the presence of polyps in the proximal part of the sinuses (Fig. 3–7).

In 22 patients with nasal polyposis, 84% showed a complete whiteout of the ethmoid sinuses, 54% of the maxillary sinuses, 44% of the frontal sinuses, and 28% of the sphenoid sinuses. In these patients, three did not have any polyp on anterior rhinoscopy but CT showed massive polyposis of the sinus cavities.[36] The MRI T_2-weighted image clearly showed the extent of massive polyposis but, because the bony structures are not visible with this imaging technique, the technique of choice for this disease remains CT. Sometimes, however, when the efficacy of a medical treatment (corticosteroid or antibiotic) needs to be evaluated, consecutive T_2-weighted MRI can be considered because no radiation load is involved, and CT can be performed before operation to evaluate the exact bony anatomy (Fig. 3–8).

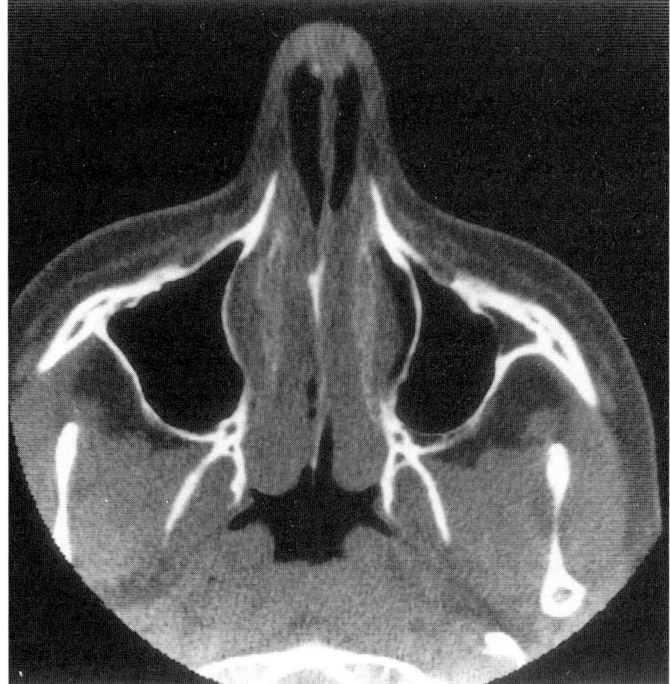

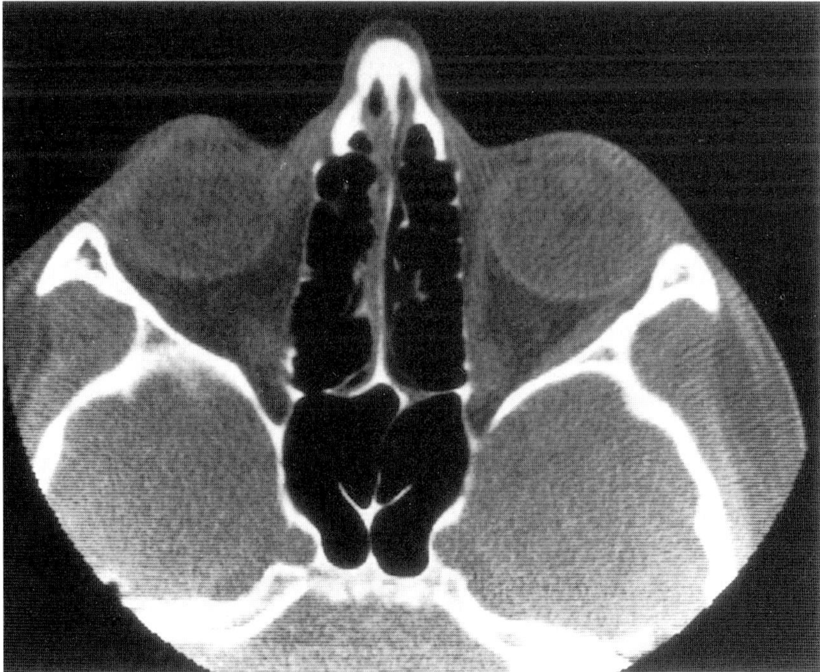

Figure 3–5. Axial computed tomography scans of a 10-year-old child with completely blocked nose because of allergy to house dust mite. *A*, Swelling of inferior turbinate blocks nose completely. Maxillary mucosa is normal. *B*, Ethmoid and sphenoid mucosa normal. Sometimes severe atopic disease can occur with extreme nasal blockade but no involvement of the sinuses.

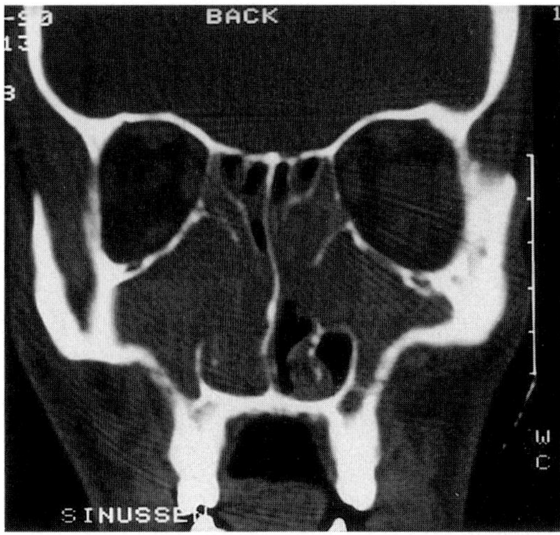

Figure 3–6. Coronal computed tomographic scan of a young adult with cystic fibrosis and massive polyposis resulting in a complete "whiteout" of paranasal sinuses.

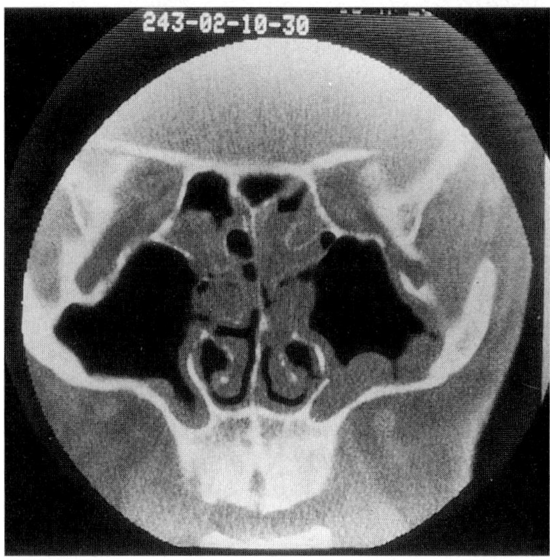

Figure 3–7. Coronal computed tomographic scan of a young adult with massive nasal polyposis in image of a "halo."

3.   *Cystic fibrosis*: In 84 patients[37] (aged 3 months to 34 years), 12% of the children had nasal obstructions due to mucopyosinusitis of the maxillary sinuses with medial displacement of the lateral nasal wall resulting in a mucopyocele (Fig. 3–9). Of the whole population, 45% had nasal obstruction due to nasal polyposis on endoscopy. In 28 patients with nasal polyposis on endoscopy, in all cases CT showed massive involvement of the anterior and middle ethmoid sinuses, maxillary sinus, and frontal sinus (if present). In 42%, the posterior ethmoid and sphenoid sinuses were free of disease.

4.   Inflammatory mucosal changes are induced mostly by chronic or recurrent inflection of the sinuses. Most of the infections are initially of viral origin followed

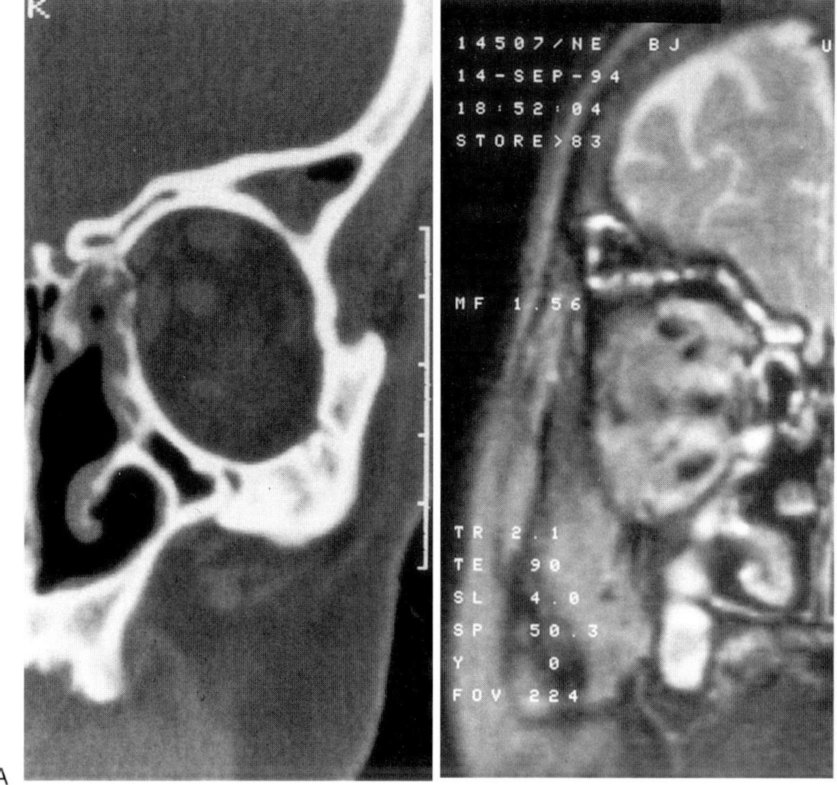

Figure 3–8.   Coronal scans of right side. *A*, Postoperative computed tomographic scan of a lateral compartment of a huge frontal sinus showing mucosal inflammation resulting in frontal pain. *B*, T$_2$-weighted magnetic resonance imaging scan of same patient after intravenous antibiotic therapy and oral prednisolone. Compartment became clear with a normal mucosa and patient had no further complaints.

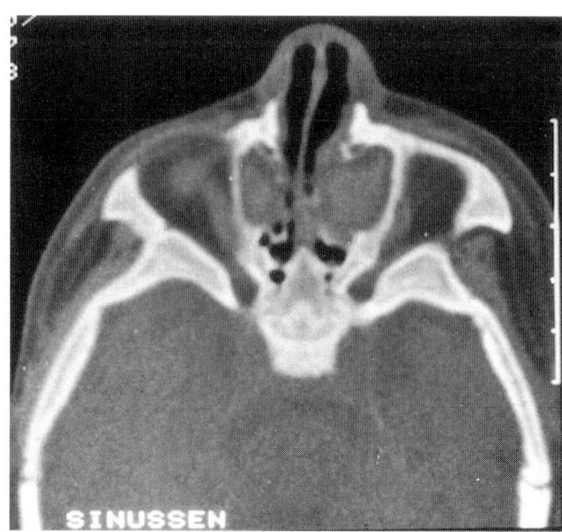

Figure 3–9.   Axial computed tomography scan of a 3-month-old infant with stridor. Total nasal blockade of the nasal airway resulted from medial displacement of lateral nasal wall due to cystic fibrosis (mucopyocele).

by a bacterial superinfection. A considerable percentage[38] of up to 10% can, however, be caused by *fungal infection* (90% by *Aspergillus fumigatus*). Sometimes CT shows the typical concrements (areas of calcification) embedded in a soft tissue mass (Fig. 3–10). If these concrements do not exist, CT does not allow differentiation between bacterial and fungal disease. On T_2-weighted MRI sequences, the fungus balls usually show signals (void areas). Although rare, there is also an invasive form of fungal disease mainly due to *Aspergillus* and *Mucormycosis*. These infections in immunocompromised patients can result in a rapid destructive process with symptoms that are not always severe enough to warrant medical attention.[27]

5. *Mechanical obstruction* also can cause chronic rhinosinusitis, but it is readily ruled out by nasal endoscopy (foreign bodies, rhinolith, prolonged intubation). Also, congenital anomalies such as choanal atresia can cause complete mechanical obstruction. Bilateral choanal atresia[39] is often diagnosed shortly after birth when a neonate shows signs of breathing and feeding difficulties. Unilateral choanal atresia is often diagnosed much later because it does not cause respiratory distress but leads to chronic rhinosinusitis. CT is not necessary for the diagnosis, but it is very helpful before operation. In particular, reformatted parasagittal CT scans clearly show the thickness of the atretic plate, the slope and thickness of the hard palate toward the skull base, and the distance between the posterior edge of the hard palate and the skull base. This is very important information before any operation can be performed. However, when the choanal atresia is accompanied by other congenital malformations (70% to 80% of cases), CT can give valuable information (Treacher Collins syndrome and other craniofacial anomalies).

6. Chronic maxillary sinusitis can be caused by *dental disease* (apical abscess, periapical infection, infected dentogenous cyst, dental filling). In these cases, most of the tissue inflammation is at the level of the floor of the maxillary sinus, decreasing toward the ostium with no or minimal involvement of the ostiomeatal complex (Fig. 3–11).

7. Although *mucoceles and other cysts* are mostly diagnosed from, or at least suspected on, CT, they are a good indication for MRI. The bony changes induced by

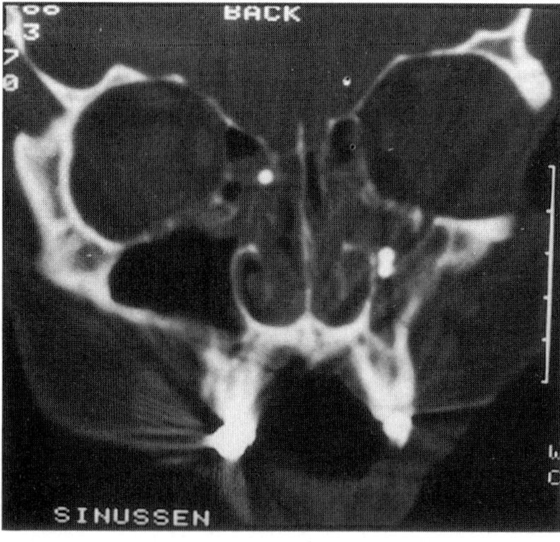

Figure 3–10. Coronal computed tomography scan of an adult with massive polyposis and concrements typical for *Aspergillus* infection.

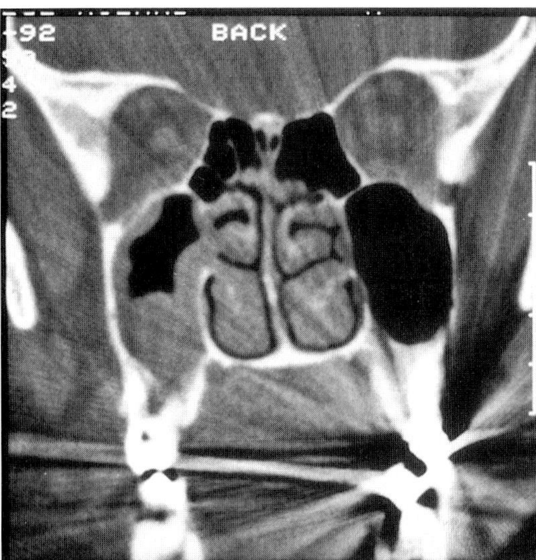

Figure 3–11. Coronal computed tomography scan of a dentogenous sinusitis.

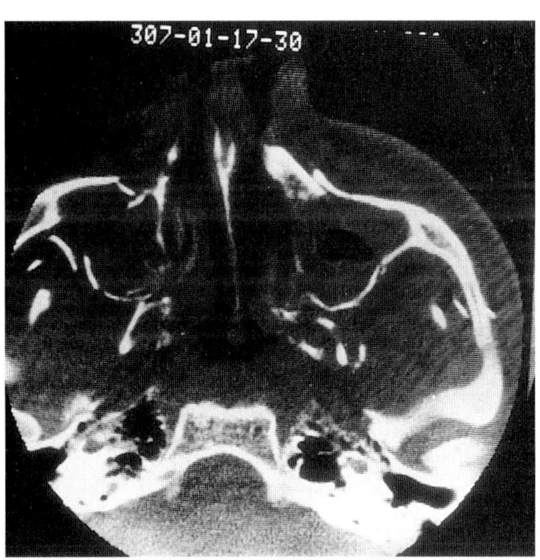

Figure 3–12. Axial computed tomography scan of extensive facial trauma with multiple fractures of maxillary sinuses and both pterygoid processes and a hematosinus on right side.

mucoceles are, of course, better diagnosed on CT; MRI, however, can differentiate between serous collections (low signal intensity on T_1-weighted scans and higher on T_2-weighted sequences) and more protein-rich fluids such as inflammatory fluid and blood (high signal on both T_1- and T_2-weighted sequences).[27]
8.   Trauma: a. *External trauma* to the head, depending on the severity, induces fractures, with or without bony displacement, resulting in bleeding, ecchymosis, hematoma, epistaxis, hematosinus, and inflammatory changes. For small fractures of the nasal bones and septum, CT scanning is not required because the diagnosis can be made easily by inspection, palpation, and rhinoscopy. For extensive frac-

tures, CT scanning is very helpful for determining the damage induced by the trauma to all facial and cranial structures (Fig. 3–12). CT scanning is superior to multidirectional tomography because the resolution and contrast are not influenced by the extent of the field to be investigated. CT scanning is very helpful for differentiating Lefort I, II, and III fractures, frontobasilar fractures (Escher types I to IV: air in the cranial fossa or subdural hematoma when posterior tabula is fractured), malar bone fractures, and blow-out fractures (fat and muscle in ethmoid or maxillary sinus). On most cases, only axial scans can be obtained because of a lack of mobility of the patient. MRI can be helpful for determining soft tissue damage, especially to the brain (T_1- and T_2-weighted images).

b. *Iatrogenic trauma* or a previous sinus operation (Fig. 3–13) is a very common indication for CT, especially after a previous Caldwell-Luc operation or limited endoscopic procedures, because it helps to establish the indications for revision operation. The most common indications for revision are closure of rhinoantrostomy

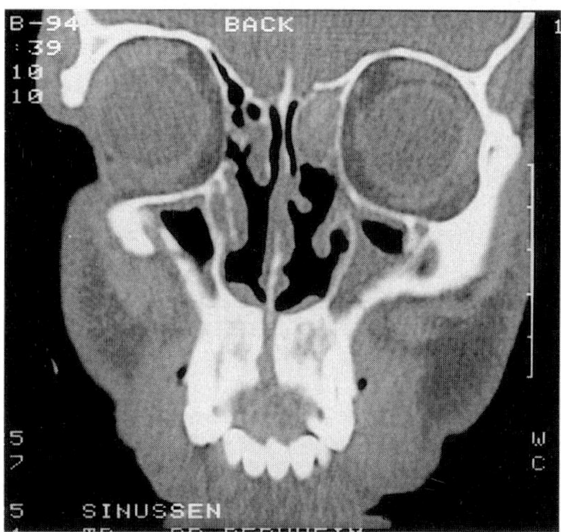

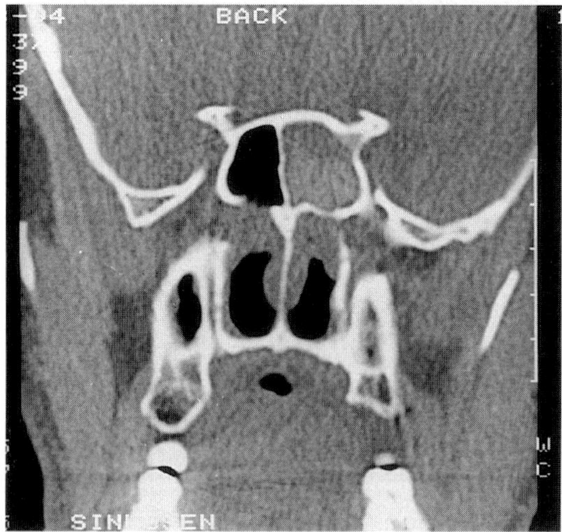

Figure 3–13. Postoperative (endoscopic sinus procedure) coronal computed tomography scans. *A*, Frontal recess on left side is not drained as well as sphenoidal sinus. *B*, Sphenoidal sinus on same side (postoperative stenosis of narrow ostium).

in the inferior meatus with or without lateralization of the inferior turbinate to this rhinoantrostomy, closure of or too small a neoostium in the middle meatus, incomplete removal of the disease in the superior cells of the ethmoidal complex (especially in the frontal recess region, inducing frontal sinus inflammation), scar formation in the previous region leading to frontal sinus disease, synechiae between the inferior border of the middle turbinate and the nasal lateral wall resulting in poor drainage and ventilation of the maxillary or frontal sinus, and closure of an insufficiently opened sphenoidal ostium.[40] Postoperatively, CT can sometimes be helpful for determining residual disease in areas that cannot be reached endoscopically (frontal sinus) or for showing the extent of recurrent disease, for instance, after operation for massive polyposis and cystic fibrosis. Normal results of endoscopy do not mean that those of CT will also be normal. During postoperative follow-up in 20 maxillary sinuses, 14 frontal sinuses, 21 sphenoidal sinuses, and 18 ethmoidal sinuses, the authors found CT signs of some abnormality (contour swelling or fibrosis, small polyps) in 55%, 14%, 23%, and 16%, respectively.

9. *The immunocompromised patient:* Any temporary or permanent immunosuppression can induce not only fungal sinusitis but also bacterial infection. This immunosuppression can be induced by cancer (such as leukemia), viral infection (such as acquired immunodeficiency virus), immunosuppressive therapy (anticancer drugs), or complications induced by drugs affecting hematopoiesis (antibiotic inducing bone narrow aplasia). The prevalence of sinusitis increases in human immunodeficiency virus (HIV)-positive patients. Actually, 30% to 68% of HIV seropositive patients experience an episode of sinusitis.[41]

10. Intracranial and intraorbital complications of sinusitis can be visualized by wide-window CT imaging for the bony lesions (osteitis, osteomyelitis) and narrow-window CT imaging with intravenous administration of contrast agent or MRI with gadolinium for the soft tissue complications (Figs. 3–14 and 3–15).

SYSTEMIC DISEASES

Some inflammatory diseases can be difficult to differentiate from tumors because they usually present both mass effect and bone destruction. This is often the case with granulomatous diseases, and even more so in the advanced stages of the diseases. All granulomatous diseases that will affect the sinonasal cavities first exhibit nasal cavity involvement that can vary from focal mucosal thickening of the nasal septum, which can be the only finding, to a localized soft tissue mass, radiologically atypical.[42] If involved, the paranasal sinuses are affected only in a later stage; maxillary and ethmoid sinuses are most often affected, whereas frontal sinuses are usually spared. Involvement of the sphenoid sinus is uncommon.

Wegener's Granulomatosis

Characterized by diffuse vasculitis and glomerulonephritis, Wegener's granulomatosis also affects the upper and lower respiratory tracts, where necrotizing granulomas are formed. The essential imaging feature of the disease at the level of the nasal and paranasal sinuses is bone destruction without the tumor mass

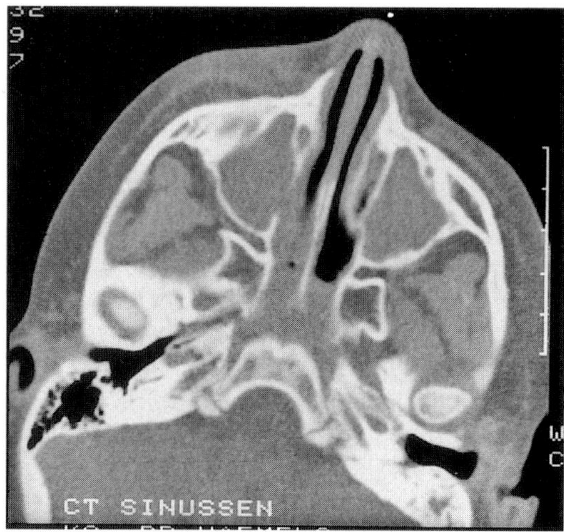

A

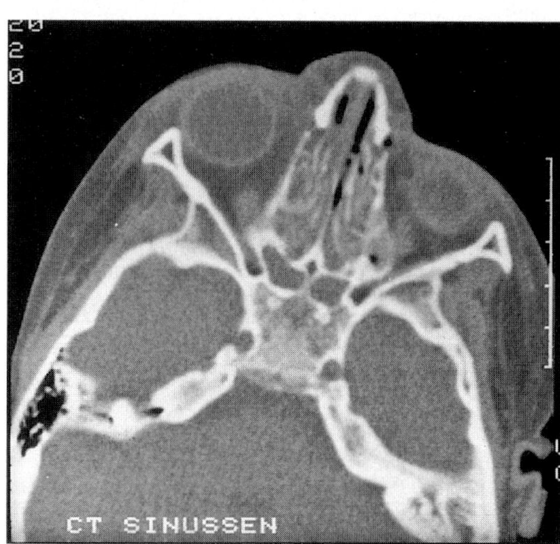

B

Figure 3–14. Axial computed tomography scans from a 9-year-old child. *A,* Bilateral maxillary sinusitis with pus under pressure on right side (bulging of posterior fontanelle region confirmed by endoscopy). *B,* Bilateral ethmoiditis and sphenoiditis with orbital phlegmone on right side.

that is to be expected in neoplastic diseases; as such, CT is more valuable than MRI.[43]

Sarcoidosis

The cause of sarcoidosis remains unclear; also a multisystem disease, it is characterized by noncaseating epithelial granulomas. Nasal involvement occurs in 3% to 20% of patients: in these cases, one may expect multiple small polypoid lesions alongside the nasal septum and turbinates.[42] The radiologic findings are totally nonspecific; still, it should be mentioned that the paranasal sinuses are seldom involved, a finding that can support the diagnosis. Rarely, sharp demarcated lytic lesions may be encountered in the facial skeleton and in the skull.

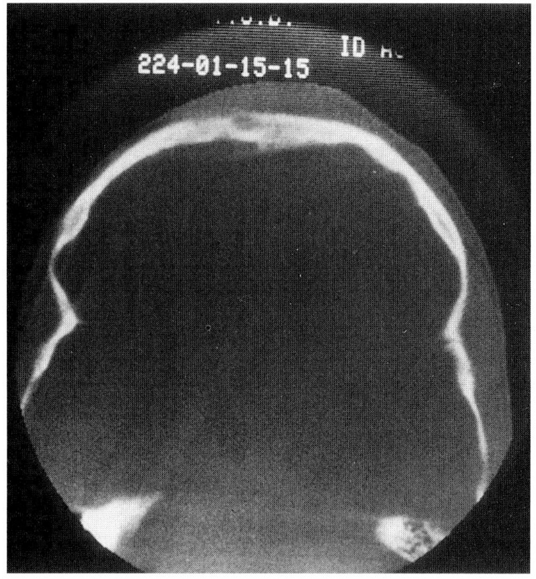

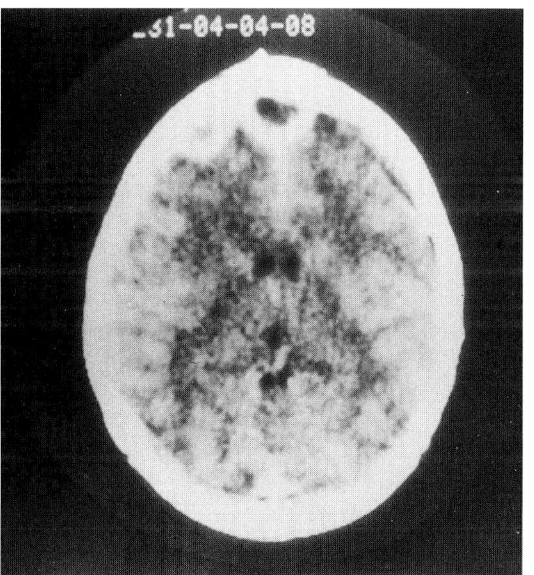

Figure 3–15. Axial computed tomography scans of a 12-year-old boy with chronic frontal sinusitis. *A,* Osteomyelitis of frontal bone (wide-window scan). *B,* Two epidural abscesses (narrow-window scan with intravenously administered contrast agent).

Other Granulomatous Diseases

These may affect the nasosinusoidal area and can be rather typical on CT. One type is lethal midline granuloma, possibly lymphoma-related and characterized by massive destruction of the nasal septum and turbinates and of the midline facial tissues. In infectious diseases such as tuberculosis and syphilis, granulomas presenting as polypoid mucosal lesions may affect the nasal cavity; both CT and MRI findings are nonspecific. Chronic exposure to irritants and especially to cocaine results first in rather nonspecific granulomas alongside the nasal septum, which may evolve into rather typical septal erosion.

TUMORS

Polyps

Even if they are not tumors, strictly speaking, polyps are in fact the most common expansile lesions in the nasal cavity. When they are multiple and packed in the nasal vault and ethmoid sinuses, they may form a conglomerate that is difficult to differentiate from bulky tumors that tend to remodel the surrounding bone as inverted papillomas or lymphomas (Fig. 3–16). On CT, polyps present with semifluid attenuation values (15 to 25 Hounsfield units), usually with a contrast-enhancing mucosal rim. On MRI, because of their rich water content, they present a high signal on T_2-weighted spin-echo sequences and a low to intermediate signal on T_1-weighted images (Fig. 3–17).

The edematous substrate of long-standing polyps may contain different cellular debris and have a higher protein content, which will lower the signal on T_2 and make the distinction between a solitary polyp and a solid tumor difficult if not impossible.

Benign Tumors

Papilloma

Three types of papillomas can be discerned in the nasosinusoidal area as a consequence of the high differentiation of the ectodermal nasal mucosa: exophytic or

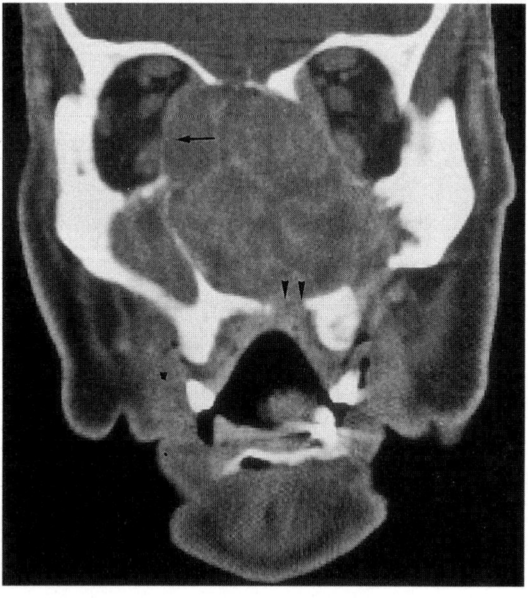

Figure 3–16. Polyposis nasi; lymphoma (coronal computed tomography image). This patient had a conglomerate of nasosinusal polyps, destruction of the maxillary sinus wall, and intraorbital extension—all suggestive of malignancy. Biopsy-proven lymphoma was found.

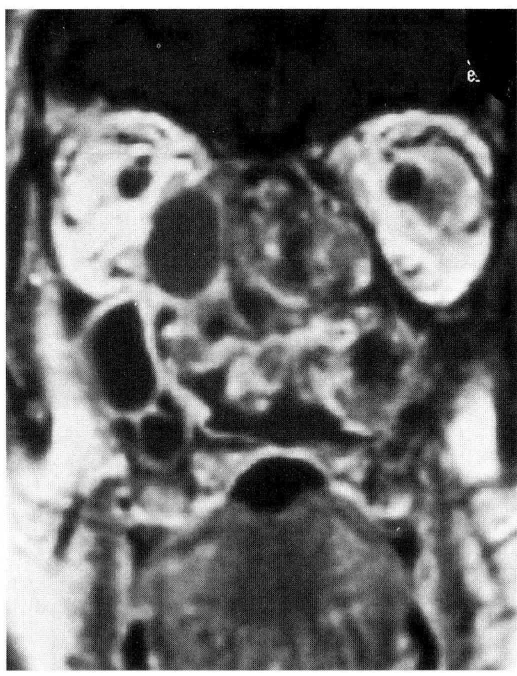

Figure 3–17. Same patient as in Figure 3–16. T_1-weighted magnetic resonance image (SE 600/15). Low to intermediate signal of the polyps with mucosal rim enhancement after intravenous injection of gadolinium-DTPA.

fungiform papillomas, endophytic or inverted papillomas, and cylindric cell papillomas.

Radiologically, we are essentially concerned with inverted papillomas because they are relatively frequent benign tumors that may become very large with massive remodeling of bone and may be confused with malignant processes. Also, cases of associated malignancy have been reported, occurring concurrently with an inverted papilloma or in patients with a previous history of inverted papilloma. The tumor usually arises from the lateral wall of the nose in the region of the middle turbinate. CT and MRI findings range from a small nasal polypoid lesion, nonspecific, to an expansile bulky mass developing near the middle turbinate with secondary extension through the maxillary ostium into the sinus cavity.[44] There can be massive bone remodeling but usually no true erosive bone lesions, which are to be expected in more aggressive malignant processes. Intralesional calcifications may be recognized on CT but will go unseen on MRI because calcium gives no MRI signal.

Angiofibroma

Consisting of highly vascular fibrous tissue, these juvenile angiofibromas affect essentially young male patients. The lesion is histologically benign, but because it is not encapsulated it may have locally aggressive growth. Angiofibromas normally arise in the nasopharyngeal wall near the pterygopalatine fossa and the sphenopalatine foramen. Most patients present with epistaxis and nasal obstruction. The first task of the radiologist is to recognize the highly vascular nature of the tumor with massive contrast enhancement on CT and to discourage any attempt at potentially dangerous biopsy before full investigation, which includes CT, MRI, and angiography. The second radiologic task is to obtain a precise mapping of the tumor, which tends to fill the entire nasopharynx and can spread intracranially; cavernous sinuses, pituitary gland, and optic chiasm should be analyzed with MRI.

Angiography is mandatory to assess the arterial supply, usually from the internal maxillary artery and ascending pharyngeal artery. Selective embolization of the nutrient vessels greatly reduces preoperative blood loss.

Angiomatous polyp

This particular polyp is thought to arise as a consequence of minor trauma. It is a fibrous nasal polyp, richly vascularized, but without the massive growth of the juvenile angiofibroma. The lesion is normally located in the nasal fossa and not in the nasopharynx, may occur at any age, and affects both male and female patients. CT contrast enhancement of the lesion can be striking, and thus differentiation from an angiofibroma is potentially difficult; still, the intranasal location and lack of extension usually indicate the diagnosis.

Hemangioma

The lesion is probably more a vascular malformation than a true neoplasm. It causes nasal obstruction and epistaxis. Most arise in the anterior septum, near Kiesselbach's plexus, are relatively small, and tend to enhance strongly after intravenous injection of contrast agent, when of the capillary type. Some hemangiomas arise more frequently from the lateral nasal wall and are usually of the cavernous type, in which case they are probably best appreciated on MRI. Hemangiomas seldom occur in the paranasal sinuses.

Solitary hemangioma of bone

Not a frequent finding in the facial skeleton, bone hemangiomas usually affect the spine; however, they have been reported in the mandible and nasal bones. They are usually incidental findings on CT, where they present as an intraosseous "honeycomb" image. Some patients are aware of a firm, nonpainful swelling, sometimes associated with a pulsating sensation. Angiography is mandatory, and selective embolization is advocated before surgical resection.

Osteoma, fibrous dysplasia, ossifying fibromas

An osteoma is a benign proliferation of bone occurring almost exclusively in the facial skeleton. It is composed of dense, mature bone and is usually found incidentally on routine CT or on plain radiography in the frontal or ethmoid sinuses and may form a mechanical obstruction to sinus drainage. Some osteomas contain mature lamellar bone but also greater amounts of intertrabecular fibrous tissue; less dense than true osteomas, these ossifying fibromas may be confused on plain radiograms with a soft tissue swelling such as a polyp or a retention cyst. High-resolution CT clearly shows the osseous nature of the lesion (Fig. 3–18).

Fibrous dysplasia is an idiopathic skeletal disorder in which medullary bone is replaced by poorly organized fibro-osseous tissue. Monostotic and polyostotic forms are recognized. When the extensive or polyostotic form is present, diagnosis of the condition usually is not difficult: different bone structures are involved with a rather characteristic "ground-glass" appearance on CT, possibly resulting in facial distortion. The diagnosis may be more difficult when only one osseous structure is involved. Depending on the amount of fibrous tissue present, the radiologic appearance varies (Fig. 3–19).

An ossifying fibroma has more highly cellular fibrous tissue and less mature osseous tissue than fibrous osteoma. On CT the lesion is expansile and usually has larger areas of fibrous tissue with lower density than fibrous dysplasia. However, in most cases the definite diagnosis has to be made histopathologically, and even the pathologist may experience difficulties in differentiating the three conditions[45] (Fig. 3–20). It is believed that an ossifying fibroma has a tendency to grow faster with possible invasion of the orbits, nasal cavity, and sinuses and to behave more aggressively than fibrous dysplasia.

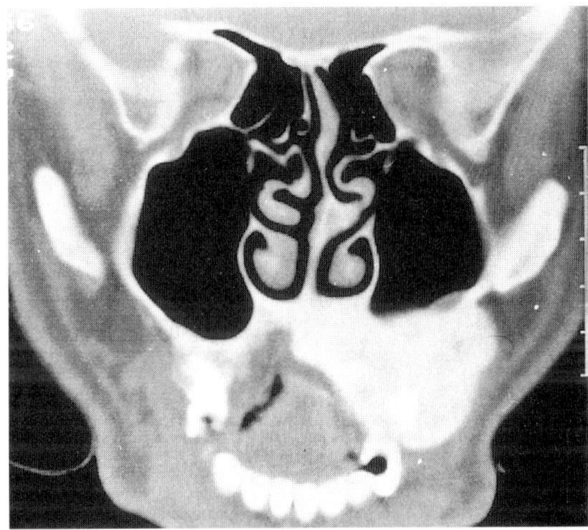

Figure 3–18. Ossifying fibroma (coronal computed tomography image). Expansile bony lesion of maxilla and alveolar ridge; computed tomography confirms osseous nature of lesion with rather characteristic "ground-glass" appearance.

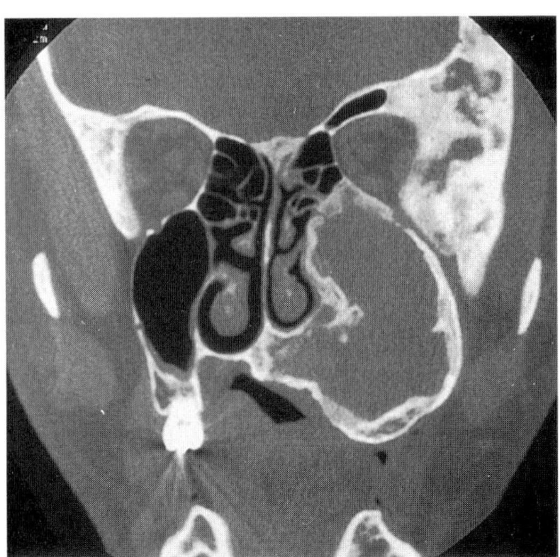

Figure 3–19. Fibrous dysplasia (coronal computed tomography image). Polyostotic form with massive involvement of facial skeleton.

Malignant Tumors

Malignant tumors of the nose and paranasal sinuses are rare and constitute less than 1% of all malignancies and 3% of all head and neck tumors. The commonest site of malignancy is the maxillary sinus, followed by the ethmoid sinuses. However, because these tumors often remain clinically "silent" for a long time, they have often reached an advanced stage when diagnosed, and thus it is often impossible to establish the exact site of origin.

Conventional plain radiography and tomography have become totally obsolete in the detection of small neoplasic lesions and are now totally replaced by CT and MRI.[46] The main objectives of current radiologic techniques are first to recognize the tumor and then to provide information on its extent. Because of their inherent different physical imaging properties, CT and MRI are complementary in the reali-

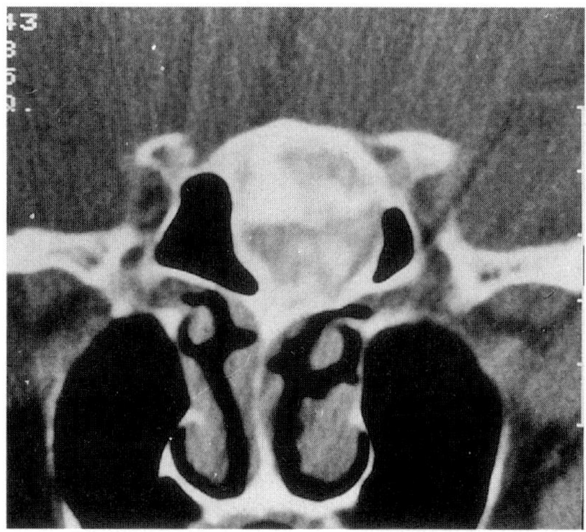

Figure 3–20. Biopsy-proven fibrous dysplasia (coronal computed tomography image). Expansile lesion involves sphenoid wing and right sphenoid sinus and has a mixed appearance with bony tissue and areas of fibrous tissue, and there is no bone destruction.

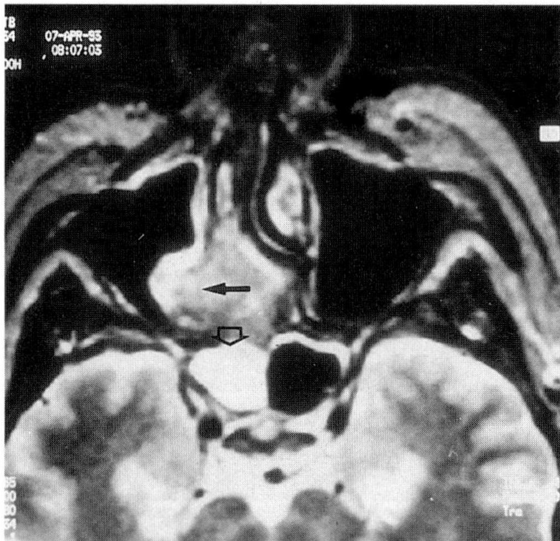

Figure 3–21. Ethmoid carcinoma (T_2-weighted magnetic resonance imaging, SE 2500/80). Solid tumor mass (*arrow*) with extension to right maxillary sinus has a lower signal than the retro-obstructive fluid (*open arrow*) in right sphenoid sinus.

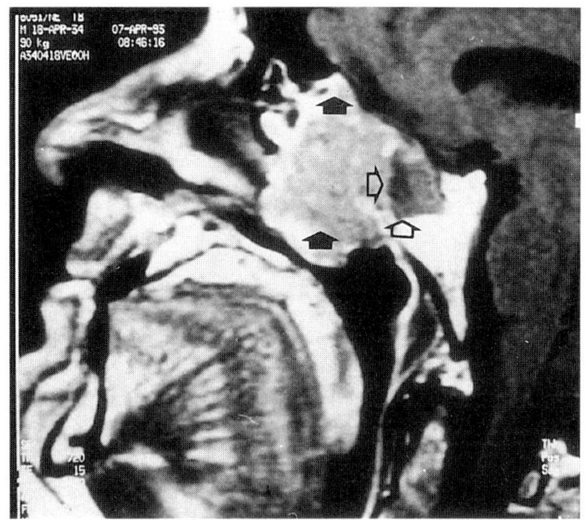

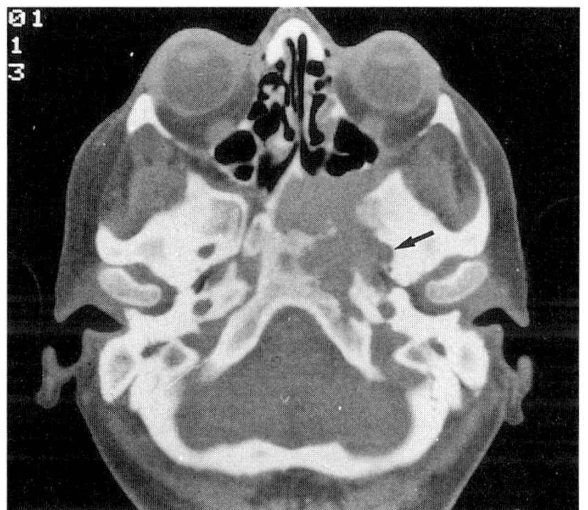

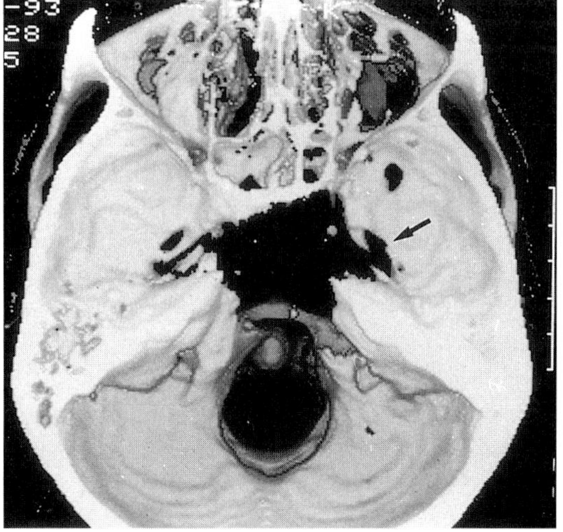

Figure 3–22. Ethmoid carcinoma. *A*, Sagittal T_1-weighted magnetic resonance imaging (SE 700/15) with gadolinium-DTPA. Massive enhancement of a huge sinonasal tumor (*arrow*). Sagittal magnetic resonance imaging allows evaluation of anterior cranial fossa. Note retro-obstructive fluid (*open arrow*) in sphenoid sinus. *B*, Axial computed tomography, high-resolution, in same patient. Evaluation of bone destruction (skull base). *C*, Three-dimensional computed tomography, in same patient, for evaluation of skull base involvement. *Arrow* on B and C refers to oval foramen.

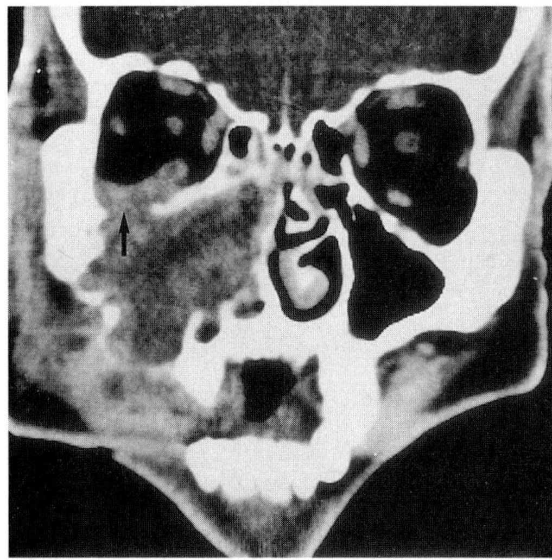

Figure 3–23. Squamous cell carcinoma of maxillary sinus (coronal computed tomography with intravenous injection of contrast agent). Heterogeneous contrast enhancement of aggressive tumor with osteolytic destruction of lateral sinus wall. Evaluation of intraorbital extent (*arrow*).

zation of this tumor mapping. CT allows a very accurate evaluation of bone destruction but has an intrinsically relatively poor density resolution. One of the main problems encountered in tumor mapping is to distinguish the tumor from adjacent inflammatory tissue. CT alone will not score very high even if an improvement in density resolution can be obtained on post-contrast CT scans. Still, the tumor margin cannot be demonstrated with certainty even after intravenous injection of a contrast medium. It is in this regard that MRI is particularly useful, essentially on T_2-weighted spin-echo sequences, in which the solid tumor has a lower signal intensity than the surrounding inflammatory edema and the retro-obstructive fluid accumulation (Fig. 3–21). Still, MRI alone is also insufficient in tumor evaluation in that cortical bone gives no signal on MRI because of a very low hydrogen content. We therefore believe that a combined approach with CT and MRI is mandatory for all malignant neoplasms (Fig. 3–22).

MRI offers the additional advantage of easy multiplanar imaging without uncomfortable repositioning of the patient. Sagittal imaging is particularly valuable in the evaluation of intracranial extent of ethmoid or sphenoid sinus carcinomas with possible growth through the cribriform plate or, in the latter case, invasion of the cavernous sinuses, not to be examined by CT alone. MRI, much better than CT, can evaluate perineural spreading. Intraorbital extension is now preferentially checked on high-resolution CT; together with a safer depiction of the fine lamina papyracea and of the orbital floor, the low attenuation values of intraorbital fat provide a very good natural contrast with the tumor mass (Fig. 3–23). The distinction beween fat and tumor is rather questionable on MRI, both tissues providing a high and very similar signal. However, improvement has been made with the development of specifically designed fat-suppression sequences. If the tumor mapping can be tolerably precise, neither CT nor MRI can distinguish the various histologic types of malignancies. Squamous cell carcinoma is by far the most frequent malignant sinonasal tumor, constituting 80% to 90% of all neoplasms, followed by

FLOW CHART OF THE IMAGING PROCEDURES OF THE NASAL AIRWAY IN PATIENTS
WITH NASOSINUSOIDAL COMPLAINTS

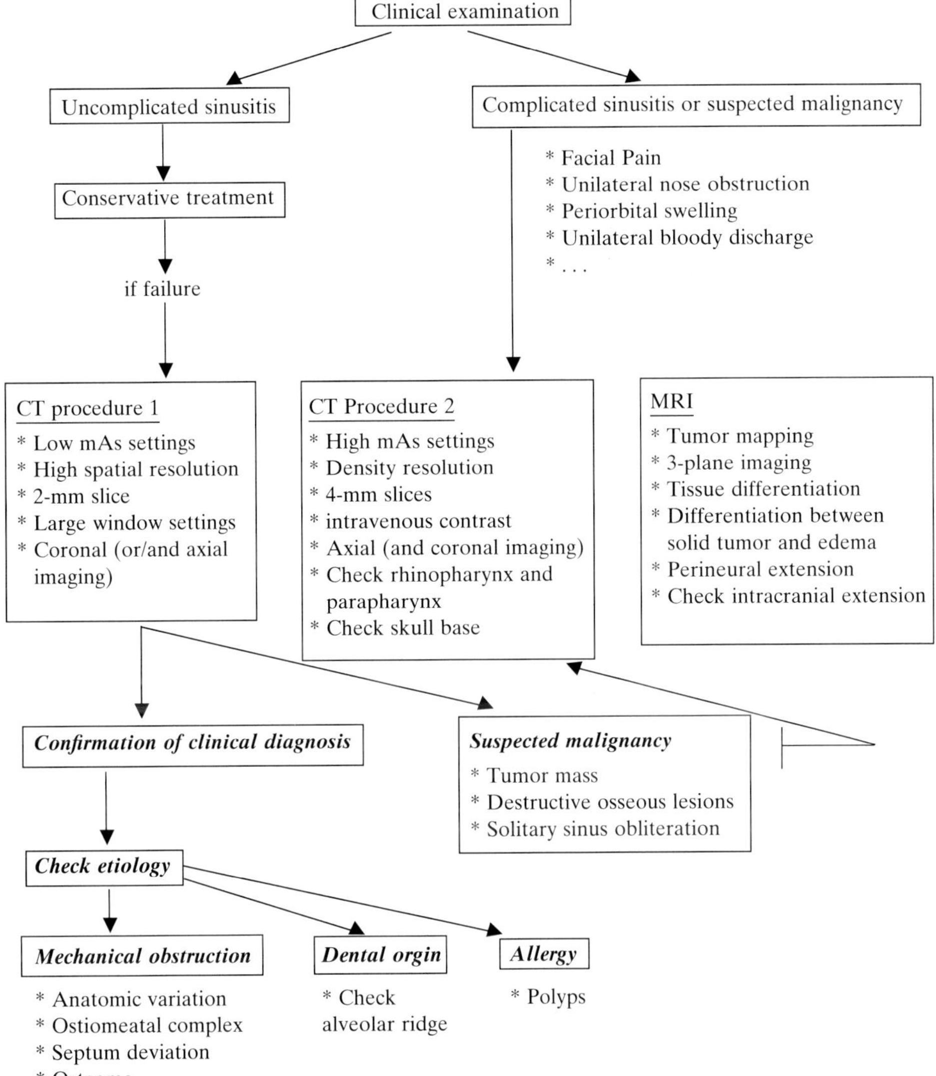

Abbreviations: CT, computed tomography; MRI, magnetic resonance imaging.

adenocarcinomas, adenoid cystic carcinomas, lymphomas, esthesioneuroblastomas, melanomas, and sarcomas.[47]

Aggressive bone destruction, demonstrated by CT, is suggestive of squamous cell carcinomas; lymphomas have more of a tendency to remodel the adjacent bone structures with less osteolysis.[48] Ethmoid carcinomas, but essentially olfactory neuroblastomas, tend to destroy the cribriform plate and to invade the anterior fossa.[49]

Nasal melanomas are unusual but may have a characteristically low signal on T_2-weighted MRI depending on their melanin content, melanin having a paramagnetic effect with lowering of the signal intensity on the T_2-weighted spin-echo sequences.[49] On the whole, it is certainly not possible to estimate the histologic nature of a malignant process on radiologic examinations because all malignant processes show a contrast-enhancing soft tissue attenuation on CT and an interme-

SUMMARY FLOW CHART

IMAGING NASAL AIRWAY   <u>1. INFLAMMATORY DISEASE</u>

Step 1:

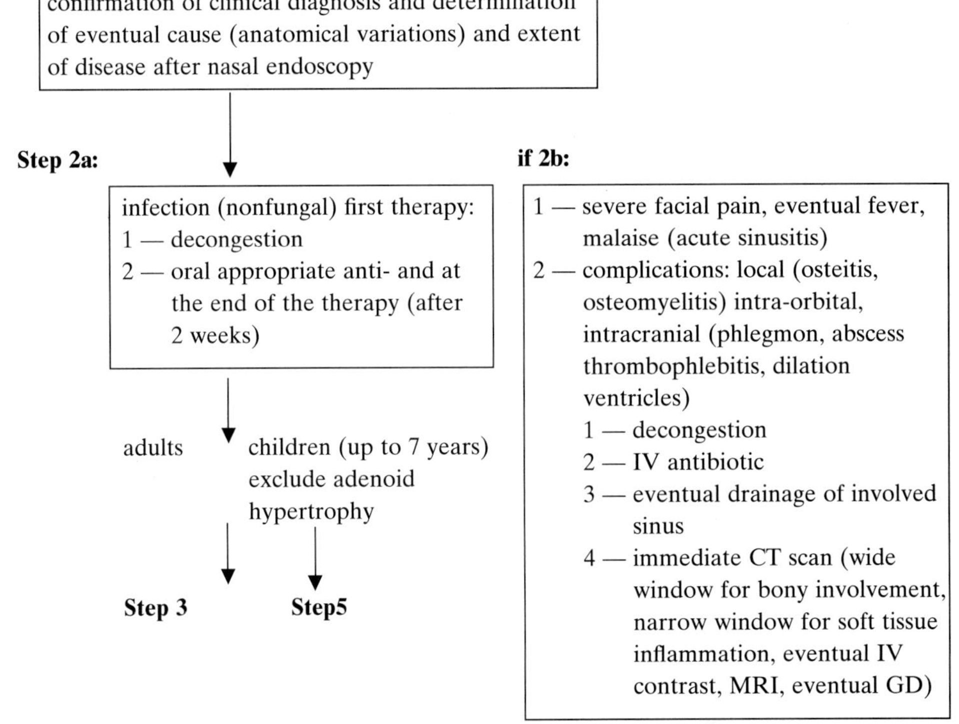

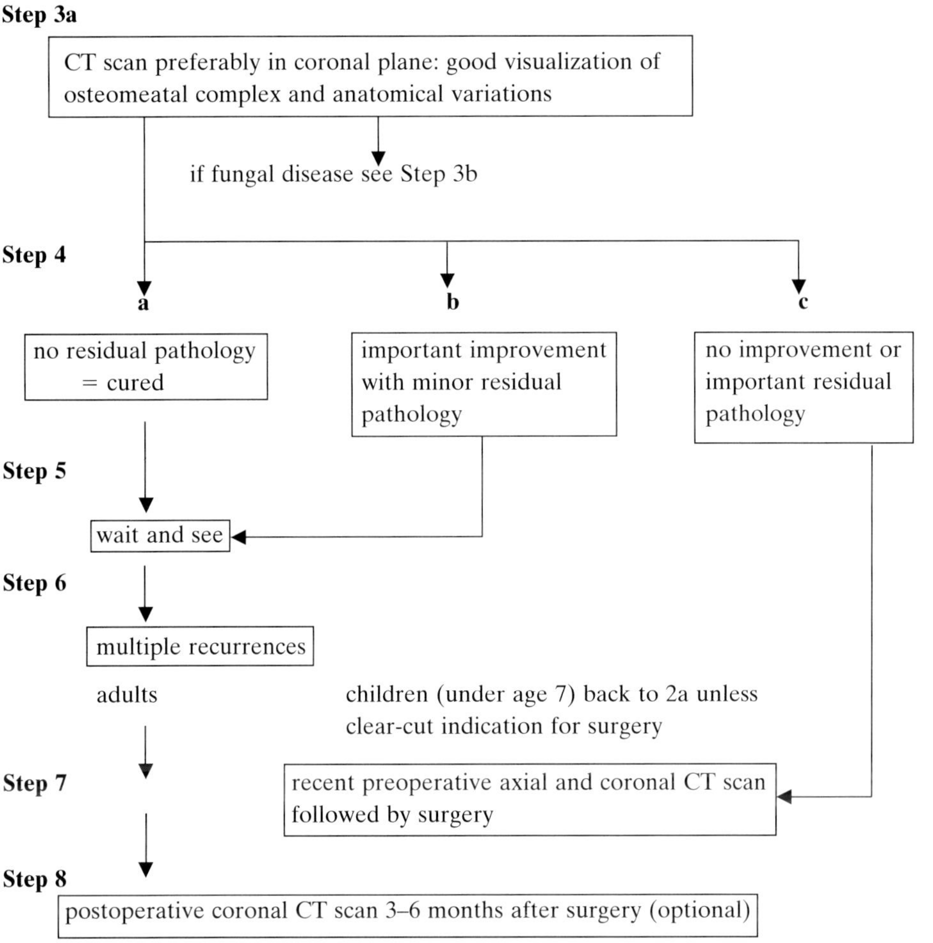

Step 3a

CT scan preferably in coronal plane: good visualization of osteomeatal complex and anatomical variations

if fungal disease see Step 3b

Step 4

a   b   c

no residual pathology = cured

important improvement with minor residual pathology

no improvement or important residual pathology

Step 5

wait and see

Step 6

multiple recurrences

adults   children (under age 7) back to 2a unless clear-cut indication for surgery

Step 7

recent preoperative axial and coronal CT scan followed by surgery

Step 8

postoperative coronal CT scan 3–6 months after surgery (optional)

Step 2c	noninfectious disease
	nasal polyposis: immediately step 3
	and—if ASA: stop NSAID
	high-dosage prednisolone therapy
	can be tried, after therapy to step 7
	—if cystic fibrosis (go to 2f)
Step 2d	allergy—proceed to step 3a + avoidance of allergen and antiallergic therapy
Step 2e	immunocompromised patients
	(immunosuppresive therapy, leukemia, AIDS)
	proceed to 2b
Step 2f	systemic disease
	—cystic fibrosis
	—immotile cilia syndrome
	(proceed to step 7)
Step 2g	dental origin—same treatment as 2a + dental care
Step 2h	mechanical obstruction
	—osteoma, rhinolith: start from 2a

	—congenital: choanal atresia: if possible CT in axial and reformatted parasagittal plane + appropriate surgery
Step 2i	mucoceles: if infected step 2a, otherwise directly step 7 and MRI helps in confirmation of diagnosis
Step 2j	trauma:—iatrogenous (= postoperative) start 2a.
	—external: fracture, intraorbital or intracranial damage immediate CT scan (wide + narrow window setting eventual + IV contrast) + eventual MRI (+GD)
Step 3b	fungal disease: diagnosis mostly made after step 3a immediately to step 7 followed by topical and general antimycotic therapy

Abbreviations: (AIDS, acquired immunodeficiency syndrome; ASA, acetylsalicylic acid; CT, computed tomography; GD, gadolinium; IV, intravenous; MRI, magnetic resonance imaging; NSAID, nonsteroidal anti-inflammatory drug.

diate, more or less homogeneous, signal on all MR sequences. We stress the importance of a baseline examination performed immediately after surgical or radiologic treatment; this is indispensable for comparison with subsequent MRI and CT examinations obtained during follow-up.

REFERENCES

1. Mittermaier R: *Otorhinolaryngologic Radiology*, ed. 3. (Translated by Hoffmann PW). Stuttgart, Georg Thieme, 1970, pp 2–180.
2. Bourjat P: *Radiodiagnostic en oto-rhino-laryngologie*, Paris, Doin. Deuxieme Partie, Nez-Sinus, 1973, pp 111–238.
3. Dodd D, Jing BS: Radiology of the Nose, Paranasal Sinuses and Nasopharynx, in Robbins LL (ed.): *Golden's Diagnostic Radiology*, Section 2. Baltimore, Williams & Wilkins, 1977, pp 57–261.
4. Potter GD: Radiology of the paranasal sinuses and facial bones, in Valvassori GE, Potter GD, Hanafee WN, Carter BL, Buckingham RA (eds.): *Radiology of the Ear, Nose and Throat*. Philadelphia, Saunders, 1982, pp 130–209.
5. Carter BL: Computed tomography, in Valvassori GE, Potter GD, Hanafee WN, Carter BL, Buckingham RA (eds.): *Radiology of the Ear, Nose and Throat*. Philadelphia, Saunders, 1982, pp 212–240.
6. Ambrose J: Computerized transverse axial scanning (tomography). Part 2. Clinical application. *Br J Radiol* 1973; 46:1023–1047.
7. Hounsfield GN: Computerized transverse axial scanning (tomography). Part 1. Description of system. *Br J Radiol* 1973; 46:1016–1022.
8. Mancuso AA, Hanafee WN: Malignant Sinus, 1 in Mancuso AA, Hanafee WN (eds.): *Computed Tomography and Magnetic Resonance Imaging of the Head and Neck*, ed. 2. Baltimore, Williams & Wilkins, 1985, pp 1–19.
9. Maatman G: *High-Resolution Computed Tomography of the Paranasal Sinuses, Pharynx, and Related Regions: Impact of CT Identification on Diagnosis and Patient Management*. Dordrecht, The Netherlands, Martinus Nijhoff, 1986.
10. Valk J: *MRI of the Brain, Head, Neck and Spine: A Teaching Atlas of Clinical Applications*. Dordrecht, The Netherlands, Martinus Nijhoff, 1987.
11. Unger IM: The nose and paranasal sinuses, in Eisenberg RL (ed.) *Head and Neck Imaging (Handbooks of Diagnostic Imaging)*. Edinburgh, Churchill Livingstone, 1987, pp 3–45.
12. Kennedy DW (ed.): *Sinus Disease: Guide to First-line Managment*. Inter Medica Partners. Health Communications, Inc., Connecticut, 1994, pp 1–48.
13. Gwaltney JM Jr, Phillips CD, Miller RD, Riker DK: Computed tomographic study of the common cold. *N Engl J Med* 1994; 330:25–30.
14. Leopold DA, Stafford CT, Sod EW, et al: Clinical course of acute maxillary sinusitis documented by sequential MRI scanning. *Am J Rhinol* 1994; 8:19–28.

15. Stammberger H, Wolf G: Headaches and sinus disease: the endoscopic approach. *Ann Otol Rhinol Laryngol* 1988; 97:3–23.

16. Messerklinger W: *Endoscopy of the Nose* (translated by J Steel). Baltimore, Urban & Schwarzenberg, 1978.

17. Kennedy DW, Zinreich SJ, Rosenbaum AE, Johns ME: Functional endoscopic sinus surgery. Theory and diagnostic evaluation. *Arch Otolaryngol* 1985; 111:576–582.

18. Kaluskar SK, Patil NP: The role of out-patient nasal endoscopy in the evaluation of chronic sinus disease (editorial). *Clin Otolaryngol* 1992; 17:193–194.

19. Vining EM, Yanagisawa K, Yanagisawa E: The importance of preoperative nasal endoscopy in patients with sinonasal disease. *Laryngoscope* 1993; 103:512–519.

20. Van der Veken P, Clement PA, Buisseret T, Desprechins B, Kaufman L, Derde MP: CAT-scan study of the prevalence of sinus disorders and anatomical variations in 196 children. *Rhinology* 1990; 28:177–84.

21. Zinreich SJ, Mattox DE, Kennedy DW, Chisholm HL, Diffley DM, Rosenbaum AE: Concha bullosa: CT evaluation. *J Comput Assist Tomogr* 1988; 12:778–784.

22. Bolger WE, Butzin CA, Parsons DS: Paranasal sinus bony anatomic variations and mucosal abnormalities: CT analysis for endoscopic sinus surgery. *Laryngoscope* 1991; 101:56–64.

23. Winzelberg GG, O'Hara K, May M: Radiology of the paranasal sinuses. Section I: Computed tomography of the paranasal sinuses, in Levine HL, May M (eds.): *Endoscopic Sinus Surgery*. New York, Thieme, 1993, pp 29–48.

24. Mehta D: *Atlas of Endoscopic Sinonasal Surgery*. Philadelphia, Lea & Febiger, 1993.

25. Vleming M: *Endoscopische Neusbijholte Chirurgie*. Thesis, Utrecht, The Netherlands, Drukkerij Elinkwijk, 1991.

26. Terrier G: *Rhinosinunasal Endoscopy*. Osnago, Marell Arti Grafiche, 1991.

27. Shakar L, Evans K, Hawke M, Stammberger H: Magnetic resonance imaging of inflammatory conditions and tumours of the paranasal sinuses, in Dunitz M (ed.): *An Atlas of Imaging of the Paranasal Sinuses*. London, The Livery House, 1994, pp 148–155.

28. Zinreich SJ, Kennedy DW, Rosenbaum AE, Gayler BW, Kumar AJ, Stammberger H: Paranasal sinuses: CT imaging. Requirements for endoscopic surgery. *Radiology* 1987; 163:769–775.

29. Clement PAR, Van der Veken P, Verstraelen J, et al: Some remarks on nasal polyposis. *Acta Otorhinolaryngol Belg* 1989; 43:267–278.

30. Weber A, May A, Von Ilberg C, Halbsguth A: The value of high resolution CT-scan for diagnosis of infectious paranasal sinuses disease and endonasal surgery. *Rhinology* 1992; 30:113–120.

31. May M, Mester SJ, Levine HL: Office evaluation of nasosinus disorders: patient selection for endoscopic sinus surgery, in Levine HL, May M (eds.) *Rhinology and Sinusology: Diagnosis, Medical Management, Surgical Approaches*. New York, Thieme Medical, 1993, pp 60–90.

32. Friedrich JP: Sinusites antérieurs: Indications et résultats de la chirurgie endoscopique. *Acta Otorhinolaryngol Belg* 1989; 43:51–58.

33. Van der Veken PJV, Clement PAR, Buisseret T, Desprechins B, Kaufman L, Derde MP: CAT-scan study of the prevalence of sinus disorders and anatomical variations in 196 children. [Dutch]. *Acta Otorhinolaryngol Belg* 1989; 43:51–58.

34. Iwens P, Clement PAR: Sinusitis in allergic patients. *Rhinology* 1994; 32:65–67.

35. Settipane GA (ed.): *Rhinitis*, ed. 2. Providence, Rhode Island Oceanside Publications, 1991, pp 173–195.

36. van Camp C, Clement PAR: Results of oral steroid treatment in nasal polyposis. *Rhinology* 1994; 32:5–9.

37. Brihaye P, Clement PAR, Dab I, Desprechins B: Pathological changes of the lateral nasal wall in patients with cystic fibrosis (mucoviscidosis). *Int J Pediatr Otorhinolaryngol* 1994; 28:141–147.

38. Stammberger H: Special problems, in Stammberger H, Kopp W, Dekornfeld TJ, Hawke M, Hasler G (eds.): *Functional Endoscopic Sinus Surgery: The Messerklinger Technique*. Philadelphia, Decker, 1991, pp 381–451.

39. Dehaen F, Clement PAR: Endonasal surgical treatment of bilateral choanal atresia under optic control in the infant. *J Otolaryngol* 1985; 14:95–98.

40. Katsantonis GP, Friedman WH, Sivore MC: The role of computed tomography in revision sinus surgery. *Laryngoscope* 1990; 100:811–816.

41. Lee KC, Tanu TA: NKO verschijnselen als gevolg van AIDS: nieuwe gegevens. *BMA* 1994; 440:5.

42. Hellquist HB: *Pathology of the Nose and Paranasal Sinuses*. London. Butterworths, 1990, pp 60–81.

43. Lloyd GAS: *Diagnostic Imaging of the Nose and Paranasal Sinuses*. London, Springer-Verlag, 1988, pp 167–168.

44. Weber AL: Tumors of the paranasal sinuses. *Otolaryngol Clin North Am* 1988; 21:439–454.

45. Harrison D, Lund VJ: *Tumours of the Upper Jaw*. London-Edinburgh, Churchill Livingstone, 1993; pp 8–224.

46. Rao VM, Flanders AE, Tom MB: *MRI and CT Atlas for Correlative Imaging in Otolaryngology,* London, Martin Dunitz, 1992.
47. Shankar L, Evans K, Hawke M, Stammberger E: *An Altas of Imaging of the Paranasal Sinuses.* London, Martin Dunitz, 1994, pp 107–121.
48. Som PM, Shugar JMA, Biller HF: The early detection of antral malignancy in the postmaxillectomy patient. *Radiology* 1982; 143:509–512.
49. Hammersmith SM, Terk MR, Jeffrey PB, Connolly SG, Colletti PM: Magnetic resonance imaging of nasopharyngeal and paranasal sinus melanoma. *Magn Reson Imaging* 1990; 8:245–253.

4

Endoscopic Diagnosis of the Nasal Airway

THOMAS V. McCAFFREY, M.D., Ph.D.

The availability of modern endoscopes has permitted detailed evaluation of intranasal structures.[1] One of the early limitations in the diagnosis and treatment of paranasal sinus disease was the difficulty in examining the narrow cleft of the nasal airway and the obscured orifices of the paranasal sinuses. The first modern endoscopic examination of the nasal airway was performed by Hirschmann, who used a modified cystoscope; however, the bulky nature of the equipment and the lack of an adequate method for illumination greatly limited the usefulness of nasal endoscopy until after World War II.[2] In the early 1950s, Hopkins greatly improved the optics used for endoscopy. The Hopkins endoscopes included bright illumination, high-contrast optics, and a large field of vision in an endoscope of very small diameter. However, the availability of high-quality endoscopes did not lead to immediate changes in the practice of nasal diagnosis and surgery. A fundamental change in the thinking about the etiology and pathogenesis of sinus disease was required. Beginning in the 1950s with the availability of the Hopkins endoscope, Messerklinger began a systematic study of the nasal airway.[3] His studies led to a fundamental change in our understanding of sinus disease. He showed that in most cases, the frontal and maxillary sinuses become involved indirectly by primary disease that originates in the lateral nasal wall and in the anterior ethmoidal sinus. This region of the nose, the ostiomeatal complex, is the common drainage pathway for the ethmoidal, frontal, and maxillary sinuses. Even minimal disease in this area is able to obstruct the normal mucociliary activity that clears the sinuses. This condition can lead to either acute or chronic sinus disease.

Over the years, Messerklinger developed surgical techniques for disease in the ostiomeatal complex region of the nose. He began using endoscopes first for diagnosis and later for surgical procedures to correct obstruction and disease in this region, because only with endoscopes could the ostiomeatal complex be delineated noninvasively. He found that very limited surgical procedures directed to the ostiomeatal complex and anterior ethmoidal sinus could correct extensive diseases

75

in adjacent sinuses. This understanding of the pathogenesis of sinus disease made it possible to correct and treat sinus disease surgically without the extensive and radical procedures previously advocated.

Messerklinger, through diligent and persistent scientific investigation utilizing newly available technology, developed a radically new approach to the treatment of sinus disease. His students and successors have expanded the application of endoscopic surgery beyond the treatment of diseases of the paranasal sinuses.[2]

ANATOMY OF THE LATERAL NASAL WALL

The detailed anatomy of the lateral nasal wall is the foundation of endoscopic nasal diagnosis, functional endoscopic sinus surgery, and related procedures. The most important aspect in the anatomy of the lateral nasal wall is the ethmoid bone. The ethmoid bone consists of a T-shaped primary structure supporting a bilateral ethmoid labyrinth (Fig. 4–1). The vertical portion of the T consists of the perpendicular plate of the ethmoid, which forms the posterior portion of the nasal septum. The horizontal limb of the T consists of the cribriform plate. Suspended from the horizontal limb of the T, the ethmoid labyrinth is a complex structure with multiple bony septa and the medial projections of the superior and middle turbinates. It is important to recognize that the middle and superior turbinates are integral parts of the ethmoid bone. The internal cells of the ethmoid labyrinth provide the drainage paths for both the frontal sinus and the maxillary sinus.[4] A secondary projection of the ethmoid bone, the uncinate process, forms a recess (the infundibulum) into which the maxillary sinus drains (Fig. 4–2). This region is critically important in both the diagnosis and the treatment of sinus disease. Because the infundibulum is

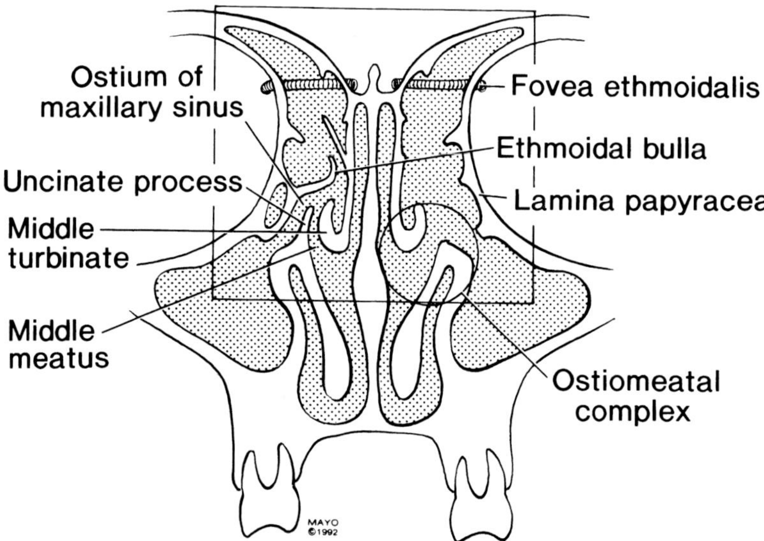

Figure 4–1.   Coronal section through mid-portion of ethmoid sinuses, showing relationships of ethmoid labyrinth, middle meatus, and ostiomeatal complex.

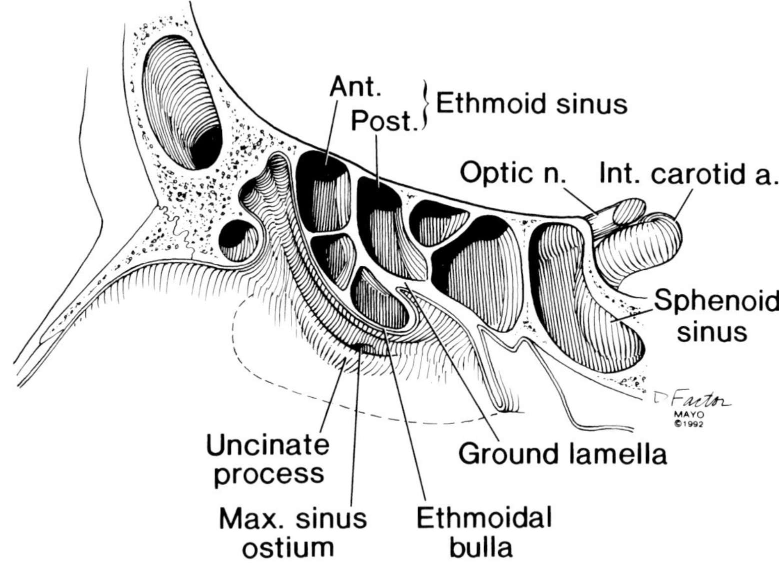

Figure 4–2.   Important structures of the lateral nasal wall.

narrow, it is likely to be obstructed, resulting in secondary disease in the adjacent maxillary sinus.

To fully understand the etiology and pathogenesis of sinus diseases, it is important to understand the function of the mucociliary transport system in maintaining the normal physiologic environment of the sinuses. The paranasal sinuses are air-filled cavities that normally communicate with the nasal airway. They are lined by pseudostratified ciliated epithelium that is covered by a thin layer of mucus. The cilia within the sinuses beat in a predetermined direction toward the natural ostia of the sinuses. Mucus produced in the sinuses is transported toward the ostia by these beating cilia and expelled into the nasal airway. Any bacterial contamination of the sinuses is effectively cleared by this mechanism. However, if the sinus ostia are obstructed, either mechanically or by edema of the closely approximated mucosa in the region of the ostiomeatal complex, mucociliary flow is interrupted. Obstruction of the sinus ostia causes the oxygen tension within the sinus to decrease and the carbon dioxide tension to increase. This relatively anaerobic high CO_2 environment within the sinus and stagnation of the mucus can facilitate bacterial growth. This in turn can further inhibit mucociliary transport by changing the viscosity of the mucus and directly inhibiting ciliary activity. This chain of events leads to the development of acute or chronic sinusitis.

It has long been common practice to treat sinus infections by surgical drainage of the sinuses. Typically, the regions of the natural ostia of the sinuses are avoided in these surgical procedures. Although such surgical procedures often result in clearing of the acute sinus infection, they are not effective in preventing reaccumulation of mucus within the sinuses. Because the normal ciliary beat transports mucus toward the natural ostium, making a new ostium in a site distant from the natural ostium fails to redirect the mucus flow to the newly created ostium.[3] The result is reaccumulation of mucus and the risk of reinfection of the sinuses. Messerklinger's observations of the patterns of mucociliary flow demonstrate this deficiency in the standard treatment of sinus disease and have led to the practice of enlarging the natural ostia of the sinuses. With the newly developed Hopkins endoscopic telescopes, highly precise dissection of the ostiomeatal complex is possible. These procedures could not have been done without this optical aid because of the inability to fully visualize this region directly.

INDICATIONS FOR NASAL ENDOSCOPY

The diagnostic workup includes diagnostic nasal endoscopy and computed tomography scanning of the paranasal sinuses in both the coronal and the axial planes. Diagnostic nasal endoscopy is performed systematically.[5] The required equipment is a nasal speculum and various Hopkins nasal endoscopes (4 mm: 0° and 30°; 2.7 mm: 30° and 70°). The nasal cavity is initially examined with conventional anterior rhinoscopy with the nasal speculum. The condition of the mucosa, the degree of congestion, and the relative patency of the nasal airway can be assessed. The nose is then decongested with topical 1% phenylephrine spray and anesthetized with topical 4% lidocaine.

After maximal decongestion is obtained, the nose is examined with a nasal telescope (Fig. 4–3). A 0° nasal endoscope is introduced into the nasal cavity and passed to the posterior of the nose along the middle meatus to obtain an overall view of the lateral nasal wall. Special attention is then turned to the middle meatus because this area of the ostiomeatal complex is most susceptible to conditions

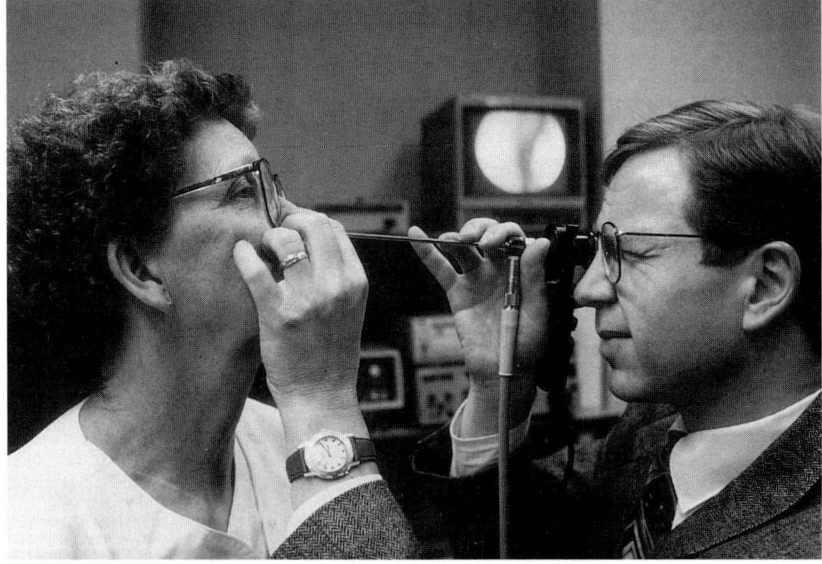

Figure 4–3.   Examination of nasal airway with an endoscope.

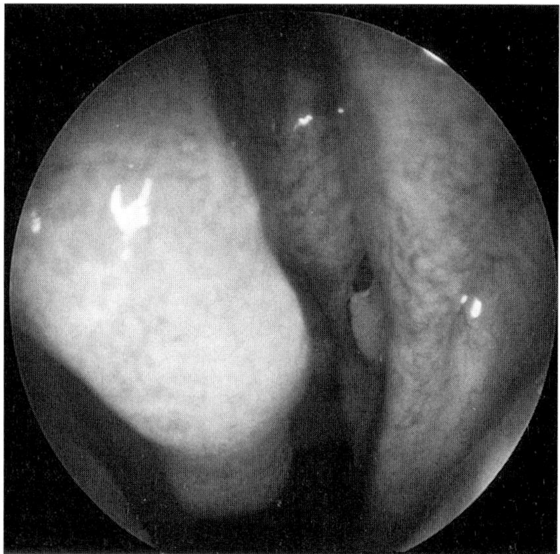

Figure 4–4. Endoscopic view of middle turbinate, ostiomeatal complex, and uncinate process.

leading to chronic sinusitis. The presence of polyps can be noted, as well as any mucopurulent material draining from the ostia of the sinuses. If the 4-mm 0° telescope does not provide adequate visualization, the 2.7-mm 30° telescope is used to obtain a better view of the recess of the middle meatus and infundibulum. The findings on nasal endoscopy are compared to computed tomography (CT) scans of the sinuses. A coronal CT scan provides optimal views of the ethmoid, maxillary, and frontal sinuses and their ostia. The uncinate process, the ostium, and maxillary sinus can be identified (Fig. 4–4). Particular attention is directed toward the ostiomeatal complex and the anterior ethmoid cells. Small cysts and congestion in this area can be the cause of more extensive obstruction of the adjacent sinuses. Pneumatization of the middle turbinate, a condition known as concha bullosa, should be noted because this may be the cause of obstructive sinus disease or it may produce a facial pain syndrome by impaction on the septum (Fig. 4–5). Evaluation of the sphenoid sinus is not always possible on coronal CT scans, and optimal examination of the sphenoid sinus is usually performed with an axial view of the paranasal sinuses.

After evaluation endoscopically and with CT, the indications for endoscopic surgical intervention can be reasonably assessed.[6] In most cases, diseases of the maxillary and frontal sinuses are associated with obstruction of the anterior ethmoid cells. Surgical opening of the anterior ethmoid cells and ostia of the frontal and maxillary sinuses will resolve these conditions. Radical exenteration of the posterior ethmoid sinuses and sphenoid sinuses is usually not necessary.

The diagnosis of nasal obstruction can also be improved by endoscopic evaluation of the nasal airway. Sites of obstruction can be qualitatively assessed, and the relative degree of obstruction can often be determined.[7] Careful endoscopic evaluation of the nasal airway can reveal the cause of nasal obstruction and sinus disease when other diagnostic procedures have failed.[8]

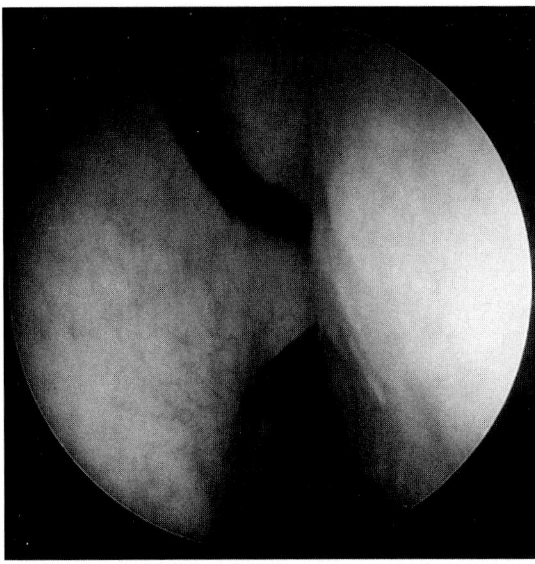

Figure 4–5. Septal impaction into middle turbinate seen through 4-mm 0° endoscope.

ENDOSCOPIC EQUIPMENT

The best endoscopic results are obtained if the equipment is properly selected for its intended use. The requirements for routine diagnostic endoscopy are different from the requirements for producing high-quality endoscopic slides or videos. The basic instrumentation and its uses and limitations are described in this section.

Endoscopes

Nasal endoscopes are available in several designs and diameters. The two major categories are flexible and rigid. Each has advantages and disadvantages and the type selected is determined by the particular needs.

Flexible endoscopes

The flexible endoscope was initially developed for bronchoscopy. It consists of two fiberoptic cables and associated optics. One cable passes light to the distal tip of the scope for illumination, and the second cable transmits the image to the observer. The outside diameter of these scopes varies from 2.5 to 4.5 mm (Fig. 4–6).

The advantages of a flexible scope are obvious. It is possible to bend the scope around obstructions and into orifices of the sinuses. The disadvantages are related to the image quality possible with a fiberoptic cable. The image produced by a fiberoptic cable is composed of an array of points produced by individual fibers within the bundle. The resolution depends on the number and size of the individual fibers. Increasing the number of fibers increases the diameter of the instrument, and decreasing the size of the fibers is limited by technical manufacturing conditions and

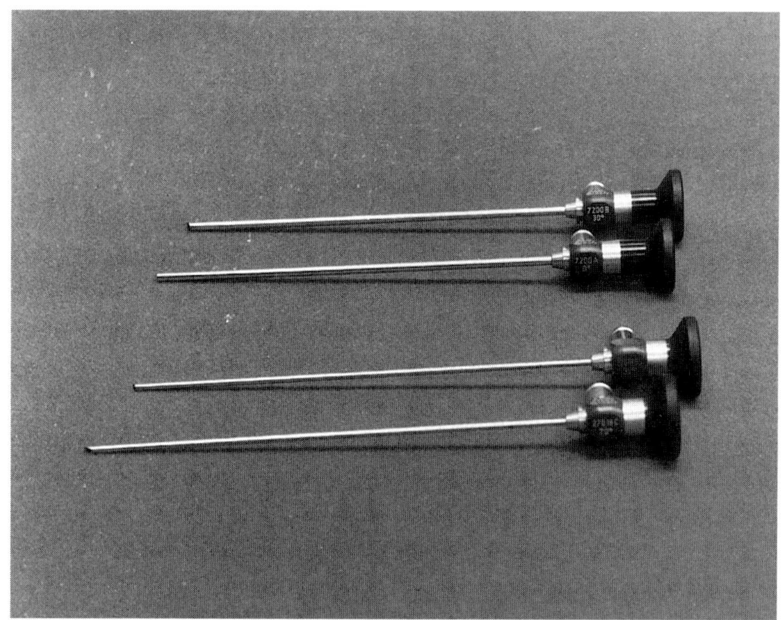

Figure 4–6. The standard endoscopes used for endoscopic diagnosis. Shown are 0° and 30° 4-mm endoscopes and 30° and 70° 2.7-mm endoscopes.

Table 4–1   Recommended Endoscopes

SCOPE	DIAMETER, MM	VIEWING ANGLE, DEGREES
Storz 7200A	4	0
Storz 7200B	4	30
Storz 27018B	2.7	30
Storz 27018C	2.7	70

cost. Even with very small fibers, a flexible scope always has less light transmission and poorer image quality than a rigid scope of equal diameter.

Despite their limitations, flexible scopes can be used effectively for diagnosis of intranasal and sinus disease.

Rigid endoscopes

Rigid endoscopes have been used for many years for the examination of body cavities and orifices. As the optics of these instruments have improved, image quality brightness and field of view have improved. The development of the Hopkins rod lens telescopes in the 1950s led to rigid endoscopes with a diameter small enough to be practically useful in the nasal cavity.

Currently, scopes of diameters down to 1.2 mm with observing angles of 0° to 120° are available. The advantages of rigid scopes are high image quality as with the flexible scope and a bright image with a wide field of view. As the diameter of the scope is reduced, the brightness and size of the image are reduced, as with the flexible scope. For practical diagnostic use in the nasal airway and sinuses, 4.0-mm and 2.7-mm scopes are most commonly used (Table 4–1). These scopes provide a good compromise between scope diameter and image size and brightness. Angled scopes of 30° and 70° are useful for examining the middle meatus sinus orifices and the roof of the nose.

Light Sources

Optical telescopes, both rigid and flexible, require intense illumination. Because the instruments provide a wide viewing angle, light falloff with distance is very rapid. Illumination from the tip of the scope can be considered a point source. The illumination decreases with the square of the distance from the light source. The imaging loss also introduces light loss, which further attenuates the brightness of the image. For this reason, intense halogen or xenon light sources are used to provide adequate illumination (Fig. 4–7). The light source with the greatest illumination should generally be used with small scopes because of the reduced light transmission. The halogen miniature light sources are adequate for viewing, but the xenon light source is necessary for still photography.

Still Photography

Photographic documentation of the nasal airway and paranasal sinuses provides a permanent record of the visual appearance of the nasal and sinus mucosa for record keeping, for transmission of documentation of referring or consulting physicians, and for comparison during and after treatment.[9]

Intranasal and intrasinus photographic documentation was difficult, if not impossible, before the wide availability of efficient endoscopes and high-intensity light sources. However, with rigid and flexible endoscopes the nasal cavity and sinuses can be visualized and photographed readily.[10] Photography places increased demands on any imaging system because photographic emulsions do not have the sensitivity and range of the human retina.

The requirements for still photography of the nasal airway are a single lens reflex camera body with a low light viewing screen, a stroboscopic light source, and a supplementary lens system to link the endoscope to the camera body (Fig. 4–8, Table 4–2). The supplementary lens system enlarges the small image produced by the optics of the endoscope and projects it onto the focal plane of the camera body. A variable focal length supplemental lens permits the image size to be expanded to fill the frame of the camera.

Usually, photodocumentation is done on slide film. Various types and speeds of films are available, and the type used depends on the light available and the quality of the image required. The highest quality image is produced by Kodachrome film. This film produces the highest color saturation with minimal graininess. The limitations of this film are its high cost of processing and the relatively slow photographic speed. The highest-speed Kodachrome film is ASA 200. Therefore, this film re-

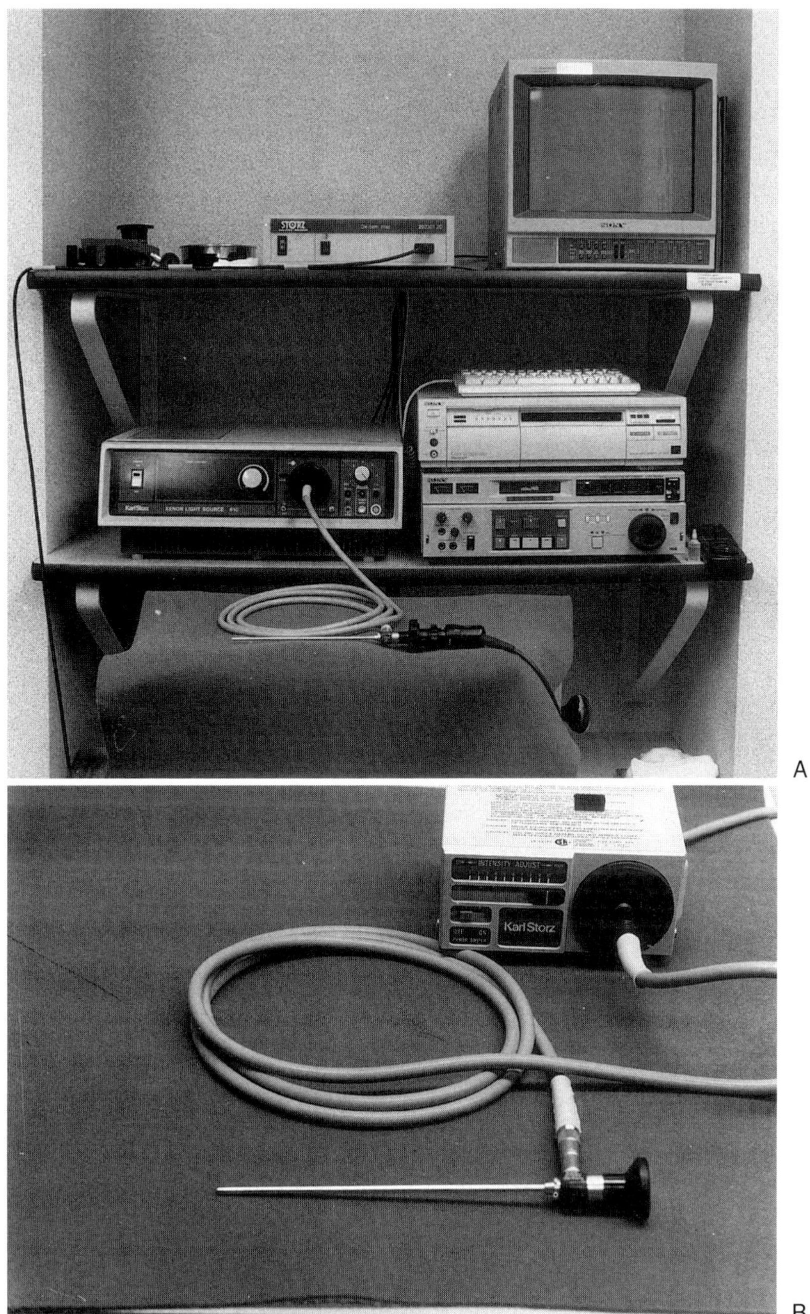

Figure 4–7. *A*, Karl Storz 610 xenon photographic light source suitable for still and video endoscopic photography. *B*, Karl Storz 481-C miniature halogen light source suitable for routine office examinations.

Table 4–2   Recommended Still Photography Equipment

ITEM	SUGGESTED MODEL
Camera Body	Nikon or Olympus OM-4
Lens	Karl Storz 593–T2
Film	Kodachrome ASA 200 or Ektachrome ASA 400
Light Source	Karl Storz Model 610

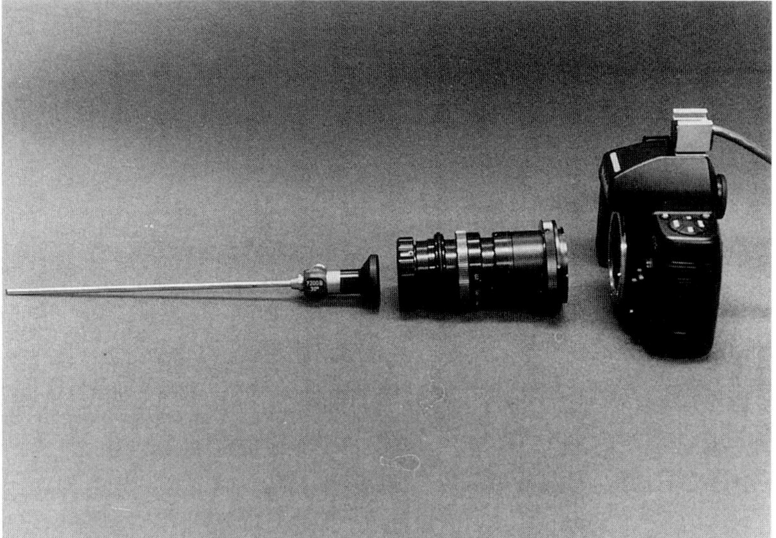

Figure 4–8.   Still photography with nasal endoscopes. Left, Nasal endoscope. Middle, Supplemental zoom lens. Right, Single lens reflex camera body.

quires bright light sources or long exposure times. High-intensity xenon strobe sources such as the Karl Storz Model 610 produces enough light for exposure of this film. Slides of suitable quality, however, can be obtained from Ektachrome film, which comes in speeds up to ASA 1600. The higher speed films tend to have increased graininess and less color saturation than Kodachrome but the advantage of the higher speed may make them more suitable in most cases.

Video Documentation

The availability of compact CCD-type video cameras has made video documentation of the nasal airway possible with endoscopes. The advantage of video documentation is the rapid acquisition of the image without the need for the photoprocessing required for still film, although the image quality is not as good with video documentation as with photography (Table 4–3).[11] Because of the small size and convenience of video cameras, the camera may be used routinely in nasal endoscopy (Fig. 4–9). The high light sensitivity of modern video systems permits their use with moderate-intensity light sources. For video recording, the available formats are VHS, sVHS, 8-mm, Hi8, and 3/4 in Umatic formats. The VHS and sVHS formats are more widely used and are best for compatibility. The 8-mm formats have the convenience of small tape size, which facilitates storage. The 3/4 in Umatic format is less common and has large cassettes, but it has the higher image quality. For most purposes, the sVHS format is a good compromise between convenient size and image quality.

With video imaging, it is now possible to rapidly produce high-quality prints of images with dye transfer imagers. These images can be used for rapid documentation of pretreatment and posttreatment findings.

Table 4–3   Comparison of Video and Photo Documentation

	VIDEO	PHOTOGRAPHY
Image Availability	Immediate	After Processing (1 day–1 wk)
Image Quality	Fair	Excellent
Initial Cost	High	Moderate
Ease of Use	High	Moderate
Major Use	Documentation	Presentation

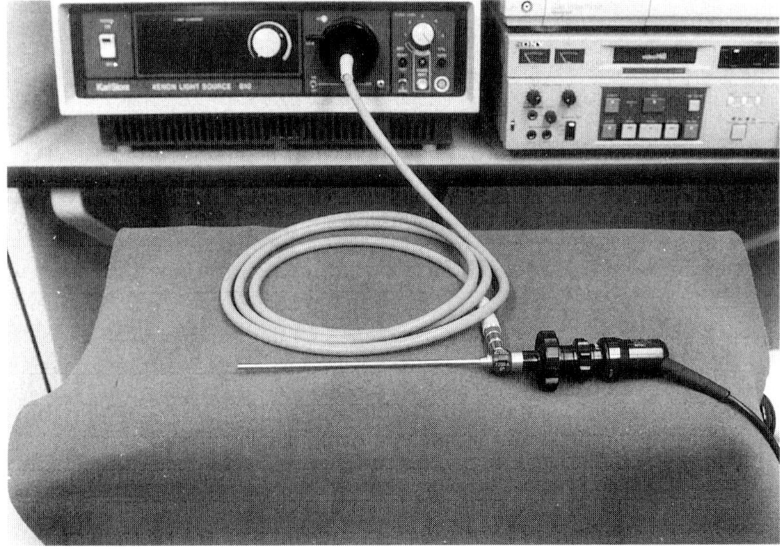

Figure 4–9. Small CCD endoscopic video camera attached to nasal endoscope.

CLINICAL CONSIDERATIONS

The clinical role of nasal endoscopy includes diagnosis, documentation, teaching, and consultation. The high-quality instruments now available permit visualization of intranasal structures that were previously inaccessible. This facilitates diagnosis of nasal obstruction, sinus infection, and neoplasms. The recording techniques of still photography and video imaging permit retention of images for later retrieval and comparison.

REFERENCES

1. Bolger WE, Kennedy DW: Nasal endoscopy in the outpatient clinic. *Otolaryngol Clin North Am* 1992; 25:791–802.
2. Stammberger H: *Functional Endoscopic Sinus Surgery: The Messerklinger Technique*. Philadelphia, Decker, 1991.
3. Messerklinger W: *Endoscopy of the Nose*. Baltimore, Urban & Schwarzenberg, 1978.
4. Lang J: *Clinical Anatomy of the Nose, Nasal Cavity, and Paranasal Sinuses*. New York, Thieme Medical Publishers, 1989.
5. Stammberger H: Nasal and paranasal sinus endoscopy. A diagnostic and surgical approach to recurrent sinusitis. *Endgoscopy* 1986; 18:213–218.
6. Vining EM, Yanagisawa K, Yanagisawa E: The importance of preoperative nasal endoscopy in patients with sinonasal disease. *Laryngoscope* 1993; 103:512–519.
7. Selner JC, Koepke JW, Staudenmayer H, et al: Assessment of nasal patency by rhinoscopic measurement of cross sectional nasal airway area: correlation with subjective nasal symptoms. *Ann Allergy* 1991; 66:43–47.
8. Levine HL: The office diagnosis of nasal and sinus disorders using rigid nasal endoscopy. *Otolaryngol Head Neck Surg* 1990; 102:370–373.
9. Gardner AP: Endoscopy and endoscopic photography in ENT. *J Audiov Media Med* 1992; 15:26–31.
10. Leopold DA: Flexible fiberoptic and rigid telescopes for intranasal photography. *Laryngoscope* 1984; 94:1509–1511.
11. Mambrino L, Yanagisawa E, Yanagisawa K, Gallo O: Endoscopic ENT photography: a comparison of pictures by standard color films and newer color video printers. *Laryngoscope* 1991; 101:1229–1232.

5

Rhinomanometry: The Application of Objective Airway Testing in the Clinical Evaluation of Nasal Obstruction

JOHN F. PALLANCH, M.D.

Rhinomanometry is an objective assessment of the nasal airway done by the simultaneous measurement of transnasal pressure and flow. This chapter describes the different methods of rhinomanometry and the equipment that is used for rhinomanometry and proposes a method for the application of objective airway testing to the clinical assessment of the patient who complains of nasal obstruction.

DIFFERENT METHODS OF RHINOMANOMETRY

Pressure Measurement

Three different methods are currently in use for measuring the pressure difference across the nose: anterior, posterior, and pernasal. In all three methods, the pressure in front of the nose is either the pressure inside a mask if the patient is wearing a mask or the atmospheric pressure in the room the patient is in.

Anterior method

In the anterior method, the pressure behind the nose is measured by sealing a tube over the nostril not being tested (Fig. 5–1). The pressure behind the nose is compared with the pressure inside a mask covering the patient's nose and thus

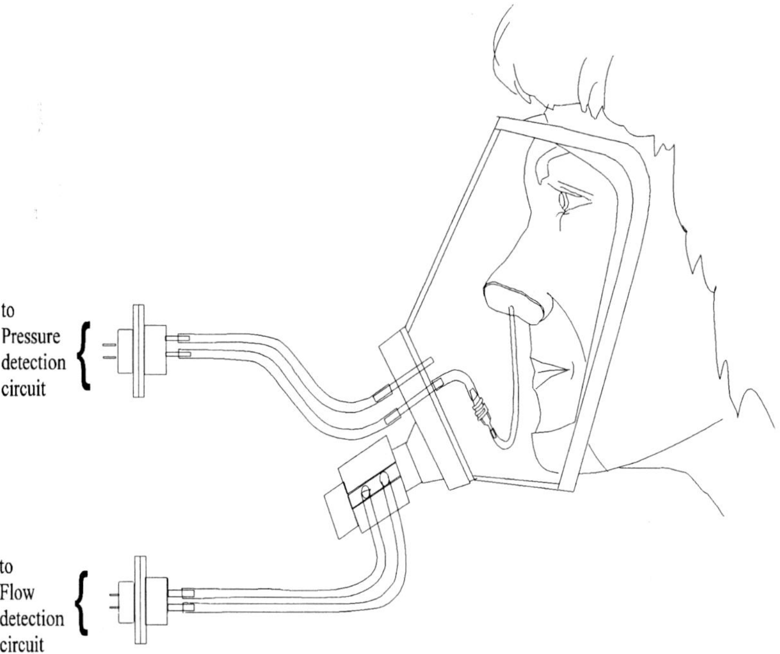

Figure 5–1.   Anterior mask rhinomanometry.

transnasal pressure is obtained. The anterior method does not require a tube inside the nose or mouth. It does not work for a patient with a septal perforation.

Posterior method

In the posterior method, the pressure behind the nose is detected with a tube positioned in the back of the patient's mouth.

The posterior method requires the most patient skill. For successful performance of the posterior method, the patient must be coached to keep both the oropharynx and nasopharynx open during the test. Failure rates up to 50% have been reported because of patient's inability to accomplish this,[1–7] including a failure rate of 15% in 5,000 patients.[8] One advantage of the posterior method is that because it is not necessary to seal one side of the nose, both sides of the nose can be measured simultaneously to assess total nasal resistance.

Pernasal method

In the third method of pressure detection, the pressure behind the nose is measured by passing a tube through one nostril to the back of the nose. Like the posterior method, this method allows direct measurement of total resistance, yet it is not difficult for the patient to learn to do. The patient can experience a bit of irritation when the catheter is passed. Cole et al.[9] found that the catheter itself did not cause any change in resistance. Of the three methods he also found that the pernasal technique provided the least variability in results.[9]

Flow Measurement

Flow can be measured in several ways. In mask rhinomanometry (Fig. 5–1), flow is measured at the outlet of a mask that is worn covering the patient's nose and a portion of the face. Flow can also be measured with a nozzle held over the opening to either nostril. When rhinomanometry is done with a head out body plethysmograph,[8] flow is measured by assessing the movement of air in and out of the closed body box the patient is sitting in. This air exchange is caused by the movement of the patient's thorax. Parker et al.[1] thought that this method was more acceptable to children than the use of a mask.

Of these different methods, a full face mask is used most commonly. The proponents of this method believe that it causes less distortion of the nasal structures than a nozzle. It is helpful if the mask is transparent so that alar movements can be observed.

Active vs. Passive Methods

Passive rhinomanometry is seldom used. In passive rhinomanometry, airflow is provided from an external source rather than from the patient. Active rhinomanometry, which uses the patient's own respiratory efforts for airflow, does not require the use of an external flow source, and it better reflects the physiologic range of respiration for each patient.

Most Commonly Used Method

Active anterior mask rhinomanometry is the most commonly used method because it has the least complicated equipment and is the easiest method to perform.

EQUIPMENT

Pneumotachograph

The actual measurement of airflow for these different methods is done with either a pneumotachograph or a calibrated orifice. These devices present a small resistance as air travels through them. The resistance is too small to be noticeable to the patient but creates a pressure difference between the two sides of the pneumotachograph. This pressure difference is measured by a sensitive pressure transducer. The output of this transducer through the appropriate electronic circuitry provides a voltage signal proportional to airflow.

Transducers

The tubes from the pressure detection sites for the front and back of the nose are connected to a pressure transducer. This is a device that converts a physical phenomenon such as pressure into an electrical signal. The pressure transducer is connected to an electronic circuit that delivers a voltage signal that varies in correspondence with changes in pressure.

Analog-to-Digital Converter and Computer

The pressure and flow signal voltages are read by a recording device, which usually is a computer. Inside the computer, an analog-to-digital converter changes the voltages into numbers. The numbers are used to generate a display on the computer screen. This real-time display of the pressure-flow data is helpful for the detection of any problems such as mask leaks that might occur during the test. The pressure and flow data are then stored for further analysis. Various parameters can be calculated from the pressure and flow data and used to report test results.

TYPICAL TEST PROCEDURE

Certain guidelines should be followed to perform the airway test with the least variability in results. The apparatus is kept in calibration according to manufacturers' standards. It is warmed up and kept stable before starting the test. The patient is allowed to sit quietly to complete a questionnaire before the test.

Routine Procedure for Test Administration

The standard test is done with the patient in the sitting position. The pressure detecting line is taped over the opening of the nose on the side not being measured (Fig. 5–1). The pressure line is connected to the connection inside the mask, and the mask is held over the face. There should be no deformation of the nostrils or alae. As the patient is breathing, the pressure-flow curve can be checked to look for any deviation from the routine sigmoid curve, which signifies a mask leak. Sometimes looping is seen at the extreme of the inspiratory curve, which corresponds with alar excursion during respiration. If patients are asked to breathe normally, they sometimes decrease their effort and the looping disappears. After successful collection of the data, the other side of the nose is measured in the same way.

A decongestant is then sprayed in each side of the nose. A consistent protocol for decongestion should be followed. In our clinical setting, spray is instilled a second time after 5 minutes. Ten minutes later, another set of measurements is collected for each side of the nose. The computer then calculates and prints the results. In addition, the pressure-flow data and the pertinent history and physical data for a patient can be stored for later reference or analysis. For children, the test is performed in a similar fashion, although a smaller face mask may be needed.

Modifications of the Test

Some patients have the chief complaint of nasal obstruction that is worse when they are recumbent or sleep disturbance attributed to a restricted nasal airway. For these patients, the study can be done in the sitting, supine, or recumbent on the right side and left side positions. For patients with suspected allergic rhinitis, nasal provocation testing can be done and the response assessed with objective airway testing.

Additional Assessment of the Anterior Nasal Airway

Additional maneuvers have been recommended to be used in conjunction with airway testing to assess the anterior nasal airway and valve area. To do this, various methods[6,10–12] can be used to hold the anterior airway open. A commercially available plastic-strip nasal dilator works well for this purpose. If the stenting results in a significant decrease in resistance, that would indicate that the nares, vestibule, or valve is the site of obstruction. If little change in resistance results, then any restriction is attributed to factors posterior to the valve area.

WHAT DATA ARE OBTAINED?

Pressure and Flow

Testing results in the simultaneous sequential assessment of the relationship of pressure and flow in the nasal airway during the course of respiration. The difference in pressure across the nose causes air to flow through the nose. This pressure difference varies through the course of respiration. An increase in pressure causes an increase in flow. If the relationship between pressure and flow was always the same in proportion, the plot of pressure and flow would be a straight line. This is not the case, however. The plot is usually curved (Fig. 5–2) in an "s," or sigmoid, shape. The amount of curvature can vary from one curve to another.

In a more obstructed airway, greater pressure is needed to generate the same amount of flow. This causes the curve to be closer to the pressure axis. The accepted standard in displaying the pressure-flow curve is to plot pressure on the x-axis and flow on the y-axis. With this arrangement, curves for data from a more obstructed airway will be rotated more toward the horizontal (x-axis) than those for less obstructed airways (Fig. 5–3).

WHAT IS REPORTED FROM THE DATA OBTAINED?

Parameters Reflecting the Pressure and Flow Relationship in the Nose for that Patient

Many different parameters have been used to represent the relationship between simultaneously measured nasal pressure and flow. Cole,[13] for example, routinely

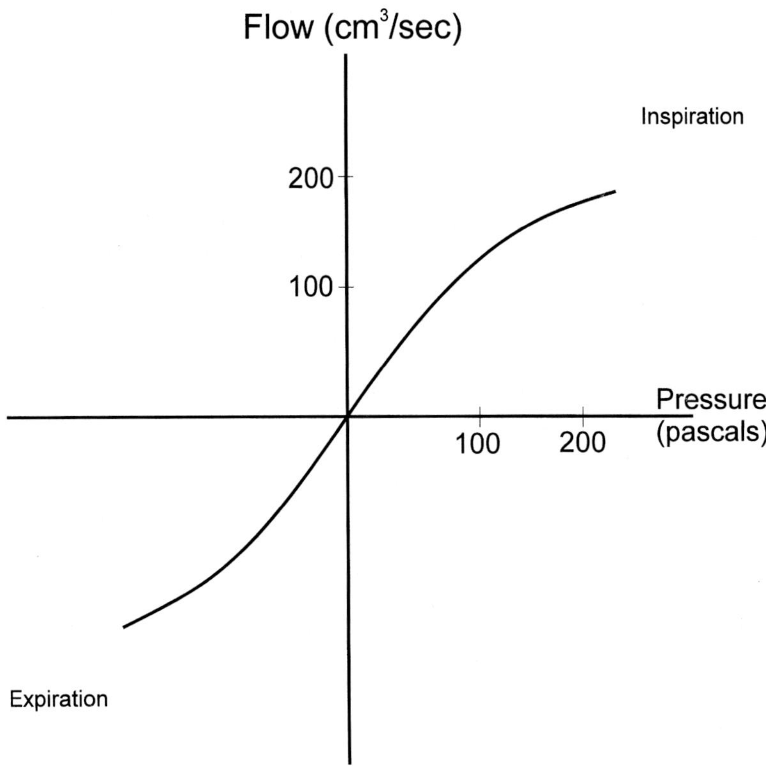

Figure 5–2. The sigmoid-shaped pressure-flow curve.

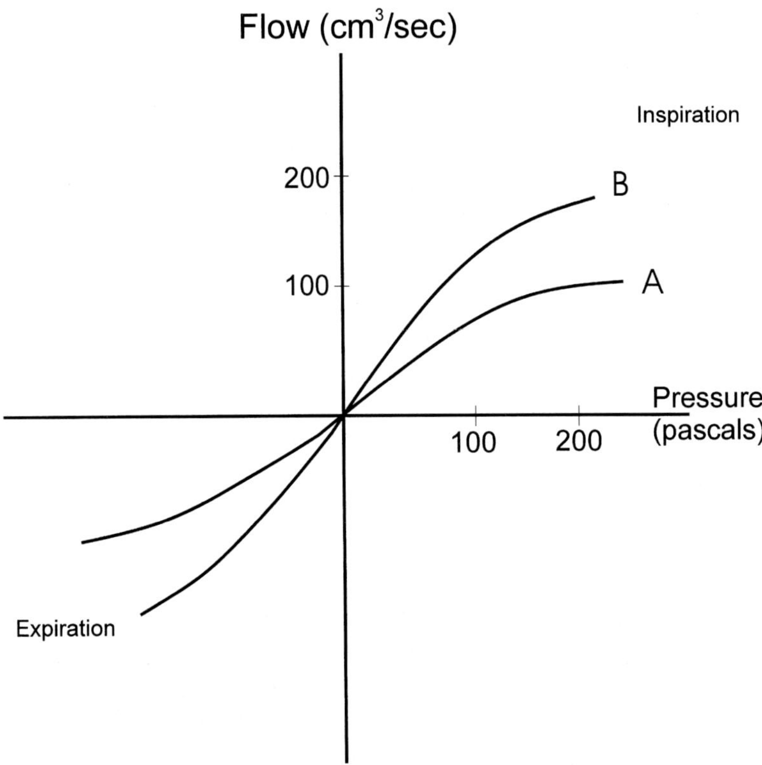

Figure 5–3. Curve **A** is the pressure-flow curve from a more obstructed nasal airway than curve **B**.

reports 14 different parameters. The most common parameter reported is resistance, or the ratio of pressure divided by flow. Conductance (the ratio of flow divided by pressure) can also be reported. Both of these vary at different points on the pressure-flow curve because the pressure-flow relationship is nonlinear. For comparison of results from a patient at different times or between different patients, a method must be used that will report the ratio from a consistent designated point on the curve.

Parameters Recognized by the International Standards Committee

Resistance or flow at a designated pressure

Resistance can be reported at a designated pressure. Reporting resistance at a pressure of 150 pascals is an international standard.[14] Voluntary increase in ventilation may be necessary for some patients to reach a pressure of 150 pascals or even 100 pascals.[15,16] In Japan, a pressure of 100 pascals is used more often because more patients can reach this value.

As an alternative to reporting resistance at a certain pressure, only the flow value corresponding to that pressure is reported.[17] This allows direct calculation of the total airway by just adding the flows from each side.

Resistance at a designated radius

Another international standard is the reporting of resistance at a designated radius. Broms[18] assigned scales to the pressure and flow axes such that $100 \text{cm}^3/\text{sec}$ on the flow axis was the same distance from the origin as 100 pascals on the pressure axis. The arc drawn between these points represents a radius of one (Fig. 5–4). Reporting the resistance value at the point where the curve crosses the arc for radius 2 is an international standard. In the international literature, the parameter v2 is used, which is the angle from the axis to this point on the arc for radius 2.[19]

OTHER PARAMETERS THAT ARE REPORTED

Maximal and Mean Resistance

Two other methods for describing the pressure-flow relationship are reporting maximal resistance[20] and reporting mean resistance.[21] Maximal resistance is calculated at the point of maximal pressure and flow reached by the patient during normal breathing (Fig. 5–4). Mean resistance is calculated by using the mean pressure and flow values. Because the computer has collected a sample at many different times, it can give an average (or mean) value for pressure and flow for each respiration. Both of these methods offer the advantage of obtaining results for all patients because it is not necessary to reach a certain point on the pressure-flow curve. Naito et al.[16] found that maximal and mean resistance results were nearly identical because near peak flows are present through most of quiet respiration.

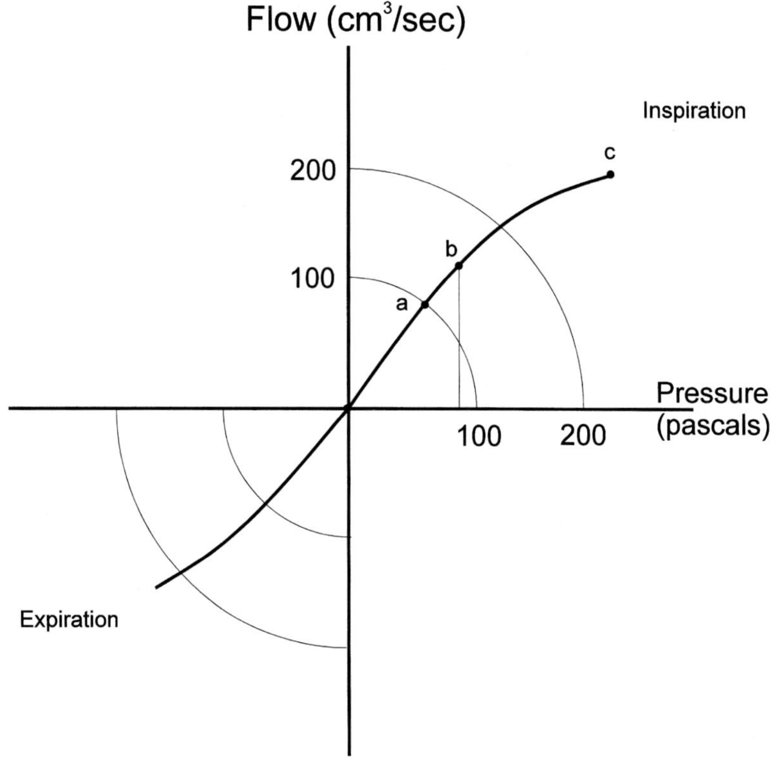

Figure 5–4. Points on the pressure-flow curve at which airway parameters are calculated. **A**, at a designated radius; **B**, at a designated pressure; **C**, at maximal pressure and flow.

Side Difference and Work Coefficient

Some currently available rhinomanometers report a number describing the difference between the airway for the two sides of the nose. Another parameter is the work coefficient, which is obtained by multiplying each pressure value times its corresponding flow value and then summing all of these. The clinical usefulness of these two parameters has not been compared with that of the more commonly used parameters.

OTHER PROPOSED PARAMETERS

Other parameters have been proposed that are not in common clinical use.

Cross-sectional Area

Cross-sectional area[3,6,22,23] is of interest because it might provide a result similar to that obtained when acoustic rhinometry is used to assess the narrowest cross-sectional area in the nose. The cross-sectional area is obtained with a specific formula that reflects the pressure-flow relationship.[6] Because of this, a ranking of clinical results based on resistance at a designated pressure is similar to one based on cross-sectional area.

Because the results obtained in calculating cross-sectional area tend to be similar along the entire curve,[6,22] it was thought to be a good way to represent the entire pressure-flow domain using a description of primarily turbulent flow through an orifice of variable area.[24]

Curve Coefficients

As one moves away from the origin on the nonlinear pressure-flow curve, the pressure-to-flow relationship becomes progressively larger as the resistance increases. This changing relationship can be described with several different mathematical models. One advantage of such modeling might be that the derived coefficients describe the entire curve and not just one point on it.

The curve fitting models that have worked the best[25] for fitting the pressure-flow data include the geometric fit[26,27] with a variable exponential power for flow, or a fixed power for flow,[28–30] a second-order polynomial fit,[31–35] and a model using polar coordinates.[18] Even a third-order polynomial fit has been used.[36]

No published study has compared the relative ability of the curve-fitting models to provide parameters that give better **clinical correlation** than simpler methods such as use of a single resistance value.

Resistance at the Origin

Resistance has been calculated by measurement of the slope at the origin of the pressure-flow curve.[7,37] Schumacher[33] pointed out that this method allows results to be obtained for all individuals, but its disadvantage is that it assesses the pressure-flow relationship at the point in the curve where the patient does not have the sensation of obstruction.

WHAT PARAMETERS ARE USED CLINICALLY?

This varies somewhat in different parts of the world. The most common parameters reported are those recommended by the International Standards Committee. If something other than the international standard is used because of historical precedent for that center, one of the international standards is usually reported at the same time.

Results for Each Side and for the Total Nose

Results are usually reported for each side of the nose and for the total nasal airway. Because the most common method used (anterior rhinomanometry) cannot directly measure the total nasal airway, these values are calculated from the unilateral results. This is based on the principle that **at a given pressure** the total flow can be obtained by summing the flow from each side.[7,38,39] Studies have shown that calculated and measured total nasal airway resistance is the same before decongestion[38] and after decongestion.[40] Another study found a small proportional difference between the calculated and measured values—the calculated total resistance was greater than the measured total resistance.[41] Because the computer has stored the flows that correspond to each pressure along the pressure-flow curve, a pressure-flow curve **for the total nose** can be obtained for the range of the pressures reached on both sides.

Results for Inspiration (vs. Expiration)

Results are reported for inspiration, and this is the recommended international standard.[14] Dvoracek et al.,[42] thought that there was more reproducibility of results during the inspiratory phase of respiration than during the expiratory phase. Connell[2] thought inspiratory data made the most sense for clinical use, stating "Have you ever heard of a patient complaining that he cannot exhale through his nose?" There has not yet been a report comparing the difference in clinical correlation between data reported for inspiration and data for expiration.

Results Before and After Decongestion

Measurements are often made before and after decongestion of the nose. Decongestion can be accomplished in most patients with either a decongestant spray or physical exercise.[43] Xylometazoline spray is more effective than drops or exercise for decongestion of the nose.[44]

SOURCES OF VARIABILITY

Due to Nasal Physiology

Several factors can explain the fact that over time there is some variability in the results obtained with any objective assessment of the nasal airway. One reason is the presence of the nasal cycle, the normal periodic alternating congestion and decongestion of the respective sides of the nose.[45,46] Although this causes a significant change in each side of the nose, the total nasal airway resistance remains relatively constant; the coefficient of variation is less than 15% over 6 hours.[47] Other sources of variability that have been described are postural changes (resistance greater when supine),[45] pressure applied to certain areas of the body (increases the resistance on that side),[48] exercise (decreases resistance),[22,28,49] hyperventilation (increases resistance),[28,50] breathing CO_2,[50] and flaring of the nostrils (decreases resistance),[51] nasal secretions and cold air (increase resistance),[52,53] and stress and anxiety (decrease in resistance thought to be mediated by the hypothalamus).[54]

Medication can affect the results. Aspirin can cause a small increase in nasal resistance.[55] In one study,[56] antihistamine treatment caused an increase in resistance in the nose when it was administered before challenge testing.

There is also some variability in results between individuals of different height[43,44,57] or anthropologic type.[58,59] There may also be a decrease in nasal resistance with advancing age in adults.[60,61]

Due to Rhinomanometric Methods

The repositioning of equipment between measurements can be a source of variability.[62] Other sources of variability that have been reported include equipment that is not consistently warmed up,[63] and mask leakage.[37,40]

Recommendations for Testing

Knowledge of the sources of variability results in the following recommendations regarding the optimal testing environment. Recommendations have included normal temperature and humidity in the testing room, a symmetric sitting position, a means of revealing mask leaks (real-time display of the pressure-flow curve works well),[64] avoidance of exercise for 30 minutes before testing,[65] explanation of the test equipment to alleviate anxiety by the patient, and no medications before testing. The variable nature of the nasal airway also means that the **most meaningful** correlation with symptoms and examination can be accomplished by obtaining the current symptoms and rhinoscopy and airway testing results as close together temporally as possible.

WHAT ARE THE CLINICAL APPLICATIONS OF RHINOMANOMETRY?

Rhinomanometry (and other objective tests for evaluation of the nasal airway) can be used for the clinical evaluation of the symptom of nasal obstruction, for pretreatment and posttreatment comparisons, and for allergy challenge testing. The remainder of this chapter describes the use of objective testing of the nasal airway for clinical evaluation of the patient with the symptom of nasal obstruction.

CLINICAL APPLICATION OF RHINOMANOMETRY FOR THE EVALUATION OF THE PATIENT WITH THE SYMPTOM OF NASAL OBSTRUCTION

Can Rhinomanometry Identify the Symptomatic Patient?

Rhinomanometry cannot identify the symptomatic patient, nor should it be expected to. Study of the normal values of resistance for a population of patients with no symptoms compared with a population with obstructive symptoms reveals a significant difference but a large area of overlap. In other words, there are many resistance values at which some patients will complain of obstruction but others will not.

Variation in Threshold of Sensation of Obstruction

Just as some patients noted to have abnormal intranasal structure have no symptoms, some patients have abnormal airway study results but do not complain of nasal obstruction. At a certain ***threshold value***, most patients change to oronasal breathing. At another threshold value short of that, many (but not all) patients complain of obstruction. An additional complexity is that this threshold value ***varies*** from one patient to another.

Some patients deny any obstruction and so are below the threshold at which they would notice obstruction, yet they can be found to appreciate a still more open airway. An example is the patient who tells the clinician that the least obstructed side of their nose is "wide open." After the clinician decongests that side or props the ala up, the patient states that it is even "more open." An additional example of this is the patient whose nose is fractured in a motor vehicle accident. The septal and external fractures are repaired. After healing the patient notes that the nasal airway is now more open than it had ever been even though they weren't "aware" of obstruction before.

There is another source of variability in the description of symptom. Patients will relate that the point of comparison that they are using in ranking symptoms of obstruction is based on the way that their nasal airway "normally" feels, for example "mild" obstruction is not a comparison with the general population but means "mild" compared with the way that side of the nose usually feels to them.

The presence of a range of thresholds at which the sensation of obstruction will be noted means that the diagnostician must give credibility to a broad range of degrees of symptoms in the course of evaluation of these patients.

Symptoms Correlate with Airway Testing Results in Patients with Obstruction Due to Airway Restriction

Unhealthy nasal mucosa (from infection, inflammatory disease, or previous radical operation) can cause the symptom of nasal obstruction even in a relatively "patent" airway. However, in patients with "nondiseased" mucosa **who complain of nasal obstruction**, a correlation **has** been found between the sensation of airflow and the results of objective testing of the airway. This is apparently due to a "sense" of the correct amount of airflow past cold receptors in the nasal airway which many patients are able to experience. This appears to be partially a learned sensation, because patients who have never known what it is like to breathe through a side of their nose often do not complain of lack of the ability to sense airflow there. Yet a patient who is familiar with the sensation and then loses that ability (for example, with a nasal fracture) often complains of significant symptoms.

If a significant number of patients do appreciate an open airway (or the lack of it), and if we had a test that could objectively measure airway patency, then that test might help in the diagnosis of nasal obstruction in that group of patients. Because one of our aims as clinicians is to improve the patient's sense of well-being, we wish to make the most accurate diagnosis so that we can choose the best therapy for a patient to accomplish this goal. We also wish to counsel the patient about the relative chance of success of various therapeutic interventions. Objective airway testing can play a role in doing so.

Can Rhinomanometry Identify the Site of Abnormality?

Rhinomanometry can distinguish the **side** with the most abnormal results. However, on a given side, unless the pressure catheter is advanced to different locations in the nose (which is not usually the case for current clinical application, though it could be done using the pernasal technique), only the results for the **smallest dimension** on that side are obtained. The modification of holding the ala open and repeating the test can give information about the relative contribution of the most anterior structures of the nasal airway. This can be done with various devices. It is a routine part of the testing done in Toronto.[13] There has not yet been a report on the clinical application of such data.

Does Rhinomanometry Provide Any Information Besides What is Known by History and Physical Examination?

Objective airway testing provides an assessment of the amount of restriction of the nasal airway. Since the patient's description of symptoms is subjective (and at varying thresholds), and since the clinician's assessment of the airway with examination is subjective, an objective assessment of the airway can provide additional information that might change the diagnosis or course of action taken in a clinical setting. An example is the case in which the degree of symptoms and pathology are different. Consequently, the clinician doesn't know which represents the true status of the airway. If the degree of airway restriction is measured and found to agree with either the symptoms or the pathology, then the answer is found. All three pieces of information can be significant in the evaluation of the patient. To demonstrate this, a clinical algorithm (flowchart) for the evaluation of the patient with nasal obstruction is described.

APPLICATION OF THE ALGORITHM

In the following description of the flowchart, the text in nonitalic print is the description of the course of action without the addition of airway testing data. The text in *italics* is the description of the additional information provided when airway testing data are available for the evaluation.

Definition of Terms Used in the Algorithm

Terms used in the description of the algorithm are as follows:

1.   Symptoms: the patient's subjective description of the sensation of obstructed nasal breathing. Symptoms can range from mild to severe. The flowchart includes only symptomatic patients. Because patients who do not have symptoms are not treated (unless a neoplasm or deleterious physiologic effect is present), application of the test to patients without symptoms is not an issue. If a patient has no symptoms on the day of evaluation, the patient should be reevaluated when symptoms are present. Some patients will have clearing of symptoms because they are nervous about being at the physician's office.

2.   Pathology: the physician's subjective description of the findings from intranasal examination which are thought to be the cause of the symptoms or which are significant enough that they would be expected to cause obstruction in some patients.

3.   Airway restriction: the amount of resistance to airflow for the nasal airway measured using rhinomanometry (or other device capable of objective assessment of the nasal airway).

4.   Decongestion: application of a decongestant spray to the patient's nasal tissues, usually done with two applications for maximal effect, using either phenylephrine or oxymetazoline (in the United States).

Following the Branches of the Algorithm

The process of clinical evaluation of the patient with nasal obstruction cannot be described without some simplifications. The use of a straightforward "yes/no" binary decision tree is desirable, but in reality clinical judgment and decisions are based on the weighting of various factors by the clinician's "neural network." In the case of the evaluation of nasal obstruction, the weighted factors that are used for this discussion are the **subjective sensation** (symptoms) noted by the patient, the **subjective observation** (pathology) of the appearance of the internal and external nose by the clinician, and **the objective airway measurements** (airway restriction). In addition, all three of these factors are considered before and after decongestion. These factors do not have a single "present or absent" status but rather a gradation of presence whose relative weights at the nodes of a decision tree can lead to a particular diagnosis and treatment. For the sake of a *workable* description of this process, the factors (symptoms, pathology, and airway results) are considered in terms of their response to decongestion (same, less, cleared) and in terms of their relevant relationships to each other in degree of presence (greater than, equal to, less than).

Other Factors that Could Play a Role in Assessment of the Patient

Other less tangible factors besides symptoms, pathology, and airway test results might also play a role in the assessment of the patient, such as the physician's observation of the general medical condition, physical conditioning, and psychological disposition of the patient, but these are not included in the algorithm except in the context of "other causes."

Goal of Evaluation is to Arrive at a Diagnosis and Select a Treatment

The **goal** in arriving at a diagnosis in evaluation of the patient with nasal obstruction is to determine when the symptoms of nasal obstruction are due to a restriction in the nasal airway which can be corrected with some form of treatment. It would also be desirable to have some idea of the relative probability of success of particular treatments for a given patient. Such information would be helpful in counseling patients regarding treatment options.

Possible diagnoses

What conditions are present which cause an airway to cross the threshold point at which nasal obstruction occurs? The possible diagnoses and modifiers used in the algorithm are listed in Table 5–1 and are described below.

Structural problem. If symptoms are present and do not improve with decongestion (assuming that the patient has nasal tissue that would respond to decongestant spray—response on the nonsymptomatic side of the nose lends credibility to this status), then the problem is considered **structural** (Fig. 5–5) and **unlikely** to respond to medical therapy and **more likely** to be corrected by **surgical therapy**.

Combined structural problem. If symptoms **decrease** with decongestion but **some symptoms persist** a contribution to the problem from both a structural problem and mucosal swelling is suggested. This type of combined problem is labeled "combined structural." (This is the first of two types of combined pathology. It is also possible to have a combined problem with **complete clearing of symptoms**. This type is referred to as "combined mucosal" and is described below.)

In the **combined structural** problem (Fig. 5–5), the addition of some mucosal swelling to an already present structural problem causes the symptoms to increase significantly in severity. In this case, the condition **might** be adequately relieved by treatment of the nasal mucosa with medical therapy, but the persistence of some symptoms even with decongestion suggests that if medical therapy is not an adequate solution for a given patient with this problem, then an operation might be warranted to modify the structure so that any mucosal congestion would be less likely to cause symptoms.

Combined mucosal problem. In this case, there is **complete clearing of symptoms** with decongestion but significant **airway resistance** is still present. In the **combined-mucosal** problem (Fig. 5–5), the addition of some mucosal swelling to an already present structural problem crosses the threshold for that patient such that the symptom of nasal obstruction is present. In this case, however, the complete clearing

Table 5–1   The Diagnoses and Diagnostic Modifiers

LABEL	DIAGNOSIS	DIAGNOSIS EXPLANATION
STRUCTURAL	Structural cause of airway restriction	Symptoms persisted despite decongestion
COMB-STRUCTURAL	Combined structural	Symptoms cleared partially with decongestion
COMB-MUCOSAL	Combined mucosal	Symptoms cleared completely but some airway resistance was still present (possibly with some pathology still noted)
MUCOSAL	Mucosal	Symptoms cleared completely with decongestant without any persistent airway restriction
?OTHER	Cause for the symptoms other than airway restriction	Symptoms due to cause other than airway obstruction. Symptoms are present but **no** significant airway restriction is present
OCCULT PATH	Occult pathology	Pathology is likely present and being missed

LABEL	DIAGNOSIS MODIFIER	DIAGNOSIS MODIFIER EXPLANATION
PATH OVEREST	Pathology overestimated	The pathology has less effect on the airway than thought
PATH UNDEREST	Pathology underestimated	The pathology has greater effect on the airway than thought—**2nd look**
HIGH THRESH	High threshold	The patient has symptoms of smaller degree than the degree of the pathology or airway restriction
LOW THRESH	Low threshold	The patient has symptoms of greater degree than the degree of the pathology or airway restriction

of symptoms with decongestion suggests that the condition might be adequately relieved by treatment of the nasal mucosa with medical therapy. If medical therapy alone does not work for a given patient with this problem, then an operation might be warranted to modify the structure so that any mucosal congestion would be less likely to cause symptoms, but there is a bit less certainty about the success of surgical intervention (particularly if it's for the "structural" part only) when the mucosal component is most significant.

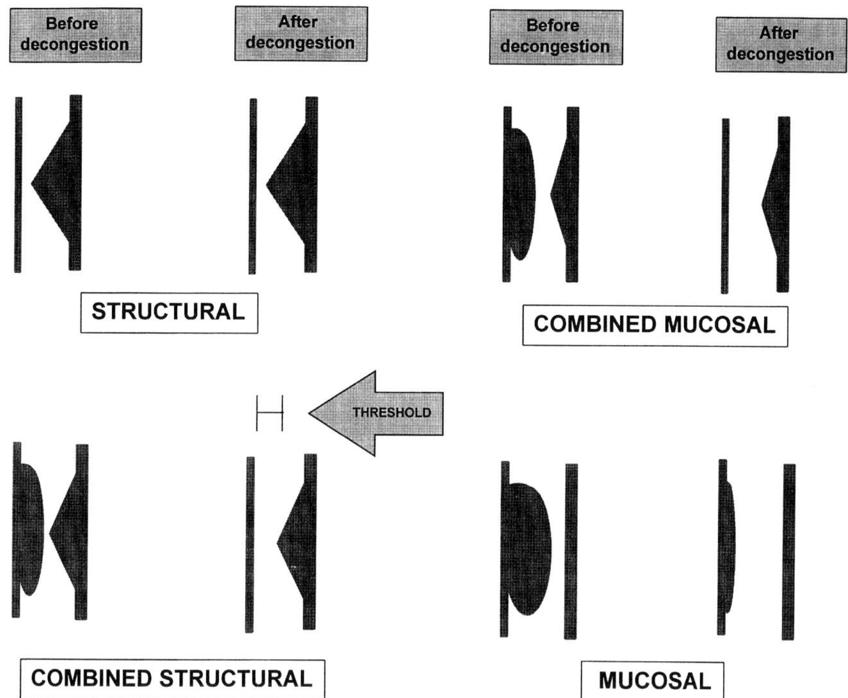

Figure 5–5. Diagrammatic representation of the different diagnoses causing nasal obstructive symptoms due to airway restriction.

Mucosal problem. In this case (Fig. 5–5), restriction is due only to mucosal congestion, and symptoms are relieved by medicine or some other treatment of the nasal mucosa. *There is no appreciable airway restriction after decongestion in a pure mucosal problem.*

Other etiology. When symptoms are present but no significant airway restriction is measured then it is concluded that the symptoms are due to a cause other than airway restriction.

Occult pathology. If **no pathology** had been noted, but **significant airway restriction** was measured, then the diagnosis **occult pathology** is suggested. This elicits another examination of the airway looking for the cause of the restriction. This examination can include both another visual exam of the intranasal appearance, and comparison of the relative opening of the airway (by patient symptom change and/or airway resistance change) when the ala are held open. The ala can be held open either with the speculum, or with an internal or external commercial dilator. The commonly available plastic strips that apply to the external nose can be used under a mask for this purpose.

Diagnosis modifiers

High threshold. Without airway testing, if the **degree of pathology** is significantly **greater than** the **degree of symptoms**, then a **high threshold** for the sensation of obstruction is suggested (though an overestimation of the pathology is possible also). *With airway testing, if the patient's symptoms are of lower degree than the airway restriction then they have a higher threshold (**HIGH THRESH**).*

An example of this is the patient who is born with a marked nasal septal deflection and is being evaluated for other problems. The clinician notes the dramatic deflection, and the patient denies being aware of it (even though the patient may be obligate mouth breathing at the time of reporting this lack of symptoms).

Another example is the patient who has some **symptoms** but they are much less severe than the dramatic **pathology** that is noted or the **airway restriction** that is measured. This situation can be due to the patient describing the symptoms not in terms of what the general population notices but rather in terms of what the patient is **accustomed to**. A patient who is accustomed to a higher level of airway restriction might say that it is causing only "mild" symptoms at a level of restriction that for another person would be "severe" obstruction.

The presence of a high threshold does not usually change the approach to treatment of symptoms because it would still be hoped that correction of the offending pathology would improve the symptoms.

Low threshold.   Without airway testing, if the **degree of symptoms** is significantly **greater than** the **degree of pathology**, a **low threshold** for the sensation of obstruction is suggested (though an underestimation of the pathology is possible also). *With airway testing, if the patient's symptoms are of higher degree than the airway restriction, then they have a low threshold (**LOW THRESH**) for the sensation of nasal obstruction.* This raises concern that the condition may be harder to treat with the same degree of success that would result from treating a patient with a normal threshold for symptoms. The reason for this is that the symptoms in a patient with low threshold have a greater chance of being due to factors other than airway restriction. One such possibility is that the symptoms are due to a sensory disturbance of the nasal mucosa (e.g., some airway tissue loses some of its sensory detection with age). Thus, some individuals might have decreased cold receptor activity and therefore, even if the airway is unrestricted they might not receive the cold receptor stimulation for the same amount of airflow and so they may feel that airflow is not adequate. If so, there is less likelihood of helping the patient's symptoms by treatment aimed at **modifying the size of the airway.**

Overestimation of pathology.   Results of airway testing are needed to determine this condition. *If the degree of airway restriction is less than the degree of the pathology, then the effect of pathology was overestimated (**PATH OVEREST**).* If the pathology is thought to be severe, the clinician might conclude that there was a high probability of success in modifying the airway so that the patient could breathe more freely. But if airway testing reveals that the restriction past that pathology is minimal, then the expectations regarding the probability of success might be tempered.

Underestimation of pathology.   Results of airway testing are needed to determine this condition also. *If airway restriction is found to be of greater degree than the* *pathology, then the effect of the pathology has been underestimated (**PATH UNDEREST**).* If the pathology is thought to be minimal, the clinician might conclude that there was a low probability of success in modifying the airway so that the patient could breathe more freely. But if airway testing reveals that the restriction past that pathology is actually quite dramatic, then the expectation about the probability of success in improving the airway by correcting the pathology would be raised.

The impact of the diagnosis modifiers.   The presence of an **underestimation** of the effect of the pathology or a **high threshold** would be supportive of increased expectations for the success of therapy aimed at increasing the diameter of the nasal airway. In other words, when the airway is actually more restricted than it appears to the clinician (**PATH UNDEREST**), then correction of the offending pathology has a greater chance of alleviating the symptoms (like a more severe conductive loss in middle ear surgery). If the magnitude of airway restriction is greater than that articulated by the patient (**HIGH THRESHOLD**), then it is more likely that improvement in the airway will have a favorable outcome. **High threshold** and **pathology underestimation** are **favorable** diagnostic modifiers. The presence of a **low threshold** would be less supportive of a successful outcome in alleviating symptoms by therapeutic intervention aimed at increasing the caliber of the airway. Overestimation of pathology does not have such an effect. If the magnitude of airway restriction is less than that described by the patient (**LOW THRESHOLD**), then it is less likely that improvement in the airway will have a favorable outcome since there is a greater possibility that factors other than decreased dimension of the airway may be playing a role. Some investigators[68] have specified a certain level of airway restriction below which the probability of success might decrease. There is not a change in the expectations for successful outcome when the airway is actually less restricted than it appears to the clinician (**PATH OVEREST**), because correction of the offending pathology can still alleviate the restriction and thus the symptoms. A **low threshold** is an **unfavorable** diagnostic modifier whereas **pathology overestimation** has a neutral effect.

Therapy

The selection of a diagnosis will lead to a corresponding option for treatment. Table 5–2 lists the treatments for nasal obstruction. The labels used in the algorithm (Fig. 5–6) are listed in boldface print with diagnoses listed in column 1 of Table 5–2. Column 2 gives the treatment label used in the algorithm. The description of each treatment is given in Column 3.

Application of the Clinical Algorithm for the Evaluation of the Nasal Obstruction

In the flowchart (Fig. 5–6), the lines and boxes that represent alternative paths with airway testing are shown in gray. All of the conditions in Table 5–3 and Figure 5–6 are **after** decongestion.

Table 5–2 Treatment Options for Nasal Obstruction

DIAGNOSIS	LABEL	THERAPEUTIC OPTIONS
STRUCTURAL	**SURG**	Surgical therapy most likely to help (medical therapy can be tried first if desired)
COMB-STRUCTURAL	**MED→SURG**	Surgery may be needed for complete relief of the symptoms, but because there was some response to the decongestant, try medical therapy first
?OTHER vs. STRUCTURAL	**SURG vs. OTHER**	Carefully consider the possibility of a non-airway cause for the symptoms before proceeding with surgery
?OTHER vs. COMB-STRUCTURAL	**MED→SURG vs. OTHER**	Try medical therapy first since there was some improvement in the symptoms with decongestion. If medical therapy does not provide adequate relief, carefully consider the possibility of a non-airway cause for the symptoms before proceeding with surgery
?OTHER	**OTHER**	Look for a cause for the symptoms other than airway restriction
?OTHER vs. MUCOSAL	**MED→OTHER**	Try medical therapy first since there was some improvement in the symptoms with decongestion. If medical therapy does not provide adequate relief, look for causes for the symptoms other than airway restriction
COMB-MUCOSAL	**MED→(SURG)**	Try medical therapy. If it fails, then the patient has the option of surgery and decides whether the symptoms are significant enough to proceed with an operation in a situation with less than maximal probability of success
MUCOSAL	**MEDICAL**	Medical therapy is the best option. Try medical therapy. *If not possible to get relief with medicine, then look for other causes. If none found, then consider turbinate treatment procedure (cautery, submucous resection, laser)*

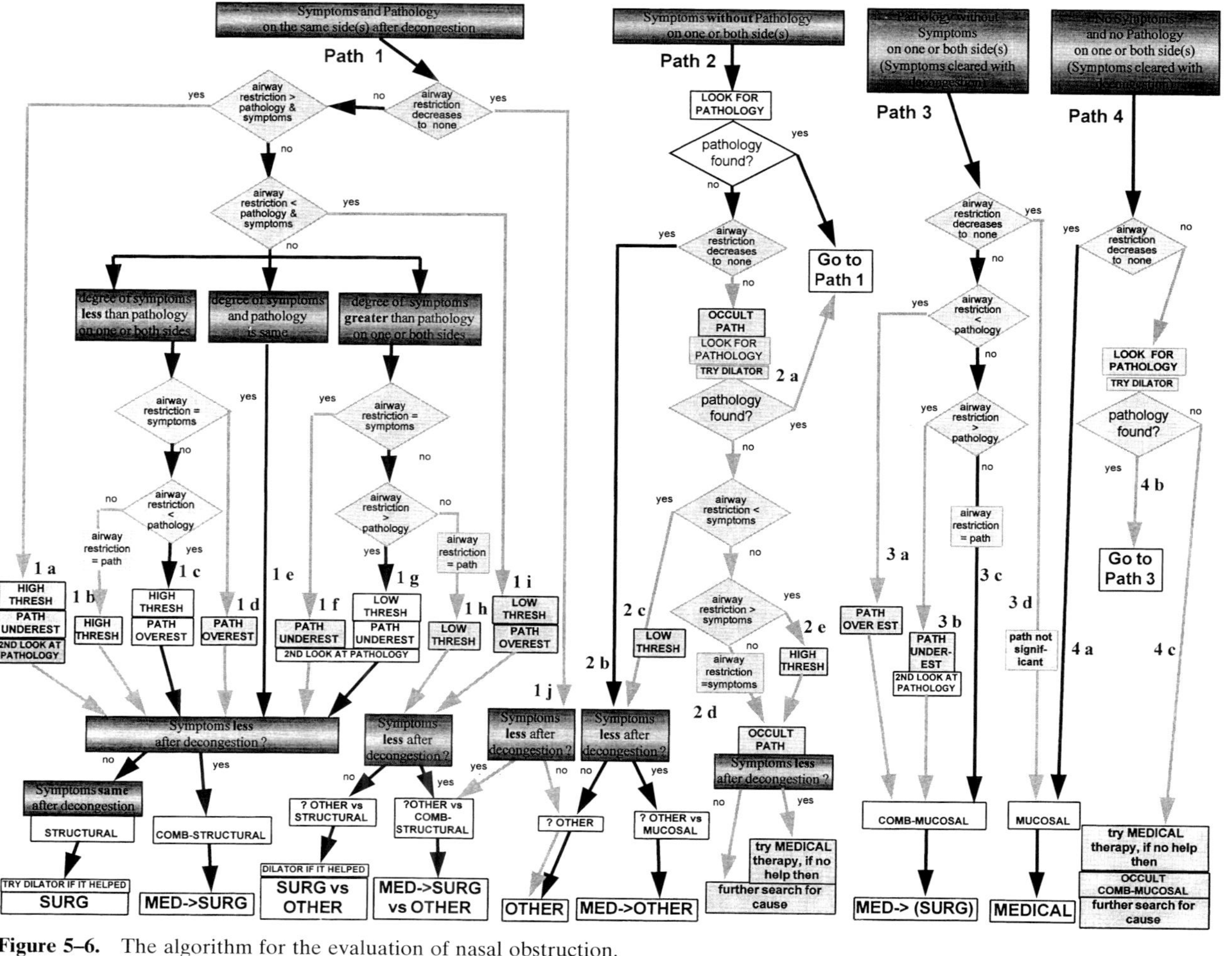

Figure 5–6. The algorithm for the evaluation of nasal obstruction.

Explanation of the Individual Paths in the Flowchart

Initial groupings—symptoms or pathology present after decongestion

Table 5–3 consists of groupings based on the persistence of symptoms or pathology after decongestion. The percentages shown are the proportion of patients in each group from a clinical sample of 50 patients selected for testing. The largest group selected for airway testing in this study were patients who had persistence of some symptoms **and** pathology after decongestion.

The following **conditions** determined the groupings:

Symptoms are still present after decongestion.   These are the patients in whom the symptoms persisted after decongestion. The symptoms could be unchanged or decreased but still present. Either the person's nasal tissues are unresponsive to spray (a minority of patients) or the symptoms are at least partially due to a non-mucosal obstruction in the airway.

Symptoms cleared after decongestion.   In most patients, the administration of a nasal decongestant spray results in vasoconstriction of nasal tissues, thus increasing the cross-sectional area of the nose and opening the nasal airway. At any given time, a significant portion of the population has relative congestion of one side of the nose compared with the other (the nasal cycle.) If the symptoms cleared completely with decongestion, then it is assumed that there has been an opening of the airway on that side of the nose (although without airway testing this occurrence cannot actually be **demonstrated** objectively). The clearing of symptoms of obstruction could be due to a decrease in the thickness of the mucosa that was swollen because of disease or because of the nasal cycle.

Pathology is still present after decongestion.   A lack of change in pathology after decongestion is attributed to the fact that the pathology does not have a mucosal component—a "structural" problem (e.g., a septal deflection, synechiae).

Pathology cleared after decongestion.   For pathology to clear with decongestion, it must have been due to a mucosal swelling. Sometimes a deformity of the septum seems to disappear after decongestion. This could be due either to **septal turbinate tissue** or to an optical illusion. This happens when there is turbinate swelling on one side of the nose and when the two sides of the nose are compared it is concluded that the septum is deflected to the side of the narrowing. Then, after decongestion, the septum appears straight and the airway looks open bilaterally. This is sometimes confirmed on a CT scan obtained to check the sinuses.

Different combinations of the conditions can be present

Table 5–3 shows that there are a number of combinations of the presence or absence of symptoms or pathology for one or both sides of the nose. The algorithm deals only with sides of the nasal airway that have symptoms at least before decongestion. Different combinations of the conditions can be present for either side of the nose.

Table 5–3 Different Groups of Conditions Encountered in Evaluation of the Nasal Airway of the Patient with Nasal Obstruction

GROUP	DESCRIPTION (AND INCIDENCE IN SAMPLE OF 50 PATIENTS)		SIDE STATUS	STARTING POINT IN FIGURE 5–6
1	**Symptoms** still **present** after decongestion Significant pathology **still noted** (56%) Pathology was **found** after decongestion (2%)	Unilateral pathology or bilateral pathology, on the same side(s) as the symptoms (34%)	Side(s) with symptoms and pathology	Path 1
		Bilateral symptoms, unilateral pathology (12%)	Side with symptoms and pathology	Path 1
			Side with symptoms only	Path 2
		Bilateral pathology, unilateral symptoms (8%)	Side with symptoms and pathology	Path 1
			Side with pathology only	Path 3
		Unilateral pathology on opposite side from unilateral symptoms (2%)	Side with symptoms only	See text
			Side with pathology only	See text
2	Symptoms still **present** after decongestion Pathology **cleared** with decongestion (4%) **No** pathology noted before decongestion (2%)		Side with symptoms only	Path 2
3	Symptoms **cleared** with spray significant pathology **still noted** (20%) Pathology was **found** after decongestion (2%)		Side with pathology only	Path 3
4	Symptoms **cleared** with decongestion Pathology **cleared** with decongestion (10%) **No** pathology was noted before decongestion (4%)		Side with **no** symptoms or pathology	Path 4

In applying the algorithm, each side of the nose can be considered first. The last column in Table 5–3 lists which of the 4 paths in the algorithm in Figure 5–6 is followed for each side of the nose for the 4 different groups. If the presence and degree of symptoms and pathology differ between the two sides of the nose then different paths of the algorithm will be followed for each side. The clinician then integrates the two results into the overall picture for that patient. The overall status of the nasal airway will lead to the predominant diagnosis and corresponding treatment.

The status of symptoms and pathology for each of the 4 paths shown in the top line of Figure 5–6 are: symptoms and pathology present on the same side (Path 1), symptoms present without pathology (Path 2), pathology present without symptoms (Path 3), and no symptoms or pathology present (Path 4).

Side of symptoms opposite side of pathology

There is one situation where consideration of the individual sides of the nose does not adequately describe the situation. If the pathology is on the side **opposite** the symptoms, this raises a question about the significance of the pathology on the one side versus the symptoms on the other. If the symptoms decrease with decongestion, then this lends evidence to an airway problem on the side of the symptoms. But if the symptoms don't change with decongestion, there's not a way to tell which side actually has an airway problem without some means of measuring the airway. Without an airway test, the clinician could believe the side of the symptoms or the pathology was the source of the problem. With airway testing, if airway restriction is present **on the side of the symptoms**, this reveals that to be the side with the airway problem and a second look is done for pathology on **that** side. If airway restriction is present **on the side of the pathology**, then symptoms the patient attributes to the opposite side could be due to the phenomenon of paradoxical nasal obstruction.[66]

Symptoms and pathology on same side(s), after decongestion (Path 1)

If both symptoms and pathology are still present after decongestion, and airway testing is not being used, then the diagnosis is based in part on the relative degree of the symptoms and pathology. If the pathology and symptoms are of the same degree then the clinician attributes the symptoms to that pathology (Fig. 5–6, Path 1e).

If no airway testing results are available and the degree of the symptoms the patient describes do **not** match the degree of the pathology noted, the clinician might either believe the degree of the patient's **symptoms** (because they are the reason for the patient coming for evaluation) or the assessment of the **pathology** since that is what the clinician can actually observe. Without objective data, however, it isn't possible to **verify** the true status of the airway.

When the degree of symptoms is less than the degree of the pathology.   Without airway testing, if the degree of the **symptoms** is **less than** that of the **pathology**, it is not known if the true condition of the airway is reflected by the symptoms (pathology overestimated, Path 1d), by the pathology (high threshold, Path 1b), or if the actual degree of the airway is between that of the pathology and the symptoms (Path 1c).

*If airway testing showed that the degree of **airway restriction** was actually the **same as** the **symptoms**, this would suggest that the **symptoms** reflected the actual state of the airway, and thus the pathology had been overestimated (Path 1d). This finding would not change the expectations regarding therapy. If the airway restriction was of smaller degree than the pathology which was in turn of smaller degree than the symptoms, then both a **high threshold** and an **overestimation of the pathology** are suggested (Path 1c). The overall effect is that this implies a more favorable prognosis. It is the same as the result without airway testing and so is marked with a black arrow. If airway testing showed that the degree of **airway restriction** was actually the **same as** the **pathology**, this would suggest that the **pathology** reflected the actual state of the airway, and the patient has a **high threshold** (Path 1b). This would result in more favorable expectations for the results of therapy.*

When the degree of symptoms is greater than that of the pathology.   If the degree of the **symptoms** is **greater than** that of the **pathology** then without airway testing the clinician might conclude that the patient has a **low threshold** for the symptom of nasal obstruction (Path 1h), that the pathology had been underestimated (Path 1f), or that both of these conditions could be true (Path 1g).

*If airway restriction was found to be of the same degree as the symptoms, then the **pathology** (which had been thought to be of lesser degree), was **underestimated** (Path 1f) and the pathology is reassessed with this additional information in mind. Credibility is given to the symptoms being due to significant pathology that could be corrected by therapy to improve the airway size. If the airway restriction was of greater degree than the pathology but less than the symptoms, then both a **low threshold and** an **underestimation** of the **pathology** are possible (Path 1g). Since these two diagnostic modifiers suggest opposite expectations as far as the outcome (low threshold—unfavorable, pathology underestimate—favorable), no effective modification of the diagnosis occurs unless it is changed by the second look at the pathology. This is also the branch followed when airway testing results are not available. If the airway restriction is of the same degree as the pathology (and thus less than the symptoms) (Path 1h), then a low threshold is present tempering the expectations for therapy that addresses the caliber of the airway.*

Degree of airway restriction greater than the degree of the symptoms and pathology.   **With airway testing**, *the persistence of **airway restriction** greater in degree than both the symptoms and the pathology suggests that the patient has a high threshold **and** that the pathology was underestimated (Path 1a). Whenever an underestimation of pathology is suggested, a second look at the pathology would be indicated. Both of the these diagnostic modifiers reinforce (enhance) the expectation that therapy addressed at increasing the diameter of the airway would be successful in alleviating the patient's symptoms.*

Figure 5–7 shows the results of airway testing in which the left nasal airway is an example of Path 1a (the right—Path 4a).

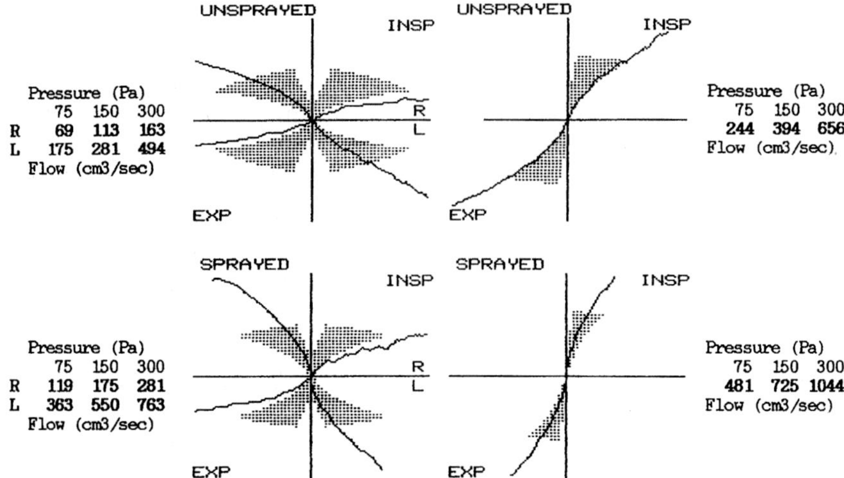

Figure 5–7. Results of nasal airway test of 37-year-old man who complained of obstruction greatest on the right side. Examination revealed a marked right-sided deflection. (R = right side, L = left side, INSP = inspiration, EXP = expiration, UNSPRAYED = prior to decongestion, SPRAYED = after decongestion. Flows are given at designated pressures of 75, 150, and 300 Pascals.) The gray shaded area is a reference area representing the 90% range for a group of 80 normal subjects. Notice that it is wider for the plots before decongestion than after. The right-sided airway restriction persists after decongestion corresponding with the persistence of significant right-sided symptoms and pathology. The left-sided airway restriction improves dramatically with decongestion (curve moves closer to the vertical-flow axis) corresponding with decrease in size of the left inferior turbinate and clearing of the symptoms on that side. The single curves on the right side of the figure show the total resistance for both sides of the nose.

A 37-year-old man complains of severe right obstruction and moderate left obstruction. After decongestion, the symptoms on the right decrease to moderate and the symptoms on the left clear.

Examination: A marked right septal deflection with some compensatory hypertrophy of the left inferior turbinate is found. After decongestion the marked septal deflection persists though it looks less dramatic but the fullness of the left inferior turbinate clears.

Airway testing: A marked restriction is present on the right before and after decongestion, consistent with the patient's symptoms and the observed intranasal pathology. On the left, some restriction is measured which clears after decongestion.

Analysis: Right side: Severe symptoms that decrease to moderate with decongestion. Severe pathology that decreases to moderate with decongestion. Airway restriction is severe even after decongestion. Path 1a. Diagnosis: **combined structural.** The moderation of symptoms and pathology despite persistence of severe airway restriction after decongestion suggests a **high threshold, path underestimated.** If medical therapy fails, then surgery. **Left** side: Moderate symptoms clear with decongestion. Moderate pathology clears with decongestion. Moderate airway restriction decreases to open. Path 4a. Diagnosis: **mucosal.**

Outcome: the patient had no relief with beclamethasone spray. The patient was much improved after septal operation.

Degree of airway restriction less than the degree of the symptoms and pathology. *If the airway restriction is **less** in degree than both the symptoms and the pathology, this suggests that the patient has a **low threshold** and that the pathology was **overestimated** (Path 1i). The low threshold raises the question of whether any other causes are contributing to the patient's symptoms and tempers the expectation for the outcome of therapy addressed at increasing the dimension of the airway.*

Selection of therapy for Path 1. If the symptoms and pathology are on the same side and there is **no change in the symptoms with decongestion**, then pathology noted after decongestion is thought to be the cause of the symptoms (**STRUCTURAL**) and surgical correction (**SURG**) would be expected to have a high probability of success in relief of the symptoms.

If the symptoms decrease (but persist) with decongestion, then the problem is thought to be due to a combination of mucosal (the part that decreased with decongestion) and structural (the part that was still causing some persistent symptoms) factors (**COMB-STRUCTURAL**) (see explanation of combined-structural pathology). Since there was a reduction in the symptoms with the decongestion, medical therapy would be tried first. If this did not provide sufficient benefit, then an operation could be done to correct the noted pathology and improve the airway (**MED→SURG**).

*For any of these cases the further substantiation of the fact that the airway is being affected in association with the symptoms implies a higher probability of success in alleviation of the symptoms with surgical intervention if medical therapy fails. Moreover, in the case of Paths 1a, 1b, 1c, and 1f where there is at least one net **favorable** diagnostic modifier, the expectations regarding the probability of success with an operation would be improved.*

*In the case of Paths 1h and 1i where there is at least one net **unfavorable** diagnostic modifier, the expectations regarding the probability of success with an operation would be tempered such that other causes should be considered before proceeding with therapy (particularly an operation). Additionally, in the case of Path 1j, if the symptoms did not change with decongestion, even though the airway restriction did, doubt is raised about the symptoms being due to an airway problem and so other causes for the symptoms are sought. In this case a different course of action is followed (no surgery) since the pathology is **not** causing any airway restriction though symptoms are still present. If the symptoms do decrease with decongestion, then there is some evidence for airway restriction playing a role in the problem and the path for therapy for a combined-structural problem is pursued with some caution.*

Symptoms present but no pathology, symptoms same after decongestion (Path 2)

If symptoms are present and pathology is **not** noted, then either pathology is being **missed** or the symptoms are from some **other** cause. *Airway testing can reveal significant restriction that would verify the presence of occult pathology, or no restriction that would verify the lack of pathology and suggest the symptoms are from other causes.*

If the patient has symptoms **without** pathology (Fig. 5–6, Path 2), there are two possibilities. Without airway testing, the clinician initially assumes the symptoms are from obstruction, and another look is done for any missed pathology. If pathology is found, then the path in the flowchart is followed for a patient with symptoms **and** pathology (Fig. 5–6, "Go to Path 1"). If pathology is **not** found, then a search is done for **other** causes (**?OTHER**) for the symptoms (Path 2b).

Some refinements can occur if nasal airway testing data are available. If there is no airway resistance after decongestion, but still significant symptoms, then other causes are looked for, and the same path is followed as when no airway data were available (Path 2b). However, for cases in which some airway restriction is evident, the clinician has stronger evidence for the presence of unseen pathology causing airway obstruction, and thus the symptoms, so another look for pathology is done (Path 2a). If no pathology is seen, an external dilator is tried to see if it reveals pathology by causing improvement in the airway. If pathology is found, then Path 1 is followed since pathology and symptoms are now both present.

*If no causative pathology can be found and the **airway restriction** is of **smaller** degree than the **symptoms**, then there is evidence of a **low threshold** and with no apparent pathology other causes are looked for (Path 2c) unless the symptoms had decreased with decongestion, in which case medical therapy would be tried first before looking for other causes. If the airway restriction is greater than (Path 2e) or equal to (Path 2d) the symptoms, this is additional supportive evidence that an airway restriction cause should be found for the significant restriction associated with the symptoms. The workup would be restarted with repeat airway testing and if a significant airway restriction was still found the clinician would continue to try to identify the offending pathology. If the symptoms had decreased with decongestion, then medical therapy would be tried before pursuing the reevaluation.*

Figure 5–8 shows the results of airway testing in which the **left** nasal airway is an example of Path 2a where occult pathology is found.

A 71-year-old man had suffered a nasal fracture 1 year earlier. He now complains of labored breathing bilaterally. He notes that he can breathe better if he tapes his nose so that the tip is elevated upward. Symptoms are the same after decongestion.

Examination: A septal deflection to the **right** in areas 2 and 3 is noted. Another otorhinolaryngologist had seen him previously and also documented a deflection to the **right** in area 2. No pathology noted on the left.

Airway testing revealed some **left-sided restriction** but the **right** side was **open**. Use of a dilator helped both the symptoms and the airflow on the **left** side.

Analysis: Left side: Moderate symptoms do not change with decongestion. No pathology seen. Mild airway restriction. Path 2a. Diagnosis: **occult pathology**. Second look unrevealing but dilator reveals anterior pathology. After discovery of pathology, go to Path 1. Degree of symptoms is greater than that of restriction or pathology, so Path 1h. Diagnosis: **?other vs. structural, low threshold**. Try dilator. If fails, option of an operation with appropriate counseling of patient regarding decreased odds of success. **Right** side: Moderate symptoms that do not change with decongestion. Mild pathology. No airway restriction. Diagnosis: **other** causes. Similar to Path 1j except no airway restriction was measured even before decongestion.

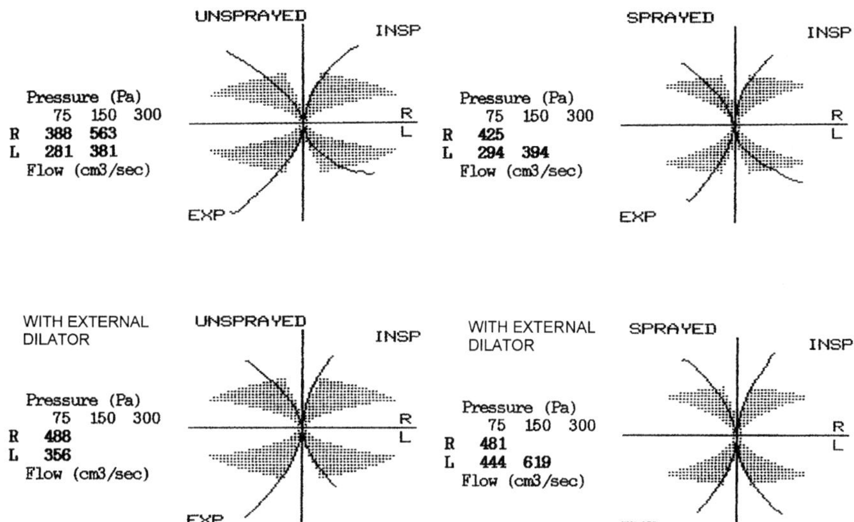

Figure 5–8.   Results in a 71-year-old man with a right nasal septal deflection noted at time of examination. He complains of mild-moderate obstruction on both sides and doesn't notice any improvement in symptoms with decongestion. Note the persistence of lower flows on the left even after decongestion (upper right). A greater restriction was present on the left than on the side where pathology was noted. The airway testing reveals no effect from the right-sided pathology, and documents the discovery of left-sided alar pathology. When the external dilator is applied, the flow markedly improves both before (lower left) and after (lower right) decongestion. (If a flow is not listed for a given pressure, it means that the airway was open enough that the pressure was not reached.)

Outcome: This patient is an example of someone with a low threshold for obstruction. He was treated with a dilator which he did not feel provided enough relief for him. The option of a rhinolift was discussed but he was also counseled regarding the odds of success in light of the suspicion that airway restriction might not be the only etiology for his symptoms.

Symptoms cleared with decongestion, pathology is still present after decongestion (Fig. 5–6, Path 3)

If **pathology is present** but the patient's **symptoms cleared** with decongestion, then the problem is thought to be either **mucosal** (**MUCOSAL**) (in which case the observed pathology was not of significance and did not enhance any effect from the mucosal pathology) or a **combination** of the observed pathology and a mucosal component that had now cleared (**COMB-MUCOSAL**) (see explanation of **combined-mucosal** problem). Without airway testing, it cannot be determined which is the case, but the clinician would generally assume that the observed pathology was a contributing factor if it is on the same side as the symptoms and might conclude that this was a combined mucosal problem (Path 3c).

*With certain airway results, the two diagnoses can be distinguished. If the airway restriction **clears** with decongestion, thus **corresponding** with the **symptoms**, then an airway cause for the symptoms is verified. Also, because the **airway** opens **completely**, the pathology that is still noted despite the open airway test result is thus found to **not** be a factor in the obstruction, and so the diagnosis of a mucosal problem*

(MUCOSAL) is made (Path 3d) and medical therapy is prescribed. **Overestimation of pathology** *is revealed if the degree of airway restriction is **less** than the pathology (Path 3a). If the airway restriction is **greater** than the pathology, then the pathology has been **underestimated** and is reassessed (Path 3b). If the airway restriction matches the pathology it confirms the presence of a persistent effect on the airway from the pathology and thus the diagnosis of a **combined mucosal** problem (Path 3c).*

Figure 5–9 shows the results of airway testing in which the **right** nasal airway is an example of Path 3a (the left—Path 1a).

A 31-year-old male with a history of nasal trauma. The patient complained of **mild right-sided** symptoms but **moderate left-sided** symptoms before spray. After decongestion, he stated that the **right** side was wide open but the **left** side still had **moderate** obstruction.

Examination: Significant-appearing septal deflection to areas 2, 3, and 4 was found on the **right**, and a **slight** caudal deflection that did not look as if it would affect the airway was noted on the **left**. Thus, symptoms were worse on the side opposite what was thought to be the most significant septal pathology. The patient noted improved airway with lifting of the ala on either side.

Airway testing confirmed that the **left** side had more airway restriction than the right, and a "second-look" examination revealed the cause of this was a left-sided valve area restriction that was not appreciated initially.

Analysis: Right side: Mild symptoms that **cleared** with decongestion. Pathology that was thought to be of clinical significance. Mild airway restriction. Path 3a, diagnosis: **combined mucosal, pathology overestimated**. Treatment is medical but the patient has the option of surgery if medical therapy does not sufficiently help.

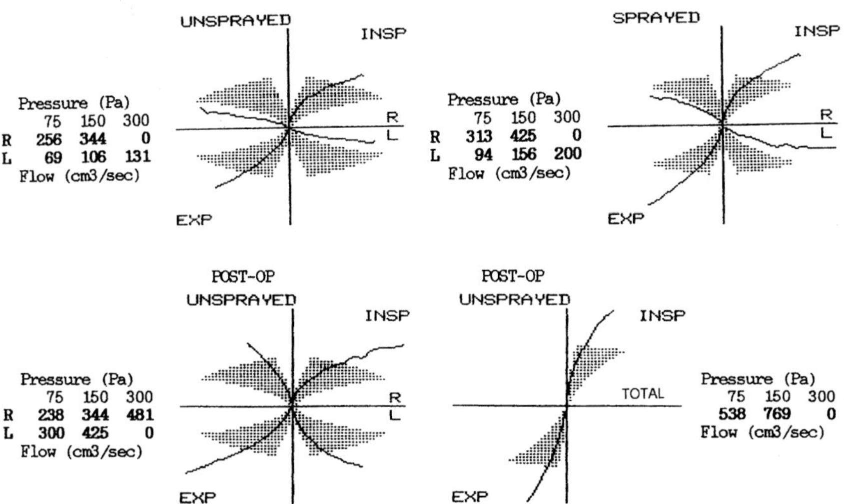

Figure 5–9. Results in a 31-year-old man. He complained of moderate left-sided symptoms that persisted after decongestion. On the right side mild symptoms cleared with decongestion. A marked right nasal septal deflection and slight left caudal deformity were noted. The airway testing shows much more impressive restriction on the left side both before (upper left) and after (upper right) decongestion. Postoperatively he had a marked improvement in the airway on the left even before decongestion (lower left). The overall effect is a significantly more open total nasal airway (lower right).

Left side: Moderate symptoms persist after decongestion. Slight pathology. Marked airway restriction. Path 1a. Diagnosis: **structural**. **Underestimate of pathology**. Reassess the pathology. Surgery.

Outcome: At the time of operation, doubled-up cartilage was found in the valve area on the left. Postoperatively, the patient now has an open airway bilaterally.

Comment: The combined mucosal problem on the right, while an example of Path 3a, becomes a secondary consideration to the overall effect on the airway of the underestimated pathology on the left side, which has the greatest symptoms.

Symptoms clear with decongestion, pathology not noted or cleared with decongestion (Fig. 5–6, Path 4)

Without airway testing, if the symptoms completely clear with decongestion and any pathology that was present disappears with decongestion (Fig. 5–6, Path 4), then the problem is thought to be due to mucosal factors (**MUCOSAL**), and medical therapy is pursued.

*If persistent **airway restriction** is demonstrated after decongestion, then one suspects a combined mucosal problem (with an occult structural component that may have been contributing to the symptoms before decongestion), and so **another look** for the pathology is warranted. If pathology is found, one pursues the path for pathology without symptoms (Fig. 5–6, Path 3). If no pathology is found then the persistent **airway restriction** suggests an underlying occult structural problem may be contributing to the overall symptoms (**COMB-MUCOSAL**) (Path 4c). This is kept in mind and if medical therapy fails to resolve the problem, reassessment is done looking for the not yet detected pathology. An example would be prominence of bony turbinate structure, not initially noted, which could be addressed with an operation if medical therapy failed.*

Figure 5–10 shows the results of airway testing in which the **right** and **left** nasal airways are examples of Path 4b.

A 29-year-old man, complains of congestion which is worst in the morning. Before decongestion, he complained of **mild** obstruction on the **right** and **moderate** obstruction on the **left**. After decongestion, he felt that both sides were **open**.

Examination: A straight septum was noted.

Airway testing showed persistent significant **restriction** even after decongestion.

Analysis: **Right** side: Mild symptoms that clear with decongestion. No pathology. Path 4b. Significant airway restriction. **Occult pathology**. Look for pathology. Pathology (prominent bone of turbinate) is found so go to Path 3c. Diagnosis: **combined-mucosal** problem. Medical therapy, if fails then option of surgery. **Left** side: Moderate symptoms that clear with decongestion. No pathology. Path 4b. Significant airway restriction. **Occult pathology**. Look for pathology. Pathology (prominent bone of turbinate) is found so go to Path 3c. Diagnosis: **combined-mucosal** problem. Medical therapy, if fails then option of surgery.

Outcome and comment: A second look reveals pathology not noted at first, bony enlargement of the turbinates. Sometimes septal pathology is focused on to a degree that the effect of the turbinates is not adequately appreciated, particularly if a very straight septum is seen. Medical therapy is pursued with the option of an

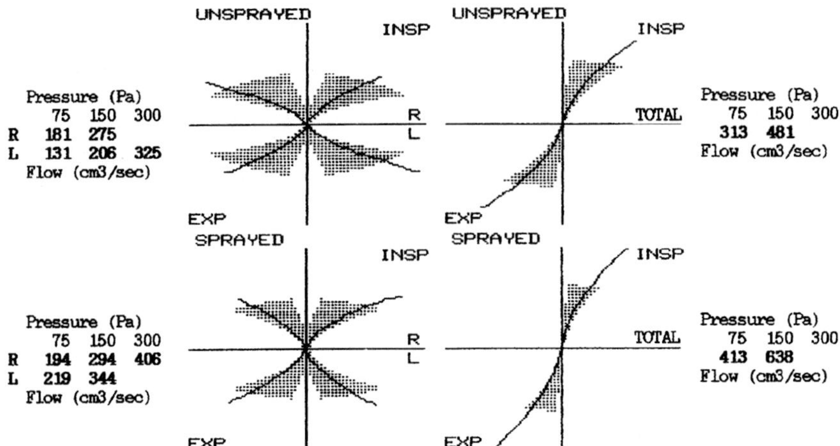

Figure 5–10.   Nasal airway test results on a 29-year-old man who complained of bilateral obstruction worst on the left. After decongestion he thought that both sides felt open. No pathology had been noted. The flow on the left side improved the most, enough to move the patient below his threshold for the sensation of obstruction so that he felt his nasal airway was open. The significant persistent airway restriction after decongestion (lower left), led to the discovery of the pathologic basis of this combined mucosal problem which was protruding bony infrastructure of the inferior turbinates bilaterally.

operation to reduce the bony protuberance of the inferior turbinates if medical therapy fails.

For all paths in the algorithm—when no airway restriction is found

An additional change in diagnosis and treatment that can result from airway testing should be mentioned because it applies to all of the paths.

*When **airway testing** data are available and **testing** reveals a widely patent, nonrestricted airway both **before** and after decongestion, it is questionable whether any symptoms are related to **nasal airway restriction** and whether any pathology that was noted is causing airway impedance because **no** airway restriction was found. A widely patent airway measurement could change any pathway action to the action of looking for other causes (**?OTHER**).*

Figure 5–11 shows a 62-year-old man who complained of nasal obstruction greater on the left side. The symptoms do not change with decongestion.

Examination: Left septal deflection was noted, and symptoms were attributed to this.

Airway testing: This showed a widely patent airway bilaterally before and after decongestion. There was **no improvement** in the airway test with use of an internal nasal **dilator.**

Outcome: *Operation on the left septal deflection was **deferred** because of lack of evidence for **airway restriction** that could be helped or that was a cause of the symptoms. Look for other causes.*

Comment: *In this case the test results showed that the patient had a widely patent airway bilaterally even though he still complained of significant symptoms. This situation is a warning that the effect of the noted pathology on the airway may have* *been overestimated, and the success of surgical correction of the septum is questionable. Some authors[67–69] have found a lower incidence of patient satisfaction if the nasal airway is widely patent on objective testing preoperatively despite the presence of symptoms. The objective test thus helps to estimate the probability of a successful outcome with operation.*

Figure 5–12 shows a 72-year-old man who had nasal trauma in a motor vehicle accident. States that since that time he has been told he has scar tissue in the left side of his nose. Before decongestion, the patient complained that the left side had

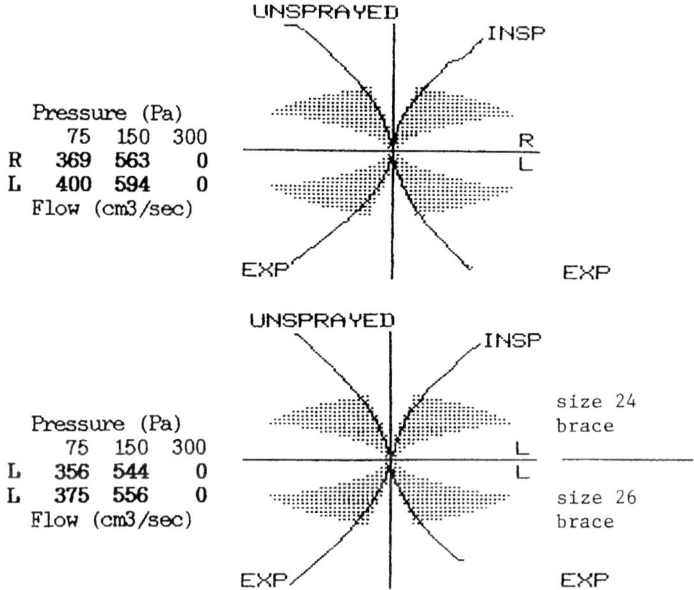

Figure 5–11. Nasal airway testing results for a 62-year-old man who complained of nasal obstruction greatest on the left side. Left septal deflection was noted on examination. No significant airway restriction was measured. (brace = commercial wire internal nasal brace that holds alae open.)

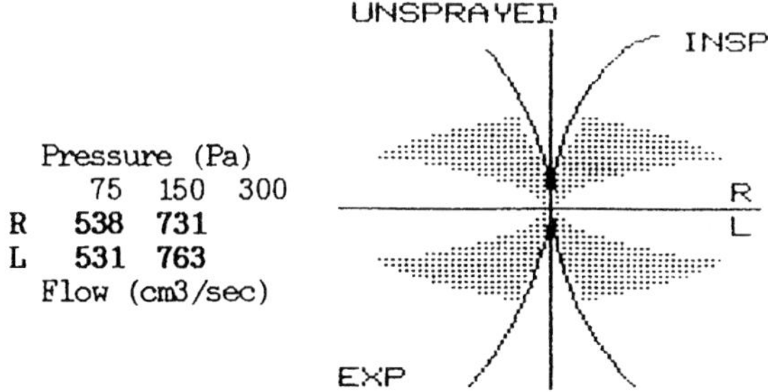

Figure 5–12. Results in a 72-year-old man with complaint of moderate to severe obstruction on the left that decreased to mild with decongestion. On the right side there was a mild restriction that opened with decongestion, though the airway still didn't feel right. No pathology was seen. The results from rhinomanometry show a widely patent airway bilaterally, even before decongestion. This doesn't deny that the patient has symptoms. It clarifies that there is no apparent airway restriction evident as an associated cause of the symptoms. The partial symptomatic improvement with decongestion could reflect a very low threshold for obstruction. The patient was found to have poor pulmonary function.

moderate to severe restriction and the right side had **moderate** obstruction. After decongestion, he stated that the left side had **mild** obstruction and the right side was open, although his nasal airway still felt "abnormal."

Examination: No pathology found before or after decongestion.

Airway testing showed **widely patent** airway bilaterally, even before decongestion.

Analysis: Right side: Symptoms clear with decongestion. No pathology. No airway restriction **even before decongestion. Left** side: Symptoms decrease to mild with decongestion. No pathology. No airway restriction **even before decongestion**. Because of the significant improvement in symptoms with decongestion, medical therapy can be tried, but look for **other** causes if it fails.

Outcome: Beclamethasone spray was tried because of symptom improvement with decongestion, but didn't alleviate the patient's problem. Since airway testing showed no restriction, this confirmed the lack of any pathology (as noted on the examination), causing airway restriction and supported looking for "other causes." In this case the patient was found to have **poor pulmonary function**. It is also possible that scarring from the trauma is causing a sensory disturbance. If patients have a mucosal or nerve ending disturbance such that the patient **feels** obstructed despite an open airway, this condition can sometimes be helped by using a menthol inhaler to stimulate the cold receptors causing a sensation of more open breathing even though the diameter of the airway doesn't change.

Comment: This example differs from the previous one in that **no** pathology was noted, and the symptoms decreased with decongestion. Since there was some symptomatic improvement with decongestion, medical therapy was tried. It did not help. Other etiologies besides airway restriction were then considered.

SUMMARY

In clinical assessment, nasal airway testing can help by verifying the diagnosis and treatment selection, modifying the diagnosis, modifying the treatment, and modifying the expectations regarding success of treatment.

Airway Testing Can Help in Verifying the Diagnosis and Increasing Confidence in a Chosen Treatment

Airway testing can reinforce the patient's description of the symptoms or the clinician's visual assessment of the intranasal airway particularly if it agrees in side and degree.

Testing of the airway can also verify the effect of changes in the airway. Airway testing results provide an objective verification of the effect of maneuvers that open the vestibule and valve area. Similarly it provides objective verification of the effect of decongestion on the airway. Testing done after surgery is another way of objectively assessing a change in the airway. When the airway restriction changes in a manner similar to the change in symptoms then there is increased confidence in a diagnosis that is based on the symptoms being caused by a decrease in airflow through the nose, and increased confidence in the probability of success of therapy that will favorably modify the nasal airway. Conversely, a change in symptoms without a corresponding change in the airway test results would raise a question about whether the symptoms were due to airway restriction.

Airway Testing Can Lead to a Clarification of the Diagnosis

*When a **high threshold** is revealed alone or in combination with an underestimation of pathology.*

This occurs when **airway restriction is greater than symptoms** (Path 1a, Path 1b, Path 2e). When airway restriction is actually greater than the degree of symptoms there might be increased confidence that a significant airway problem is present but this does not change the treatment.

*When an **underestimation of pathology** is revealed alone or in combination with a high threshold.*

This occurs when airway restriction is greater than the degree of pathology (Path 1a, Path 1f, Path 3b). When **airway restriction is greater than the pathology** it implies that the pathology may have more effect on the airway than was anticipated and a second look at the degree of pathology is warranted, but the treatment would still address that pathology.

Airway Testing Can Lead to a Change in Diagnosis and Treatment

If **no pathology** had been noted, but **significant airway restriction** was measured, then the diagnosis changes to one of **occult pathology**. This leads to another examination of the airway looking for the cause of the restriction and **changes** in **diagnosis** and **therapy** if such pathology is found.

For **Path 1**, the diagnosis of structural vs. combined-structural (Paths 1a–1g) is based on the response to decongestion and that would determine the treatment. If the degree of airway restriction is less than that of the symptoms (low threshold alone or with pathology overestimation, Path 1h and Path 1i), then **other** causes of the symptom of obstruction should be considered before surgery is pursued. The patient might also be counseled that the odds of success in alleviating the symptoms might not be as optimal as the other branches in Path 1. If there is **no** airway restriction (Path 1j), and no response to decongestion, then no medical or surgical therapy is pursued and other causes are considered.

In **Path 2**, if the airway testing leads to the discovery of pathology, the diagnosis changes from "other causes" to structural or combined-structural and the corresponding treatment is then pursued. If pathology is not found but there is a **degree of airway restriction** that is greater than or equal to the **degree of the symptoms** (Paths 2d and 2e) then further investigation is pursued looking for the cause of the airway restriction.

In **Path 3**, if airway testing shows no restriction (Path 3d), then the diagnosis is a mucosal problem rather than a combined-mucosal problem, which means an operation that would modify intranasal structure is no longer considered an option for treatment if medical therapy fails, since there is no **structural** airway restricting pathology to correct.

In **Path 4**, if airway testing leads to the discovery of pathology, the diagnosis could change from **mucosal** to **combined-mucosal**, and an operation on intranasal structure would then be one of the treatment options.

Airway Testing Can Modify the Prediction of the Probability of Success of a Treatment

*When a **low threshold** is revealed by itself or in combination with an overestimation of pathology.*

This occurs when **airway restriction is of a smaller degree than the symptoms** (Paths 1h, 1i, 2c). When airway restriction is less than the degree of symptoms there might be decreased confidence that treatment of the airway will improve the symptoms.

*When an **overestimation of pathology** is revealed alone or in combination with a low threshold.*

This occurs when the degree of airway restriction is **less** than the degree of pathology (Paths 1d, 1i, 3a). This implies that the pathology may have less effect on the airway than was thought and so there is less confidence that correction of the pathology will improve the airway as much as was expected in trying to improve the airway.

The probability of success of **treatment that modifies the nasal airway** is related to the amount of certainty that the patient's **symptoms** are due to **pathology** that is causing **airway restriction**. Because airway testing can objectively assess the amount of airway restriction, it can play a role in helping to determine the probability of success of treatment aimed at relief of airway restriction. This information is useful both in treatment planning and in counseling the patient about therapeutic options.

CONCLUSIONS

Rhinomanometry can be used for objective assessment of the nasal airway. The clinical algorithm for evaluation of the patient with the symptom of nasal obstruction without and with the information obtained by objective testing of the nose was described. The instances in which diagnosis and treatment course can be refined by having this additional information demonstrates the clinical utility of objective testing of the nasal airway.

REFERENCES

1. Parker LP, Crysdale WS, Cole P, Woodside D: Rhinomanometry in children. *Int J Pediatr Otorhinolaryngol* 1989; 17:127–137.
2. Connell JT: Rhinometry: measurement of nasal patency. *Ann Allergy* 1982; 49:179–185.
3. Foxen EH, Preston TD, Lack JA: The assessment of nasal air-flow: a review of past and present methods. *J Laryngol Otol* 1971; 85:811–825.

4. Gordts F, Clement PA, Derde MP: Nasal provocation with histamine: a comparison of the determination of the threshhold of reactivity by three methods of rhinomanometry. *Rhinology* 1989; 27:263–269.
5. Schumacher MJ: Rhinomanometry. *J Allergy Clin Immunol* 1989; 83:711–718.
6. Rivron RP: Cross-sectional area as a measure of nasal resistance. *Rhinology* 1990; 28:257–264.
7. Georgitis JW: The applicability of rhinomanometry in nonatopic children: comparison of three techniques. *J Allergy Clin Immunol* 1985; 75:614–620.
8. Cole P: Rhinomanometry 1988: practice and trends. *Laryngoscope* 1989; 99:311–315.
9. Cole P, Ayiomanimitis A, Ohki M: Anterior and posterior rhinomanometry. *Rhinology* 1989; 27:257–262.
10. Berkinshaw ER, Spalding PM, Vig PS: The effect of methodology on the determination of nasal resistance. *Am J Orthod Dentofacial Orthop* 1987; 92:329–335.
11. Haight JS, Cole P: The site and function of the nasal valve. *Laryngoscope* 1983; 93:49–55.
12. Guillette BJ, Perry CJ: Use of nasal valve stent with anterior rhinomanometry to quantitate nasal valve obstruction. *Ann Otol Rhinol Laryngol* 1990; 99:175–178.
13. Cole P (ed.): *The Repiratory Role of the Upper Airways: A Selective Clinical and Pathophysiological Review*. St. Louis, Mosby Year Book, 1993.
14. Clement PA: Committee report on standardization of rhinomanometry. *Rhinology* 1984; 22:151–155.
15. Cole P, Havas TE: Resistance to respiratory airflow of the nasal passages: comparison between different common methods of calculation. *Rhinology* 1986; 24:163–173.
16. Naito K, Cole P, Chaban R, Humphrey D: Computer averaged nasal resistance. *Rhinology* 1989; 27:45–52.
17. Bachmann W: The present status of rhinomanometry. *Rhinology* 1976; 14:5–9.
18. Broms P, Jonson B, Lamm CJ: Rhinomanometry. II. A system for numerical description of nasal airway resistance. *Acta Otolaryngol (Stockh)* 1982; 94:157–168.
19. Wihl JA, Malm L: Rhinomanometry in routine allergen challenge. *Clin Otolaryngol* 1985; 10:185–189.
20. McCaffrey TV, Kern EB: Clinical evaluation of nasal obstruction. *Arch Otolarngol* 1979; 105:542–545.
21. Cole P, et al: Computer-aided rhinometry. A research rhinometer for clinical trial. *Acta Otolaryngol* 1980; 90:139–142.
22. Hoshino T, Togawa K, Nishihira S: Statistical analysis of changes of pediatric nasal patency with growth. *Laryngoscope* 1988; 98:219–225.
23. Reeves HM, Wright WK, Novakovic M: Quantitative measurement of nasal-airway resistance. *Arch Otolaryngol* 1970; 92:573–575.
24. O'Neill G, Tolley NS: Theoretical considerations of nasal airflow mechanics and surgical implications. *Clin Otolaryngol* 1988; 13:273–277.
25. Pallanch JF: Nasal resistance: a comparison of the methods used for obtaining normal values and a comparison of proposed models of the transnasal pressure-flow curves. Thesis, Mayo Graduate School of Medicine (University of Minnesota), Rochester, 1984.
26. Clement PA, Marien J: The use of a mathematical model in rhinometry. *Rhinology* 1980; 18:197–207.
27. Enzmann H: Luftdruck und Volumenflus in der Nase—Darstellung im doppeltlogarithmischen System. *Laryngol Rhinol* 1975; 54:200–235.
28. Dallimore NS, Eccles R: Changes in human nasal resistance associated with exercise, hyperventilation and rebreathing. *Acta Otolaryngol (Stockh)* 1977; 84:416–421.
29. Eichler J, Lenz H: Comparison of different coefficients and units in rhinomanometry. *Rhinology* 1985; 23:149–157.
30. Spoor A: A new method for measuring nasal conductivity. *Int Rhinol* 1965; 3:27–35.
31. Cockcroft DW, MacCormack DW, Tarlo SM, et al: Nasal airway inspiratory resistance. *Am Rev Respir Dis* 1979; 119:921–926.
32. Craig AB Jr, Dvorak M, McIlreath FJ: Resistance to airflow through the nose. *Ann Otol Rhinol Laryngol* 1965; 74:589–603.
33. Schumacher MJ: Advances in tests for the evaluation of rhinitis. *Immunol Allergy Clin North Am* 1987; 7:15–35.
34. Solomon WR, Stohrer AW: Considerations in the measurement of nasal patency. *Ann Otol Rhinol Laryngol* 1965; 74:978–990.
35. Speizer FE, Frank NR: A technique for measuring nasal and pulmonary flow resistance simultaneously. J Appl Physiol 1964; 19:176–178.
36. Schumacher MJ, Gaines JA, Bescript B: Computer-aided rhinometry: analysis of inspiratory and expiratory nasal pressure-flow curves in subjects with rhinitis. *Comput Biol Med* 1985; 15:187–195.
37. Solow B, Greve E: Rhinomanometric recording in children. *Rhinology* 1980; 18:31–42.

38. Jones AS, Lancer JM, Stevens JC, Beckingham E: Rhinomanometry: do the anterior and posterior methods give equivalent results? *Clin Otolaryngol* 1987; 12:109–114.

39. Unno T, Naitoh Y, Sakamoto N, Horikawa H: Nasal resistance measured by anterior rhinomanometry. *Rhinology* 1986; 24:49–55.

40. Cole P, Naito K, Chaban R, Ayiomamitis A: Unilateral and bilateral nasal resistances. *Rhinology* 1988; 26:209–216.

41. Naito K, Cole P, Humphrey D: Unilateral and bilateral nasal resistances: a supplement. *Rhinology* 1990; 28:91–95.

42. Dvoracek JE, Hillis A, Rossing RG: Comparison of sequential anterior and posterior rhinomanometry. *J Allergy Clin Immunol* 1985; 76:577–582.

43. Broms P: Rhinomanometry. III. Procedures and criteria for distinction between skeletal stenosis and mucosal swelling. *Acta Otolaryngol (Stockh)* 1982; 94:361–370.

44. Jessen M, Malm L: Use of pharmacologic decongestion in the generation of rhinomanometric norms for the nasal airway. *Am J Otolaryngol* 1988; 9:336–340.

45. Hasegawa M, Kern EB: Variations in nasal resistance in man: a rhinomanometric study of the nasal cycle in 50 human subjects. *Rhinology* 1978; 16:19–29.

46. Heetderks DR: Reaction of normal nasal mucous membrane. *Am J Med Sci* 1927; 174:231–244.

47. Cole P, Fastag O, Forsyth R: Variability in nasal resistance measurements. *J Otolaryngol* 1980; 9:309–315.

48. Haight JS, Cole P: Unilateral nasal resistance and asymmetrical body pressure. *J Otolaryngol* 1986; 15 Suppl 16:1–31.

49. Forsyth RD, Cole P, Shephard RJ: Exercise and nasal patency. *J Appl Physiol* 1983; 55:860–865.

50. McCaffrey TV, Kern EB: Response of nasal airway resistance to hypercapnia and hypoxia in man. *Ann Otol Rhinol Laryngol* 1979; 88:247–252.

51. Strohl KP, O'Cain CF, Slutsky AS: Alae nasi activation and nasal resistance in healthy subjects. *J Appl Physiol* 1982; 52:1432–1437.

52. Cole P, Forsyth R, Haight JS: Effects of cold air and exercise on nasal patency. *Ann Otol Rhinol Laryngol* 1983; 92:196–198.

53. Salman SD, Proctor DF, Swift DL, Evering SA: Nasal resistance: description of a method and effect of temperature and humidity changes. *Ann Otol Rhinol Laryngol* 1971; 80:736–743.

54. Eccles R, Lee RL: The influence of the hypothalamus on the sympathetic innervation of the nasal vasculature of the cat. *Acta Otolaryngol* 1981; 91:127–134.

55. Jones AS, Lancer JM, Moir AA, Stevens JC: Effect of aspirin on nasal resistance to airflow. *Br Med J (Clin Res Ed)* 1985; 290:1171–1173.

56. Havas TE, Cole P, Parker L, et al: The effects of combined H1 and H2 histamine antagonists on alterations in nasal airflow resistance induced by topical histamine provocation. *J Allergy Clin Immunol* 1986; 78:856–860.

57. Pallanch JF, McCaffrey TV, Kern EB: Normal nasal resistance. *Otolaryngol Head Neck Surg* 1985; 93:778–785.

58. Ohki M, Naito K, Cole P: Dimensions and resistances of the human nose: racial differences. *Laryngoscope* 1991; 101:276–278.

59. Stocks J, Godfrey S: Nasal resistance during infancy. *Respir Physiol* 1978; 34:233–246.

60. Cole P: Toronto rhinomanometry: laboratory, field and clinical studies. *J Otolaryngol* 1988; 17:331–335.

61. Hasegawa M, Kern EB, O'Brien PC: Dynamic changes of nasal resistance. *Ann Otol Rhinol Laryngol* 1979; 88:66–71.

62. Hardcastle PF, White A, Prescott RJ: Clinical and rhinometric assessment of the nasal airway—do they measure the same entity? *Clin Otolaryngol* 1988; 13:185–191.

63. Sandham A: Rhinomanometric method error in the assessment of nasal respiratory resistance. *Rhinology* 1988; 26:191–202.

64. Jones AS, Lancer JM, Stevens JC, Beckinham E: Nasal resistance to airflow (its measurement, reproducibility and normal parameters). *J Laryngol Otol* 1987; 101:800–808.

65. Cole P: Stability of nasal airflow resistance. *Clin Otolaryngol* 1989; 14:177–182.

66. Arbour P, Kern EB: Paradoxical nasal obstruction. *Can J Otolaryngol* 1975; 4:333–338.

67. Broms P, Jonson B, Malm L: Rhinomanometry IV. A pre- and postoperative evaluation in functional septoplasty. *Acta Otolaryngol* 1982; 94:523–529.

68. Mertz JS, McCaffrey TV, Kern EB: Objective evaluation of anterior septal surgical reconstruction. *Otolaryngol Head Neck Surg* 1984; 92:308–311.

69. Sipila JI, Suonpaa JT, Kortekangas AE, et al: Rhinomanometry before septoplasty: an approach to clinical material with diverse nasal symptoms. *Am J Rhinology* 1992; 6:16–22.

6

Acoustic Rhinometry

HEINRICH G. LENDERS, Ph.D.

Acoustic rhinometry (AR) is a recently introduced method[1] to evaluate nasal geometry by an acoustic reflection technique. It is especially useful for evaluating the geometry in the anterior and middle thirds of the nasal cavity. In the nasopharynx, AR computes cross-sectional areas (CSA), which varies because of the dynamic variations of the soft palate (see Fig. 6–29). Therefore, the clinical application of AR in this part of the upper airway is limited. If breathing is quiet, all age groups, including premature infants, can have measurements obtained within seconds. AR curves can be interpreted only in connection with the rhinoscopic findings of each patient. The geometric assessment of the nasal structures is of interest for both clinicians and researchers. Rhinosurgeons, for instance, want to document objectively the nasal pathology and the efficacy of surgical therapy. Allergologists are interested in the response of the nasal mucosa to allergens and antiallergic drugs. Pediatricians need a noninvasive technique to evaluate nasal patency and the geometry of the nasopharynx in children. The dilemma of this technique is the lack of standardization, different presentation of measured results, and insufficient data on normal values for different populations.

HISTORICAL NOTES

There has been a long-term interest in estimating airway dimensions in the field of speech research. Various workers have attempted to correlate upper airway tract measurements with the sound being produced. The description of fast Fourier transformation (FFT) by Cooley and Tukey in 1965[2] and the recent explosive growth in computer technology induced a huge swing from analog to digital analysis techniques. Physical models of the upper airway have largely been replaced by mathematical models. The main reason for this development has been the increase in power and the reduction in cost of FFT analyzers. The early work of acoustical experiments was done in the frequency domain.[3–6] Sondhi and Gopinath[7] began using time domain reflectometry in 1971. In 1977, Jackson et al.[8] introduced a system to investigate the geometry of excised tracheas and lungs. In 1980, Fredberg et al.[9] developed the acoustic reflection technique for use with humans; this equipment is currently used by respiratory clinicians.[10–13] Hilberg et al.,[1] in 1989, utilized this technique to study the geometry of the nasopharyngeal airway.

125

TECHNIQUE

The principle of acoustic reflectometry or acoustic rhinometry (AR) is simple. It is a method of measuring the CSA of the nasal cavity as a function of distance from the nostril. An acoustic signal is produced by a source transducer in the distal end of a wave tube, and this signal passes down the wave tube into the measured object (Fig. 6–1). As the sound waves travel through the respiratory airways, they are partially reflected whenever there is a change in the CSA of the airways. The transmitted signal and the reflection from the measured object are recorded by a microphone and digitized by a computer system. Computer analysis of the reflected signal leads to a reconstruction of the impedance and area profile of the measured object. The results can be visualized and plotted as an area-distance-function or can be mathematically integrated to obtain values of volumes within the nasal cavities. The object being measured is considered as a series of discrete cylinders (100 to 200), each having the same length (L). Because the acoustic impedance (Z) of a cylinder is inversely proportional to its CSA, the object is represented as a series of impedance sections. Data acquisition and analysis assume the following ideal model: (1) single duct, (2) one-dimensional propagation, (3) infinite measurement bandwidth, (4) very large wall inertiance, (5) lossless gas, (6) uniform gas composition, (7) infinite computational accuracy, (8) infinite signal-to-noise ratio, and (9) zero discretization error. Although none of the possible errors associated with these idealizations can be disregarded, the most important ones are discussed.

1. In practice, the most relevant branching is at the choana between the nasal cavity and nasopharynx. Because the algorithm cannot recognize branching, the calculation of area beyond the choana is influenced by the geometry of the

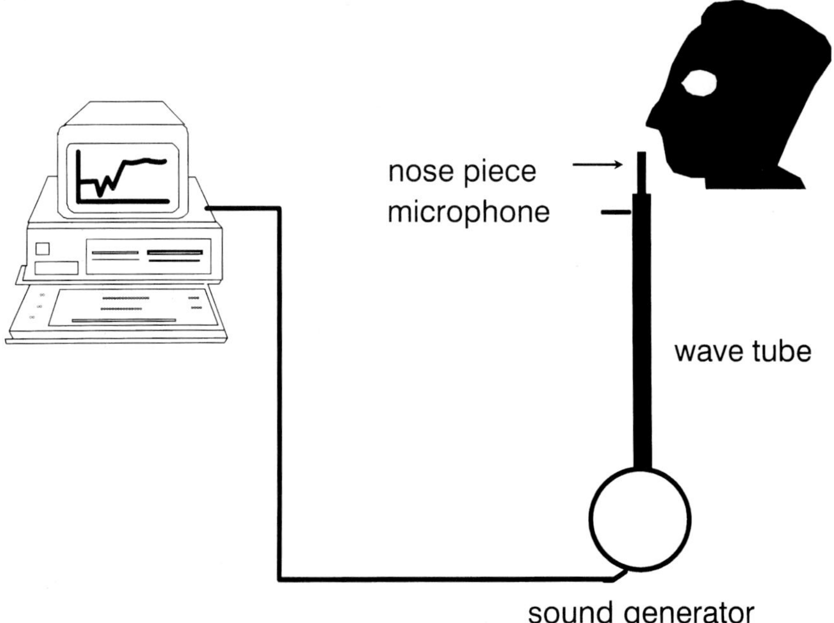

Figure 6–1. Apparatus for acoustic rhinometry.

nasopharynx itself and the contralateral nasal cavity. Furthermore, videoendoscopic and AR studies show involuntary movements of the velum, which result in quick changes of CSA in the nasopharynx. Therefore, the amount of information regarding CSA in the nasopharnyx is clearly reduced.

2. In long, straight, rigid ducts, cross-modes begin to propagate at frequencies:

$$f = \sqrt{\_} c_o / (2d)$$

> $f = Frequency$
> $c_o = speed\ of\ propagation$
> $d = maximal\ diameter$

The problem with using a broadband signal is that cross-modes may be induced in the object, violating the assumption of one-dimensional plane wave propagation. To avoid cross-modes, the transmitted signal should be limited to frequencies, the wavelength of which is less than twice the maximal diameter of the object. Cross-modes would theoretically form first in the nasopharynx because this is the part of the airway with the largest diameter. Because the geometric profile of the nasal cavity contains a small CSA in the vestibule and a relatively large CSA in the nasopharynx, cross-modes do not arise in the nasal cavity and therefore do not influence the calculated CSA within the nasal cavity. In contrast, AR via the oral route may lead to cross-modes and interference with planar wave propagation because of the relatively large transverse dimension of the oral cavity.

3 and 4. The best working bandwidth depends on the lower limit by wall inertiance and at the upper limit by formation of cross-modes. Walls of the human airway behave dynamically at frequencies less than about 800 Hz. Therefore, and to avoid cross-modes, the working bandwidth should be between 0.8 kHz and 6 kHz (see paragraph 2 above).

5 and 6. The effects of other idealizations such as lossless gas and nonuniform gas compositions are not well documented.[14-16]

7, 8, and 9. The calculation of CSA as an approximate reconstruction of the real geometry deals with infinite computational accuracy, infinite signal-to-noise ratio, and zero discretization error. The accuracy and stability of calculated data depend on the combination of program code and compiler, on the floating processing unit, and the AD-converter. The acoustic rhinometer should be tested as a system by using calibration tubes.

Despite these limitations, very accurate values of CSA can be obtained in measured objects.

The design and performance of an acoustic rhinometer depend on the kind of sound used. Principally, a click or a continuous sound can be used. The kind of the transmitted signal determines the characteristics of detectors and estimators. The method using continuous sound needs much more time for one measurement than the pulse method. When CSA is constant in the measured object, the values of CSA are identical for both methods. In measured objects with dynamic variations of CSA, such as the nasopharynx, only the pulse method is able to demonstrate these variations. The time consumption is usually 0.1 s for the pulse method (measurement frequency up to 10 Hz) and 2 to 30 s for the continuous sound method (measurement frequency up to 0.5 Hz). Commercially available acoustic rhinometers use continuous sound or the pulse method.

DATA FROM NASAL MODELS

As a means for comparison of AR with measurements made on the intact nasal cavity, dimensions have been estimated with water displacement, rhinomanometry (RM), and computed tomography (CT). The obtained dimensions correlate well with acoustic estimations (coefficients, 0.90 to 0.96). However, RM and CT were based on CSA at given distances within the nasal cavity. Furthermore, water displacement estimations disregard the interesting anterior part of the nasal cavity, and CT estimations are based on arbitrarily chosen planes of the scanning gantry. Large differences in the CSA by CT[1] occur just by changing the upper limit of adsorption coefficients of air or by changing the convolution kernels from a smooth to a relatively hard borderline projection. RM has its special problem of reproducibility.[17] Using the Cavalieri principle in cadavers, Mayhew and O'Flynn[18] focused on volumes.

Only nasal models provide the possibility of unbiased and direct estimations of CSA and volumes inside the nasal cavities, including their experimental modifications. Therefore, the author has used nasal models made of different materials, which were taken from casts of human cadavers. To simulate the real conditions of the nose as far as possible, some nasal models were coated with bovine mucosa.

First, the accuracy and reproducibility of CSA within nasal models were determined. In the nasal models, defined changes of anatomical structures (turbinates, septal deviation, polyps of the middle meatus, adenoid) were correlated with the rhinometric curves before and after changes. Figure 6–2 presents an example of simulating turbinate hypertrophy. Rhinometric measurements were made before and after changes in the nasal model. The volume in the anterior third of the nasal cavity (between 1 cm and 6 cm from the nostril) was defined as standard volume ($V_{standard}$). The added or resected volume was called $V_{diffreal}$, and the calculated

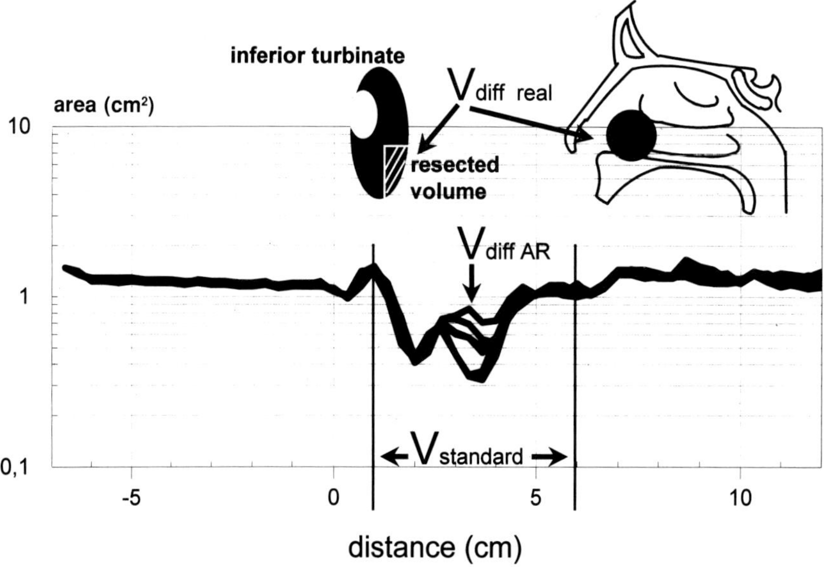

Figure 6–2. Simulation of turbinate hypertrophy of different sizes in a nasal model.

**Table 6–1   Absolute Values of Volume Measured in
Simulation of Turbinate Hypertrophy of Different Sizes
(Fig. 6–2)**

VOLUME, mL				
$V_{standard}$*	1.89	2.06	2.30	2.65
$V_{diffreal}$†	0.2	0.3	0.6	0.8
$V_{diff\ AR}$‡	0.17	0.33	0.57	0.76

*Volume in anterior third of nasal cavity.
†Added as resected volume.
‡Calculated difference of volume by acoustic rhinometry.

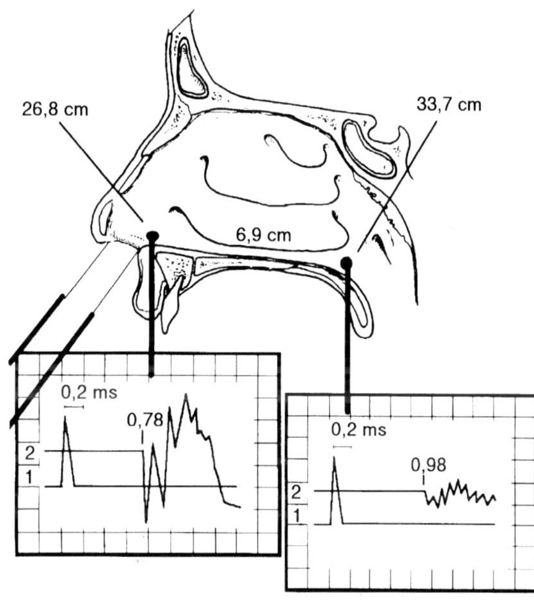

Figure 6–3. The propagation of sound through the nasal cavity. Two sound probes, 26.8 cm and 33.7 cm from the microphone in the wave tube. The measurement pulse and the signal at both measurement points are plotted. The reduction in intensity with distance and the effect of reflections are visible.

difference of volume by AR was called V_{diffAR}. Table 6–1 presents the absolute values of Figure 6–2. All the experimental data showed differences between $V_{diffreal}$ and V_{diffAR} in the range of 5% to 15%. Thirty different series (at different locations within the nasal cavity; 50 measurements for all variations) with four steps of 0.2 m $V_{diffreal}$ were made. The calculated mean value was 0.2 m (SD, 0.016 m; range, 0.17 to 0.22 m). The test of reproducibility (30 measurements on 30 following days) showed differences of absolute values less than 1% in the nasal models.

Second, we tried to determine the plane of the measured CSA. The isotemporal layers of the acoustic pulse through the nasal cavity were measured. The propagation of the acoustic signal through the nasal cavity (Fig. 6–3) was measured with subminiature microphones for the lateral wall and a perforated septum for the medial wall. The isotemporal layers were found to be oriented nearly parallel to the

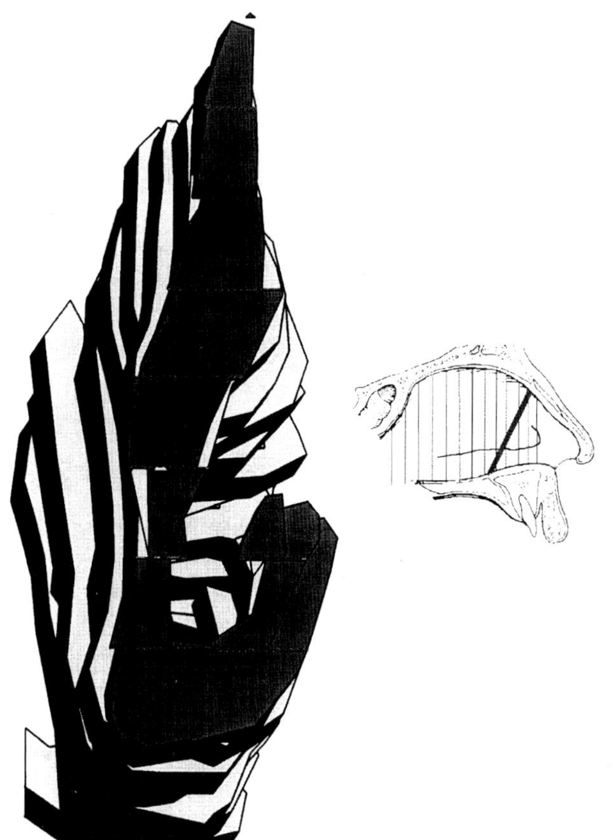

Figure 6–4. Screen dump from ACAD 12. Pictogram of the nose and reconstruction of a left nasal cavity after digitizing cuts from a nasal model.

nasal valve. Then, the acoustically measured CSA was correlated with the CSA of cuts from our nasal models. After these cuts were digitized, ACAD-software (ACAD® V 12) allowed reconstruction of the nasal cavity and calculations of CSA in all orientations and distances (Fig. 6–4). The best correlation of CSA was found in orientation parallel to the nasal valve. The difference between the measured and calculated CAS was up to 3% in the nasal cavity and up to 17% in the nasopharynx. The hypothesis—that the measured CSA is located nearly parallel to the nasal valve—was confirmed.

The acoustic conditions of the nose may influence the calculated CSA. Therefore, some of the cylindrical and nasal models with known dimensions were coated with bovine mucosa. Figure 6-5 shows the rhinometric curves of a cylindrical tube with a closure at 20 cm distance; curve 1 represents the model coated with mucosa. Models with the same dimensions built up by Silastic (curve 2) and acrylic (curve 3) resulted in different data. Accurate estimations of CSA can be obtained only in objects, the walls of which behave rigidly or in which the loss of signal is known. To measure this loss is very difficult or impossible in experiments. Therefore, we adjusted the correcting factor in the algorithm to estimate correct areas in the models coated with mucosa (Fig. 6–6). The arrows in the figure indicate the real

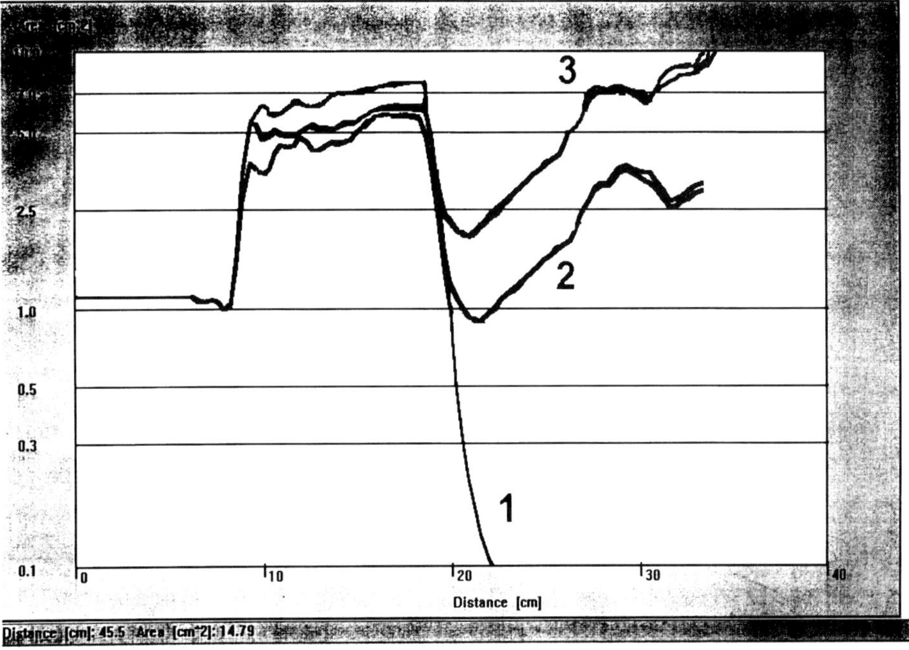

Figure 6–5. Effect of different materials on calculated cross-sectional area in acoustic rhinometry. Model coated with mucosa (curve 1), built up by Silastic (curve 2), and built up by acrylic (curve 3).

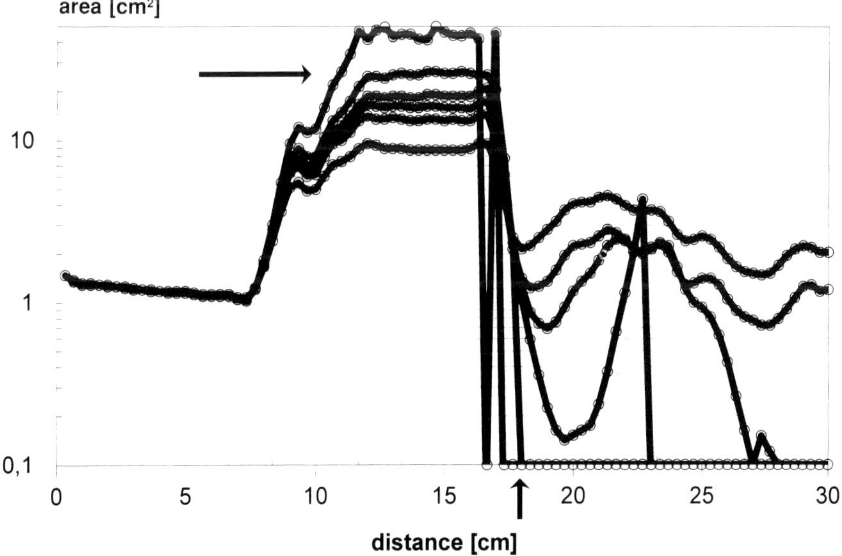

Figure 6–6. Adjustment of the correcting factor in the algorithm to estimate correct cross-sectional area in the model coated with mucosa. The arrows indicate the real dimensions of the model.

dimensions of a cylindrical tube with a closure at 13.5 cm distance. Under the condition that the loss of signal is larger than presented in the algorithm, the calculation results in error of too small a CSA and too large distances. The closure at the end of the tube cannot be detected.

Because accurate estimations of areas can be obtained only in objects whose acoustic conditions are presented in the algorithm, an empirical correction for the object nose was done. The problem in application of this technique to study the geometry of the nasal cavity is that the area beyond a severe constriction may not be accurately estimated. In the nose, there is a rather severe reduction of CSA in the anterior third. We determined this—$C_{ross-sectional}A_{rea\ critical}$ (CA_{crit})—in nasal models. Stepwise, the CSA at the head of the inferior turbinate was reduced by simulating turbinate hypertrophy in different sizes of nasal models. Figure 6–7 presents data with a CA_{crit} of 0.3 cm² at 2.9 cm distance from the nostril. Our results indicate that, in general, the CA_{crit} is not an absolute value. It depends on the dimensions and geometry of the areas beyond the severe obstruction. With use of nasal models with dimensions of children and adults, the CA_{crit} in the anterior third of the nose ranged from 0.16 to 0.22 cm² for children and from 0.35 to 4.0 cm² for adults.

THE NOSEPIECE, A CRITICAL PART OF THE EQUIPMENT

Because the nosepiece (adapter to connect the nose with the rhinometer) is part of the measured object, acoustic conditions of the adapter may influence the calculated CSA. The profile and dimensions of the adapter may bias the geometry of the

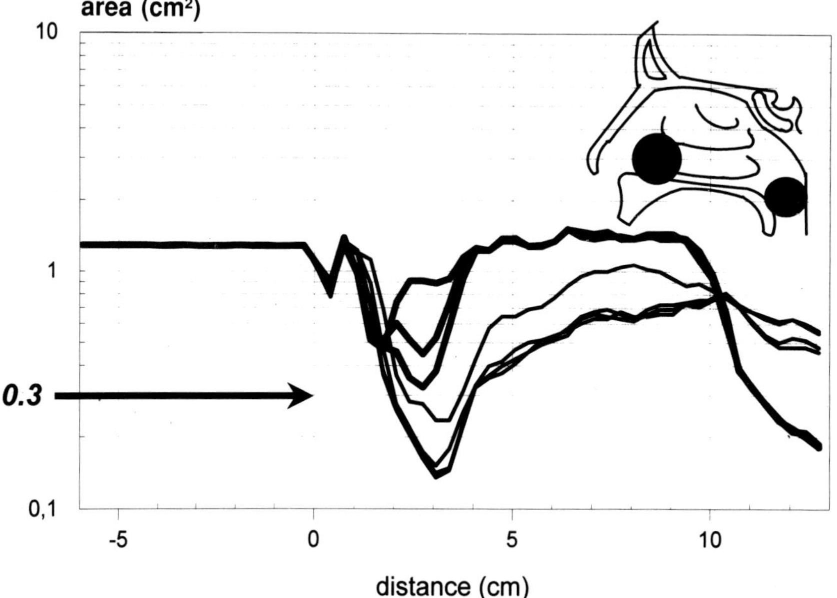

Figure 6–7. Determination of CA_{crit} (in this situation, 0.3 cm²) by simulating turbinate hypertrophy of different sizes.

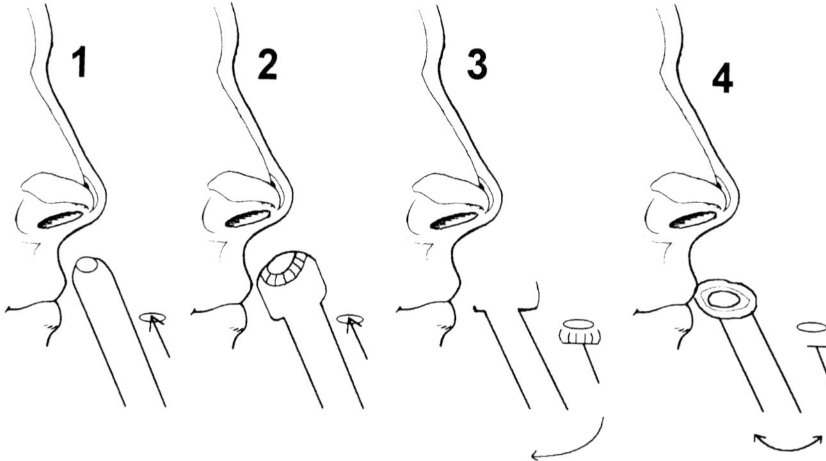

Figure 6–8.   Four different types of adapters.

anterior nose, and acoustic leakage at the areas of connection may result in incorrect measurements. Therefore, we studied the influence of the adapter on the calculated CSA obtained by AR. Measurements were made on nasal models and in probands.

Nasal models were connected to the rhinometer by cylindrical adapters with constant diameter over the whole length. The adapters were made of copper, brass, acrylic, or polyphen. Four nosepieces of different shapes were used for measurements in human noses: a conical adapter (Fig. 6–8–1), a modified conical type (Fig. 6–8–2), an alar type (Fig. 6–8–3), and an anatomically conformed adapter (Fig. 6–8–4). The conical adapters were made of copper, brass, acrylic, or polyphen; adapters 2 through 4 consisted of polyphen. All adapters had an inner diameter of 13 mm, and the thickness of the wall ranged from 0.5 to 2.5 mm. The conical adapter was designed in seven different sizes and had a concave opening at the connecting area from 0.4 to 1.2 cm². The anatomically conformed adapter (Fig. 6–8–4) was designed from casts of 122 nasal lobules of healthy white controls and patients. The adapter was connected to the nostril from the outside. According to the shape of the lobule, we choose the most similar type from seven different adapters of the anatomically conformed type. Each anatomically conformed adapter had a groove in the connecting surface (Figs. 6–8 and 6–9), which was filled with petrolatum to fit the adapter tightly to individual noses.

In nasal models the adapter was coupled by sticky wax. In probands, the adapter was placed under visible control into or to the individual nostril, and an effort was made not to deform the nasal lobule. Video documentation of the outer nose with the adapter and of the endoscopic view through the nasal adapter was obtained.

Different materials of the adapter (polyphen, acrylic, metal; thickness of wall greater than 1 mm) with a length up to 10 cm are not critical.

In regard to the connection between the wave tube and adapter, any acoustic leak in the system may result in discrepancies in AR measurements. After a short time of usage, a simple adapter led to minimal changes of the inner geometry with acoustic leakage. This acoustic leak resulted in a small overestimation (range, 3% to 10%) of the CSA of the adapter at the nasal end. This phenomenon may be even

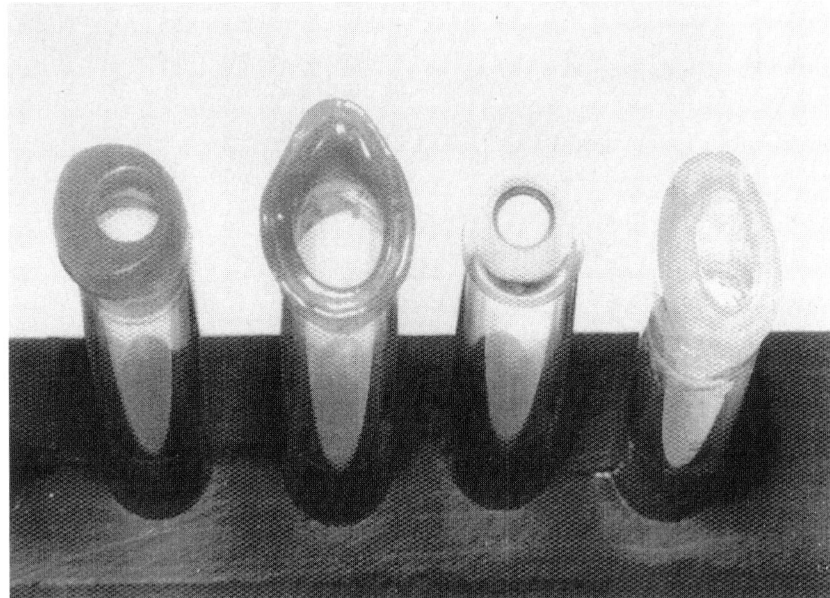

Figure 6–9. Four different types of adapters. Left, Adapter for children. Middle left, Anatomically conformed adapter. Middle right, Conical adapter. Right, Modified conical type.

more pronounced in clinical measurements, because the deviation increases with distance. In nasal models, the overestimation of CSA ranged from 5% to 106%, and the overestimation of distance from 0% to 6%. Therefore, we recommend use of a screw-mounting with a rubber sealing O-ring for coupling the adapter to the wave tube without any acoustic leak. The use of this coupling unit guarantees measurements without acoustic leak between the wave tube and adapter.

The influence of the angle between adapter and nasal cavity axis on the nasal CSA was evaluated with nasal models and in probands. The angle between the nosepiece and the horizontal plane of the ostium externum was changed by ±30 degrees in 5-degree steps. Vertically, the angle was changed by ±45 degrees in 5-degree steps. The change of angle did not influence the results obtained by AR. In probands, an anatomically conformed adapter was used. The angle between the plane of the connecting surface and the adapter axis was changed by ±30 degrees in steps of 10 degrees horizontally and vertically. This procedure was performed with a total of 49 adapters. Figure 6–10 shows the result of measurement in a proband. As in the model, the change of angle did **not** influence the result.

In regard to the connection between the adapter and the nose, it is very important that the connection between the rhinometer and the nose does not distort the valve area. The influence of the nosepiece in distorting the valve area was compared with different types of adapters. We measured 56 adults (27 males, 29 females, aged 17 to 68 years) with different nasal abnormalities and 23 normal controls (12 males, 11 females, aged 28 to 59 years) with adapter types 1 through 4. In the probands, measurements were defined as correct when three repeated measurements within 2 minutes, revealed a standard deviation of <3% from mean values for every measurement point within the first 3 cm of the nasal cavity by the anatomically conformed adapter. In addition, the analysis of the videotape showed no distortion of the valve area.

With use of two different conical adapters (1.0 and 1.2 cm outer diameter, as used by Grymer et al.[19]), only 28% of the probands had correct measurements of the CSA in the anterior third of the nose. The use of seven different nosepieces (0.4 to 1.2 cm outer diameter, with choice of the adequate one for the individual nose) improved the result of correct measurements to 73%. The anterior nose can be distorted by the conical type of nosepiece in two ways. First, incorrect measurements may result from a widening in the anterior nose (Fig. 6–11 Left). Second, the compression with bending of the lateral cartilage by the conical adapter can result in an obstruction in the valve region (Fig. 6–11 Right).

The modified conical adapter showed the same result as the conical and had no advantage. With use of the alar type, only 37% of the probands had correct mea-

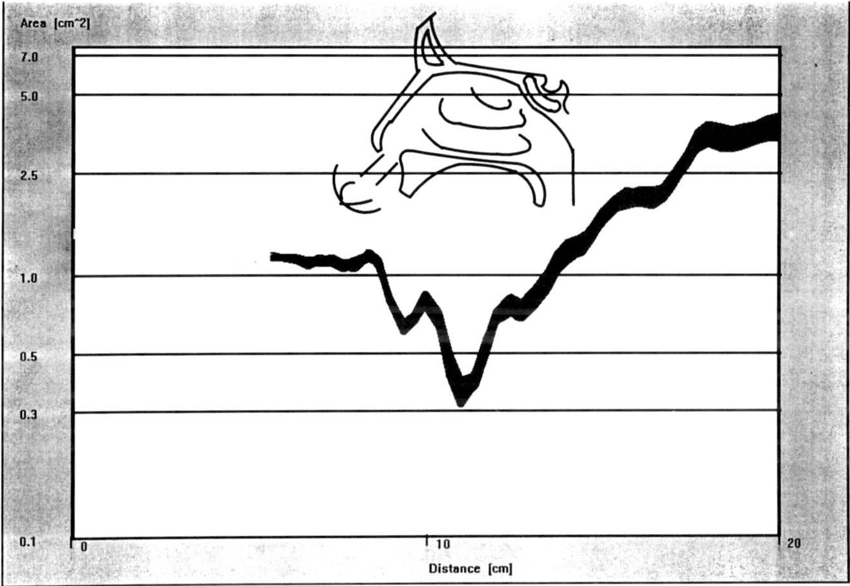

Figure 6–10. Angulation between adapter axis and nasal cavity in a proband: 49 different angles did not influence the calculated cross-sectional area within the nasal cavity.

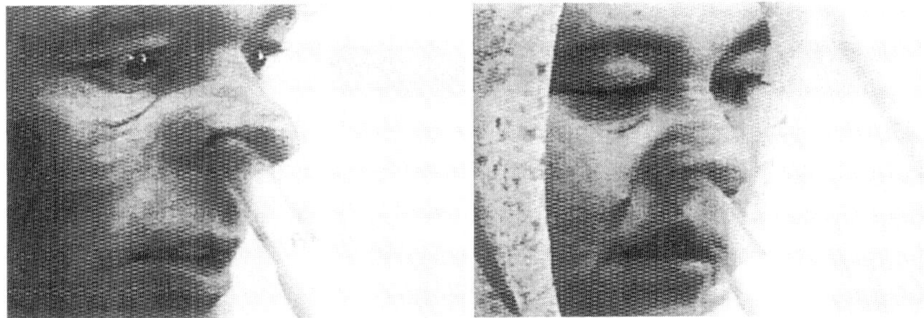

Figure 6–11. Left, Widening of the anterior nose by the conical adapter (top), and no change in the geometry of the nose by the anatomically conformed adapter (bottom). Right, Valve area deformed by the conical adapter (top), and no deformation by the anatomically conformed adapter (bottom).

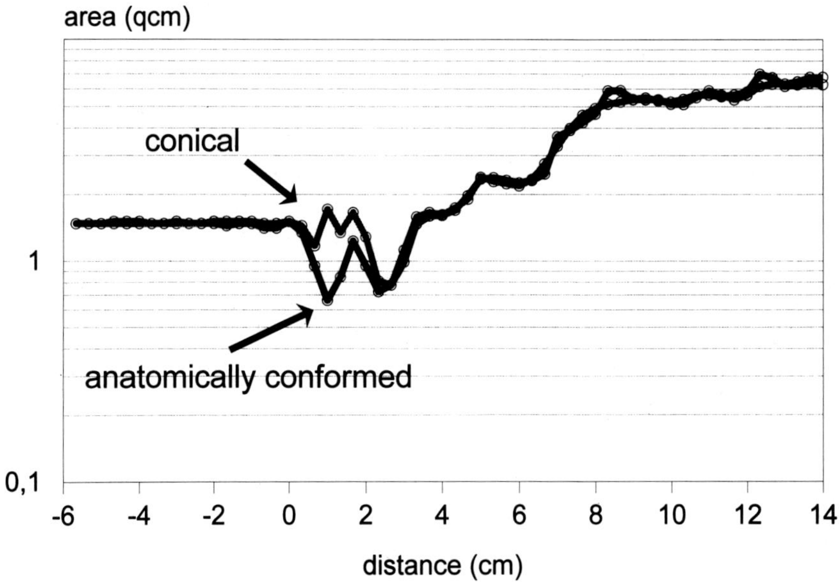

Figure 6–12.   Acoustic rhinometry data from Figure 6–11, Left.

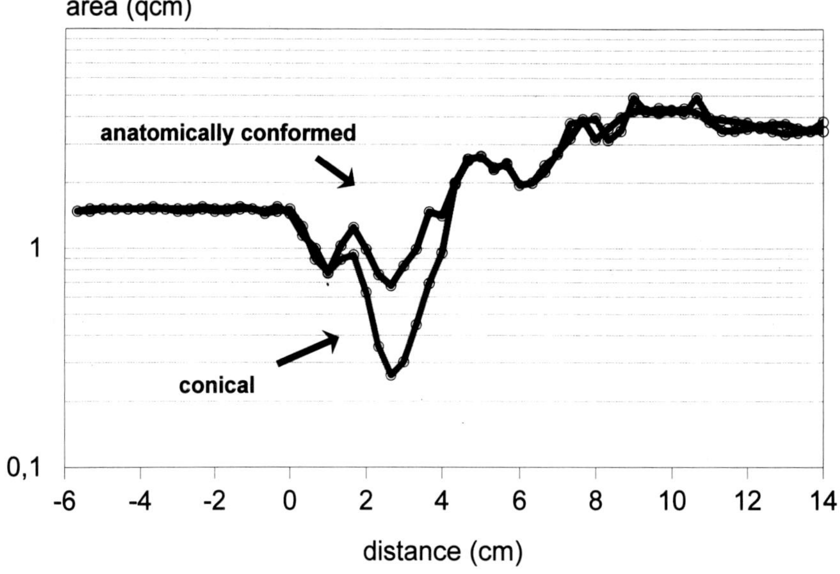

Figure 6–13.   Acoustic rhinometry data from Figure 6–11, Right.

surements of CSA in the anterior third of the nose. In 63% of the probands, the compression with bending of the lateral wall by the adapter resulted in an artificially obstructed valve area. The measured data in Figure 6–11 were similar to this. Only the anatomically conformed type of nosepiece allowed correct measurements— 94% of all probands. The essential feature of our new type of nosepiece is that it does not distort the entrance of the nose (Figs. 6–12 and 6–13).

We can conclude that the use of adapters of different shape and material, leads to different data from the same measured object. The result may explain some of the discrepancies of AR measurements reported in the literature. Because the highest rate of accurate measurements is obtained with the anatomically conformed adapter, clinically routine AR and further studies in AR should be performed only with anatomically conformed adapters.

ERRORS

We can differentiate errors of instrumentation, errors of the adapter, and errors in procedure. The most frequent errors of instrumentation are detected by the examiner. Acoustic leaks are possible at the distal end of the wave tube, at the microphone connection, and at the proximal end of the wave tube between the adapter and the tube. Calibration procedures with occluded adapters will show these leaks. Acoustic leaks between the adapter and the nose are detectable by the acoustic sound during measurement. To avoid these acoustic leaks, the use of petrolatum is recommended to couple the adapter and nose. Problems about the correct type of adapter are discussed above. Disturbances by breathing sounds can be detected by analyzing the dimensions of the nosepiece at the beginning of each curve. Increasing or decreasing the CSA in the adapter segment of the curve clearly indicates acoustic disturbances during measurement. For use of AR to test nasal function, we recommend investigation conditions as developed for RM.[17,20]

NORMAL NASAL ANATOMY

The appearance of the normal nose depends on racial, developmental, and environmental differences, which provide a wide range of skeletal and mucosal variations within the nose.

Data on CSA in a large group of normal white controls are available from two studies.[19,21,22] Both studies were performed with the conical type of adapter.

Grymer et al.[19] used only two different conical nosepieces (10 mm and 12 mm). Normal values were calculated from 82 individuals, defined by the following inclusion criteria: normal feeling of nasal patency and no gross structural changes. They found that the minimal cross-sectional area (MCA) was located anteriorly in the nasal cavity; it was located at the head of the inferior turbinate in some subjects and more anteriorly at the nasal valve in other subjects. They found that the MCA nondecongested was 0.73 cm² on the right side and 0.72 cm² on the left side. After decongestion, MCA moved even more anteriorly. Beyond the MCA, the dimension of the nasal cavity increased, with the maximal effect of decongestion at 4 cm from the nostrils. Decongestion increased the total volume of the nasal cavity by 35%; the MCA was 0.92 cm² at the right side and 0.95 cm² at the left side.

Apart from Grymer et al.,[19] we[21,22] used 12 different polyphen nosepieces (inner diameter, 1.5 cm; length, 7 cm) with a concave opening at the nostril measuring from 0.4 to 1.5 cm outer diameter. The normal controls were 134 white subjects, 74 men and 60 women, aged 21 to 60 years, defined by the following inclusion criteria: no

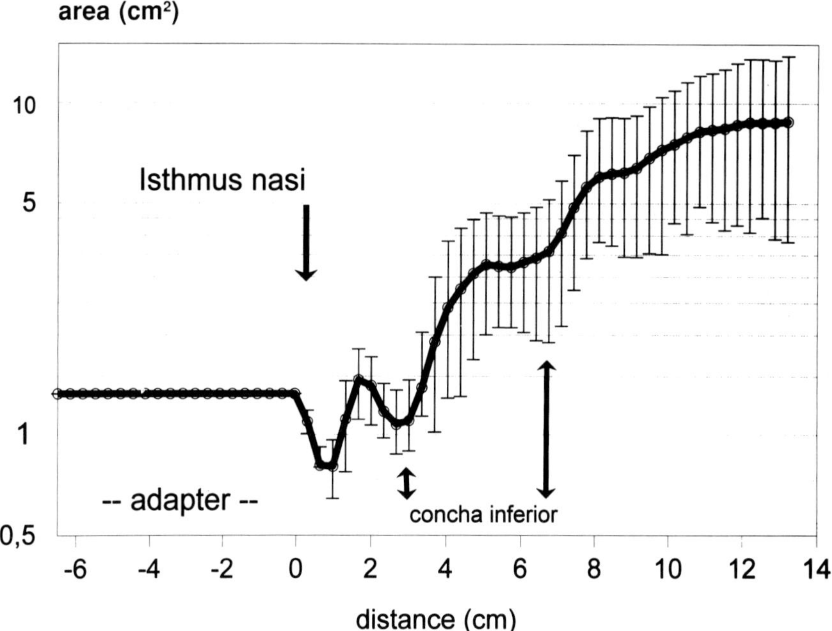

Figure 6–14.   Distance function obtained with acoustic rhinometry. Mean curve and standard deviation of cross-sectional area in 134 normal controls.

history of nasal problems, normal feeling of nasal patency, no midfacial abnormalities, no significant septal deformities, and no turbinate hypertrophy. The CSA of the nasal cavity was obtained as a function of distance from the nostril. Figure 6–14 shows the mean curve to the 134 normal controls with the standard deviation. The range of standard deviations is mainly a result of the interindividual differences of the measurements. The first centimeters (straight line) of the curve reflect the dimension of the nosepiece and allow the self-test of the system. The following part of the curve (first notch = I-notch) is the MCA with $0.73 \pm 0.2\,\mathrm{cm}^2$ at 1.3 cm distance from the nostril, corresponding to the functional isthmus nasi. Repeated measurements in the same patient under constant conditions revealed that the standard deviation of the mean CSA in the nasal cavity was always less than 7%. The second notch (C-notch) after a small peak with CSA of $1.46 \pm 0.41\,\mathrm{cm}^2$ at 3.3 cm corresponds to the head of the inferior turbinate and anterior part of the septal body. The pattern of curve in Figure 6–2—termed "climbing W"—with the MCA at the isthmus nasi and a second minimum at the region of the anterior inferior turbinate, was observed in all of the 134 normal controls.

Figure 6–15 shows superposition of mean curves measured before decongestion (lower curve) and after decongestion (upper curve) in the 134 controls. There is a significant difference for both curves in the region of the inferior turbinate at distances of 3.5 cm and 5.5 cm from the nostril (for 3.5 cm, $p < 0.01$; for 5.5 cm, $p < 0.01$). For better comparison, standard deviations are not shown. The values are nearly in the same range with respect to the congested and decongested state. These two curves are identical at the isthmus nasi, reflecting the anatomical fact that nasal mucosa cannot be found in the isthmus nasi. The curves separate in

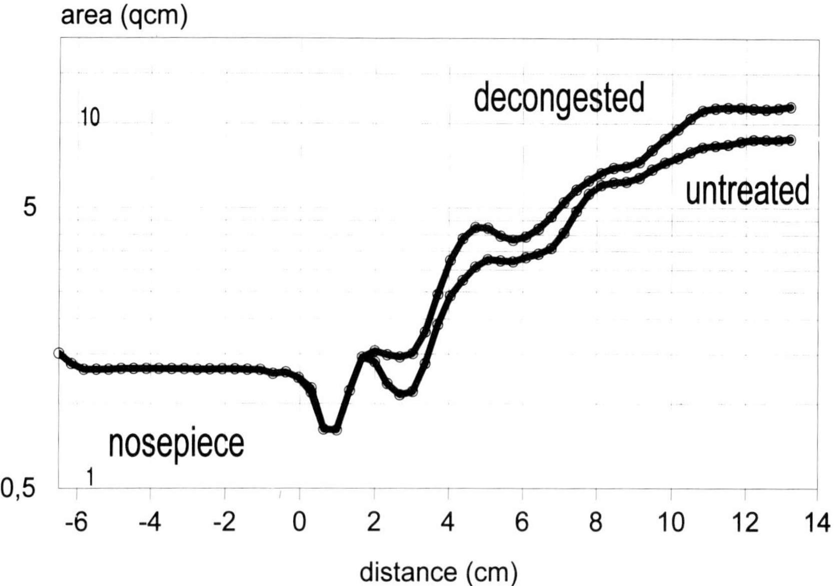

Figure 6–15. Mean curves in 134 normal controls before and after decongestion.

the beginning of the anterior inferior turbinate, because of the congestive capacity of the nasal mucosa.

In all our normal controls, both before and after decongestion, the MCA was located in the region of the valve (I-notch). The second narrowest CSA was found around the head of the inferior concha (C-notch). The MCA was 0.73 cm^2 and was constantly located at the region of the nasal valve (I-notch). This area favorably corresponds to the isthmus nasi, which has been previously reported by Legler[23] and by Bachmann,[24,25] by means of casts of the anterior nose, to be 0.8 cm^2 in men and 0.71 cm^2 in women. Measuring the nasal resistance in normal controls by different methods, Masing,[26] Legler,[23] Fischer,[27] and Bachmann,[24,25] and more recently Haight and Cole,[28] showed that the most resistive segment is localized in the region between the valve and the head of inferior turbinate. AR allows a more detailed analysis of this most resistive segment, which is built up of two compartments.

In normal controls, it contains two MCA, the I-notch at 1.3 cm and the C-notch at 3.6 cm distance from the nostril ("climbing W" pattern). We found that in normal controls the first notch (I-notch) always represents the minimum of the CSA of the whole nasal cavity.

The different inclusion criteria and different use of adapters may explain the discrepancies in normal values in both studies. Further studies in different racial populations performed with anatomically conformed adapters are necessary.

TURBINATE HYPERTROPHY

Turbinate hypertrophy occurs in allergic and vasomotor rhinitis. We studied 130 patients (54 men, 76 women, aged 18 to 61 years) with allergic or vasomotor rhinitis

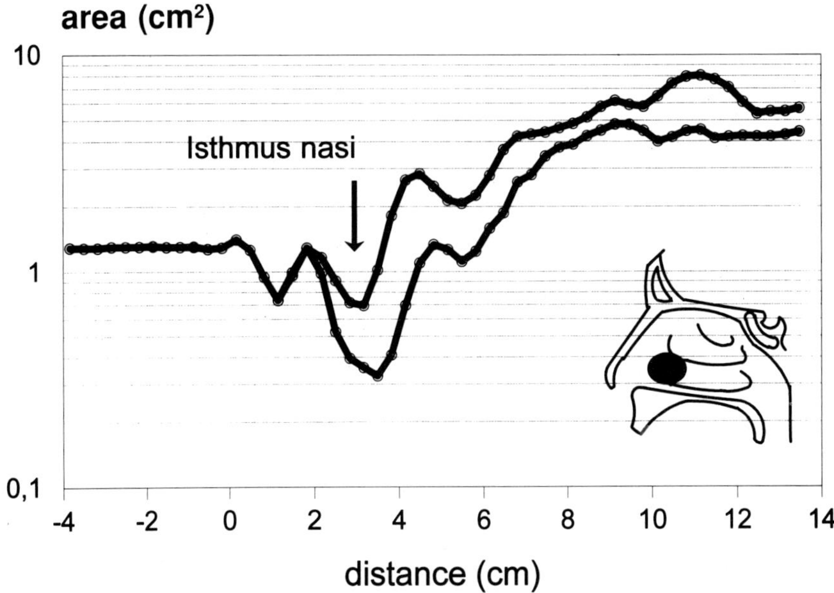

Figure 6–16.   Acoustic rhinometry curves of one nasal cavity in a patient with turbinate hypertrophy, before and after decongestion.

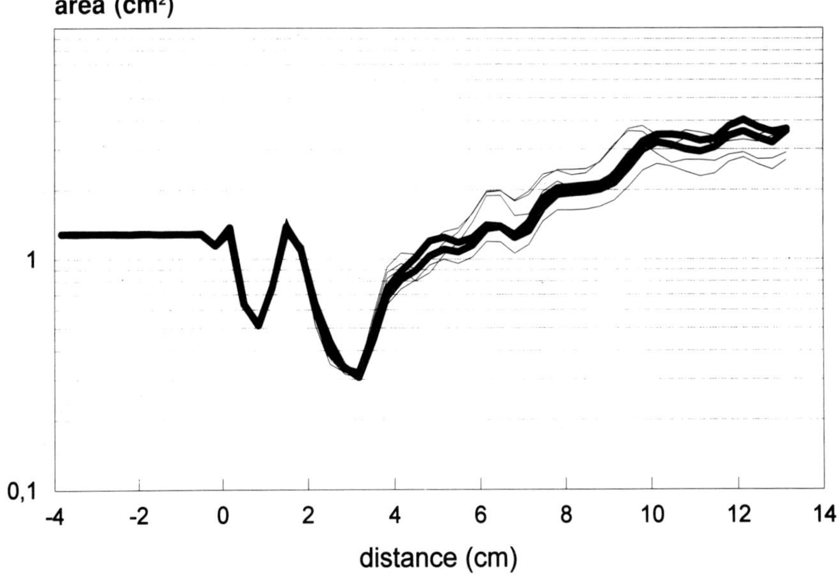

Figure 6–17.   Area-distance function obtained by acoustic rhinometry: negative reaction to allergic challenge in a patient with turbinate hypertrophy.

and a mainly straight septum. All the subjects were assessed by the same otolaryngologist. Vasomotor rhinitis was defined as chronic nasal obstruction and nasal hypersecretion, with hypertrophy of both inferior turbinates and negative reactions to allergic tests. Patients with positive reactions to allergy tests were the allergic group.

In patients with turbinate hypertrophy, especially those with vasomotor rhinitis (Fig. 6–16), AR demonstrated that the MCA was located 3.0 to 4.0 cm (mean, 3.6 ± 0.4) distant from the nostril (C-notch). This corresponds to the region of the head of the inferior turbinate. We called this pattern of rhinometric curves the "descending W."[21] Decongestion remarkably increases the CSA in the C-notch. The I-notch is not changed; thus, the MCA is now at the I-notch. Most patients with turbinate hypertrophy have a widening of CSA at the C-notch after decongestion. However, the value of the CSA in the C-notch ($0.65\,cm^2$ in the patient in Fig. 6–17) does not reach the range in normal controls without decongestion (mean value, $0.73\,cm^2$). The curve in Figure 6–17 shows that the value of isthmus nasi (I-notch) remains unchanged.

AR was used in the follow-up of patients before and after anterior turbinoplasty, a resection of the anterior 2 cm of the bone and the lateral mucosa of the head of the inferior turbinate. Preoperative and postoperative CSA values at the isthmus nasi were identical. In contrast, surgical treatment resulted in a widening of the region of the head of the inferior anterior turbinate (C-notch). Thus, AR can show that reduction surgery of the anterior inferior turbinate has improved breathing conditions, with values comparable to those in controls. The MCA is situated at the isthmus nasi 6 months postoperatively (I-notch).

ALLERGIC RESPONSE

Figure 6–17 shows the negative result of a nasal challenge with house dust in a patient with turbinate hypertrophy. The curves before challenge and 15 and 30 minutes after challenge show almost identical patterns. AR demonstrated the MCA was $0.31\,cm^2$ at 3.5 cm (Fig. 6–18) from the nostril before challenge with house dust.

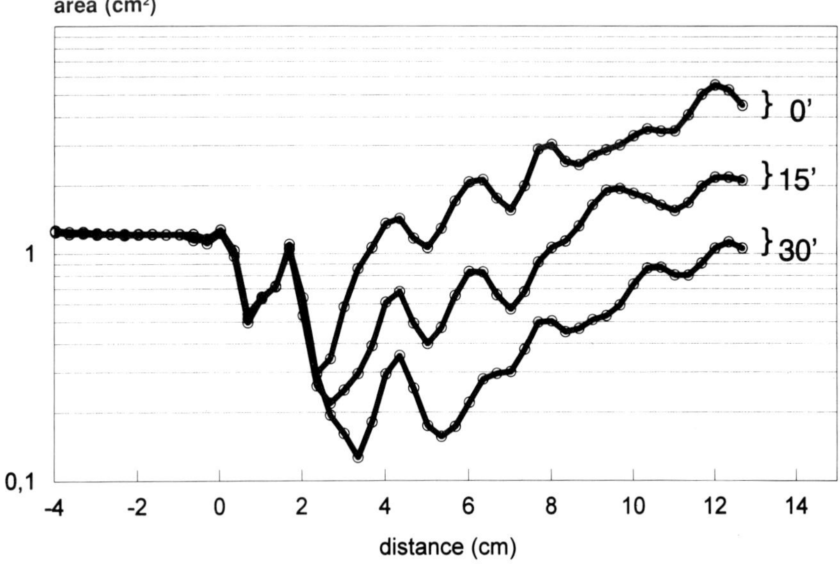

Figure 6–18. Acoustic rhinometry curve of a remarkable response to allergic nasal challenge in a patient with turbinate hypertrophy.

This stable condition for the CSA in the nasal cavities corresponded with the patient's feeling that nothing had changed in his nose.

In contrast, Figure 6–18 represents the positive response after intranasal challenge in a patient with allergy to house dust. The MCA was increasingly reduced during the observation period of half an hour. Before the exposure to house dust, the MCA was 0.3 cm^2 at 2.3 cm from the nostril in the region of the inferior turbinate ("descending W" pattern). At 15 minutes after challenge, the area was reduced to 0.2 cm^2 at 2.8 cm from the nostril. At 30 minutes after challenge, this area was almost blocked, with a CSA of 0.15 cm^2. Similar data were confirmed by RM: 0 min, 216 mLs^{-1}; 15 min, 126 mLs^{-1}; 30 min, 82 mLs^{-1} at 150 Pa. Note that the reduction of the CSA was not limited to the head of the inferior turbinate, where the allergen solution was applied, but also included the areas behind this point.

A paradoxical response was recorded in a patient with vasomotor rhinitis (Fig. 6–19). This patient initially reacted with a widening of the CSA in the C-notch after challenge with an allergen solution, instead of a reduction as observed in another patient (Fig. 6–18). Before the testing, the MCA was 0.53 cm^2 at 3.2 cm, corresponding to the head of the inferior turbinate. At 15 minutes after the allergen solution had been applied to the mucosa of the anterior inferior turbinate, the patient reported nasal hypersecretion and itching with normal nasal breathing. AR showed that this secretion was paralleled by a localized widening of the CSA in the C-notch (0.9 cm^2 at 3.8 cm). A control measurement 30 minutes later indicated that the condition of the nasal mucosa had returned to the previous status (0.53 cm^2). This was paralleled by the patient's report that the nasal secretion had ceased. With anterior rhinoscopy and RM, this type of reaction cannot be detected.

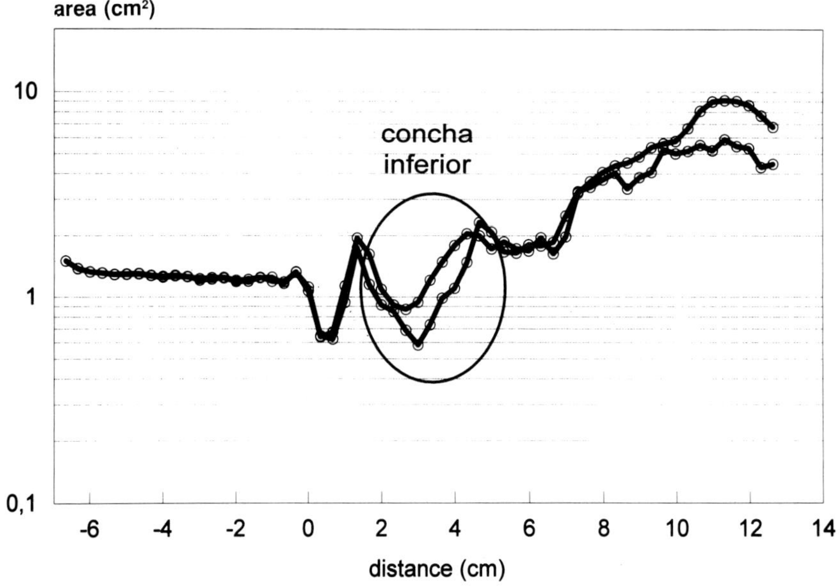

Figure 6–19.   Paradoxical response to allergic challenge in a patient with turbinate hypertrophy. At 15 minutes after application of allergen solution, a strictly localized widening of the cross-sectional area was registered. At 30 minutes after application, the area returned to the previous values.

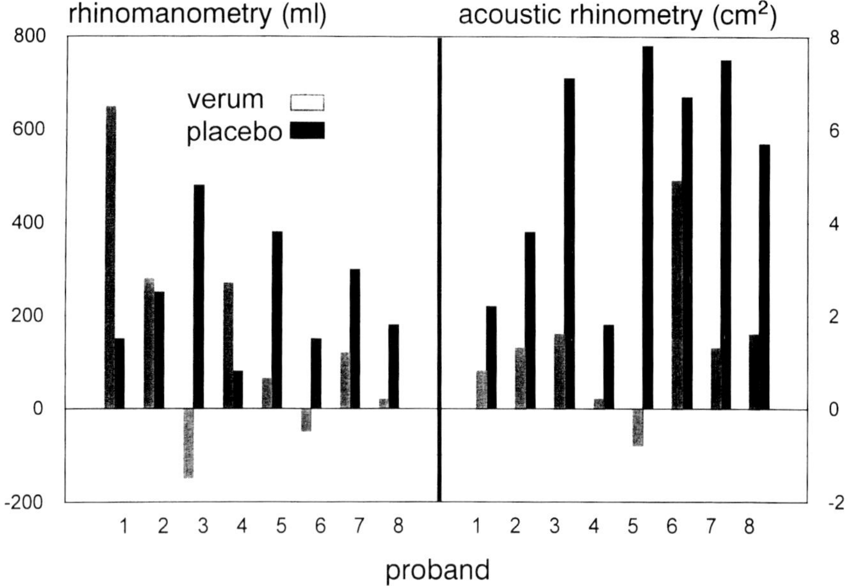

Figure 6–20.   Data obtained with acoustic rhinometry and rhinomanometry used to compare the estimation of allergic reaction of blocked mucosa to antihistamine.

Within the context of a placebo-controlled, randomized, double-blind, two-way crossover study, data of active anterior RM (Rhinotest mP) and AR were compared concerning the estimation of allergic reaction. Eight patients with hay fever, symptom-free at time of inclusion, were examined. In two study periods for 3 days, each of the subjects was treated three times daily in a randomized sequence with a commercial antihistaminic agent or placebo. One drop of a specific allergen solution was applied with a needle on the head of the inferior turbinate. Figure 6–20 presents the data obtained with AR and RM. The AR data show the volume differences between the first 5 cm within the nasal cavity before and 10 minutes after challenge. The RM data were calculated as volume differences at 150 Pa before and 10 minutes after challenge. AR exactly showed the protecting effect of the antihistaminic agent. In every proband, the congestion of mucosa was significantly more with placebo than with antihistamine treatment. RM was not able to demonstrate these significant differences in reaction, which were confirmed by the visual analog scaled information of nasal patency by the probands. Thus, AR seems to be more sensitive for measuring the swelling reaction than RM.

SEPTAL DEFORMITY

To evaluate septal deformities, the acoustic rhinometric curves after decongestion of both nasal cavities are compared. Grymer et al.[29] reported data on 21 patients with septal deformities who were measured preoperatively and postoperatively by AR. The values were compared with those of 21 normal control subjects. The MCA was located in the anterior part of the nose and shifted anteriorly after decongestion. It is difficult to interpret the data of Grymer et al.[29] because there is no strict separation of data after septoplasty alone and after septoplasty in combination with turbinate operation. To analyze the size and location of the obstructing septum, we found that AR was very useful after having studied 121 consecutive patients who underwent only septoplasty, whereas the turbinates remained untouched.[15] Thus, AR proved to be a good tool to evaluate the efficacy of septal reconstruction. Figure 6–21 presents data about an anterior septal deformity (upper curves) and a vomeral spur (lower curves). In contrast to RM, AR in connection with rhinoscopy reveals the size and location of the septal deformity.

NASAL CYCLE

The human nasal mucosa undergoes cyclical fluctuations in congestion and decongestion, which results in a rhythmic alternating pattern in up to 80% of adults.[30] This was first convincingly demonstrated with calibrated bellows by Kayser in 1885.[31] Since then, various methods have been utilized to characterize this phys-

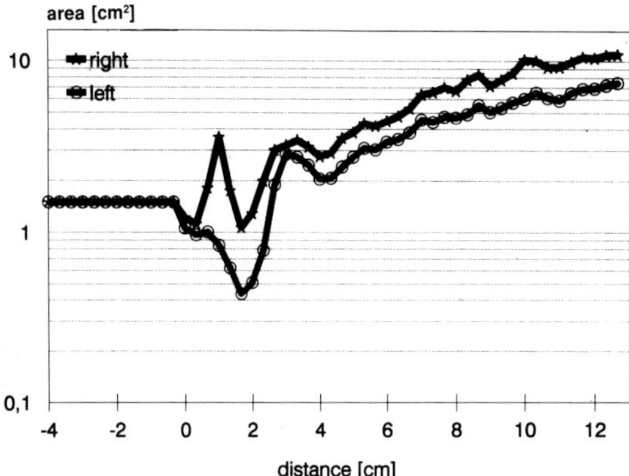

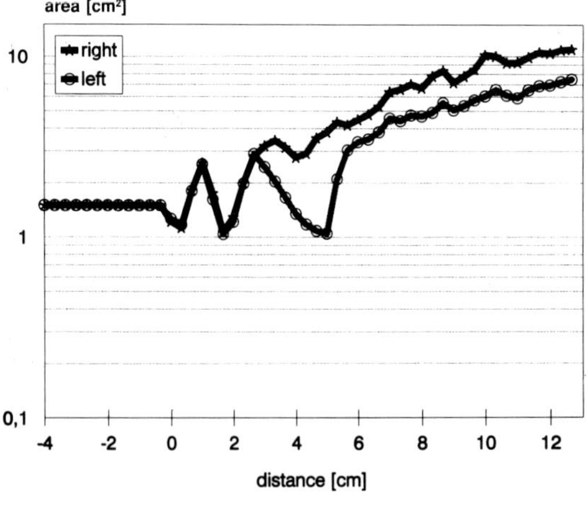

Figure 6–21. Acoustic rhinometry data about two examples of septal deformities. *Top,* Septal deviation in the anterior part of the left nasal cavity. *Bottom,* A vomeral spur in the left nasal cavity.

iologic phenomenon.[32] These include simple anterior rhinoscopy,[30] rhinomanometry, elaborate optical devices,[33] a forced random-noise technique,[34] thermography,[35] and, most recently, magnetic resonance.[36] However, each of these techniques has disadvantages in terms of time, expense, reproducibility, requirement for cooperation by the patient, or a need for airflow to occur during the assessment. Therefore, we applied AR to a small series of 10 children aged 0.5 to 13 years to test its value for investigating the physiology of the nasal cycle.

We measured the acoustic rhinometric curves in 10 healthy children (4 boys, 6 girls), every 15 minutes, from 9 AM to 4 PM. The children were kept under basic conditions. One 8-year-old boy with a well-defined nasal cycle was, at the same time, assessed by active anterior RM at 20-minute intervals over a period of 7 hours (modified Rhinotest mP). RM and AR were performed in a sitting position. For AR, six measurements were taken from each nostril at each assessment. The C-MCA (MCA in the C-notch) was chosen as the critical parameter when compared with nasal resistance.

Four children (5 to 13 years) had a classic alternating nasal cycle that was demonstrable with AR. Five children (0.5 to 13 years) presented a regular pattern of fluctuations of CSA. It was, however, not an alternating cycle as seen in adults. The fluctuations of CSA of both nasal cavities were in the same direction and not contrary (alternating). One 5-year-old boy had no cycle. A graphic demonstration of the cyclical changes in C-MCA is shown in Figure 6–22. The corresponding changes in nasal resistance as measured by RM are displayed for the same child in Figure 6–23. Furthermore, AR shows that the changes in nasal geometry are spread throughout the nasal cavity and are not confined to the region of the anterior portion of the inferior turbinate (C-notch of the AR curve). The periodicity of the

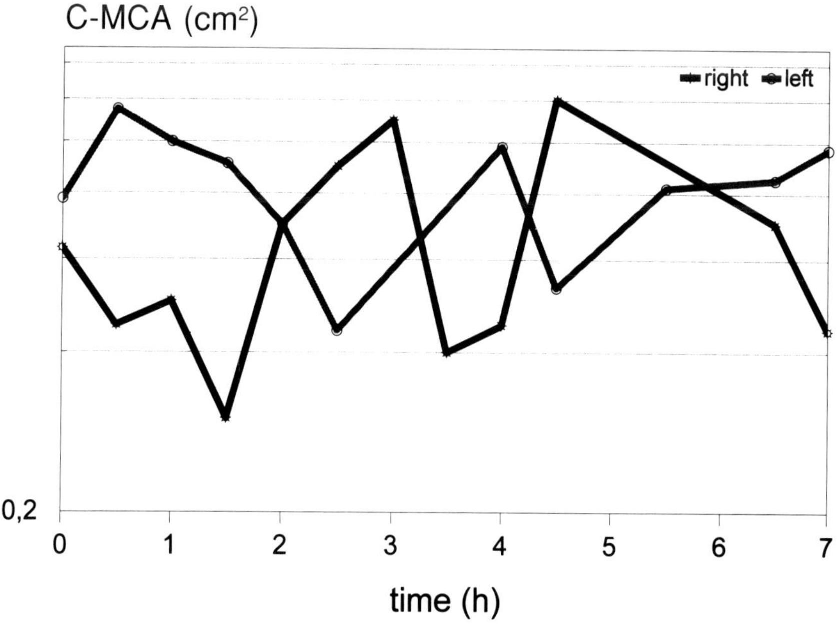

Figure 6–22.   Nasal cycle: C-MCA measured in an 8-year-old boy over 7 hours.

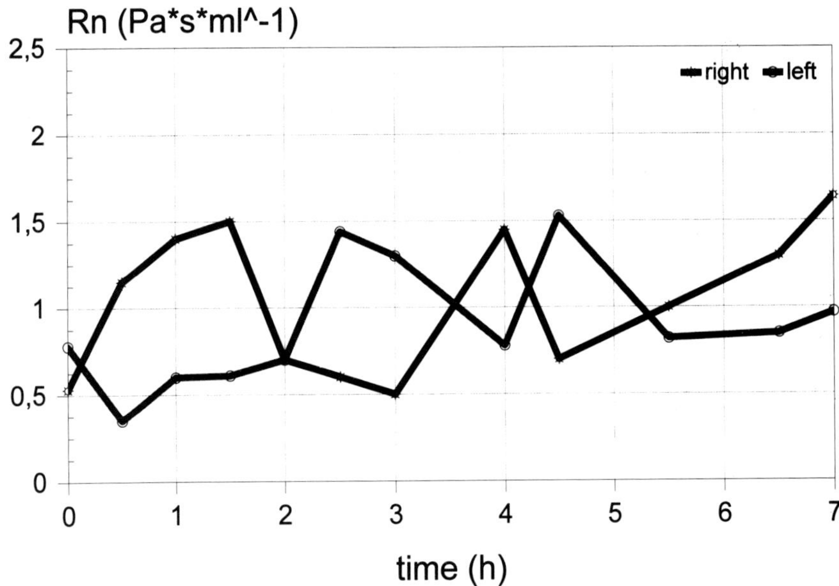

Figure 6–23.   Nasal cycle: Nasal resistance (R_n) measured at the same time as the C-MCA in an 8-year-old boy over 7 hours (same child as in Fig. 6–22).

nasal cycle varied from 50 minutes to 2.5 hours and showed a positive correlation between cycle duration and age.

AR does not provide geometric information as extensive as that with MRI or CT, but it allows analysis of the whole nasal cavity and is thus superior to RM for studying the nasal cycle. AR also requires only minimal cooperation, is rapid (less than 1 minute for six measurements for both sides), is reproducible, is not loading, and does not depend on nasal airflow.

EVALUATION OF ADENOID SIZE AND TUMOR RECURRENCE IN NASAL CAVITY

AR is an excellent method to evaluate the geometry of the anterior nose and the response of the nasal mucosa. However, on the basis of our findings, AR is not able to answer questions that arise in connection with the adenoids and the recurrence of tumors within the nasal cavities.

In a series of 20 children, Elbrønd et al.[37,38] demonstrated changes in the volume of the nasopharynx after adenoidectomy. The relation between the volume of the adenoid and the calculated change of volume in the nasopharynx was proportional and highly significant (P = 0.0005). Elbrønd et al.[37,38] concluded that AR gives a reliable, objective measurement of the amount of adenoid tissue in the naso-pharynx. They speculated that these results may help to reduce the number of unnecessary adenoidectomies.

In a series of 26 children (4 to 12 years), the changes in the volume of the nasopharynx before and after adenoidectomy were measured.[15] The relation be-

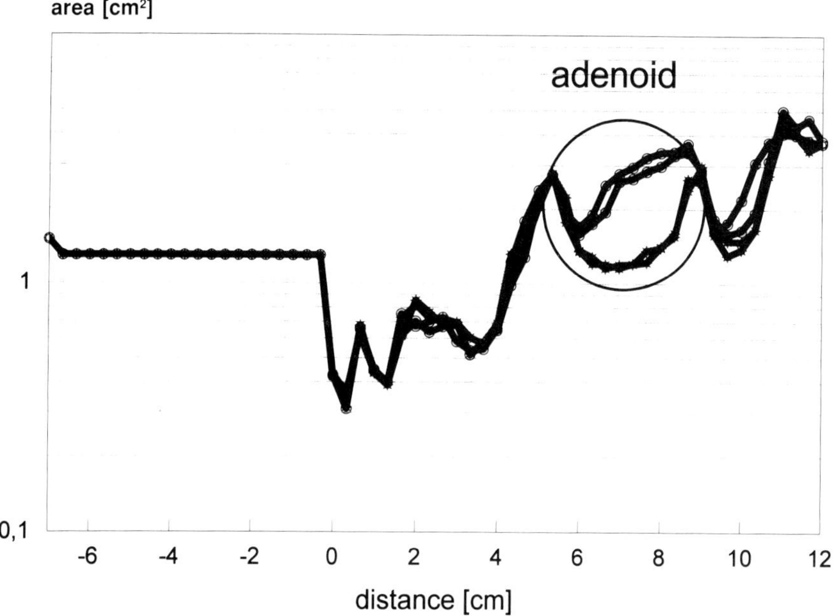

Figure 6–24.   Area-distance function of the decongested left nasal cavity: 4-year-old boy with adenoid (within circle) before and after adenoidectomy.

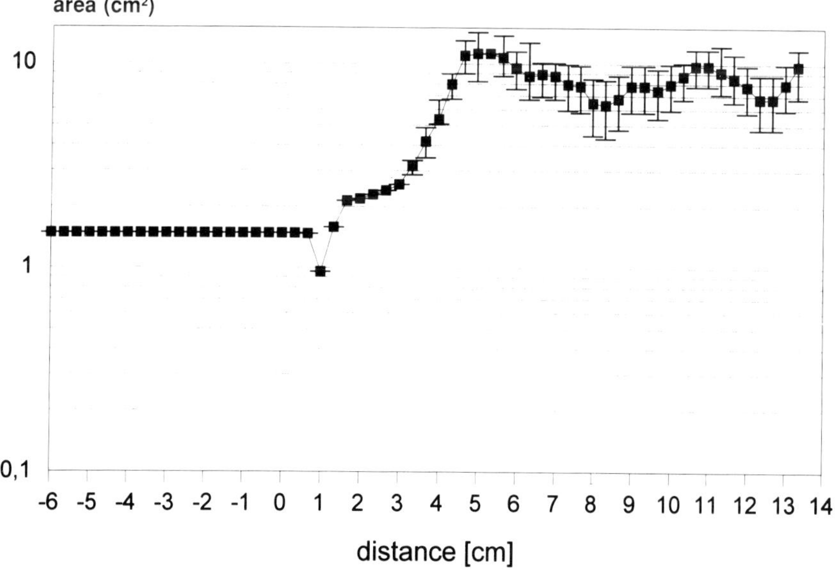

Figure 6–25.   Mean curve and standard deviations of 12 subsequently measured traces during normal breathing. The increase of standard deviations 5 cm distant from the nostril to the nasopharynx represents the changes of cross-sectional area due to movements of the soft palate.

tween the volume of the resected adenoid and the calculated change of volume (Fig. 6–24) in the nasopharynx was found to be proportional and highly significant (r = 0.87, P = 0.001). However, there is no significant correlation between the clinical relevance of the adenoid size or the amount of the removed adenoid tissue and the nasopharyngeal CSA or volumes. Therefore, AR gives a reliable, objective measurement of the amount of the resected adenoid tissue in the nasopharynx. However, AR has no predictive value for adenoidectomy because the volumes of adenoids were calculated postoperatively. In addition, as mentioned earlier, information on CSA in the nasopharynx is reduced to the physical properties of the nasopharynx and due to dynamic variations of the velum (Fig. 6–25).

Concerning the evaluation of tumor recurrence in the nasal cavity, two factors limit the value of AR. First, operation for tumor usually changes the geometry of the nasal cavity, to a large extent creating a larger cavity that is influenced in its posterior part by the dynamic variations of the velum. Second, the recurrent tumor often develops submucosally and produces only small changes in the volume, which are masked by the variations in volume caused by the velum, nasal secretions, and crusts. Although a very small increase of volume can be demonstrated in nasal models, in clinical practice this small increase of volume cannot be detected. This has been shown in a study of 17 patients with inverted papilloma of the nasal cavities who underwent surgical treatment.[39]

These patients were examined with nasal endoscopy, CT, and AR to study the changes in the geometry of the nasal cavities before and after surgical treatment. Four to five weeks postoperatively, when epithelialization of the operated nasal cavity was completed, CT, videoendoscopy, and AR of the decongested nasal cavity were repeated. The nasal cavity was decongested by spraying a solution of

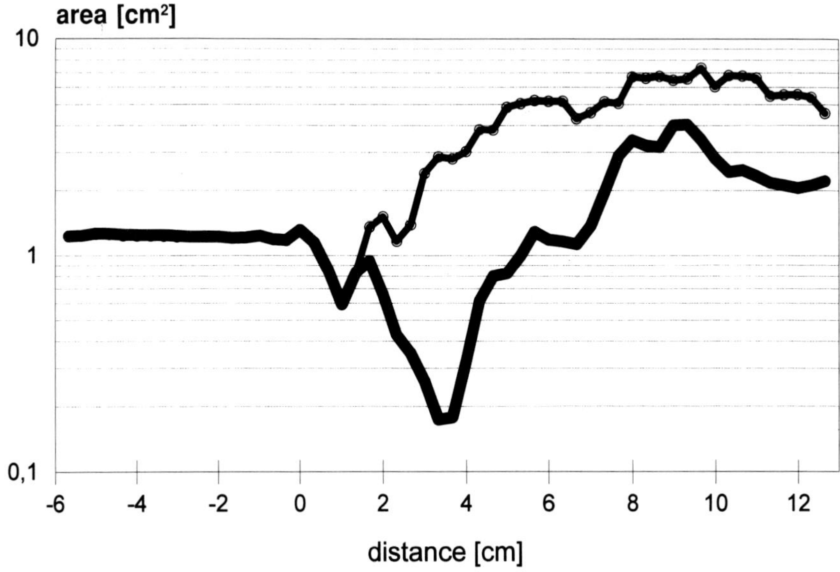

Figure 6–26.   Case 17: Superimposed acoustic rhinometry curves of the preoperative state. *Upper curve,* Area-distance function of the healthy decongested right nasal cavity. *Lower curve,* Cross-sectional area of left decongested nasal cavity filled with inverted papilloma.

xylometazoline 0.05% into the inferior and middle nasal meatus. The same examinations were repeated every 4 to 6 months to detect recurrences. With these follow-
up studies, three recurrences were found, mainly by videoendoscopy.

The problems in the detection of tumor recurrence with AR will be discussed
in the context of the clinical findings in the 17 patients and experiments in nasal
models. In Figure 6–26, the preoperative AR curves of one patient (case 7) are
depicted. There are two curves separating at 2 cm from the nostril. The upper curve
shows the CSA of the healthy decongested right nasal cavity. The lower curve
represents the CSA of the left decongested nasal cavity filled with inverted
papilloma. The first centimeters (straight line) of the curves reflect the dimension of
the nosepiece. The following dip of the curves is the I-notch, which represents the
MCA with 0.61 cm², corresponding to the functional isthmus nasi. The second dip
(C-notch) of the upper curve with a CSA of 1.2 cm² corresponds to the head of the
inferior concha and the septal concha. The second notch of the lower curve with
MCA of 0.2 cm² corresponds to the obstructing tumor masses 3.5 cm behind the
nostril.

Figure 6–27 compares the AR curves of the healthy nasal cavity (lower curve)
with the state 3 months after lateral rhinotomy (upper curve) in case 7. This comparison clearly demonstrates that the CSA of the operated nasal cavity is markedly
widened as a consequence of the surgical procedure. The MCA, which
preoperatively was in the second notch, is now located in the unchanged isthmus
nasi (I-notch). Figure 6–28 presents the AR curves measured during three follow-up
studies within 6 months in intervals of 8 weeks in case 5, during which there was no
tumor recurrence. On each follow-up, three measurements were recorded. Therefore, this bundle of acoustic rhinometric curves is composed of 12 single curves. All
these curves are nearly identical within the period of 6 months.

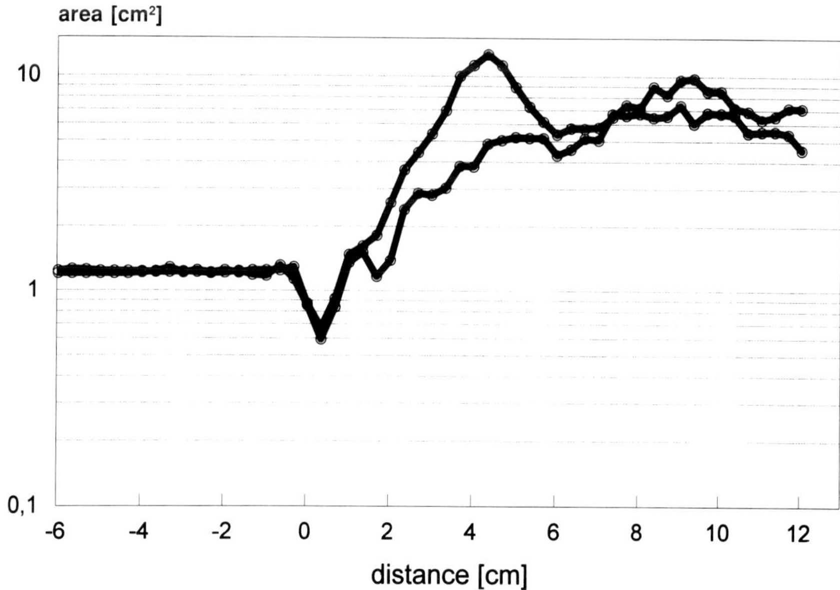

Figure 6–27. Case 17: Superimposed acoustic rhinometry curves of the healthy nasal cavity (lower
curve) and 3 months after lateral rhinometry of the diseased nasal cavity (upper curve).

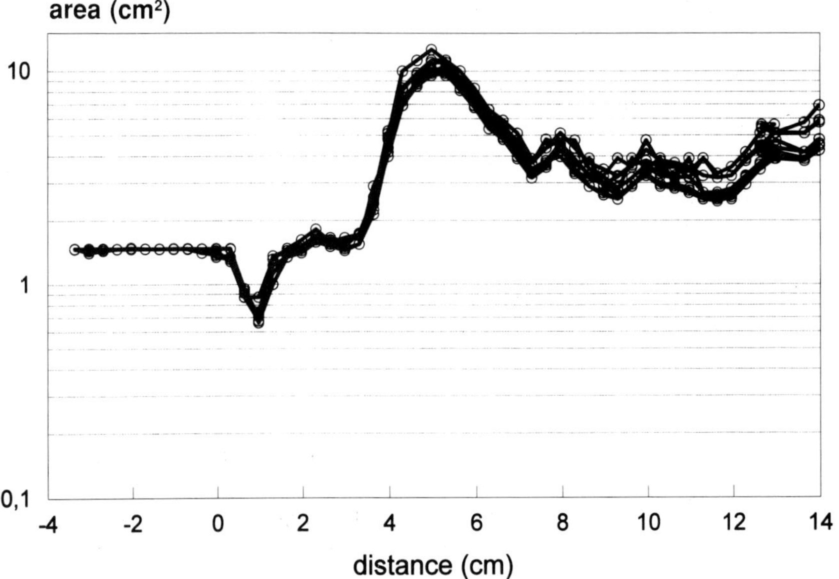

Figure 6–28.   Case 5: Four assessments during follow-up within 6 months. All 12 curves are nearly identical within the period.

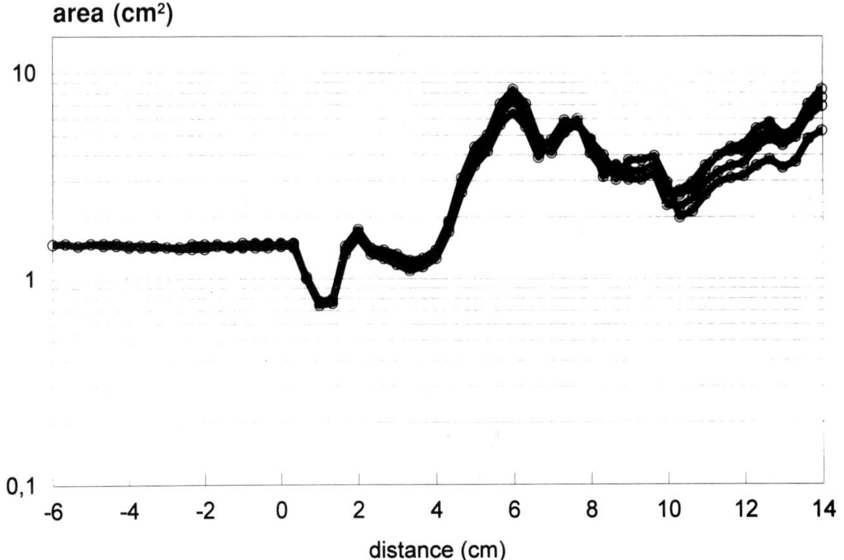

Figure 6–29.   Case 2: Acoustic rhinometry curve after limited surgical procedure is more similar to that of a healthy nasal cavity (compare with Fig. 6–27, lower curve) than to the curve after radical surgical procedure (compare with Fig. 6–28).

AR allows determination of whether only the ethmoidal cells had been removed or whether the whole lateral nasal wall including the inferior turbinate had been resected. One patient (case 2) had a small papilloma in an initial stage and underwent only endonasal ethmoidectomy and partial reduction of the middle turbinate with preservation of the inferior turbinate. The pattern of the AR curve

(Fig. 6–29) after this limited surgical procedure is similar to the pattern of a healthy nose (compare with Fig. 6–27, lower curve). The curve in Figure 6–29 was taken from the nasal cavity of case 2 after lateral rhinotomy with resection of the inferior turbinate and the whole lateral nasal wall (compare with Fig. 6–27, upper curve).

In regard to the interpretation of AR curves, two observations in our patients should be pointed out. In serial measurements (for instance, 10 shots within 3 s) in a normally breathing patient, we could record changes in CSA (Fig. 6–25) as a result of movements of the soft palate. Figure 6–25 shows the mean curve and standard deviations of 10 subsequently measured curves. The increase of standard deviations 5 cm from the nostril onward represents the changes of CSA. When the same patient was asked to stop breathing during the measurements, 10 nearly identical curves, such as in Figure 6–28, could be recorded.

Presentation of AR measurements in a logarithmic scale eliminates small changes of CSA in the nasopharynx. Small changes of CSA are normal and in most cases without clinical significance. However, in follow-up examinations, such small changes of CSA are interesting because they can be an early sign of tumor growth. Because the logarithmic scale presentation makes these small alterations invisible, AR is not the adequate tool to show early recurrences in follow-up tumors.

COMPARISON WITH RHINOMANOMETRY

AR measures CSA within the nasal airway. CSA builds up the nasal resistance measured by active anterior RM. In this regard, four questions arise: 1. Is it possible to gain the same information about nasal patency from both methods? 2. Can we calculate the MCA from the RM data? 3. Is it possible to calculate nasal resistance from the measured CSA of AR? 4. What is the significance of both methods in functional rhinologic diagnosis?

To answer these questions, we examined 59 probands with both methods. RM measurements were obtained as active computerized anterior RM according to the evaluation method described by ICSR.[20] Five to seven pairs of flow-pressure curves were recorded. Each RM value was related to 150 Pa and also expressed as Flow INC from 75 to 150 Pa respectively from 150 to 300 Pa. All AR and RM measurements were performed on awake subjects in a seated position during normal breath-

**Table 6–2   Criteria for Classification of Nasal Breathing in
Rhinomanometry and Acoustic Rhinometry**

	RHINOMANOMETRY			ACOUSTIC RHINOMETRY
No obstruction	$850\,\mathrm{m\,s^{-1}}$*	Respiratory flow increase	>35%	$\beta = 1$
Minor	$700–850\,\mathrm{m\,s^{-1}}$*	Respiratory flow increase	35–25%	$\beta = 2$
Moderate	$500–700\,\mathrm{m\,s^{-1}}$*	Respiratory flow increase	<25%	$\beta = 3$
Severe	$<500\,\mathrm{m\,s^{-1}}$*			$\beta = 4$

*At 150 Pa.
β = sum of obstruction class factors ($\beta_I + \beta_C$).

**Table 6–3   Relation Between Obstruction Class Factor and
Cross-Sectional Area Measured by Acoustic Rhinometry**

CSA IN % FROM MEAN VALUE	OBSTRUCTION CLASS FACTOR β
80%	1
65%	2
55%	3
54%	4

ing. To study the influence of nasal mucosa, patients had AR and RM before and 15 minutes after decongestion with 0.5% tramazoline.

On the basis of data from our normal controls,[21] nasal breathing has been placed (Table 6–1) into four classes. To quantify the nasal obstruction in the most resistive segment of each patient, we calculated separate obstruction class factors β from 1 to 4 in I-notch (β_I) and C-north (β_C). The degree of obstruction increases from 1 to 4. The relation between obstruction class factor and CSA is shown in Tables 6–2 and 6–3. We added the obstruction class factors for I-notch and C-notch, $\beta = \beta_I + \beta_C$. β-values larger than 4 were categorized into β-class 4. Using AR and based on these calculations, we found four groups (Fig. 6–3) concerning the severity of nasal obstruction in the most resistive segment of 59 patients: 2 patients (3%) had no obstruction, 13 patients (22%) had minor obstruction, 24 patients (41%) had moderate obstruction, and 20 patients (34%) had marked obstruction. Concerning the nasal resistance measured by RM, four groups of 59 patients were evaluated: 4 patients (7%) showed normal nasal resistance, 14 patients (24%) had a minor increase, 23 patients (39%) had moderate increase, and 18 patients (31%) showed a marked increase of nasal resistance. The maximal difference in obstruction classes was one for each patient. The data show that the information of an obstruction class (normal to marked) can be evaluated with both methods. Furthermore, the result confirms the data of Haight and Cole,[28] that the most resistive segment in the anterior third of the nose determines the nasal resistance. RM measures the amount of the nasal resistance, and AR can clearly determine the exact size and location of the different constrictions in the nasal cavity which contribute to the increased nasal resistance.

Concerning the second and third question, MCA_{rhin} was calculated by the formula[15]:

$$MCA_{rhin} = k_1 \frac{V}{\sqrt{k_2 \tilde{N} P}}$$

Linear regression analysis of MCA_{rhin} and MCA_{AR} revealed a correlation coefficient of r = 0.263042, P = 0.2727. This poor correlation is explained by the fact that AR does not give any information about the shape of the measured CSA, although AR is able to evaluate the geometry of the nasal cavity.

To calculate nasal resistance from the CSA, we need information about the shape of a given CSA. However, AR does not provide this information. Therefore, nasal resistance cannot be calculated from AR data and MCA cannot be calculated from RM data.

From answers of questions 1 through 3, the methods are not exchangeable. To estimate nasal patency, RM is needed, and to examine the geometry of the nasal cavity, AR is the appropriate method.

REFERENCES

1. Hilberg O, Jackson AC, Swift DL, Pedersen OF: Acoustic rhinometry: evaluation of nasal cavity geometry by acoustic reflection. *J Appl Physiol* 1989; 66:295–303.
2. Cooley JW, Tukey JW: An algorithm for the machine calculation of complex Fourier series. *Math Computation* 1965; 19:297–301.
3. Mermelstein P: Determination of the vocal-tract shape from measured forman frequencies. *J Acoust Soc Am* 1967; 41:1283–1294.
4. Schroeder MR: Determination of the geometry of the human vocal tract by acoustic measurements. *J Acoust Soc Am* 1967; 43:1002–1010.
5. Paige A, Zue VW: Computation of vocal tract area functions. *IEEE Trans Audio Electroacoust* 1970; AE-18:7–18.
6. Stansfield EV, Bogner RE: Determination of vocal-tract-area function from transfer impedance. *Proc IEE* 1973; 120:153–158.
7. Sondhi MM, Gopinath B: Determination of vocal-tract shape from impulse response at the lips. *J Acoust Soc Am* 1971; 49:1867–1873.
8. Jackson AC, Butler JP, Millet EJ, Hoppin FG Jr, Dawson SV: Airway geometry by analysis of acoustic pulse response measurements. *J Appl Physiol* 1977; 43:523–536.
9. Fredberg JJ, Wohl ME, Glass GM, Dorkin HL: Airway area by acoustic reflections measured at the mouth. *J Appl Physiol* 1980; 48:749–758.
10. Hoffstein V, Zamel N: Tracheal stenosis measured by the acoustic reflection technique. *Am Rev Respir Dis* 1984; 130:472–475.
11. Hoffstein V, Zamel N, Phillipson EA: Lung volume dependence of pharyngeal cross-sectional area in patients with obstructive sleep apnea. *Am Rev Respir Dis* 1984; 130:175–178.
12. Rivlin J, Hoffstein V, Kalbfleisch J, McNicholas W, Zamel N, Bryan AC: Upper airway morphology in patients with idiopathic obstructive sleep apnea. *Am Rev Respir Dis* 1984; 129:355–360.
13. Rubinstein I, McClean PA, Boucher R, Zamel N, Fredberg JJ, Hoffstein V: Effect of mouthpiece, noseclips, and head position on airway area measured by acoustic reflections. *J Appl Physiol* 1987; 63:1469–1474.
14. Fredberg JJ: Acoustic determinants of respiratory system properties. *Ann Biomed Eng* 1981; 9:463–473.
15. Lenders, H: Akustische Rhinometrie: Eine Analyse der methode und ihrer klinischen Anwendung. Habilitationsschrift, Universität, Ulm, 1992.
16. Marshall I, Rogers M, Drummond G: Acoustic reflectometry for airway measurement. Principles, limitations and previous work. *Clin Phys Physiol Meas* 1991; 12:131–141.
17. Jones AS, Lancer JM, Stevens JC, Beckingham E: Nasal resistance to airflow (its measurement, reproducibility and normal parameters). *J Laryngol Otol* 1987; 101:800–808.
18. Mayhew TM, O'Flym P: Validation of acoustic rhinometry by using the Cavalieri principle to estimate nasal cavity volume in cadavers. *Clin Otolaryngol* 1993; 18:220–225.
19. Grymer LF, Hilberg O, Pedersen OF, Rasmussen TR: Acoustic rhinometry: values from adults with subjective normal nasal patency. *Rhinology* 1991; 29:35–47.
20. Clement PA: Committee report on standardization of rhinomanometry. *Rhinology* 1984; 22:151–155.
21. Lenders H, Pirsig W: Diagnostic value of acoustic rhinometry: patients with allergic and vasomotor rhinitis compared with normal controls. *Rhinology* 1990; 28:5–16.
22. Lenders H, Pirsig W: Acoustic rhinometry: normal values in adults, in Sacristàn T, Alvarez-Vincent JJ, Bartual J, Antolì-Candela F (eds.): Proceedings of the XIV World Congress of ORL and Head and Neck Surgery, Madrid, Spain, 10–15 Sept. 1989. Amsterdam, Kugler & Ghediri, 1990; pp 1533–1538.
23. Legler U: Beitrag zur Morphologie, Physiologie und Klinik des Vestibulum nasi vermittels eines neuzeitlichen Abdruckverfahrens. *Z Laryngol Rhinol Otol* 1967; 46:482–487.
24. Bachmann W: Untersuchungen über Morphologie und Funktion des vorderen Nasenabschnittes.

Kritische Analyse der derzeitigen Rhinomanometrie und Vorschlag zu ihrer Standardisierung. Habilitationsschrift, Universität, Heidelberg, 1973.
25. Bachmann W: Die Funktionsdiagnostik der be hinderten Nasenatmung. Berlin, Springer, 1982.
26. Masing H: Experimentelle Untersuchungen über die Strömung im Nasenmodell. *Arch Klin Exp Ohren Nasen Kehlkopfheilkd* 1967; 189:59–70.
27. Fischer R: Die Physik der Atemströminginder Nase Habilitationsschrift. Berlin, Universität, 1969.
28. Haight JS, Cole P: The site and function of the nasal valve. *Laryngoscope* 1983; 93:49–55.
29. Grymer LF, Hilberg O, Elbrond O, Pedersen OF: Acoustic rhinometry: evaluation of the nasal cavity with septal deviations, before and after septoplasty. *Laryngoscope* 1989; 99:1180–1187.
30. Heetderks DR: Reaction of normal nasal mucous membrane. *Am J Med Sci* 1927; 174:231–244.
31. Kayser R: Die exakte Messung der Luftdurchgängigkeit der Nase. *Arch Laryngol* 1885; 3:101.
32. Lund VJ: Objective assessment of nasal obstruction. *Otolaryngol Clin North Am* 1989; 22:279–290.
33. Juto JE, Lundberg C: Human nasal mucosa reaction during chilling of the feet. *Rhinology* 1985; 23:131–136.
34. Fullton JM, Drake AF, Fischer ND, Bromberg PA: Frequency dependence of effective nasal resistance. Ann Otol Rhinol Laryngol 1984; 93:140–145.
35. Canter RJ: A non-invasive method of demonstrating the nasal cycle using flexible liquid crystal thermography. *Clin Otolaryngol* 1986; 11:329–336.
36. Kennedy DW, Zinreich SJ, Kumar AJ, Rosenbaum AE, Johns ME: Physiologic mucosal changes within the nose and ethmoid sinus: imaging of the nasal cycle by MRI. *Laryngoscope* 1988; 98:928–933.
37. Elbrønd O, Felding JU, Hilberg O, Pedersen OF, Andersen OB: Acoustic rhinometry used as a method to demonstrate changes of the volume in the epipharynx after adenoidectomy. *Rhinology* 26 Suppl. 1 1988; 26:111.
38. Elbrønd O, Hilberg O, Felding JU, Blegvad AO: Acoustic rhinometry, used as a method to demonstrate changes in the volume of the nasopharynx after adenoidectomy. *Clin Otolaryngol* 1991; 16:84–86.
39. Lenders H, Pentz S, Brunner M, Pirsig W: Follow-up of patients with inverted papilloma of the nasal cavities: computer tomography, video-endoscopy, acoustic rhinometry? *Rhinology* 1994; 32:167–172.

7

Mucociliary Transport

SVEN LINDBERG, M.D., Ph.D.

The mucociliary system constitutes the first line of the airway defense against noxious stimuli and other agents in the environment. Inhaled particles, bacteria, and viruses are trapped in the mucus that covers the airways and are transported by the beat of the cilia to the pharynx, where they are either swallowed or coughed up. The mucous membranes in the nose, paranasal sinuses, and the tubal part of the middle ear are all covered by a ciliated epithelium, and cells of the same type are found in the bronchi and trachea. Nasal cilia are approximately 6μm in length, and each ciliated cell has 50 to 200 cilia beating continuously.[1] Determinants of ciliary beat frequency, and the composition of the airway secretions, regulate the efficiency of transport of mucus.

Because examination of ciliary ultrastructure is crucial to the diagnosis of diseases of the mucociliary system, a brief preliminary recapitulation is warranted. A cilium consists of an axoneme surrounded by a cell membrane, which is part of the ciliated cell membrane. Within the axoneme, nine peripheral double microtubules encircle the two central microtubules, the peripheral and central microtubules being connected by radial spokes and the peripheral microtubules by nexin links. These structures provide the structural rigidity of the axoneme. Of clinical importance is the fact that one microtubule in each peripheral doublet is furnished with an inner and an outer dynein arm. Figure 7–1 shows a schematic cross-section of a cilium. The dynein arms contain most of the ATPase activity of the axoneme and are important in releasing energy for the sliding and bending of the microtubules when the cilia beat. In healthy persons, the central microtubules are parallel in adjacent cilia.[2] The direction of ciliary beat is at right angles to a line between the two central microtubules. Ciliary beat consists of an effective stroke propelling mucus followed by a recovery stroke. In the base of the axoneme, where the cilia connect to the cell body, is a basal body with a spur aligned with the direction of the effective stroke. The beat in adjacent cilia is coordinated, forming a metachronous wave.[3] Because the ultrastructure of cilia is common to different species, it may be regarded as a primitive recurrent structure that has survived thousands of millennia of evolution. The sperm tail has the same ultrastructure as cilia.

155

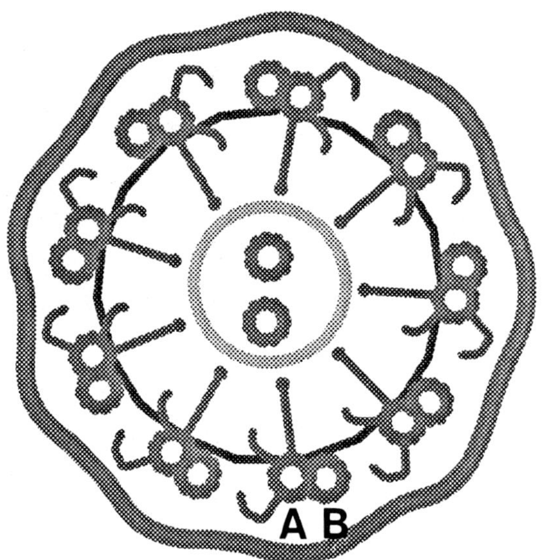

Figure 7–1.   Schematic representation of ciliary ultrastructure. Two central microtubles are surrounded by nine double peripheral microtubules, marked A and B. Two dynein arms from the A microtubule project toward the B microtubule in the next doublet. The cilia move by repeated binding of the dynein arms to the neighboring microtubule doublet. By successive dissolution of this bond, the doublets slide along each other. The peripheral doublets are connected with nexin links. Each peripheral doublet is connected to the central microtubules by a radial spoke. The central microtubules are encompassed by a sheath.

Knowledge of the relevance of the mucociliary system to health increased considerably with the description in 1976 of a genetically determined disease initially named immotile cilia syndrome, a designation referring to the inability of cilia to beat because of a structural defect. However, as was later discovered, in several cases the cilia did in fact beat, although insufficiently and without coordination. The term "immotile cilia syndrome" was abandoned and superseded by "primary ciliary dyskinesia" (PCD).

PCD denotes conditions of a genetically determined structural origin. The most common aberration in PCD is deficiency of outer or inner dynein arms and randomly oriented central microtubules.[4] Even as infants, patients with PCD are characterized by problems with increased secretion and stagnation in the airways, initially manifested as persistent purulent rhinorrhea and later as recurrent otitis media. A common symptom is chronic cough, and many affected children manifest lobular pulmonary atelectasis on chest radiography. On bronchoscopy, which is usually performed because a foreign body cannot be excluded as a cause of the atelectasis, bronchitis is found in association with edema and secretion.[5] As the child ages, chronic sinusitis emerges, and later recurrent bronchitis and pneumoniae occur with development of bronchiectasis. Almost all men with this disease are sterile, whereas women have reduced fertility. Exceptional cases have been reported of men with normal sperm ultrastrucure and motility despite manifest defects in the airway epithelial cells; thus, a sperm specimen should always be analyzed before a patient is told that he is sterile.[6] Half of patients with PCD

Table 7–1 Indications for Investigation of the Mucociliary System

AGE GROUP	INDICATION
Children and Adolescents	Protracted purulent rhinitis
	Recurrent serous and purulent otitis media not improved by treatment, and results of immunologic investigations are normal
	*Chronic sinusitis not associated with cystic fibrosis
	Protracted cough of unknown cause
	*Lobular pulmonary atelectasis of unknown cause
Adults	Chronic sinusitis not improved by treatment
	Recurrent bronchitis and chronic bronchitis in nonsmokers
	*Bronchiectasis
	Reduced fertility

*Very strong indication for investigation, including electron microscopy.

also manifest dextrocardia (situs inversus) and thereby fulfill the criteria for Kartagener's triad (chronic sinusitis, bronchiectasis, and situs inversus).[7] The rotation responsible for the heart being situated on the left and the liver on the right, which normally occurs when the embryo is 20 days old, has not taken place. Instead, the embryonic gut is randomly bent to the left or the right. An alternative explanation is that the dynein molecule is in itself asymmetrical, and the defect causing situs inversus is present in cytoplasmic rather than in ciliary dynein.[8] Clinical experience of patients with PCD has resulted in the demonstration of acquired defects in the function and ultrastructure of cilia in other categories of patients with similar symptoms. These defects are usually caused by infections or toxic influences. The indications for investigation of mucociliary function are listed in Table 7–1.

The typical features of diseases of the mucociliary system are not dramatic symptoms, but persistence of disease despite treatment and pulmonary involvement in almost all cases. Sinus and sputum cultures grow typical airway pathogens such as *Haemophilus influenzae* or *Streptococcus pneumoniae*, whereas *Pseudomonas* species, which are common among patients with cystic fibrosis, rarely occur.[9,10] Patients with genetic conditions may have a family history of chronic pulmonary disease. PCD is considered an autosomal recessive disease, although the existence of exceptional cases with a new dominant mutation cannot be excluded.[11]

Clinical investigation of these conditions should include function tests and morphologic study. It may be appropriate to investigate cilia from the lower airways, because the most serious symptoms of diseases of the mucociliary system originate from the lungs. However, not only are the ultrastructural morphologic findings identical in the upper and lower airways in cases of PCD but also correlation exists between recordings of the ciliary beat frequency in samples from the nose and the trachea.[12] It is therefore feasible to start all investigations of the mucociliary system in the nasal mucosa. A flowchart for the recommended investigations is given at the end of this chapter. The diagnostic workup can be divided into a basic investigation, which can be done at most hospitals, and a more sophisticated investigation, which is performed at research centers.

BASIC INVESTIGATIONS

Mucociliary Transport

The transport rate can be measured by using small particles of saccharine or radiolabeled particles. Radioisotope measurements yield a more accurate estimation of the transport rate than the saccharine test because it can be followed continuously, but they are marred by the possible effects of gamma radiation on the mucous membranes and have therefore been abandoned for use in investigations in children or for repeated investigations in adults.

The routine method used is the saccharine test. A small particle of saccharine is placed on the nasal mucosa and the time elapsed before the patient feels the intensely sweet taste of saccharine is measured. The saccharine particle is placed in the nasal cavity, which, owing to the nasal cycle, has the best passage of air. Because taste is subjective, the particle is first immersed in a dye powder such as indigo blue, and the investigator can then verify the occurrence of a blue color in the nasopharynx after the patient has sensed the taste of saccharine. As with investigations using radiolabeled particles, the flaw with the saccharine test is the great variation of the results and the poor reproducibility. One possible reason for this is that the particle is placed in the nose under nonstandardized conditions. To minimize this problem, the author and colleagues have developed a technique in which a 0.5-mm (diameter) particle of saccharine is dipped in indigo blue and placed in a plastic pipette. When the pipette is compressed, the particle is ejected without the investigator touching the mucosa (Fig. 7–2). The particle is placed on the septal mucosa in the middle meatus at the level of the anterior end of the middle turbinate, which is done during inspection with an endoscope (Panoview Plus 4mm, Richard Wolf GmbH, Knittlingen, Germany). The reason for choosing the septum instead of the turbinates is that the septal mucosa has less vasoactive tissue than the turbinates. If the effects of pharmacologic substances or airway irritants on the mucociliary transport are investigated, they may produce a swollen edematous mucosa, which in turn may affect transport. Some diseases that may affect the mucociliary system are

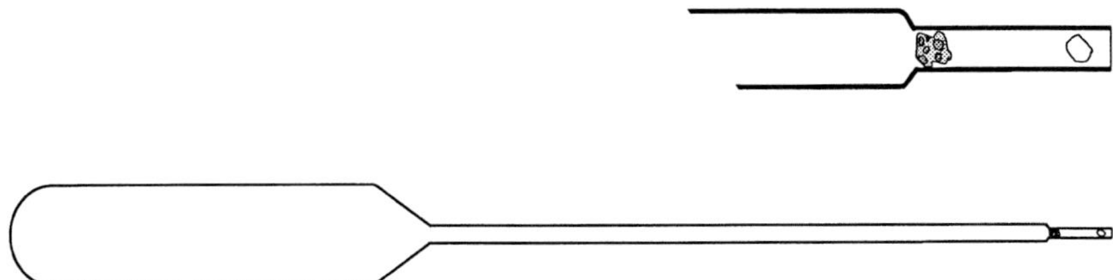

Figure 7–2.   Plastic pipette suitable for applying a particle of saccharine on the nasal mucosa. Pipette contains a piece of foam rubber, which hinders particle from entering more than 5mm into the pipette. When pipette is compressed, airstream ejects the particle. Pipette was modified by Associate Professor Rauf Khan, ASTRA-Draco, Lund, Sweden.

prone to engage the middle meatus (such as chronic sinusitis or nasal polyposis), and they may introduce a mechanical hindrance to transport which has less significance for the septal than for the turbinate mucosa. Patients are instructed to swallow once a minute, and the time until the patient senses the sweet taste is recorded.

At the author's institution, the reference value for healthy adults is 22 ± 7 min (mean ± SD). In an earlier study in which the saccharine method was compared with transport of resin particles labeled with ^{99m}Tc, the saccharine time was reported to be somewhat longer, 30 ± 13 min,[13] perhaps because the particles had been placed more anteriorly. This difference emphasizes that all laboratories investigating mucociliary transport rate need to establish their own reference figures based on standardized placement of the particles used. If more than 1 hour elapses without the patient sensing a sweet taste, the experiment is interrupted and the nasopharynx is examined for color. A particle of saccharine is placed on the tongue so that the investigator may acertain that the subject in fact is able to sense the taste of saccharine.

The author and colleagues have sometimes found that the saccharine time is shorter than normal during upper airway infections or exposure to allergens, when the subject has a watery secretion in the nose. The cause of this decreased time is probably dissolving of the saccharine particle in the secretion, and the subject then transfers the saccharine molecules to the nasopharynx by sniffing. It is therefore important that the patient be told not to sniff during the test.

Not only the placing of the saccharine particle but also the test environment should be standardized. Temperature and humidity should be controlled and noted in the test protocol. The patient should be acclimatized to the test room for 30 minutes before the test commences. If the result of the saccharine test is suspected to be pathologic, it should be repeated after 4 weeks. If repeated saccharine tests show slow or no transport, the test result is considered pathologic. Common virus infections in the upper airways may affect both morphology and function in the nasal epithelium, a finding indicating that the investigation should be postponed for at least 4 weeks if there is any sign of an acute upper airway infection.[14,15]

Ciliary Beat Frequency In Vitro

Because the beat of the cilia provides the motive force for the transport of mucus, it is of substantial interest to investigate ciliary beat frequency (CBF) and possible disturbances of its metachronous coordination. The easiest way to collect specimens for this purpose is to use cup forceps to take a superficial biopsy from the septal mucosa in the middle meatus. Alternatively, a cytology brush can be carefully introduced into the middle meatus and then gently swept to and fro and rotated for 5 s to collect a specimen.[16] The biopsy specimen is placed in sterile buffer. We prefer to use a HEPES buffer of the following composition (values in mmol/liter): NaCl 135, KCl 4.6, MgSO$_4$ 1.2, CaCl$_2$ 1.5, glucose 11, and HEPES (N-2-hydroxyethylpiperazine-N′-2-ethane-sulfonic acid) 10. If a biopsy specimen is used, it is placed on a coverslip, a drop of HEPES buffer is added, and the coverslip is inverted and placed on a microscopy slide with a shallow well. If a brush specimen is used, imprints are made in a 5- by 12-mm well on a slide, the well being immediately filled with HEPES buffer and covered with a coverslip. Independent of the type of sample, it is important to use a closed system because the cilia are susceptible to changes in ambient humidity.

It is essential to control the temperature during recordings of CBF because CBF has been shown to be approximately a linear function of temperature in the range of 20° to 40°C.[17,18] The measurements should be determined at 32° to 33°C, because this is the temperature at the surface of the nasal mucosa.[19,20] The sample is placed on a thermostat-controlled platform, and the preparation is observed through a microscope. We use a phase contrast microscope (Nikon Diaphot TMD, Nikon Corporation, Tokyo, Japan) at a magnification of ×400, but phase contrast is not a necessity.

Reported values for CBF in healthy persons vary somewhat. At the author's laboratory, the reference value for healthy adults (at 33°C) is 11.1 ± 1.1 Hz, whereas it is 9.2 ± 2.2 Hz to 10.6 ± 2.3 Hz at a Dutch laboratory,[21] 11.3 ± 1.0 Hz has been reported by an American team,[20] and an Israeli group obtained values of 12.2 ± 1.7 Hz for adults and 13.6 ± 1.5 Hz for a group of 10 to 19 year-olds at 35°C.[12] At testing, the CBF usually manifests an initial increase but returns to the baseline level after 30 to 60 minutes.[20] This initial increase in CBF is probably caused by the release of inflammatory mediators in response to trauma to the ciliated cell at harvesting, in that many of these mediators are known to accelerate mucociliary activity.[22] Accordingly, no measurement of CBF should be obtained until this reponse has subsided (after about 60 minutes).

CBF can be measured by photometric or high-speed video techniques. The photometric technique is simpler and faster and is preferred for routine use. The beam of light from the microscope passes through the specimen, and variations in the light intensity produced by the beating cilia are picked up by a sensitive photodetector. The best signals derive from cells viewed tangentially, that is, their ciliated brush border is seen clearly. The photodetector replaces one of the oculars, or is attached with an adaptor. The electrical current produced by the photodetector is processed for calculation of the CBF. As a means to reduce the risk of artifacts from movements in the environment or movements within the ciliated cells themselves, the processing includes the use of fast Fourier transformation of the signals. Fast Fourier transformation of a signal of varying frequency produces a spectrum of frequencies in which the relative power at each frequency is calculated (Fig. 7–3). The peak with the highest power is considered to be the predominant CBF in the sample. To obtain a representative CBF for a specimen, cilia from different cells are analyzed, each cell being represented by a median value of 10 consecutive calculations. The mean of measurements from at least five different cells is then considered representative for the specimen examined.

When is the CBF pathologic? Available reference values have been derived from healthy adults, and few corresponding investigations have been done in children. The lowest reported mean value for adults, 9 Hz with a standard deviation (SD) of 2 Hz, implies that a sample mean diverging by more than two SD (that is, outside the range of 5 to 13 Hz) in multiple specimens and repeated biopsy specimens from an adult patient is pathologic, although possibly this range is too wide. If the average CBF reported by several investigators of approximately 11 Hz with an SD of 1.5 Hz is assumed to be more appropriate, then a sample mean less than 8 Hz

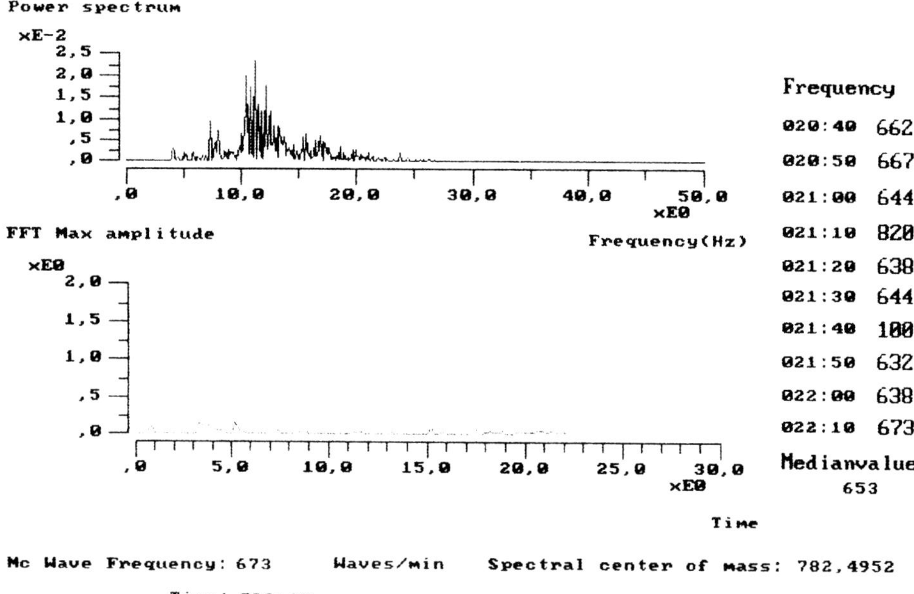

Figure 7–3. Fast Fourier transformation (FFT) of ciliary beat frequency (CBF) in a sample from human nasal mucosa. The illustration is a screen dump from the software View-DAC used for the analysis. The highest peak represents the predominant CBF. The table to the right shows the latest 10 FFT calculations of CBF and their median value.

may be pathologic. It is obvious that laboratories dealing with disorders of the mucociliary system need to establish their own reference values. Whether an increased CBF represents a pathologic condition is not known. One noteworthy reported observation is that the CBF was significantly higher in patients with unspecific chronic rhinitis than in healthy persons.[23] CBF values obtained in biopsy specimens and brush specimens from normals and from patients with various airway diseases are given in Table 7–2.

Efficient transport of mucus requires coordination of ciliary beat, not only among cilia in a given cell but also between cilia in adjacent cells. In a study using high-speed video technique, ciliary coordination was found to be defective in PCD, ciliary movement being described as rotational and vibratile instead of manifesting an effective forward and recovery stroke.[25] In another study using a video technique, a Dutch group assessed ciliary function in terms of a semiquantitative aggregate score derived from evaluation of three variables, as follows: CBF rated on a scale of 0 to 3 (0 representing totally immotile cilia, and 3 a CBF too high to be counted with the naked eye); ciliary coordination rated on a scale of 0 to 2 (0 representing totally immotile or randomly beating cilia, and 2 uniform direction, frequency, and amplitude of beat in a given cell); and finally, ciliary beat amplitude rated on a scale of 0 or 1 (0 representing vibratile movement only, and 1 a normal pattern with an effective forward and recovery stroke). The median aggregate scores for the groups studied manifested clear-cut differences, being only 1.3 for patients with PCD, 8.0 for healthy persons, and 7.6 for patients with airway infections of unknown causes, the last two groups not differing significantly from each other.[26]

Table 7–2   Nasal Ciliary Beat Frequency in Healthy Persons and in Certain Diseases

TEMPERATURE °C	CATEGORY	CILIARY BEAT FREQUENCY, Hz*	TYPE	REFERENCE
32–33				
	Normals n = 30	11.3 ± 1.0 (FFT)	Brush	Phillips et al.[20]
	Normals n = 11	9.2 ± 2.2 (FFT)	Biopsy	Ingels et al.[21]
	Normals n = 7	10.6 ± 2.3 (FFT)	Biopsy	Idem.
	Normals n = 8	13.3 ± 1.4	Brush	Lindberg and Runer[23]
	Normals n = 10	11.1 ± 1.1 (FFT)	Biopsy	Lindberg et al. unpublished data
	Polyposis n = 5	11.9 ± 2.4 (FFT)	Biopsy	Idem.
	Adenoids n = 7	11.8 ± 1.9 (FFT)	Biopsy	Idem.
35–37				
	Normals n = 10	12.2 ± 2.3	Brush	Rutland and Cole[16]
	Normals n = 45	12.2 ± 1.7 (FFT)	Brush	Roth et al.[12]
	Normals n = 35 (10–19 years old)	13.6 ± 1.5 (FFT)	Brush	Idem.
	Normals n = 10	14.6 ± 0.9	Brush	Rutland et al.[24]†
	Cystic fibrosis n = 16	13.7 ± 0.9	Brush	Idem.
	Bronchiectasis n = 15	12.9 ± 1.1	Brush	Idem.
	Primary ciliary dyskinesia n = 15	6.0 ± 4.6	Brush	Idem.
	Normals n = 55	12.5 ± 1.8	Brush	Rossman et al.[25]‡
	Chronic rhinitis n = 10	15.3 ± 1.2	Brush	Idem.
	Cystic fibrosis n = 15	12.7 ± 1.5	Brush	Idem.
	Primary ciliary dyskinesia n = 9	7.9 ± 3.2	Brush	Idem.

* In older studies, the measurements were obtained without the use of fast Fourier transformation (FFT) for signal analysis; whether FFT was used is stated within parentheses.
† The results of Rutland et al.[24] (1983) were originally published as a diagram; the values given here were extrapolated by the author.
‡ Rossman et al.[25] used high-speed video, instead of a photometric technique, for the measurements.

It has been suggested that lack of coordination between ciliated cells also can be recognized when the photometric technique is used.[27] However, no single objective variable such as the CBF has been convincingly presented, and more research is needed before this question is settled.

The equipment needed for automatic analysis of CBF is a microscope with sufficiently high magnification ($\times 400$ is recommended) and a photodetector. Commercially available photodetectors are expensive, but the technology required is well known, and most medical technical departments are capable of constructing one. The electrical current produced by the photodetecor needs to be amplified and filtered to minimize the effect of the AC disturbances in the building where the laboratory is located. The signals are digitized by an A/D converter (ADC) installed in the computer before processing the data to calculate CBF. The ADC used in the author's institution is a DAS-1401 (Keithley, Taunton, MA, USA), and the FFT analysis is performed by the software Viewdac (version 2.1) from the same manufacturer.

Ultrastructure

When there is reason to suspect a serious disease in the mucociliary system (Table 7–1) or repeated pathologic results have been obtained with the saccharine test or recording of CBF, ciliary ultrastructure is investigated with electron microscopy. The best sample is a brush specimen harvested with the same technique used for measurements of CBF. The brush is placed in a fresh solution of 2% glutaraldehyde containing 2 mM magnesium sulfate in 0.1 M sodium cacodylate buffer (pH 7.2) with 0.1 M sucrose. This solution has a refrigerated storage life of 10 days, but it should be discarded after that time. The specimen should be transported to the electron microscopy laboratory as soon as possible. Specimens mistakenly placed in formaldehyde can never be used for meaningful investigations of ciliary ultrastructure.

At least 50 cross-sectioned cilia should be examined, the items studied being the occurrence of dynein arms, nexin links, radial spokes between peripheral and central microtubules, the orientation of central microtubules and basal spurs, and transpositions of microtubules. Some cilia should be longitudinally sectioned, because disease associated with extra-long cilia has been reported.[28] Deficiency of dynein arms is a finding of major clinical relevance in that it supports the diagnosis of PCD.[25,29] Because the nexin links are often hard to discern even in normal cilia, their apparent absence is of less clinical pertinence. By contrast, deficiency of the radial spokes linking the peripheral and central microtubules is important because the radial spokes are less numerous in patients with PCD than in healthy persons or in patients with acquired diseases of the mucociliary system.[29] Transpositions (the central microtubules have been replaced by one of the peripheral doublets) occur in both PCD and acquired conditions.[29,30] Deficient orientation of the central microtubules (more than 25° deviation for adjacent cilia) has been reported as the only ultrastructural finding in PCD, but it also occurs in acquired disease.[9,31] The direction of beat is orthogonal to the line between the two central microtubules, but the direction of the effective stroke is also shown by the basal body spur where the cilia connect to the cell body. The direction of the basal spur has been suggested to be more representative of the direction of the beat than the localization of the central microtubules, because the risk of preparation artifacts is greater in the axoneme than in the cell body. Other aberrations, such as compound cilia where more than one axoneme is found in a common membrane, occur at low frequencies in healthy persons and in patients with PCD or acquired conditions and so are of little value for differential diagnosis.[25] Cases have been reported of total aplasia of ciliated cells in multiple biopsy specimens from different locations in the airways, but the condition is usually regarded as acquired rather than genetic because occasional intact cilia and basal bodies also are found.[32] However, in exceptional cases, total ciliary aplasia may constitute a genetic defect; in one study, cultured specimens from three patients manifested no sign of ciliogenesis.[33]

At a workshop in 1992, organized to reach consensus regarding the ultrastructural diagnosis of PCD and acquired conditions, it was emphasized that extreme care must be taken to avoid misinterpretation of acquired changes as representing genetic abnormalities. The result of investigations of a genetic disease must show both persistence and universality; the following criteria must be fulfilled:

1. Demonstration of a specific abnormality affecting all cilia in a given sample
2. Demonstration of the same abnormality in cilia collected from at least one additional site
3. Demonstration of the same abnormality in cilia collected on at least one additional point in time.[32]

Approximately 5% of cilia from healthy persons manifest ultrastructural changes. At least 40% to 50% of the cilia need to be affected before clinical symptoms develop.[25] In contrast to genetic diseases, acquired conditions are typically focal and transient. The most common finding is extra microtubules. The number of radial spokes may be reduced. Occasional dynein arm defects are also common, but the finding is of doubtful clinical significance. Figures 7–4 and 7–5 show typical samples from a patient with PCD and a patient with an acquired condition, respectively.

Cases of a PCD-like disease, but with normal ciliary ultrastructure, have been reported. The diagnosis was based on a classic history, including bronchiectasis, reduced CBF in repeated biopsy specimens, impaired coordination between adjacent cilia, and no transport of mucus in the nose as measured with labeled particles.[26] Whether this condition is an irreversible but acquired disease or a genetically determined functional disturbance in the mucociliary system is not known. This condition, which is probably very rare if stringent criteria are adopted, should be clearly distinguished from PCD, which is diagnosed by repeated ultrastructural examinations. To avoid confusion between these two conditions, another term might be adopted to designate cases with normal ultrastructure, for example, "irreversible functional ciliary dyskinesia."

There has been a promising development in investigations of CBF and ultrastructure during recent years. Culturing of ciliated cells in a suspension

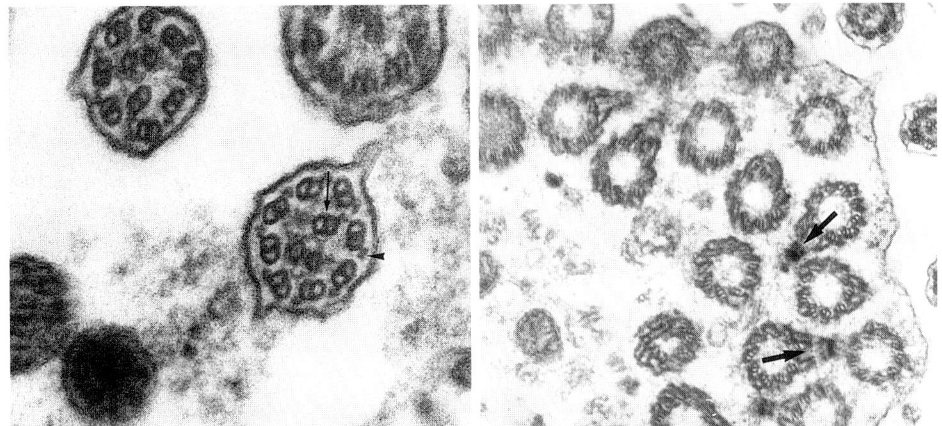

Figure 7–4.   Electron micrographs of cilia from a 13-year-old boy with primary ciliary dyskinesia. The patient had recurrent otitis media and chronic sinusitis. The outer dynein arms are longer than normal (arrowhead), whereas the inner arms are missing. Translocations in which one of the peripheral doublets is centrally displaced are also seen (long arrow), and the radial spokes are deficient (A). The basal spurs are randomly oriented (arrows) (B).

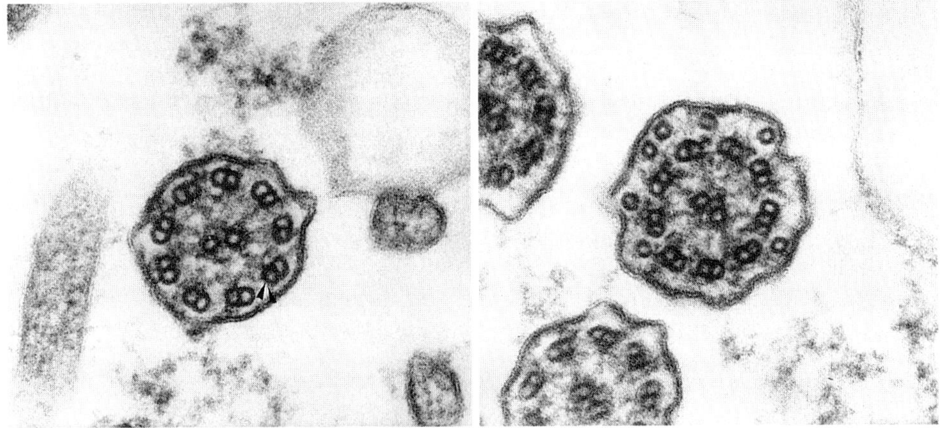

Figure 7–5.   Electron micrographs of cilia from a 2-year-old boy with an acquired disorder of the mucociliary system. The patient had recurrent bronchitis. Dynein arms are missing, but only in 20% of the cilia (arrowhead) (A). Many of the cilia manifest aberrant numbers of microtubules, whereas other cilia manifest a normal ultrastructure (B).

culture may induce ciliogenesis and help to distinguish between genetic and acquired diseases, in regard to both morphology and measurements of CBF. Thus, in patients with cystic fibrosis after culture of cells from nasal polyps in flasks for 4 weeks, both ultrastructure and CBF were indistinguishable from those of control tissue.[34]

ADVANCED DIAGNOSTIC METHODS

In Vivo Recordings of Mucociliary Activity in the Nasal Mucosa

In vitro measurement of CBF with the photometric technique uses light passing through the preparation, whereas in vivo methods for measurements of mucociliary activity use reflected light. The cilia beating beneath the mucous layer produce a flickering light reflection if a light beam of any kind is directed at an angle against the mucosa. Variations in the light reflection are picked up by a photodetector and transformed into electrical signals that are processed for calculations of mucociliary wave frequency, the result representing an averaged CBF for cilia on many adjacent cells. In principle, is it possible to use the same equipment as in in vitro investigations.

Previous research was confined to animal models. The author and colleagues have used the rabbit maxillary sinus as a model, whereas an American group has investigated mucociliary activity in the canine trachea with a sophisticated laser technique.[35,36] The main drawback to use of experimental animals is the mandatory need of anesthesia, which may dampen important airway reflexes known to affect mucociliary function.[37] Moreover, a direct effect of the anesthesia on CBF cannot be excluded. Also, surgical trauma in itself affects CBF.[38] For these reasons, it was considered urgent to develop a method for recording mucociliary activity in vivo from the human nasal mucosa.

A probe was developed in the shape of a rigid tube of stainless steel which contained the following optical system. Light from a cold light source (Wolf 4510, Richard Wolf Gmbh, Knittlingen, Germany) is transmitted to the mucosa by an optic fiber with an inner diameter of 100 μm. The reflected light is transmitted through a glass-covered window (approximately 1.5 mm in diameter) at the side of the tube. The tube houses a mirror of polished stainless steel and a lens. The optical axis of the mirror and lens is 35° vis-à-vis the incident light, which corresponds to the angle of incident and reflected light in the rabbit maxillary sinus model. To increase the focal depth of the system, a lens with a diameter of 1.8 mm and a focal length of 15 mm is used. An optic fiber with a diameter of 100 μm is positioned in the middle of the focal plane produced by the lens. This arrangement allows the recording of variations in reflected light from a surface area of 100 μm in diameter, because the image in the focal plane is neither magnified nor reduced (Fig. 7–6).

The probe is introduced, without the use of local anesthesia, with the help of the same endoscope used in the saccharine test (Wolf Panoview Plus 4 mm, Richard Wolf Gmbh, Knittlingen, Germany). Visual control of the light reflex in the mucosa is obtained by mounting the optic fiber in the center of a transparent Plexiglas window. The image around the detector fiber is transmitted through another lens (f, 15 mm; diameter, 8.2 mm), which produces a new focal plane approximately 120 mm from the mucosal surface with a magnification of ×1.7. This image is observed by the optic fibers of a gastroscope allowing visual control of the light reflex, the detector fiber being seen as a black spot in the center. Light variations transmitted by this fiber are picked up by a sensitive photodiode and analyzed by a

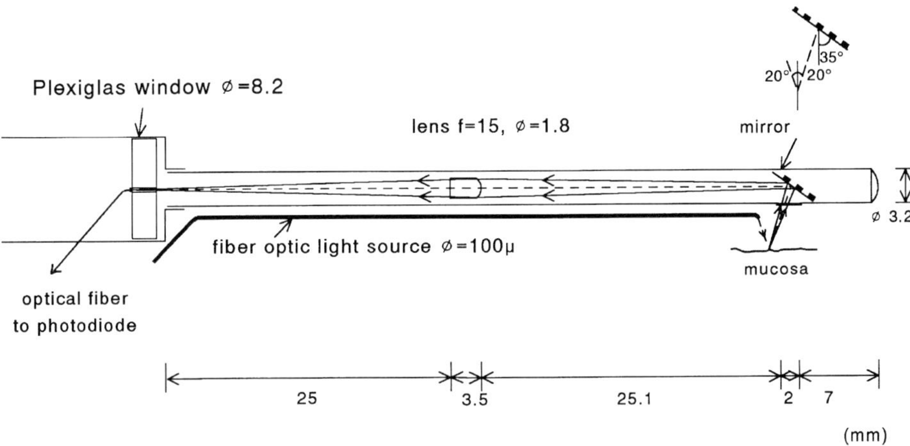

Figure 7–6. Probe developed for in vivo measurements of mucociliary activity in human nose. Light is reflected by nasal mucosa, and path through probe is indicated by dashed line. Arrows indicate direction of light. Details of optical system, including the lenses, are given in the text. (Reprinted with permission from reference 23.)

computerized frequency calculator that computes the mucociliary wave frequency in waves per minute every 10 seconds during the experiments.

Any movement affecting the mucosa can compromise the recordings of mucociliary activity and so should be minimized. Stable fixation of the volunteer's head is accomplished by modifying a stand intended for corneal microscopy which provides support for the forehead and the lower jaw. The upper jaw is fixed by a plastic cast of the subject's upper jaw teeth. A steel rod embedded in the cast is screwed to the stand. The experimental setup is shown in Figure 7–7.

One of the aims of the human experiments is to investigate the effects of drugs on the mucociliary system. Diseases involving the mucociliary system are common, and because many people are reported sick (or "absent from work") for this reason, better mucociliary defense against infection is of significance both to the individual and to the community. A methodologic problem for in vivo mucociliary research is the administration of drugs. In the animal models, this problem is solved by intra-arterial injection of the compounds to be investigated. This route of administration could not be used in humans, and some sort of local administration had to be chosen. The use of drops was infeasible not only because they can change the rheologic properties of the mucus but also because mechanical load is known to stimulate CBF.[39]

To standardize the local application of drugs and to limit the effect on the mucociliary system resulting from this route of administration, a jet nebulizer (Up-Draft II Neb-U-Mist Nebulizer, Hudson, Temecula, CA, USA) was modified and a magnetic valve with a timer was added, allowing delivery of aerosols at constant intervals. The cup containing the fluid to be nebulized and the connecting tube are supplied with a thermostat-controlled heater to keep the aerosol temperature at 33°C. The size of the particles delivered by the nebulizer has been investigated with a laser diffraction technique. At a flow rate of 6 liters/min and a temperature of

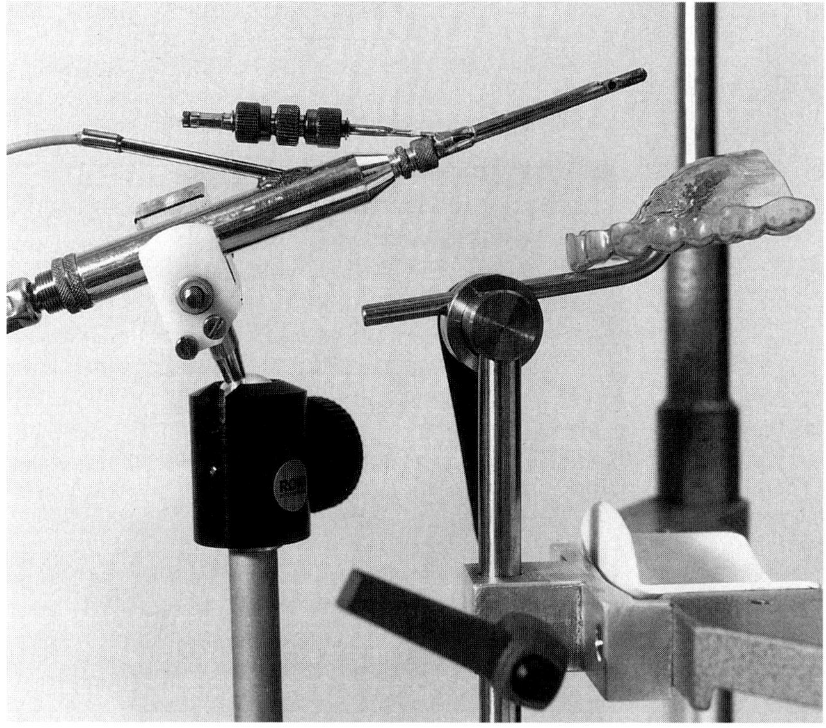

Figure 7–7.   Setup for in vivo studies of mucociliary activity. Subject's lower jaw and forehead are supported by a frame taken from a corneal microscope stand, and upper jaw is fixed by a plastic cast of the subject's teeth, affixed to the stand. Probe and optic fiber system are in center. (Reprinted with permission from reference 23.)

33°C, the mass median diameter is 3.56 + 0.26 µm; thus, if the subject holds his or her breath during the nebulization, the major part of the spray is deposited in the nasal cavity.

Mucociliary activity was investigated in nine healthy volunteers, all men between 29 and 42 years old. All were nonsmokers, and none had a history of chronic sinusitis or of rhinosurgical or medical treatment. They had no signs of an upper airway infection during the 3 weeks preceding the investigation. Mucociliary wave frequency was found to vary spontaneously. The coefficient of variation during a 10-minute interval was 13.4% between subjects and 8.3% to 14.3% within subjects. Correlation between two consecutive 5-minute recordings was good ($r = 0.87$), and correlation between measurements at different sites was acceptable ($r = 0.72$), as was the correlation between measurements made on different days ($r = 0.58$).[23]

To investigate artifacts in the photoelectrical signals produced by inevitable movements despite the fixation to the corneal microscopy stand, the experimental setup has been connected to a computer that analyzes the mucociliary wave frequency with FFT of the signals each 10 seconds during the experiments. The sample frequency is 100 Hz, implying that every FFT analysis is based on 1,000 raw data points. The spectrum of frequencies analyzed was set to 0.5 to 40 Hz. The author and colleagues compared recordings from the nasal septum with reflections of light produced by aluminum foil placed on the nasal dorsum. Recordings from the septum and from the aluminum foil manifested similarities in the lower frequency spectrum. This finding is probably explained by artifacts from the pulse at approximately 1 Hz, and also peaks at 2 to 3 Hz may represent duplicates of the pulse. However, there was a distinct difference between the two measurements at frequencies of more than 5 Hz (usually around 7 to 8 Hz), the mucociliary recordings from the septum manifesting a distinct peak not usually seen in the aluminum foil experiments. The average mucociliary wave frequency on the septal mucosa in six healthy persons, aged 31 to 44 years, was 7.8 ± 1.6 Hz, which is lower than CBF measurements in vitro. This difference may be due to a different composition of the mucus layer in vitro, because the samples are washed in HEPES-buffer, and the cilia beat in this buffer instead of in their original environment. An alternative explanation is that the trauma caused by harvesting ciliated cells may induce a release of cilia-stimulant factors which is sustained for more than 60 minutes.

Although the development of an in vivo method for recording mucociliary activity in the unanesthetized human nose is a major advance, the method has limitations. For instance, restraint by the experimental stand was found awkward by most volunteers after about 30 minutes. Introduction of the probe and selecting a light reflection on the nasal mucosa takes approximately 10 minutes; thus, only 15 to 20 minutes remain for experiments. Because challenge with pharmacologic substances is therefore limited to baseline recordings during 5 minutes and to 10 minutes after challenge, only one concentration could be tested each time. In practice, unlike animal experiments, the human setup is not feasible for obtaining full dose-response curves of various drugs. The limited observation period that is possible also hampers continuous recording of subchronic effects of drugs and irritants. Alternatively, chronic effects could be followed on a day-to-day basis because of the reproducibility of repeated measurements.

In addition to pharmacologic studies, the method will be of use in patients with certain diseases of the upper airways, such as nasal polyposis and chronic sinusitis, and in cases of occupational exposure to airway irritants.

Measurements of Mucociliary Transport With Isotope Techniques

In contrast to the saccharine test, radioactive isotopes can be used for continuous measurements of mucociliary transport in the nose. The method enables recording of time courses and of the direction of transport to be monitored. Either a ^{99m}Tc-labeled albumin-colloid, applied as droplets with a volume of 10 µL on the mucosa, or ^{99m}Tc-labeled resin particles in the form of very small spheres (usually 50 to 350 µm in diameter) can be used. The radioactivity is applied at standardized sites on the mucosa. We prefer to use the septal mucosa in the middle meatus at the level of the anterior end of the middle turbinate (that is, the same site used in the saccharine test or in harvesting of ciliated cells). Transport of mucus can be followed with either of two techniques. The most convenient is to use a gamma camera equipped with a pinhole-collimator, which works as a camera obscura and monitors emitted gamma rays in a matrix where a picture is taken each minute for 60 minutes. Alternatively, multicollimator detectors can be used, which have two or three slits, positioned at a fixed distance from each other. The transport rate can be calculated by following the increase of radioactivity at each slit. Multicollimator detectors are less expensive than the gamma camera, but they are marred by the disadvantage that transport can be measured in only one direction, and thus the results constitute only a minimal estimate of the true transport rate. In many cases, transport in the nose is directed at an oblique angle to the direction of the nasal cavity, and in the anterior part of the nose even an anteriorly directed transport has been reported.[40]

Two variables can be measured if radiolabeled albumin-colloid is used, but this cannot be done when resin spheres are used. On one hand, residual radioactivity could be measured with correction for the half-life of ^{99m}Tc (approximately 6 hours), by analogy with measurements of mucociliary clearance from the lung. On the other hand, the rate at which the tracer frontline moves can be quantified. Studies in the nose have been confined to movements of the tracer frontline. Reported reference values for this rate in healthy persons have varied, probably for the same reason as the variation in reports of time measured in the saccharine test (see above). A French group reported a transport rate of 3.3 ± 3.5 mm/min (range, 0 to 13.9 mm/min),[13] Japanese investigators reported 7.5 ± 4.3 mm/min (range, 1.1 to 15.2 mm/min),[41] and a Finnish group found an average transport rate of 9.0 mm/min (range, 5.8 to 13.5 mm/min) in healthy subjects.[42] An example of a measurement with ^{99m}Tc-labeled albumin-colloid is shown in Figure 7–8.

A Danish study of nasal transport illustrates the problem of the great variations reported for this kind of measurement. In 56 healthy volunteers investigated in a climate chamber at 23°C and 68% relative humidity, the mean transport rate was 8.4 mm/min (range, 2.3 to 23.6 mm/min); only 32 manifested unequivocal transport, and the other 24 had either a very slow transport or no transport at all.[40] In further studies of healthy volunteers by the same investigators, irrespective of whether radiolabeled or saccharine particles were used, approximately 80% of the subjects manifested transport rates of 3 to 25 mm/min, whereas the remaining 20% manifested very slow transport or no transport at all.[43]

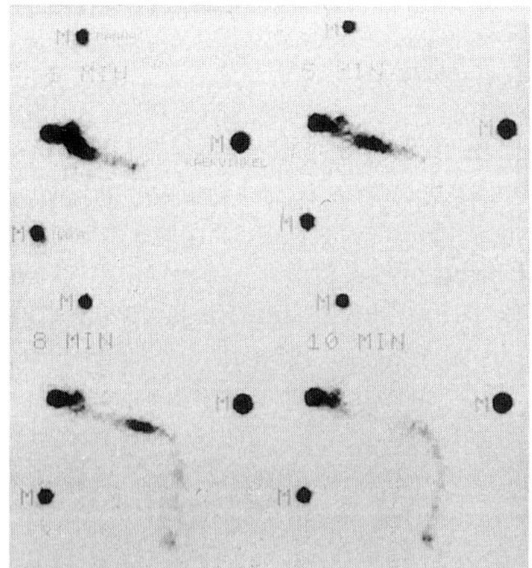

Figure 7–8. Recording of mucociliary transport in septal mucosa in a healthy person manifesting a fast transport rate. Three separate spots of radioactivity are external cobalt markers, which are used for calculations of transport rate of tracer frontline. Experiment was done with 10 µm ^{99m}Tc-labeled albumin-colloid. A substantial part of the applied radioactivity is retained at site of application.

Repeated measurements in the same subject have shown poor reproducibility in transport studies. The French investigators reported a correlation coefficient of $r = 0.25$ for repeat measurements 24 hours later,[13] and a corresponding calculation in the Danish study, in which a repeat measurement was done 2 hours later, yielded a correlation coefficient of $r = 0.33$ (Spearman's rho, calculation by the author based on published raw data).[43] The great variation in results indicates that a finding of no or very slow transport should be followed by repeat investigation after an interval of at least 4 weeks, before mucociliary transport can be regarded as impaired. One reservation is that because the older studies were performed before the modern endoscopic technique was developed, a more standardized application of the tracer might yield better reproducibility.

A possible explanation for the reduced transport rate found in many healthy persons is that upper respiratory tract infections, usually caused by virus, are very common. Viruses cause damage to the epithelium in the nose which lasts for several weeks after the infection.[15] This hypothesis derives support from a finding in the Danish study, in which a greater proportion of subjects in the nil or slow transport group had had a common cold during the 2 weeks preceding the investigation. Members of the same group also developed a cold within days after the study more frequently than volunteers in the group with unequivocal transport.[40] Whether subclinical virus infections in the nose affect the mucociliary activity in the upper airways is not known.

The isotope technique was compared with the simple saccharine test in the same healthy subjects.[13] Unexpectedly, reproducibility was slightly better for the saccharine test, the respective correlation coefficients being $r = 0.46$ and $r = 0.25$ for repeat measurements after a 24-hour interval. When the results of the two methods were checked for correlation, a significant correlation was found ($r = -0.59$), a finding that supports the view that the saccharine test is useful for clinical routine work. The correlation coefficient was negative because the saccharine time was correlated with transport rate (that is, the faster the transport rate, the shorter the corresponding saccharine time). Attempts have been made to calculate the transport rate also with the saccharine test, by measuring the distance to the nasopharynx on radiographs, but it is doubtful whether this calculation contributes to the precision of the test.

FUTURE DEVELOPMENTS

In view of the major progress made during recent years in efforts to investigate the motive force of the mucociliary system, the ciliated cell and its cilia, in all likelihood future developments will focus on the product of ciliary function, mucociliary transport. It is hoped that new methods will be developed for measurement of the mucociliary transport rate which are more precise than the saccharine test and demand less investment in expensive equipment than the isotope techniques. The radioactive load on the mucosa, which prevents use of the techniques in children and in repeated experiments in adults, also may be avoided by the development of new techniques. The second line of development is to focus on the airway mucus. It has long been known that the cilia need a layer of mucus before any transport can

Flow Chart for Mucociliary Investigations

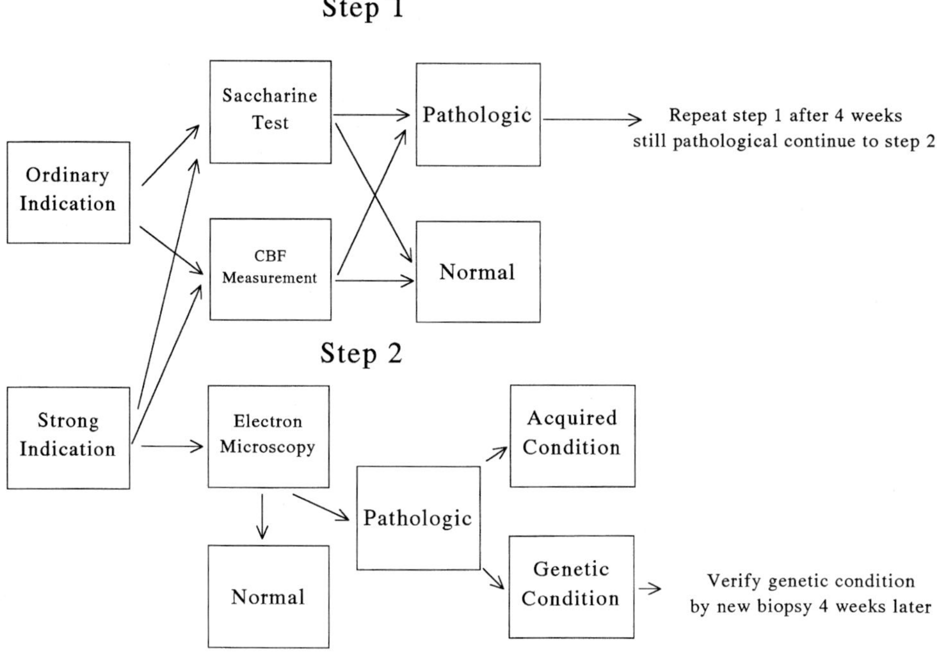

be established, and quantitative elucidation of the properties of mucus is of substantial interest. There is an ideal range of viscosity and elasticity for optimal function of mucociliary transport. If the viscosity of the medium in which the cilia beat in vitro is manipulated, the CBF is changed.[44,45] If samples of mucus can be obtained from the upper airways in various conditions and diseases, and the viscoelastic properties are investigated in parallel with measurement of CBF, our knowledge regarding the significance of these diseases for the mucociliary system may be substantially improved. Finally, genetic counseling of patients could be improved if the gene aberrations causing the dynein arm defect in PCD could be identified.

SUMMARY

The technique for clinical investigation of the mucociliary system in the nose by recordings of CBF in biopsy and brush specimens is well established. Mucociliary transport can be studied with the saccharine test. Mucociliary research may benefit from new techniques for the measurement of mucociliary wave frequency in vivo on the same mucosa, and transport can be measured more precisely with the isotope techniques than with the saccharine test. Because of the great variation in healthy persons, findings of impaired mucociliary function, such as a reduced CBF or transport rate, must be verified by repeat investigation after an interval of at least 4 weeks. Results of functional investigations must be supplemented with those of ultrastructural studies before any conclusion can be drawn regarding the significance of the mucociliary system for the patient's symptoms and disease.

Acknowledgments—The author thanks his coworkers at the mucociliary research laboratory, Department of Otorhinolaryngology, Head and Neck Surgery, University Hospital, Lund: Anders Cervin, Charlotte Cervin-Hoberg, Jan Dolata, Samuel Leino, Ulf Mercke, and Thomas Runer. The electron micrographs were kindly provided by Birgitta Carlén, Department of Pathology, University Hospital, Lund, who is an expert on the ultrastructural diagnosis of mucociliary disorders. A debt of gratitude is also due to Associate Professor Rauf Khan of ASTRA-Draco, Lund, who has given me much good advice regarding the measurements of CBF in vitro and the saccharine test, and to Professor Per Wollmer of the Department of Clinical Physiology, Malmö General Hospital, for fruitful collaboration regarding measurements of mucociliary transport with the isotope technique.

The work at the mucociliary research laboratory is supported by the Swedish Medical Research Council (project nos. 7940, 10609, and 11021), the Torsten Söderberg and Ragnar Söderberg Trusts, and the Medical Faculty of the University of Lund.

REFERENCES

1. Jafek BW: Ultrastructure of human nasal mucosa. *Laryngoscope* 1983; 93:1576–1599.
2. Sleigh MA: The nature and action of respiratory tract cilia. *Lung Biol Health Dis* 1977; 5:247–288.
3. Sanderson MJ, Sleigh MA: Ciliary activity of cultured rabbit tracheal epithelium: beat pattern and metachrony. *J Cell Sci* 1981; 47:331–347.
4. Afzelius BA: A human syndrome caused by immotile cilia. *Science* 1976; 193:317–319.
5. Ernstson S, Afzelius BA, Mossberg B: Otologic manifestations of the immotile-cilia syndrome. *Acta Otolaryngol (Stockh)* 1984; 97:83–92.
6. Escudier E, Escalier D, Pinchon MC, Boucherat M, Bernaudin JF, Fleury-Feith J: Dissimilar expression of axonemal anomalies in respiratory cilia and sperm flagella in infertile men. *Am Rev Respir Dis* 1990; 142:674–679.
7. Kartagener M: Zur Pathogenese der Bronchiektasien: Bronchiektasien bei Situs viscerum inversus. *Beitr Klin Tuberk* 1933; 83:489–501.
8. Brown NA, McCarthy A, Wolpert L: Development of handed body asymmetry in mammals. *Ciba Found Symp* 1991; 162:182–196.
9. Rutland J, de Iongh RU: Random ciliary orientation: a cause of respiratory tract disease. *N Engl J Med* 1990; 323:1681–1684.
10. Perraudeau M, Scott J, Walport M, Oakley C, Bloom S, Brooks D: Late presentation of Kartagener's syndrome: consequences of ciliary dysfunction. *BMJ* 1994; 308:519–521.
11. Rott H-D: Genetics of Kartagener's syndrome. *Eur J Respir Dis Suppl* 1983; 127:1–4.
12. Roth Y, Aharonson EF, Teichtahl H, Baum GL, Priel Z, Modan M: Human in vitro nasal and tracheal ciliary beat frequencies: comparison of sampling sites, combined effect of medication, and demographic relationships. *Ann Otol Rhinol Laryngol* 1991; 100:378–384.
13. Puchelle E, Aug F, Pham QT, Bertrand A: Comparison of three methods for measuring nasal mucociliary clearance in man. *Acta Otolaryngol (Stockh)* 1981; 91:297–303.
14. Pedersen M, Sakakura Y, Winther B, Brofeldt S, Mygind N: Nasal mucociliary transport, number of ciliated cells, and beating pattern in naturally acquired common colds. *Eur J Respir Dis Suppl* 1983; 128:355–365.
15. Winther B, Brofeldt S, Christensen B, Mygind N: Light and scanning electron microscopy of nasal biopsy material from patients with naturally acquired common colds. *Acta Otolaryngol (Stockh)* 1984; 97:309–318.
16. Rutland J, Cole PJ: Non-invasive sampling of nasal cilia for measurement of beat frequency and study of ultrastructure. *Lancet* 1980; 2:564–565.

17. Mercke U, Håkansson CH, Toremalm NG: The influence of temperature on mucociliary activity. Temperature range 20 degrees C-40 degrees C. *Acta Otolaryngol (Stockh)* 1974; 78:444–450.
18. Ingels KJAO, Kortmann MJW, Nijziel MR, Graamans K, Huizing EH: Factors influencing ciliary beat measurements. *Rhinology* 1991; 29:17–26.
19. Åkerlund A, Bende M: Nasal mucosal temperature and the effect of acute infective rhinitis. *Clin Otolaryngol* 1989; 14:529–534.
20. Phillips PP, McCaffrey TV, Kern EB: Measurement of human nasal ciliary motility using computerized microphotometry. *Otolaryngol Head Neck Surg* 1990; 103:420–426.
21. Ingels KJ, Meeuwsen F, van Strien HL, Graamans K, Huizing E: Ciliary beat frequency and the nasal cycle. *Eur Arch Otorhinolaryngol* 1990; 248:123–126.
22. Dolata J, Lindberg S, Mercke U: The effects of prostaglandins E1, E2 and F2 alpha on mucociliary activity in the rabbit maxillary sinus. *Acta Otolaryngol (Stockh)* 1989; 108:290–297.
23. Lindberg S, Runer T: Method for in vivo measurement of mucociliary activity in the human nose. *Ann Otol Rhinol Laryngol* 1994; 103:558–566.
24. Rutland J, Cox T, Dewar A, Cole P: Screening for ciliary dyskinesia—a spectrum of defects of motility and structure. *Eur J Respir Dis Suppl* 1983; 127:71–77.
25. Rossman CM, Lee RM, Forrest JB, Newhouse MT: Nasal ciliary ultrastructure and function in patients with primary ciliary dyskinesia compared with that in normal subjects and in subjects with various respiratory diseases. *Am Rev Respir Dis* 1984; 129:161–167.
26. van der Baan S, Veerman AJP, Wulffraat N, Bezemer PD, Feenstra L: Primary ciliary dyskinesia: ciliary activity. *Acta Otolaryngol (Stockh)* 1986; 102:274–281.
27. Ingels KJ, van Strien H, Graamans K, Smoorenburg G, Huizing EH: A study of the photoelectrical signal from human nasal cilia under several conditions. *Acta Otolaryngol (Stockh)* 1992; 112:831–838.
28. Afzelius BA, Gargani G, Romano C: Abnormal length of cilia as a possible cause of defective mucociliary clearance. *Eur J Respir Dis* 1985; 66:173–180.
29. van der Baan S, Veerman AJP, Bezemer PD, Feenstra L: Primary ciliary dyskinesia: quantitative investigation of the ciliary ultrastructure with statistical analysis. *Ann Otol Rhinol Laryngol* 1987; 96:264–272.
30. Sturgess JM, Chao J, Turner JAP: Transposition of ciliary microtubules: another cause of impaired ciliary motility. *N Engl J Med* 1980; 303:318–322.
31. Boat TF, Carson JL: Ciliary dysmorphology and dysfunction—primary or acquired? (editorial) *N Engl J Med* 1990; 323:1700–1702.
32. Mireau GW, Agostini R, Beals TF, et al: The role of electron microscopy in evaluating ciliary dysfunction: report of a workshop. *Ultrastruct Pathol* 1992; 16:245–254.
33. DeBoeck K, Jorissen M, Wouters K, et al: Aplasia of respiratory tract cilia. *Pediatr Pulmonol* 1992; 13:259–265.
34. Jorissen M, Van der Schueren B, Van den Berghe H, Cassiman JJ: In vitro ciliogenesis in respiratory epithelium of cystic fibrosis patients. *Ann Otol Rhinol Laryngol* 1991; 100:366–371.
35. Hybbinette JC, Mercke U: A method for evaluating the effect of pharmacological substances on mucociliary activity in vivo. *Acta Otolaryngol (Stockh)* 1982; 93:151–159.
36. Wong LB, Miller IF, Yeates DB: Stimulation of ciliary beat frequency by autonomic agonists: in vivo. *J Appl Physiol* 1988; 65:971–981.
37. Lindberg S, Dolata J, Mercke U: Nasal exposure to airway irritants triggers a mucociliary defence reflex in the rabbit maxillary sinus. *Acta Otolaryngol (Stockh)* 1987; 104:552–560.
38. Wong LB, Yeates DB: Stimulation of tracheal ciliary beat frequency by localized tissue incision. *J Appl Physiol* 1990; 68:411–416.
39. Sanderson MJ, Dirksen ER: Mechanosensitivity of cultured ciliated cells from the mammalian respiratory tract: implications for the regulation of mucociliary transport. *Proc Natl Acad Sci USA* 1986; 83:7302–7306.
40. Andersen I, Lundqvist GR, Proctor DF: Human nasal mucosal function in a controlled climate. *Arch Environ Health* 1971; 23:408–420.
41. Sakakura Y, Ukai K, Majima Y, Murai S, Harada T, Miyoshi Y: Nasal mucociliary clearance under various conditions. *Acta Otolaryngol (Stockh)* 1983; 96:167–173.
42. Kärjä J, Nuutinen J, Karjalainen P: Radioisotopic method for measurement of nasal mucociliary activity. *Arch Otolaryngol* 1982; 108:99–101.
43. Proctor DF, Andersen I: *The Nose: Upper Airway Physiology and the Atmospheric Environment.* Amsterdam, Elsevier Biomedical Press, 1982, pp 245–278.
44. Chen TM, Dulfano MJ: Mucus viscoelasticity and mucociliary transport rate. *J Lab Clin Med* 1978; 91:423–431.
45. Majima Y, Sakakura Y, Matsubara T, et al: Rheological properties of middle ear effusions from children with otitis media with effusion. *Ann Otol Rhinol Laryngol Suppl* 1986; 124:1–4.

8

Mucosal Cytology

FUAD M. BAROODY, M.D.

The cellular constituents of nasal secretions and the mucosa are useful indicators of underlying pathologic processes of the nose. Different methods of sampling these cells are available, and the types of cells seen differ depending on the underlying pathologic process. Some of these underlying processes include allergic rhinitis, nonallergic rhinitis, nonallergic rhinitis with eosinophilia (NARES), and viral and bacterial upper respiratory tract infections. Cytologic nasal changes in seasonal and experimentally induced allergic rhinitis are better documented and more studied than changes in other pathologic conditions of the upper airway.

This chapter details the different techniques available for sampling nasal cells and describes expected changes in different disease processes. This information will aid in diagnosis when evaluating patients with rhinitis. Needless to say, nasal cytology is only an adjunctive tool in the diagnosis, and other methods such as history, physical examination, allergy skin tests, and in vitro serum antibody determinations remain the mainstay of diagnosis of diseases of the nose.

SAMPLING AND PROCESSING METHODS

There are several methods of obtaining nasal cells, and different techniques sample different compartments of the nasal mucosa and, consequently, different types of nasal cells. Many of these techniques are more useful for research than for clinical purposes, especially because some of the instruments needed for processing, such as centrifuges, are not available in a regular clinical setting. However, some of these techniques are simple, and nasal cells can be quantitated quickly in an office setting equipped with a microscope.

Blown Secretions

This consists of blowing nasal secretions onto wax paper or a plastic film, and the secretions are later placed on a glass slide. The cells obtained are only those present in nasal secretions, and this technique does not sample the epithelium or other layers of the nasal mucosa. Another disadvantage of this sampling technique is that

175

it is dependent on the presence of nasal secretions at the time of specimen acquisition. Thus, patients with scant nasal secretions will not be able to provide an adequate specimen for examination.

Nasal Smears

These are usually obtained with cotton-wool swabs moved along the nasal mucosa from the anterior to the posterior part of the nasal cavity. The swab is then smeared over a glass slide, and the specimen is fixed and stained. This technique samples cells from nasal secretions and the superficial portion of the nasal mucosa. The cellular yield is usually small and varies considerably; therefore, results should be interpreted with great care.[1] The best use for this technique is to determine the presence or absence of a specific cell type as a relative proportion of total cells.

Nasal Scrapings

For this technique, a specimen of nasal secretions and surface epithelium is obtained by using a plastic curette (Rhinoprobe, Apotex Scientific, Arlington, TX) to scrape the nasal mucosa under direct vision. The specimen is usually obtained from the medial surface of the inferior turbinate, and the procedure is relatively well tolerated without anesthesia. The scraping is then smeared on a slide, fixed, and stained. The advantages of this technique are the specificity of sampling site, ease of repetition, and adequacy of sampling in different disease states. The disadvantage is that the technique samples the epithelial layer but does not provide information about deeper layers of the nasal mucosa. The cell type of interest is quantitated as a percentage of the total cells counted.

Imprints

Initially, specimens were obtained by applying small, rounded glass slides on the nasal mucosa, but this method yielded very few cells.[2] The method was subsequently improved by using small, thin, plastic strips painted with 1% albumin to increase the adherence of cells.[3] These are introduced into the nasal cavity under direct vision and are gently pressed over a nasal mucosal surface, usually the septum. The strips are then fixed, stained, and examined under the microscope. A reasonable number of cells is usually obtained with this technique, and they are representative of nasal secretions and the epithelium. Disadvantages include the need to be manually dextrous and the presence on the slide of mucus from nasal secretions. Mucus is also present when smears and blown secretions are used, and it might hamper the interpretation of cellular elements because the mucopolysaccharides in the mucus are usually stained along with the cells.

Brush

Cells are harvested with a small brush made of plastic-coated steel wire with nylon bristles. This is introduced into the nasal cavity, under direct vision, between the nasal septum and the inferior turbinate and is rotated while being removed. The brush is then dipped into a buffer solution and carefully shaken so that the harvested cells are now in suspension. Because the volume of the suspension is known, the total number of cells can be determined with a hemocytometer. The cells are then cytocentrifuged (600 rpm for 6 minutes) on slides, fixed, and stained. The percentage of each cell type is then counted, and because the total number of cells is available, the total number of each cell type can be determined. Depending on the cellular yield, multiple slides can be obtained from this technique, and this allows staining with multiple reagents to enumerate different cell types (for example, one slide could be stained with a modified Wright's stain to enumerate eosinophils and polymorphonuclear cells and the other with alcian blue to enumerate mast cells and basophils). Cells can also be used for biochemical analysis, such as measurement of the histamine content of the cell pellet. Cells sampled by this technique are from nasal secretions, and the epithelial layer and the proportions of cells recovered in a study of asymptomatic allergic subjects were 45% epithelial cells, 38% granulocytes, 16% mononuclear cells, and 1% eosinophils with a coefficient of variation of the order of 40% for the proportions of cells harvested.[4] Mild, but very transient, discomfort is a disadvantage of this technique, and the number of cells obtained is limited by the capacity of the brush.

Nasal Lavage

This is performed by introducing 2.5 mL or 5 mL of buffer in each nostril while asking the patient to tilt the head back and close the soft palate against the posterior pharyngeal wall. Patients are asked to keep the solution in the nose for about 10 seconds, after which they bend the head forward and expel the lavage solution in a plastic receptacle. The recovered lavage is usually about 80% of the volume that was originally introduced into the nose[5] and contains both cells and biochemical mediators sampled from nasal secretions. The volume of the lavage is recorded, and the total number of cells is counted with a hemocytometer, thus it is possible to obtain the total number of cells collected. The lavage is then placed on ice until centrifugation at 5,000 rpm for 15 minutes at 4°C. The supernatant is decanted for the measurement of different biochemical mediators, and the cell pellet is resuspended in an adequate volume of buffer and cytospun onto one or more slides depending on the total number of cells. The cells are then dried, fixed, and stained with different reagents to allow enumeration of different types of cells. The percentage of each cell type is counted, and because the total number of cells is known, the total number of each cell type can be obtained. This technique has been described in detail[5] and used extensively as a research tool to elucidate changes in mediators[5–9] and cells[8,10] after nasal allergen provocation and during natural allergen exposure.[11] We use Ringer's lactate solution for the lavage and processing of cells because cellular morphology is better preserved with this buffer. Other physiologic buffers can also be used.

This technique samples cells in nasal secretions and offers the advantage of ease of performance, a high yield of cells, the possibility of measuring biochemical mediators, and the ease of repetition such that measurements can be undertaken at frequent intervals to follow the kinetics of cellular changes. Harvested cells can also be used for ex vivo studies. Nasal lavage does not allow sampling of deeper layers of the nasal mucosa and does not provide information about the localization of the obtained specimen because this technique samples both nasal cavities and the nasopharynx.

Biopsy

The most common site for nasal biopsy is the anterior, inferior edge of the inferior turbinate. This site is easily accessible, facilitating both the biopsy process and control of post-biopsy bleeding. Because the lining of the nasal mucosa changes from squamous epithelium most anteriorly to pseudostratified columnar ciliated respiratory epithelium in the middle and posterior parts of the nasal cavity, it is important to obtain biopsy specimens from similar anatomic sites when comparing biopsy specimens from different persons or when attempting to compare changes due to certain treatments in the same person. In preparation for the biopsy, the nasal mucosa is anesthetized by topical application of a decongestant (phenylephrine, oxymetazoline) followed by a local anesthetic (lidocaine, tetracaine). Further anesthesia is achieved by injecting the biopsy site with a solution of 1% lidocaine and 1:100,000 epinephrine. The biopsy specimen is obtained with a punch forceps, and post-biopsy bleeding is controlled with local application of silver nitrate. The tissue is preserved in various ways (embedded in medium and frozen, preserved in formaldehyde and embedded in paraffin, preserved in glutaraldehyde), depending on what staining procedure is going to be used (immunohistochemistry, hematoxylin-eosin stain, orcein-Giemsa stain) or what type of examination will be performed (light or electron microscopy). The major advantage of biopsy is that all the layers of the nasal mucosa are sampled from the superficial epithelium, basement membrane, and submucosa with the superficial vessels to the deeper layers that contain glands and larger vessels. Disadvantages include discomfort to the patient and the need for anesthesia, limitation of the number of specimens that can be obtained from the same person, and possible complications such as post-biopsy bleeding, pain, and synechiae formation.

Comparison of Different Sampling Techniques

Nose blowing and mucosal scraping were compared in adults with allergic rhinitis.[12] An adequate specimen could be obtained in 100% of the cases with the scraping technique but in only 60% to 66% of the cases with nose blowing. The concordance for the presence of eosinophils as assessed by the two methods was fair (67%), but basophils were noted more frequently in the scrapings than in the blown specimens (70% vs. 4%). Cellular findings from nasal mucosal scrapings have also been compared to those obtained from nasal lavages.[13] In patients with allergic rhinitis after allergen challenge, both techniques correlated significantly for increased percentage of eosinophils and neutrophils. In nonallergic patients, or allergic patients provoked with an irrelevant allergen, the correlation was not as good, probably due to the decreased number of cells collected. Nasal lavage and biopsy specimens obtained from allergic and nonallergic subjects 24 hours after allergen challenge have also been compared.[14] Although both techniques showed significant increases in the number of eosinophils in allergic subjects compared with subjects who had nonallergic rhinitis, mononuclear cells increased significantly in biopsy specimens but not lavage, and polymorphonuclear cells increased significantly in lavage but not in biopsy specimens. Furthermore, the predominant cell type in the nasal biopsy specimens from the allergic subjects was the mononuclear cell, but eosinophils and polymorphonuclear cells predominated in nasal lavages. This finding suggests that nasal secretions (sampled by lavage) and the nasal mucosa (sampled by biopsy) are two distinct compartments with different cellular predominance. Hence, it is always important to remember what is being sampled by the specific technique used, keeping in mind that different compartments of the nasal mucosa might have different functions.

Processing of Sample

Depending on the sampling technique used, cells are transferred onto glass slides directly, by smearing, or by cytospinning. Once the specimen is on a glass slide, it can be fixed with various reagents, including acetone, buffered formalin, methyl alcohol, and 95% ethyl alcohol. A specific stain is then used depending on the cell type that the investigator is interested in enumerating. Some of the commonly used stains are Hansel's (eosinophils), Wright's (basophils), Wright-Giemsa (eosinophils, neutrophils, and basophilic cells), toluidine blue (basophilic cells), and alcian blue (basophilic cells).

In a research setting, the author uses a modified Wright stain kit, which is available commercially (Diff-Quik Stain Set, Baxter Healthcare Corporation, Miami, FL) and consists of a fixative solution and two other dye solutions. Dried slides are immersed in each of these three solutions 5 times (each dip is 1 second in duration) and then rinsed with distilled or deionized water. The total duration of the staining is about 15 to 20 seconds. The slides are then allowed to dry, covered with a coverslip, and read with a light microscope under oil immersion and 1,000× magnification. Eosinophils are easily distinguished with this stain by their blue nucleus and cytoplasm and their red to red-orange cytoplasmic granules. Epithelial cells are easily identifiable because they are larger than granulocytes and have a dark-blue nucleus and an abundant light-blue cytoplasm. Polymorphonuclear cells are characterized by a dark-blue, multilobulated nucleus, pale-pink cytoplasm, and reddish lilac granules that are usually smaller than eosinophilic granules. It is usually difficult to distinguish between lymphocytes and monocytes because the differentiation is based on purely morphologic criteria. We have found it easier to lump all mononuclear cells into one category, and these cells usually have a violet nucleus and blue cytoplasm.

Cellular Quantitation

When nasal secretions are sampled from blown secretions, smears, scrapings, and imprints, the total number of cells cannot usually be obtained and the cell types are quantitated as a percentage of cells counted. Under 1,000× magnification, the examiner should count at least 100 cells (if more cells are available, one can count up to as many as 500) and assign a cell type to each of the cells counted. The result for each cell type is therefore a percentage. A semiquantitative method of evaluating nasal specimens is to count the different cells in each of 10 high-power fields (HPF) under 1,000× magnification and obtain the mean number of each cell type per HPF. Many investigators evaluate nasal specimens qualitatively and grade them on a scale from 0 to 4+ (Table 8–1). With the brush and lavage techniques, the cells are suspended in solution, and therefore the total number of cells harvested can be accurately estimated. The cells are then cytocentrifuged onto slides, 100 to 500 cells are counted, and the percentage of each cell count is obtained. In addition to percentage information, and because the total number of cells is known, the total number of each cell type harvested can be obtained. This information is important because although the percentage of a specific cell type might be different between two specimens, the total number of cells from this type might be unchanged because the total number of cells harvested was different between the two specimens. In nasal biopsy specimens, the total number of cells in a specific area of the submucosa should be counted. Grids and computer-assisted programs are available to enable an accurate estimate of the area counted. The cell types are then reported as number per unit of area (can be $0.5\,mm^2$ or $1\,mm^2$). For enumeration of intraepithelial cells,

Table 8–1   Qualitative Evaluation of Nasal Cytograms

CELL TYPE	ANALYSIS	GRADING
Eosinophils & neutrophils	None or rare	0
	Few scattered cells or small clumps	1+
	Moderate number of cells and larger clumps	2+
	Even larger clumps, but do not cover entire field	3+
	Large clumps of cells that cover the entire field	4+
Basophils	None or rare	0
	Few scattered cells	1+
	Moderate number of cells	2+
	Many cells easily seen	3+
	Large number of cells, up to 25 per high-power field	4+
Bacteria	None or rare	0
	Occasional clump	1+
	Moderate number	2+
	Many easily seen	3+
	Large numbers covering the entire field	4+

the number of cells in a certain length of epithelium is counted, and the cells are reported as number per length of epithelium (0.5 mm or 1 mm).

NASAL MUCOSAL CYTOLOGY IN DIFFERENT CLINICAL CONDITIONS

Normal Subjects

The mucosal cytology of normal subjects consists of numerous epithelial cells with a moderate number of neutrophils and possibly a few bacteria.[15,16] There are usually no, or very few, eosinophils and basophilic cells. Cohen et al.[17] examined samples obtained by scraping the anterior portion of the inferior turbinates of 22 asymptomatic infants whose ages ranged from 2 days to 12 months. Occasional basophils were found in 2 of 22 specimens and occasional eosinophils in 3 of 22. Fifty percent of the subjects had neutrophils in their cytology specimens, and an equal percentage had bacteria identified. The authors explained the presence of neutrophils and bacteria by contamination due to anterior sampling or by the fact that these findings are a reflection of the normal nasal flora. When sampling is from the most anterior portion of the nasal cavity, this is not a surprising finding.

Allergic Rhinitis

Nasal mucosal cytology has been studied extensively in patients with allergic rhinitis, both after allergen provocation and during natural pollen exposure. Sampling techniques used include nasal scrapings, smears, lavages, brush samples, and biopsies.

Cellular changes after allergen provocation

Bascom et al.[10] collected nasal secretions by nasal lavage hourly for several hours after antigen provocation and noted a slight initial increase in eosinophils within 1 to 2 hours of challenge, which was followed by a peak 6 to 8 hours later. Alcian blue-positive cells were also recovered in small (1% of recovered cells) but significantly increased numbers during the hours after allergen provocation; 68% of these cells were classified as basophils by light microscopic criteria. Polymorphonuclear cells and mononuclear cells also increased hours after allergen provocation (Fig. 8–1). Juliusson et al.[18] examined nasal inflammatory cellular influx by both lavaging of the nasal cavities and obtaining brush samples from the nasal mucosa hours after antigen challenge. They observed a rapid and significant increase in the number of eosinophils in the nasal mucosa of allergic subjects which was noted as early as 2 hours after challenge in the lavage specimens and 4 hours after challenge in the brush samples. There was an increase in the percentage of activated eosinophils (as assessed by cytoplasmic vacuolization) in brush samples which reached a peak 8 hours after provocation, and the basal values of eosinophils correlated significantly with symptoms of congestion, sneezing, and rhinorrhea observed after challenge. Metachromatic cells increased significantly 8 to 10 hours after allergen provocation

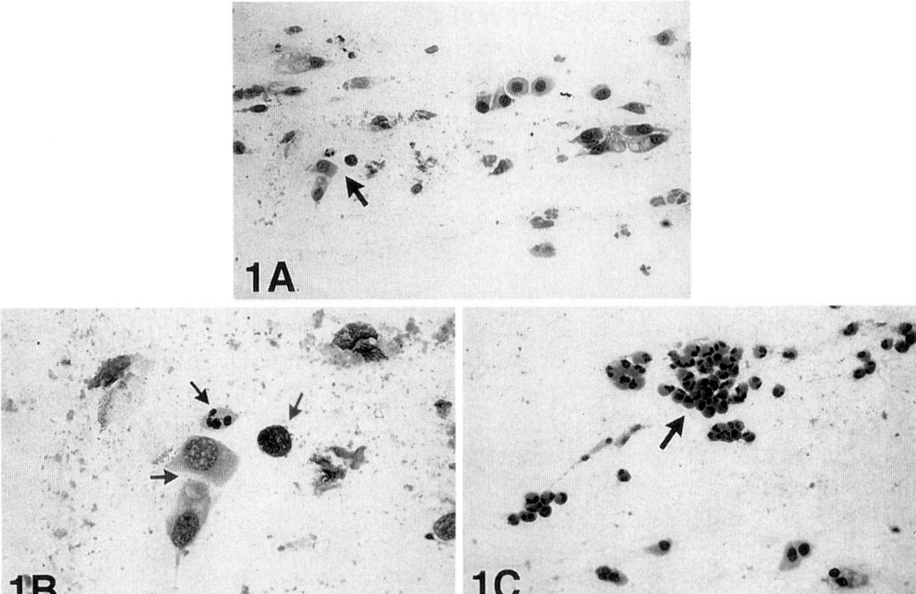

Figure 8–1.   This is a nasal cytologic specimen obtained by the scraping technique using a plastic curette. In this instance, specimen was obtained from an allergic individual 24 hours after allergen provocation. Panel A is seen under light microscopy with x80 magnification and shows several epithelial cells characterized by a large nucleus and a pale cytoplasm. The arrow points to a cluster composed of an eosinophil, a polymorphonuclear cell and two epithelial cells which are seen with greater detail in panel 1B. In panel 1B, the cells mentioned previously are now seen under x225 magnification using light microscopy. The arrow to the right points to an eosinophil characterized by a bilobed dark nucleus and multiple red granules in the cytoplasm. The arrow in the center points to a polymorphonuclear cell characterized by a multilobed nucleus and a lightly stained cytoplasm. Often times the cytoplasm of polymorphonuclear cells will have very light red or pink granules that are much less intensely stained and much fewer in number than the eosinophil granules. The arrow to the left points to two epithelial cells with the large nucleus and the pale cytoplasm. Panel 1C is seen under x128 magnification and shows a cluster of eosinophils as identified by the arrow. Some epithelial cells are seen in the lower right hand corner of the panel.

in brush samples and 8 to 12 hours after provocation in lavages of the nasal mucosa, with more metachromatic cells obtained by the brush technique. Light microscopic morphology and ultrastructural observations indicated that these cells were mast cells rather than blood basophils. Furthermore, the basal number of metachromatic cells in the nasal mucosa correlated significantly with sneezes and symptoms of congestion after antigen provocation, a finding suggesting that baseline metachromatic cell content of the nasal mucosa was a predictor of the extent of clinical symptoms generated after antigen provocation.

Nasal biopsy has also been used in investigations of cellular changes in subjects with allergic rhinitis after allergen provocation. Lim et al.[14] obtained biopsy specimens of the inferior turbinate before and 24 hours after challenging allergic subjects with allergen. There were significant increases in the number of eosinophils and mononuclear cells in nasal biopsy specimens of allergic subjects 24 hours after nasal provocation when compared with nonchallenged allergic subjects and normal, nonallergic controls (Fig. 8–2). Mononuclear cells were the predominant cells in the nasal mucosa of nonallergic subjects and allergic subjects both before and

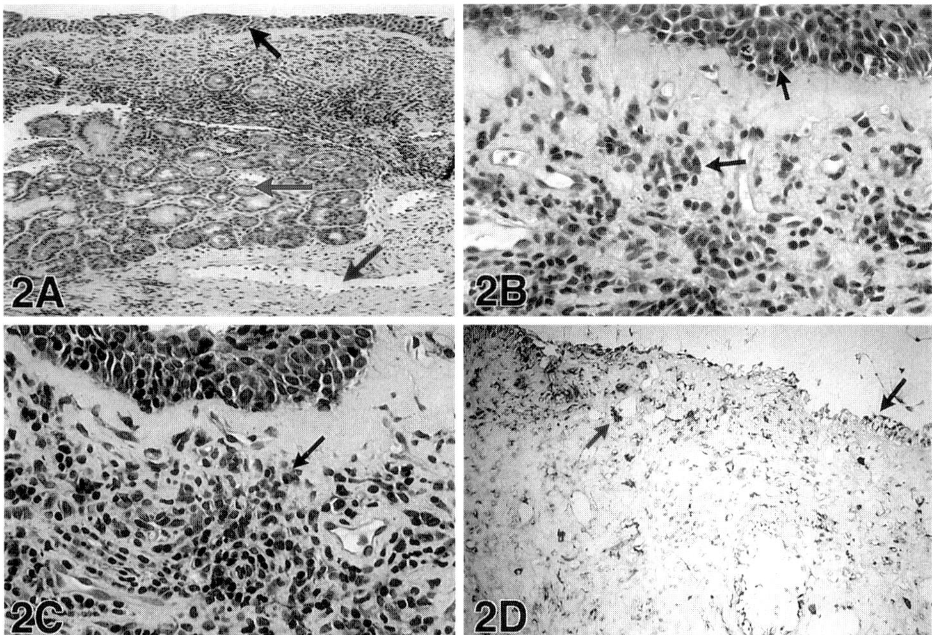

Figure 8–2. This figure shows biopsy specimens obtained from different allergic subjects 24 hours after allergen provocation and stained using different techniques. Panel 2A shows a biopsy specimen stained with hematoxylin and eosin (H&E) and examined using light microscopy at x40 magnification. The arrow at the top of the panel points to the superficial epithelial layer, the arrow in the middle to the glandular layer and the bottom arrow to the deepest layer of the mucosa which is rich in large blood vessels, one of which is seen at the tip of the arrow. The lamina propria is seen between the epithelial layer and the glandular layer and is notable for an abundant inflammatory cellular infiltrate. Panel 2B shows a similarly stained (H&E) specimen at x128 magnification. The top arrow points to an eosinophil within the epithelial layer. This is identified by red granules in the cytoplasm. The deeper arrow points to an eosinophil within the lamina propria. Other inflammatory cells seen are mononuclear cells with a single lobed nucleus and relatively scanty cytoplasm. These cells are either lymphocytes or monocytes and are the most abundant cell type in the nasal mucosa. Panel 2C shows a biopsy stained using the Orcein Giemsa stain which is also useful to visualize eosinophils. This specimen is examined under x128 magnification. Note several eosinophils in the lamina propria identified by red cytoplasmic granules (appearing darker than other cells in this picture). The arrow points to a representative cell. Panel 2D is stained using immunohistochemical techniques and an antibody against EG2 which identifies activated eosinophils. The specimen is examined using light microscopy and x100 magnification. Note the partially destroyed epithelial layer, a remnant of which is delineated by the top arrow. It is common for the epithelial layer not to be well preserved by freezing of the specimens prior to immunohistochemical staining. Also note that the specimen morphology is not as well delineated as in the other panels, a finding common with frozen specimens and immunohistochemical staining. Multiple activated eosinophils (EG2[+]) are seen in the lamina propria and a representative cell is delineated by the arrow to the left of the panel. The cytoplasm of these cells stain darker than other cells in the submucosa.

after allergen provocation. To examine the different types of mononuclear cells found in the nasal mucosa after antigen provocation, Varney et al.[19] used immunohistochemical staining to analyze nasal biopsy specimens obtained from allergic subjects 24 hours after challenge with either diluent or the relevant antigen. There were significant increases in the numbers of CD4[+] (T-helper) lymphocytes, CD25[+] (IL-2 receptor-bearing) cells, eosinophils (MBP[+]), and neutrophils (neutrophil elastase positive) after antigen challenge compared with challenge with the diluent solution. No significant changes were found in the numbers of CD45[+] cells (total leukocytes), CD3[+] cells (total lymphocytes), CD8[+] (T-suppressor) cells,

CD68[+] cells (macrophages), HLA-DR-positive cells, or tryptase-positive mast cells. The number of IL-2-receptor-bearing cells (CD25[+]) correlated positively with the numbers of CD3[+] and CD4[+] cells, a finding suggesting that CD25[+] cells were activated lymphocytes. To further support these observations, Hamid et al.[20] used double immunofluorescent staining to show that 60% to 100% of CD25[+] cells identified in the nasal mucosa 24 hours after antigen challenge were also CD3[+].

Cytokines are important proinflammatory substances in allergic diseases and have multiple functions that range from enhancing IgE synthesis to increasing recruitment and survival of inflammatory cells into sites of allergic inflammation. Durham et al.[21] obtained nasal biopsy specimens from allergic subjects 24 hours after local nasal provocation with either allergen or diluent and processed the tissues by in situ hybridization using RNA probes for IL (interleukin)-2, IL-3, IL-4, IL-5, granulocyte macrophage-colony stimulating factor (GM-CSF), and interferon-γ (IFN-γ) and by immunohistochemistry using a monoclonal antibody against EG2 to identify activated eosinophils. When the biopsy specimens obtained after allergen challenge were compared with those obtained at the site of diluent challenges, there were significant increases in cells bearing mRNA for IL-3, IL-4, IL-5, and GM-CSF but not for IL-2 and IFN-γ. Activated eosinophils (EG2+) increased significantly after allergen challenge (Fig. 8–2), and their numbers correlated positively with mRNA expression for IL-5, IL-4, GM-CSF, IL-3, and IL-2 but not IFN-γ. Ying et al.[22] developed a method of simultaneous immunocytochemistry and nonradiolabeled in situ hybridization and determined that most IL-5 mRNA[+] cells were also CD3[+] (83%) and the rest were positive for tryptase (16.4%). This finding suggests that T lymphocytes are a major contributor to IL-5 in nasal allergic reactions. This cytokine profile observed after allergen provocation supports the involvement of T_{H2}-type lymphocytes in the allergic reaction. Because IL-5 promotes the differentiation,[23] vascular adhesion,[24] and in vitro survival[25] of eosinophils and enhances histamine release from basophils,[26] and because IL-4 is a mast cell growth factor[27] and also promotes the switching of B cells to the production of IgE,[28] T_{H2}-like T cells are thought to be particularly important in allergic disease.

Bradding et al.[29] used immunocytochemistry with a monoclonal antibody against human IL-4 to identify this cytokine in nasal biopsy specimens obtained from patients with perennial allergic rhinitis. They detected positive staining for IL-4 in nasal mucosal cells and showed that 78% to 100% of the IL-4-positive cells were mast cells (tryptase positive). These data suggest that IL-4 is localized to mast cells in the nasal mucosa of subjects with perennial allergic rhinitis, but they do not provide solid proof that mast cells themselves are responsible for secretion of IL-4, because they could simply be storing the cytokine. The authors hypothesized that mast cells provide the initial burst of IL-4 that will enhance other cells such as T lymphocytes to keep on secreting this cytokine, thus perpetuating the inflammatory allergic reaction. Therefore, the important role of cytokines in allergic diseases is being increasingly recognized and supported by in vivo cytologic observations.

Cellular changes during natural allergen exposure

In separately conducted studies, Bryan and Bryan[30] and Okuda and Otsuka[31] observed basophilic cells in nasal secretions during seasonal pollen exposure of allergic persons. Ultrastructural and light microscopic studies of these cells suggested that most of them are identical to blood basophils.[32–34] In contrast to nasal secretions, which represent the most superficial compartment of the nasal mucosa, examination of nasal mucosal scrapings[34,35] or biopsy specimens,[34,36] which sample deeper layers, showed that most metachromatic cells in these compartments were mast cells. The mast cells were divided into two subpopulations, one located in the epithelium and the other located deeper, in the lamina propria.[37] Unlike allergic subjects in season, nonallergic subjects had fewer basophilic cells in nasal secretions and few mast cells in the mucosa.[33,34]

Enerback et al.,[36] using biopsy specimens and cytologic imprints to examine the cellular content of the nasal mucosa during the birch pollen season in Sweden, showed a seasonal increase in mast cell number on the surface of the nasal epithelium after 4 or 5 days of pollen exposure. Because the overall number of mast cells in the nasal mucosa remained unchanged, they suggested that seasonal exposure led to migration of mast cells from the deeper layers of the lamina propria to the epithelium. Bentley et al.[38] reported a similar significant increase in intraepithelial tryptase-positive mast cells in nasal biopsy specimens obtained from allergic subjects during the pollen season compared with preseasonal biopsy specimens and nonallergic controls. They also observed significant seasonal increases in total (MBP^+) and activated ($EG2^+$) eosinophils in the submucosa of these allergic patients. The consensus of most studies is that basophils predominate in nasal secretions, whereas mast cells are more abundant in the epithelium and lamina propria of allergic subjects exposed to antigen either experimentally or naturally. Unlike changes after antigen provocation, there were no significant increases in $CD45^+$, $CD3^+$, $CD4^+$, $CD8^+$, $CD25^+$, or $CD68^+$ cells or neutrophils in the nasal submucosa during the season in the study by Bentley et al. This finding might be related to the lower dose of antigen that allergic patients are exposed to during the season compared with the amount used during experimental provocation.

From the above-described studies, it is clear that eosinophils and basophilic cells increase in nasal secretions and the submucosa of allergic patients after exposure to allergen and that mononuclear cells increase in the nasal mucosa. Because most clinically useful sampling techniques involve examining nasal secretions, an increase in eosinophils and basophilic cells is going to be of most help in detecting patients with allergic rhinitis in a clinical setting. Indeed, studies sampling nasal secretions and examining them for eosinophilia have shown variable detection rates in allergic subjects: 50%,[39] 69%,[40] 81%,[41] 90%,[42] and 100%.[43] Depending on the area of the nasal mucosa sampled, basophilic cells can represent either basophils (in nasal secretions) or mast cells (in the submucosa). These cells are also frequently found in subjects with allergic rhinitis, although to a lesser extent than eosinophils, and their number correlates well with nasal eosinophilia in allergic rhinitis.[31]

Nonallergic Rhinitis

This term can be applied to any chronic condition of the nose characterized by nasal obstruction, sneezing, and rhinorrhea without evidence of an allergic cause. Affected patients have negative skin tests or radioallergosorbent test (RAST), and their symptoms are not related to exposure to any identifiable allergen. One must also exclude several other reasons for rhinitis, including pregnancy, the rebound congestion induced by prolonged use of intranasal decongestants (rhinitis medicamentosa), mechanical causes of nasal obstruction (septal deviation), systemic medication intake (vasodilator antihypertensives, reserpine, oral contraceptives, and antidepressants), topical ophthalmic treatment with β-adrenergic blockers, and the triad of aspirin sensitivity, asthma, and nasal polyposis. Patients with none of these conditions and rhinitis are often labeled as having vasomotor rhinitis and can have exacerbation of their symptoms due to climatic changes or exposure to irritants. Most of these patients will have no increases in either eosinophils or basophilic cells in nasal specimens.[44]

About one-fourth of patients with nonallergic chronic rhinitis have characteristic eosinophilia in their nasal secretions; this condition is termed the "nonallergic rhinitis with eosinophilia syndrome" (NARES). This can occur in patients of any age and presents with chronic nasal symptoms and marked eosinophilia in nasal secretions but no identifiable allergic cause. Jacobs et al.[45] described 52 patients with symptoms of paroxysms of sneezing, and a clear, watery rhinorrhea was dominant in more than 75%. There was no identifiable seasonal pattern, and the symptoms were usually perennial with no prolonged symptom-free periods. Intradermal skin tests were negative in 95% of the patients, and no patient had a positive intradermal skin test to any perennial allergen. All patients demonstrated more than 20% eosinophilia on nasal smears. Nasal secretions and nasal lavages were also collected, and the eosinophil percentages ranged from 19% to 66% in nasal secretions and from 7% to 74% in nasal lavage samples. The presence of eosinophilia in nasal secretions warrants treatment with intranasal steroids, which are usually more effective than in nonallergic rhinitis without eosinophils.

Rhinitis Induced by Exposure to Irritants and Environmental Pollutants

Several environmental irritants can induce symptoms in otherwise healthy subjects and can aggravate symptoms of existing allergic or nonallergic rhinitis. Certain patients complain of cold air-induced rhinitis, and this condition is often referred to as skier's nose. Togias et al.[46] mimicked this response in the laboratory by challenging cold air-sensitive subjects with cold-dry air for 15 minutes: They reported increases in symptoms and levels of inflammatory mediators in these subjects as opposed to non-cold-air-sensitive persons. These patients have a significant increase in the number of epithelial cells in nasal lavages after challenge, a finding suggesting that the stimulus leads to epithelial cell dessication and detachment.[47] Formaldehyde, another upper airway irritant, leads to occasional epithelial metaplasia and dysplasia.[48] Challenging healthy volunteers with 0.4 ppm ozone with exercise for 2 hours resulted in a significant increase in the number of neutrophils in nasal lavage immediately after exposure and 18 hours later.[49]

Rhinosinusitis

Several studies have been conducted to evaluate the effect of bacterial rhinosinusitis on the nasal mucosa, and some of these have also attempted to address the usefulness of nasal cytology in the diagnosis of the disorder. Petruson and Hansson[50] obtained nasal biopsy specimens from 12 children with severe and frequent respiratory tract infections and continuous nasal drainage and examined mucosal changes by transmission and scanning electron microscopy. Secretions obtained from the nasal floor and nasopharynx in these children showed a combination of *Haemophilus influenzae, Branhamella catarrhalis*, and *Streptococcus pneumoniae* in 9 of the 12 children. The main finding of the study was the high frequency of damage, not only to the epithelium (decreased ciliated cells, discontinuous epithelial layer, missing epithelial cells) but also to the basement membrane (thicker basement membrane than normal) and underlying structures (increased vascularization and submucosal glands, clusters of bacteria and inflammatory cells penetrating the basal membrane and extending into the submucosa). The dominant inflammatory cells in most biopsy specimens were lymphocytes and plasma cells. The study therefore suggests a significant alteration in the nasal mucosa and submucosa of patients with recurrent bacterial infections as visualized by electron microscopy. However, these changes might be too subtle for detection by the more crude methods of nasal cytology, which mostly examine surface secretion cells under light microscopy.

Several studies have evaluated the role of nasal cytology in predicting the presence of sinusitis as gauged by abnormal radiographs. Wilson et al.[51] reported a 79% correlation between nasal cytologic findings (nasal scraping considered positive if there was more than 1 neutrophil/HPF with bacteria present) and radiographic findings (positive in the presence of asymmetry, mucoperiosteal thickening, opacification, or air-fluid levels as assessed by the radiologist) in 55 patients with acute and chronic sinusitis. When the cytologic examination showed more than 6 neutrophils/HPF, the radiograph was positive in 90% of cases. In another study, nasal cytologic results and sinus radiographs, obtained at the time of initial clinical evaluation, were correlated in 300 children and adults with allergic rhinitis.[52] Radiographs were significantly more likely to be positive when nasal cytologic specimens contained more than 5 neutrophils/HPF or more than 5 eosinophils/HPF. The presence of 25 neutrophils/HPF was 86% sensitive and 40% specific for predicting radiographic abnormalities. Although the cytologic findings were sensitive, they were not very specific as predictors of radiologic disease; therefore, the authors concluded that nasal cytology should not be considered an adequate alternative to sinus radiography.

Meltzer et al.[53] recently obtained nasal scrapings from 51 allergy clinic patients 14 years of age or older who had sinusitis defined by symptoms and positive radiographic findings (at least 6 mm of maxillary mucosal thickening, opacification or an air-fluid level). The nasal scrapings showed eosinophils in 78%, basophilic cells in 41%, neutrophils in 90%, and bacteria in 24% of the patients. The percentage of eosinophils, basophilic cells, and bacteria were not different from those in patients with seasonal or perennial allergic rhinitis, and this finding was not surprising because the majority of the patients studied had allergic rhinitis. However, the high frequency of neutrophils in these patients (90%) was higher than that found in subjects with allergic rhinitis (60% to 70%).

Among the different inflammatory cells, the number of neutrophils in nasal secretions seems to be most significantly correlated with the diagnosis of sinusitis, as is the presence of bacteria. However, these studies should be interpreted with caution for several reasons: (1) plain sinus radiographs were used to establish the diagnosis of sinusitis, and it is now well known (from comparisons with computed tomography scans) that plain radiographs can often give false positive or false negative results, especially in the pediatric age group; (2) none of the studies included a control group for comparison; (3) neutrophils are also increased in the nasal secretions of subjects with allergic rhinitis and after exposure to irritants; and (4) many patients with clinically and radiographically confirmed sinusitis do not have bacteria in their nasal specimens.[53] Therefore, nasal cytology should be considered only an adjunctive tool in the diagnosis of sinusitis, and it certainly should not replace proper history, physical examination, and radiographic tests.

In viral infections affecting the nasal mucosa, ciliated epithelial cells undergo destructive changes (ciliocytophthoria), which include clumping of nuclear chromatin and margination of the pyknotic chromatin mass, halo formation around the nucleus, increased granulation of the cytoplasm, constriction of the ciliated cell, and separation of the nucleus-containing basal portion from the ciliated apical portion.[54] Winther et al.[55] examined scrape biopsy specimens from rhinovirus-infected volunteers and compared the changes to these in sham-inoculated individuals. The number of polymorphonuclear leukocytes in the nasal epithelium of the infected subjects was significantly increased early in the course of the cold compared with the baseline number before infection and with the number in sham-infected subjects. In their studies, polymorphonuclear leukocytes increased in nasal secretions in both the virus-infected and the sham-inoculated groups as a result of the repeated trauma during sampling, and therefore no conclusions could be drawn relating to cellular changes in nasal secretions. Naclerio et al. challenged volunteers with rhinovirus and obtained nasal lavages at 4-hour intervals for 5 days after challenge. Subjects who became infected (shed virus in nasal secretions or had a fourfold or more increase in serum antibody titer) and symptomatic had a significant increase in the number of neutrophils in nasal lavages compared with the number in the control group.[56]

Cytologic Changes in Therapeutic Intervention

In addition to its importance in the diagnosis of different nasal disorders, nasal cytology is often useful for evaluating and documenting response to treatment, especially in the context of clinical studies. This use has been largely true for patients with allergic rhinitis. Among the treatments available for allergic rhinitis, antihistamines and anticholinergic agents have no effect on nasal cytologic findings of increased eosinophils and basophilic cell.[57–60] Cromolyn sodium treatment results in significant reductions in the numbers of eosinophils but not basophilic cells or neutrophils.[59,61] Treatment with topical intranasal steroids leads to significant reduc-

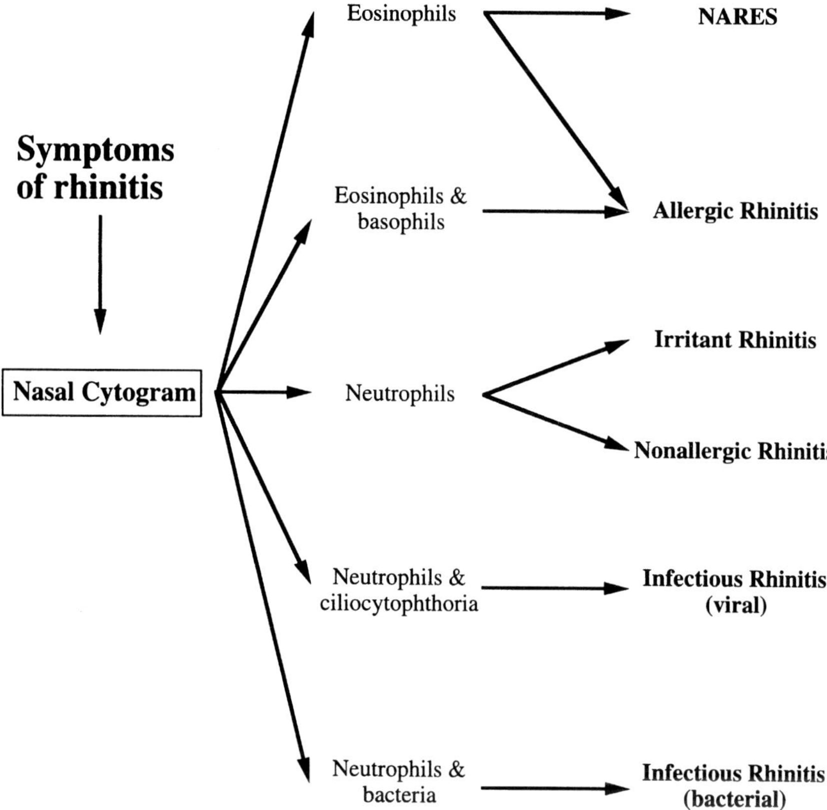

Figure 8–3.   A guide to the diagnosis of rhinologic disorders using nasal cytology. The cytogram is usually obtained by the scraping, brush, smear, or blown secretion methods. The cells listed are the distinctive cell types for each disease. Most cytograms, especially if obtained by scraping, brush, or smear techniques, have a large proportion of epithelial cells. The distinctive cell types, however, guide the clinician to favor one diagnosis over the others. Nasal cytology alone is not considered sufficient to establish any of these diagnoses, and a history, physical examination, and other laboratory tests (such as in vivo and in vitro allergy tests) are essential. For example, the diagnosis of nonallergic rhinitis with eosinophilia syndrome (NARES) cannot be made until IgE-mediated allergic causes have been ruled out by skin testing or in vitro serum IgE determinations.

tions in eosinophils, neutrophils, and basophilic cells in nasal secretions during the late-phase response after allergen challenge[10] and during natural allergic exposure.[41,61–63]

CONCLUSION

Nasal cytology is a useful tool in the study of nasal disorders. Information can be obtained with different sampling techniques, which should be carefully selected depending on the aim of the investigation. In a clinical setting, nasal swabs, scrapings, and blown secretions are probably the least traumatic and therefore preferred methods of sampling. Several stains can then be easily and rapidly performed to obtain information about the types of inflammatory cells in nasal secretions (Fig. 8–3). This technique is most useful in the acutely ill patient in whom the differential diagnosis includes allergic or infectious rhinitis. Numerous eosinophils help the clinician make the diagnosis of allergic rhinitis, and numerous polymorphonuclear cells suggest an infectious cause. Treatment can then be delivered accordingly. Another use in the clinic is in the patient with NARES, in whom a skin test for common allergens will be negative but a nasal smear will demonstrate numerous eosinophils. It is important to identify patients with this disorder because they will respond well to intranasal corticosteroids. The use of nasal smears might be helpful in the diagnosis of sinusitis, but it by no means replaces careful history and physical and radiographic examinations.

In a research setting, obtaining information about the cellular infiltration of different compartments of the nasal mucosa with the different sampling techniques described can prove very useful. In addition to elucidating pathophysiologic mechanisms, it can provide information on the effects of different available treatments on nasal inflammation and help gauge their efficacy.

REFERENCES

1. Pipkorn U, Enerback L: Nasal mucosal mast cells and histamine in hay fever: effect of topical glucocorticosteroid treatment. *Int Arch Allergy Appl Immunol* 1987; 84:123–128.
2. Mygind N, Thomsen J: Cytology of the nasal mucosa. A comparative study between a replica-method and a smear-method. *Arch Klin Exp Ohren Nasen Kehlkopfheilkd* 1973; 204:123–129.
3. Pipkorn U, Enerback L: A method for the preparations of imprints from the nasal mucosa. *J Immunol Methods* 1984; 73:133–137.
4. Pipkorn U, Karlsson G, Enerback L: A brush method to harvest cells from the nasal mucosa for microscopic and biochemical analysis. *J Immunol Methods* 1988; 112:37–42.
5. Naclerio RM, Meier HL, Kagey-Sobotka A, et al: Mediator release after airway challenge with allergen. *Am Rev Respir Dis* 1983; 128:597–602.
6. Baumgarten CR, Nichols RC, Naclerio RM, Proud D: Concentration of glandular kallikrein in human nasal secretions increases during experimentally induced allergic rhinitis. *J Immunol* 1986; 137:1323–1328.
7. Creticos PS, Peters SP, Adkinson NF Jr, et al: Peptide leukotriene release after antigen challenge in patients sensitive to ragweed. *N Engl J Med* 1984; 310:1626–1630.
8. Bascom R, Pipkorn U, Proud D, et al: Major basic protein and eosinophil-derived neurotoxin concentrations in nasal-lavage fluid after antigen challenge: effect of systemic corticosteroids and relationship to eosinophil influx. *J Allergy Clin Immunol* 1989; 84:338–346.
9. Shin MH, Averill FJ, Hubbard WC, et al: Nasal allergen challenge generates 1-O-hexadecyl-2-lyso-sn-glycero-3-phosphocholine. *Am J Respir Crit Care Med* 1994; 149:660–666.
10. Bascom R, Wachs M, Naclerio RM, Pipkorn U, Galli SJ, Lichtenstein LM: Basophil influx occurs after nasal antigen challenge: effects of topical corticosteroid pretreatment. *J Allergy Clin Immunol* 1988; 81:580–589.
11. Pipkorn U, Karlsson G, Enerback L: The cellular response of the human allergic mucosa to natural allergen exposure. *J Allergy Clin Immunol* 1988; 82:1046–1054.
12. Welch MJ, Meltzer EO, Kemp JP, Orgel HA, Ostrom NK, Jalowayski AA: Comparison of two different techniques for obtaining specimens for nasal cytology: nose-blowing vs nasal mucosal scraping (abstract). *J Allergy Clin Immunol* 1991; 87:144.
13. Piacentini GL, Kaulbach HC, Scott T, White MV, Kaliner MA: Correlation between inflammatory cell responses in nasal mucosal scrapings and lavages after allergen challenge (abstract). *J Allergy Clin Immunol* 1991; 87:145.
14. Lim MC, Taylor RH, Naclerio RM: The histology of allergic rhinitis and its comparison to cellular changes in nasal lavage. *Am J Respir Crit Care Med* 1995; 151:136–144.
15. Bryan MP, Bryan WTK: Cytologic diagnosis in allergic disorders. *Otolaryngol Clin North Am* 1974; 7:637–666.
16. Bickmore JT: Nasal cytology in allergy and infection. *J Cont Educ ORL Allergy* 1978; 40:39–46.
17. Cohen GA, MacPherson GA, Golembesky HE, Jalowayski AA, O'Connor RD: Normal nasal cytology in infancy. *Ann Allergy* 1985; 54:112–114.

18. Juliusson S, Pipkorn U, Karlsson G, Enerback L: Mast cells and eosinophils in the allergic mucosal response to allergen challenge: changes in distribution and signs of activation in relation to symptoms. *J Allergy Clin Immunol* 1992; 90:898–909.

19. Varney VA, Jacobson MR, Sudderick RM, et al: Immunohistology of the nasal mucosa following allergen-induced rhinitis: identification of activated T lymphocytes, eosinophils, and neutrophils. *Am Rev Respir Dis* 1992; 146:170–176.

20. Hamid Q, Barkans J, Robinson DS, Durham SR, Kay AB: Co-expression of CD25 and CD3 in atopic allergy and asthma. *Immunology* 1992; 75:659–663.

21. Durham SR, Ying S, Varney VA, et al: Cytokine messenger RNA expression for IL-3, IL-4, IL-5, and granulocyte/macrophage-colony-stimulating factor in the nasal mucosa after local allergen provocation: relationship to tissue eosinophilia. *J Immunol* 1992; 148:2390–2394.

22. Ying S, Hamid Q, Barkans J, Moqbel R, Durham SR, Kay AB: Phenotype of cells expressing interleukin-5 mRNA in the nasal mucosa after local allergen provocation (abstract). *J Allergy Clin Immunol* 1993; 91:252.

23. Clutterbuck EJ, Hirst EMA, Sanderson CJ: Human interleukin-5 (IL-5) regulates the production of eosinophils in human bone marrow cultures: comparison and interaction with IL-1, IL-3, IL-6, and GM-CSF. *Blood* 1989; 73:1504–1512.

24. Walsh GM, Hartnell A, Wardlaw AJ, Kurihara K, Sanderson CJ, Kay AB: IL-5 enhances the in vitro adhesion of human eosinophils, but not neutrophils, in a leucocyte integrin (CD 11/18)-dependent manner. *Immunology* 1990; 71:258–265.

25. Lopez AF, Sanderson CJ, Gamble JR, Campbell HD, Young IG, Vadas MA: Recombinant human interleukin-5 is a selective activator of human eosinophil function. *J Exp Med* 1988; 167:219–224.

26. Hirai K, Yamaguchi M, Misaki Y, et al: Enhancement of human basophil histamine release by interleukin 5. *J Exp Med* 1990; 172:1525–1528.

27. Saito H, Hatake K, Dvorak AM, et al: Selective differentiation and proliferation of hematopoietic cells induced by recombinant human interleukins. *Proc Natl Acad Sci USA* 1988; 85:2288–2292.

28. Del Prete G, Maggi E, Parronchi P, et al: IL-4 is an essential factor for the IgE synthesis induced in vitro by human T cell clones and their supernatants. *J Immunol* 1988; 140:4193–4198.

29. Bradding P, Feather IH, Howarth PH, et al: Interleukin 4 is localized to and released by human mast cells. *J Exp Med* 1992; 176:1381–1386.

30. Bryan WTK, Bryan MP: Significance of mast cells in nasal secretions. *Trans Am Acad Ophthalmol Otolaryngol* 1959; 63:613–627.

31. Okuda M, Otsuka H: Basophilic cells in allergic nasal secretions. *Arch Otorhinolaryngol* 1977; 214:283–289.

32. Okuda M, Kawabori S, Otsuka H: Electron microscope study of basophilic cells in allergic nasal secretions. *Arch Otorhinolaryngol* 1978; 221:215–220.

33. Hastie R, Heroy JH III, Levy DA: Basophil leukocytes and mast cells in human nasal secretions and scrapings studied by light microscopy. *Lab Invest* 1979; 40:554–561.

34. Okuda M, Ohtsuka H, Kawabori S: Basophil leukocytes and mast cells in the nose. *Eur J Respir Dis* 1983; Suppl 128:7–14.

35. Otsuka H, Denburg J, Dolovich J, et al: Heterogeneity of metachromatic cells in the human nose: significance of mucosal mast cells. *J Allergy Clin Immunol* 1985; 76:695–702.

36. Enerback L, Pipkorn U, Granerus G: Intraepithelial migration of nasal mucosal mast cells in hay fever. *Int Arch Allergy Appl Immunol* 1986; 80:44–51.

37. Okuda M, Sakaguchi Y, Suzuki F, et al: Ultrastructural heterogeneity of the basophilic cells in the allergic nasal mucosa. *Ann Allergy* 1985; 54:152–157.

38. Bentley AM, Jacobson MR, Cumberworth V, et al: Immunohistology of the nasal mucosa in seasonal allergic rhinitis: increases in activated eosinophils and epithelial mast cells. *J Allergy Clin Immunol* 1992; 89:877–883.

39. Vaheri E: Nasal allergy with special reference to eosinophilia and histopathology. *Acta Allergol* 1956; 10:203–211.

40. Miller RE, Paradise JL, Friday GA, et al: The nasal smear for eosinophils: Its value in children with seasonal allergic rhinitis. *Am J Dis Child* 1982; 136:1009–1011.

41. Meltzer EO, Orgel HA, Bronsky EA, et al: A dose-ranging study of fluticasone propionate aqueous nasal spray for seasonal allergic rhinitis assessed by symptoms, rhinomanometry, and nasal cytology. *J Allergy Clin Immunol* 1990; 86:221–230.

42. Kaufman HS, Rosen I, Shaposhnikov N, Wai M: Nasal eosinophilia. *Ann Allergy* 1982; 49:270–271.

43. Lans DM, Alfano N, Rocklin R: Nasal eosinophilia in allergic and nonallergic rhinitis: usefulness of the nasal smear in the diagnosis of allergic rhinitis. *Allergy Proc* 1989; 10:275–280.

44. Elwany S, Bumsted R: Ultrastructural observations on vasomotor rhinitis. *ORL J Otorhinolaryngol* 1987; 49:199–205.

45. Jacobs RL, Freedman PM, Boswell RN: Nonallergic rhinitis with eosinophilia (NARES syndrome): Clinical and immunologic presentation. *J Allergy Clin Immunol* 1981; 67:253–262.

46. Togias AG, Naclerio RM, Proud D, et al: Nasal challenge with cold, dry air results in the production of inflammatory mediators: possible mast cell involvement. *J Clin Invest* 1985; 76:1375–1381.

47. Cruz AA, Naclerio RM, Proud D, et al: Epithelial cell detachment is observed during the nasal reaction to cold, dry air (CDA) (abstract). *J Allergy Clin Immunol* 1991; 87:147.

48. Boysen M, Zadig E, Digernes V, et al: Nasal mucosa in workers exposed to formaldehyde: a pilot study. *Br J Indust Med* 1990; 47:116–121.

49. Graham DE, Koren HS: Biomarkers of inflammation in ozone-exposed humans. Comparison of the nasal and bronchoalveolar lavage. *Am Rev Respir Dis* 1990; 142:152–156.

50. Petruson B, Hansson HA: Nasal mucosal changes in children with frequent infections. *Arch Otolaryngol Head Neck Surg* 1987; 113:1294–1300.

51. Wilson NW, Jalowayski AA, Hamburger RN: A comparison of nasal cytology with sinus x-rays for the diagnosis of sinusitis. *Am J Rhinol* 1988; 2:55–59.

52. Gill FF, Neiburger JB: The role of nasal cytology in the diagnosis of chronic sinusitis. *Am J Rhinol* 1989; 3:13–15.

53. Meltzer EO, Orgel HA, Jalowayski AA: Cytology, in Mygind N, Naclerio RM (eds.): *Allergic and Non-allergic Rhinitis. Clinical Aspects.* Copenhagen, Munksgaard, 1993, pp 66–81.

54. Bryan WTK, Bryan MP, Smith CA: Human ciliated epithelial cells in nasal secretions. Morphologic and histochemical aspects. *Ann Otol Rhinol Laryngol* 1964; 73:474–487.

55. Winther B, Farr B, Turner RB, et al: Histopathologic examination and enumeration of polymorphonuclear leukocytes in the nasal mucosa during experimental rhinovirus colds. *Acta Otolaryngol (Stockh)* Suppl 1984; 413:19–24.

56. Naclerio RM, Proud D, Lichtenstein LM, et al: Kinins are generated during experimental rhinovirus colds. *J Infect Dis* 1988; 157:133–142.

57. Klementsson H, Andersson M, Pipkorn U: Allergen-induced increase in nonspecific nasal reactivity is blocked by antihistamines without a clear-cut relationship to eosinophil influx. *J Allergy Clin Immunol* 1990; 86:466–472.

58. Howarth PH, Wilson SJ, Brewster H: The influence of cetirizine on symptom generation and nasal eosinophilia in seasonal allergic rhinitis (abstract). *J Allergy Clin Immunol* 1991; 87:151.

59. Orgel HA, Meltzer EO, Kemp JP, et al: Comparison of intranasal cromolyn sodium, 4%, and oral terfenadine for allergic rhinitis: symptoms, nasal cytology, nasal ciliary clearance, and rhinomanometry. *Ann Allergy* 1991; 66:237–244.

60. Meltzer EO, Orgel HA, Bronsky EA, et al: Ipratropium bromide aqueous nasal spray for patients with perennial allergic rhinitis: a study of its effect on their symptoms, quality of life, and nasal cytology. *J Allergy Clin Immunol* 1992; 90:242–249.

61. Okuda M, Otsuka H, Sakaguchi K, et al: Effect of anti-allergic treatment on nasal surface basophilic metachromatic cells in allergic rhinitis. *Allergy Proc* 1989; 10:23–26.

62. Holopainen E, Malmberg H, Tarkiainen E: Experiences of treating allergic rhinitis with intra-nasal beclomethasone dipropionate: short-term trials and long-term follow-up. *Acta Allergol* 1977; 32:263–277.

63. Orgel HA, Meltzer EO, Kemp JP, Welch MJ: Clinical, rhinomanometric, and cytologic evaluation of seasonal allergic rhinitis treated with beclomethasone dipropionate as aqueous nasal spray or pressurized aerosol. *J Allergy Clin Immunol* 1986; 77:858–864.

9

Nasal Allergy Testing

HOLLY H. BIRDSALL, M.D., Ph.D.

Allergy testing can provide the clinician with very useful information regarding atopic disease, that is, disease mediated by IgE antibodies. Allergy tests measure the sensitivity of patients to specific allergens. Either in vitro or in vivo methods can be used. In vitro tests can measure the total quantity of IgE in the serum and circulating IgE antibodies specific for allergens. Allergens also can be added to patient blood samples to determine whether basophils release histamine in vitro. In vivo tests use specific allergenic substances to elicit physiologic responses. Two types of responses are measured: cutaneous reaction to allergens introduced into the superficial skin or provocation of allergic rhinitis symptoms by allergens introduced into either the nose or the gastrointestinal tract.

There are two reasons for performing allergy tests: patient education and immunotherapy. The physician should not pass up the opportunity to point to a floridly positive skin test on the patient's arm and discuss what the same allergen is doing to the upper respiratory tract each day. The ways in which the physician plans to use the information from allergy tests largely dictates when testing will be used and which mode of testing will be selected. This chapter discusses how the different tests are performed, how they are interpreted in the clinical setting, and how one selects among the different methods available.

TESTING TECHNIQUES

In Vitro Methods

Total serum IgE

Even though IgE levels may be elevated in significant numbers of patients with multisystem atopic disease, and a markedly elevated serum IgE level in a sympto-matic child may predict atopic disease,[1] the usefulness of total IgE measurements is limited. The normal range for adults is wide, and normal values for children are highly age-dependent. IgE levels are elevated in only 30% to 40% of adults with symptomatic allergic rhinitis,[2] and there is no clear diagnostic "cutoff" for those with allergic disease.

Allergen-specific IgE

RAST (radioallergosorbent test), MAST (multiple allergosorbent test), and FAST (fluoroallergosorbent test) are but some of the names given to tests that measure allergen-specific IgE in serum. The underlying principle is the same in all of the tests (Fig. 9–1). The allergen is immobilized on some surface, such as a polystyrene bead, a paper disk, a thread, or a plastic dish. Dilute serum is added, and specific IgE

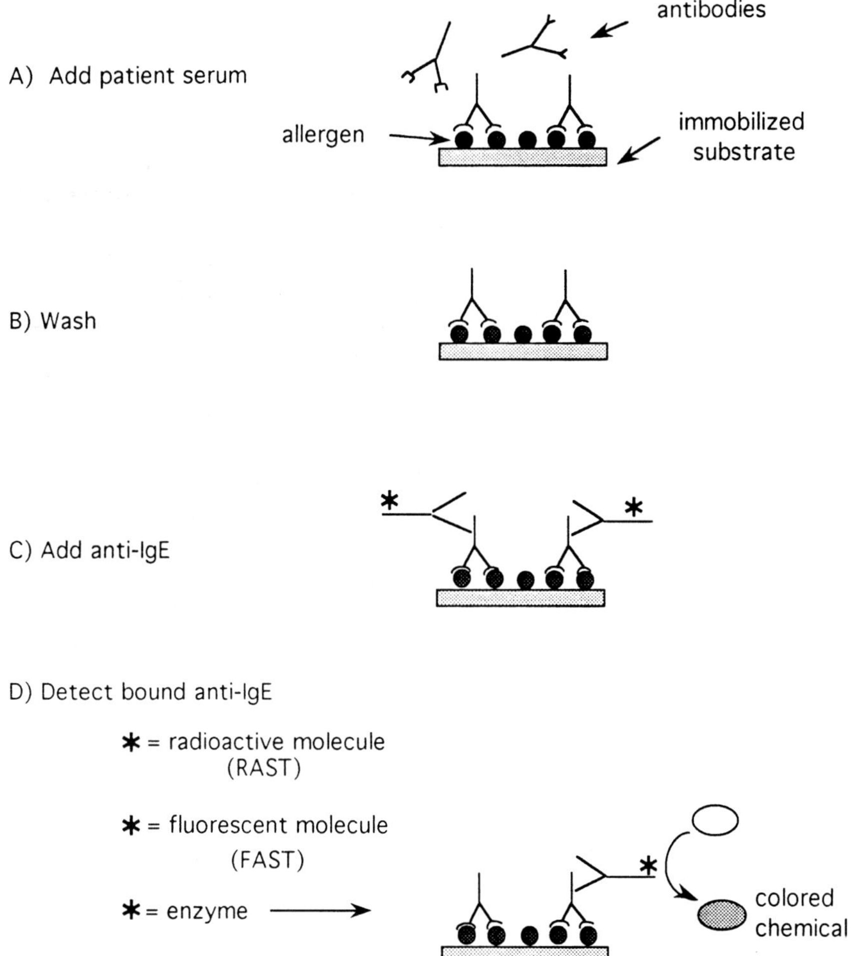

Figure 9–1. In vitro tests for specific IgE antibodies. *A*, Serum is added to allergen immobilized on a substrate; specific antibodies bind to the allergen. *B*, Nonspecific immunoglobulin is washed away. *C*, A secondary antibody specific for human IgE reacts with IgE antibodies that have bound to the allergen. The anti-IgE antibody has been chemically linked to a radioactive molecule, a fluorescent molecule, or an enzyme so that it can be quantified. *D*, Enzyme-linked anti-IgE antibodies are detected by addition of a substrate that changes color when acted on by the enzyme.

molecules are allowed to bind to the allergen. The surface is then washed to remove unbound IgE, and a secondary antibody specific for human IgE, which has been prepared in mice, goats, or rabbits, is then added. These anti-IgE antibodies attach to the patient's IgE antibodies bound to the immobilized allergen. The uptake of these secondary anti-IgE antibodies can be detected because these antibodies have been tagged with a radioactive element, a fluorescent molecule, or an enzyme that converts a substrate into a colored reagent. The commercially available tests seem to have similar accuracy[3-7] for most but not all allergens. Accuracy may vary among laboratories,[8] but a voluntary interlaboratory proficiency survey conducted by the College of American Pathologists found good agreement among the participating laboratories.[9]

Patients with greatly elevated quantities of total IgE may have enough nonspecific binding of IgE that their test results are weakly positive for specific allergens. In the survey of commercial testing laboratories,[9] the area of greatest inconsistency was the tendency of some laboratories to report weakly positive RAST results in sera that had high total IgE but lacked specific IgE antibodies for the test allergen.[9] Specific IgG antibodies that appear during immunotherapy may compete against the IgE antibodies and falsely lower the estimate of specific IgE antibody levels.[10] Experimental manipulations to increase the sensitivity of the assay will, by necessity, be accompanied by some increase in nonspecific background and a greater potential for false-positive results. Test results are compared against negative and positive controls. In a study in which aliquots of the same sera were tested in vitro by a laboratory 17 times in 12 months, sera with results that were at least 2.5-fold of the negative control were consistently positive, whereas samples in the borderline zone (1.5- to 2.5-fold of the negative control) gave more erratic results.[11]

Basophil histamine release

This test measures the ability of the basophils to respond to various allergenic extracts and, among the in vitro tests, it comes the closest to measuring the whole biologic response to an allergen. The test is not universally applicable because not all basophils release histamine in vitro.[12] The histamine release test currently is primarily a research tool because it requires extremely fresh samples of blood and may show considerable variation among laboratories.[13]

In Vivo Methods for Allergy Testing

Overview of skin tests

The general principle of skin testing is to introduce allergenic extracts into the superficial skin and observe the formation of a wheal at the site within 15 to 20 minutes. A sample of saline diluent is always included as a negative control. A dilute histamine solution is used as a positive control. If no reaction is seen with the histamine control, interference from antihistamines must be suspected, and testing should be repeated at a later date. Many persons show a small wheal with saline alone, and any reaction that is no larger than the saline control is still considered to be negative. If the wheal induced by saline is large and approaches the reaction seen

Grading the cutaneous response

Results are interpreted after 15 to 20 minutes. Some clinicians record erythema as well as wheal size, but most practitioners consider only the wheal size in evaluating the response. Two approaches are used for grading the results. The cutaneous reaction can be quantified in an objective manner, such as measuring the largest diameter, taking the product of the widest diameter and the diameter at right angles, or tracing the wheal on paper, cutting it out, and weighing the paper. The threshold for positive is defined either as a predetermined size in millimeters or as a ratio that uses the size of the histamine positive control. The potential flaws in relying on an absolute diameter are that: (1) certain individuals may have a greater wheal reaction to one vs. another stimulus, (2) not all allergen extracts have the same quantity of allergenic material, (3) it is difficult to deliver a standard quantity of allergen in an absolutely consistent manner, and (4) skin reactivity varies between sites, such as the upper and lower back.[16] For prick tests in particular, the size of the wheals is greatly influenced by the type of device used to abrade the skin.[16] An easier and equally valid approach is to assign the saline control as negative and the histamine control as 3+. All other reactions are then graded on a scale of negative to 4+. Wheals notably larger than the histamine reaction, especially those with pseudopods, receive a 4+. A 1+ designation is given to any reaction that is larger than the saline control, and a 2+ reaction is intermediate in size between the 1+ reaction and the 3+ histamine control.

Interference from medications

Patients must stop taking antihistamines before skin testing. Use of some of the longer-acting antihistamines must be stopped several weeks in advance

Table 9–1   Interference from Medications

ANTIHISTAMINE	REPORTED DURATION OF INHIBITION, DAYS	CUSTOMARY DRUG-FREE INTERVAL BEFORE SKIN TESTING, DAYS	REFERENCE
Astemizole	30–60	21	Ghys and Rihoux,[17] Almind et al.[18]
Terfenadine	3–10	3	Ghys and Rihoux,[17] Almind et al.[18]
Loratidine	3–10	3	Ghys and Rihoux,[17] Almind et al.[18]
Cetirizine	3–10	3	Ghys and Rihoux,[17] Almind et al.[18]
Clemastine	1–10	1	Phillips et al.[19]
Chlorpheniramine	1–3	1	Galant et al.[20] Long et al.[21]
Diphenhydramine	1–3	1	Galant et al.[20] Long et al.[21]

(Table 9–1). There is no interference from nasal steroids, systemic steroids, decongestants, cromolyn sodium, or nonsteroidal anti-inflammatory drugs. Patients should not undergo skin testing or immunotherapy while receiving β-adrenergic blockers because they would interfere with the use of epinephrine should it become necessary.

Intramuscular injections

It has been suggested that clinically relevant hypersensitivity reactions can be detected by injecting dilute solutions of allergens intramuscularly and monitoring the patients for development of symptoms. The interpretation under these circumstances is usually more subjective than that of the other tests. The patient self-reports symptoms, such as fatigue or headache, that cannot be verified by the observer. There may be clinical situations in which subjective tests are the only alternative; however, the clinician must be scrupulously careful that the tests are conducted in blinded fashion so that neither the patient nor the person administering the test knows which reagents are used. There must be negative controls and, if possible, positive controls introduced in a random fashion.[22] In contrast to the potential subjectivity of intramuscular tests, cutaneous and nasal provocation tests are easily evaluated in an objective manner and the functional basis of the test is clearly related to the pathophysiology of the nasal symptoms.

Nasal provocation

This is perhaps the most direct assay of nasal response to aeroallergen. Potential allergens are introduced into the nasal cavity, and the response is detected from changes in airway resistance and accumulation of proteins and eicosanoids in the nasal secretions which represent mast cell-derived mediators and serum proteins that have escaped through leaky blood vessels.[23] This test is largely restricted to research settings and is more fully discussed in Chapter 10.

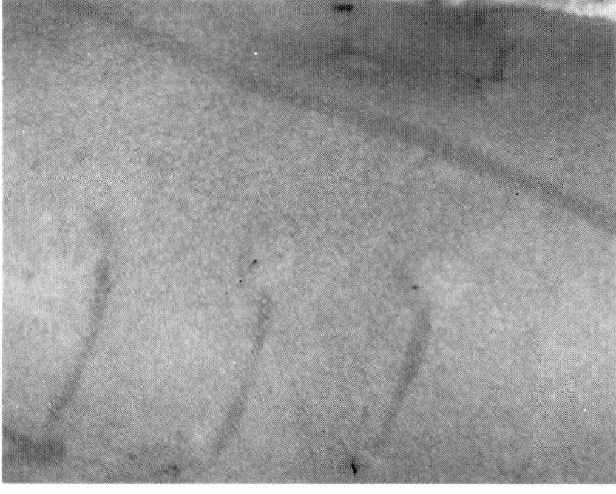

Figure 9–3. Evaluation of the wheal response in skin testing. Diameter of indurated area of wheal is estimated in comparison with the negative saline and the positive histamine controls. Wheal size is best evaluated by viewing the skin from a slight angle (see wheals at the top of the figure) and by palpating the area lightly with a gloved finger.

Oral provocation

The standard for identifying food sensitivity is the double-blind placebo-controlled food challenge.[24] The suspected foods are removed from the diet for 2 weeks before the test. Dried food powders are placed in opaque capsules in doses ranging from 20 to 2,000 mg, depending on estimates of the patient's sensitivity. Foods, intermixed with placebo items, are given to patients in random order so that neither the patient nor the examiner knows which items are being tested at a particular time. The patient should be observed for about 2 hours to determine whether the suspected symptoms develop. If no reaction occurs, the dose can be doubled each day until the challenge dose contains the amount of material in a typical serving of hydrated food. If the symptoms are of a subjective nature and cannot be independently verified by the examiner, the testing should be repeated on at least three occasions to rule out chance associations.

INTEGRATION OF ALLERGY TEST INTO THE CLINICAL DIAGNOSIS

The Allergy History

Allergy tests all have a potential for false-positive and false-negative results. Consequently, test results must be interpreted in the context of the patient's clinical history. A careful history will often reveal whether a patient is atopic. A comprehensive allergy history systematically follows the patient through a normal day to identify when and where symptoms occur. Sneezing, itchy and watery eyes, and scratchy throat are the symptoms most closely associated with allergic rhinitis. Nasal drainage may be clear or mucoid, but it is usually less voluminous than that associated with vasomotor rhinitis. Nasal congestion, popping ears, itchy ears, and headache also may occur. Some patients relate that their symptoms are reminiscent of the prodromal stage of a "cold" that never resolves.

The allergens that provoke the patient's symptoms may be associated with the workplace. Thus, it is important to ask whether the symptoms are better or worse on workdays compared with non-workdays and holidays. Other helpful questions include whether symptoms are more prominent when the patient is in the house or outside. Insight can be gained as to the cause if patients report that their symptoms improve when they travel to sites where different pollens prevail or where the housing results in reduced exposure to dust mites or cockroaches. The major categories of allergens to be considered are pets, pollens, molds, and house dust.

Specific Allergens

Pets

Allergies to pets are easiest to diagnose when patients relate their symptoms directly to times when they are in contact with animals. Cats, dogs, and feathers are the most common source of epidermal allergens. Horses and goats may be a consideration for patients in rural locales or for weekend farmers. Because of its small size, the allergen in cat dander may remain airborne for long periods.[25] Thus, patients may report symptoms shortly after entering a house where a cat has been even if the cat is not physically present. Cat dander also can be transported on clothing to schools, where it may cause symptoms in allergic children.[26] Dog dander, by contrast, is large and settles quickly; thus, patients may not report symptoms until they are in contact with the animal. Some persons are sensitive only to certain canine breeds, whereas others react to all breeds.

Pollens

Pollen sensitivity usually follows a seasonal pattern, with symptoms peaking in the spring or fall. The major culprits are grasses, weeds, and trees whose tiny pollen grains are distributed by the wind. Many newspapers print local pollen counts, and patients may have noted that their symptoms are worse, for example, in the ragweed season. The prevalent allergenic plants and their exact pollinating seasons vary throughout the United States, and physicians need to become familiar with the patterns in their community. Floristic zone charts, listing the prevalent plants in different geographic areas, are available from several sources. However, because these maps often divide the United States into broad regions and overlook local variations, they may not be helpful in certain locations. Companies that market allergy test reagents are a helpful source of information regarding selection of allergens for a particular geographic area. State agricultural extension services also may provide information regarding local flora. Along the humid, warm, semitropical southern border of the United States, pollination of many grasses continues year-round. Thus, allergic rhinitis due to pollen may be perennial in this area. Symptoms that increase when a patient mows the grass, works in the garden, walks around a golf course, or goes on a hunting trip may be due to exposure to either pollens or mold spores.

Molds

The major allergenic molds are distributed fairly uniformly throughout the United States with little geographic variation. Molds are a particularly severe problem in humid areas. Short torrential rains may stir up pollens and spores, whereas prolonged rainfall may clear the air. However, the first sunny day after a rainstorm can be a prime time for release of mold spores. Moist garden soil and damp leaves are common sites for mold growth outdoors. Damp wall boards, flooring or carpeting, filters on air conditioners (especially window units), and houseplants all can be sites for growth of mold inside the home.

House dust

Patients whose symptoms are worse when they are indoors may be sensitive to dust or cockroaches. One of the major allergenic substances in house dust comes from the dust mite and its fecal pellets. Dust mites proliferate when the humidity is above 50%. Thus, in the northern United States, mite allergy symptoms are lower in the winter when indoor heating dries the air. In warm and humid regions, dust mite allergies may be perennial. Dust mites feed on skin dander that commonly accumulates in bedding and carpets. Symptoms may be worse at night because the nose is close to contaminated bedding. Regular laundering of bedding in hot (>55°C) water kills the dust mite and denatures the allergenic proteins.[27] To ensure a barrier to dust mite exposure in bedding, mattresses may be enclosed in allergen-proof covers. Pillows can be enclosed in allergen-proof covers or the pillow itself must be washed in hot water every 2 weeks. Feather pillows present a special problem both because they cannot be laundered and because many persons are allergic to feathers. Foam-rubber pillows can harbor not only dust mites but also molds if they become damp.

A detailed inquiry about the furnishings of the bedroom can be very informative, because the patient is likely to spend at least 8 hours a day in that room. Other "dust traps" to look for are books, stuffed animals, throw pillows, drapes, cluttered shelves that are dusted infrequently, and, worst of all, carpeting (Fig. 9–4). Symptoms of patients with dust allergies often improve in the hospital because the floors are not carpeted and bedding either is covered in plastic or is disposable. Symptoms that increase while vacuuming the carpet provide an excellent clue that the person has dust allergies because the dust mite allergens are transiently made airborne during the process. Vacuum cleaners that have water or HEPA filters may remove dust mite allergens from the discharged air. However, cat allergen is highly water-soluble, and vacuum cleaners with water filters may actually increase the concentration of this allergen in the air.[28] Cockroaches are also a prominent allergen.

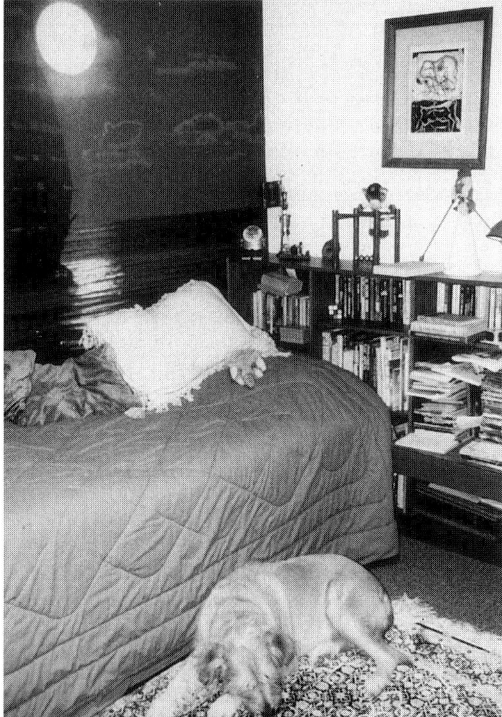

Figure 9–4. The allergy history. This bedroom contains many potential sites for allergens to which the patients will be exposed all night. The carpeted floor, thick bedspread, throw pillows, and stuffed animals are sites for dust mites. Books and cluttered shelves accumulate dust and cannot be cleaned easily. Pets sleeping in the bedroom disperse dander.

Distinguishing between sensitivity to cockroaches and sensitivity to dust mites may be difficult on the basis of the history.

What Do Allergy Tests Really Measure?

Specific IgE and mast cell degranulation

In vitro tests measure specific circulating IgE antibodies, but it is the IgE antibodies that are bound to the surface of mast cells that are responsible for atopic disease. Allergens impacting on the nasal mucosa may bind to specific IgE molecules displayed on the surface of submucosal mast cells. It has been suggested that atopic persons may have a higher density of mast cells in their nasal mucosa.[29] When antigens crosslink membrane-bound IgE, a transmembrane signal results in the release of mediators of inflammation from cytoplasmic granules. Among the preformed mediators are histamine, which triggers sneezing, itching, and arteriolar vasodilation, various proteolytic enzymes, and other hydrolases whose function is not well understood. The activated mast cell also produces derivatives of arachidonic acid metabolism, including prostaglandins and leukotrienes. These cause mucosal vasodilation, increase the production of mucus, provide chemotactic stimuli to promote influx of inflammatory cells, and induce bronchoconstriction. These mediators can be measured as part of nasal provocation studies. When an allergen is introduced into the skin, the physiologic response to the inflammatory mediators from mast cells results in the wheal that is the parameter measured in skin testing.

The late-phase response

The acute-phase response occurs within 15 minutes of the initial exposure to allergen. Three to 8 hours later, even with no further exposure, many atopic persons experience the same symptoms again. The soluble mediators released during the late-phase reaction are generally the same as those released in the acute-phase reaction. The exception is prostaglandin D_2, which is not found during the late-phase reaction. Because basophils release virtually the same mediators as mast cells except for prostaglandin D_2, it has been suggested that the late-phase reaction probably is mediated by basophils.[30,31] The late-phase reaction should be kept in mind when taking an allergy history because patients may display symptoms many hours after their initial exposure. Although the late-phase response may contribute to the patient's symptoms, there are no readily available tests to evaluate the late-phase response. The basophil histamine release test measures the reactivity of circulating basophils, but there are no studies that evaluate the correlation between basophil histamine release and the development of the late-phase response. Only a third to a half of persons with an immediate response to nasal allergen challenge will have a late-phase reaction.[23] The magnitude of the nasal response to histamine challenge is predictive of the appearance of a late-phase reaction after nasal challenge with ragweed in allergic patients.[32] However, the appearance of a late-phase reaction after cutaneous challenge with allergen does not predict those in whom a late-phase reaction will develop after nasal challenge with allergen.[33,34]

Hyperresponsiveness of atopy

The upper respiratory tract of atopic persons also may show an exaggerated response to histamine or methacholine. For example, patients with asthma are known to have a very sensitive bronchospastic response to methacholine. Even patients with allergic rhinitis and no clinical symptoms of asthma may have an exaggerated bronchospastic response when challenged with methacholine.[35,36] The hyperresponsiveness of atopic persons may influence nasal provocation studies but is not directly addressed in either skin tests or in vitro tests.

False-Negative Results in Allergy Testing

Etiology

Allergenic extracts are usually prepared as aqueous extracts according to a standardized formula. All allergen extracts contain many, perhaps dozens of, different proteins. Dust extract, for example, is the aqueous extract of vacuum cleaner bags, collected in low-pollen seasons, from the homes of persons who do not keep pets. This dust contains fabric fibers, cleansers, and dirt, in addition to dust mite proteins and dust mite feces.

Despite the complexity of the mixtures, false-negative results can and do occur. The particular allergen to which a patient is sensitive may not be represented in the extract. For in vitro tests in which the allergen is immobilized on some substrate such as a thread, polystyrene bead, or paper disk, there is the additional uncertainty as to whether the proteins in an aqueous extract bind to the substrate in a conformation recognized by the specific IgE antibodies in patient sera.

Clinical implications

Depending on how convincing the patient's history of sensitivity might be, the physician should still counsel the patient to avoid a particular substance even if the test results are negative. With potentially life-threatening situations such as a history of an anaphylactic reaction to an insect bite, patients should be counseled to carry epinephrine for self-administration, even if tests for stinging insect venoms yield a negative result. But under no condition should patients receive immunotherapy with an allergen extract toward which there has been no significant test response. Immunotherapy should be reserved for situations in which there is an appropriate history of sensitivity together with a positive cutaneous test to that allergen.

False-Positive Results in Allergy Testing

Etiology

Depending on the type of test used, false-positive results also can be obtained. A false-positive result is usually defined as a positive result in a patient who shows no clinical evidence of hypersensitivity to that allergen and has no history of symptoms when exposed to that substance. Skin tests often are cited as the reference standard for confirmation of in vitro tests, and nasal or oral provocation tests are ultimate standards for both. False-positive results may reflect the use of allergen extracts that were too concentrated for in vivo testing, or sera that contained very high levels of IgE for in vitro tests.

Clinical implications

There are also data to suggest that some persons may show some reactivity with allergens years before the development of clinically apparent symptoms. Hagy and Settipane[37] found that 18.2% of 1,352 college students with a positive result of skin testing but no clinical symptoms developed atopic symptoms to specific allergens up to 3 years after their initial positive cutaneous reactions. Only 1.7% of those unreactive to a panel of immediate hypersensitivity tests developed atopic disease. There is no way to determine whether apparently false-positive results are predictive in the case of a specific individual, and it would be highly inappropriate to begin immunotherapy with any allergen in the absence of clinical symptoms.

WHICH ALLERGY TEST SHOULD BE USED?

Nasal Provocation or Skin Tests?

The principal advantage of in vivo allergy testing is that it measures a biologic response to the allergen and thereby takes into account the distribution of IgE on mast cells, the sensitivity of the mast cells to a given stimulus, and the vascular response to the mediators released. Skin testing does make the assumption that cutaneous mast cells are coated with the same types of IgE and respond in the same way to allergens as do mast cells in the mucosa of the upper respiratory tract. Indeed, there appears to be good correlation between cutaneous reactivity and response to nasal provocation with specific allergens.[33] This is fortunate because nasal provocation is not easily accomplished outside a research setting, nor is it amenable to test multiple allergens in a timely fashion.

Prick or Intradermal Skin Tests?

Because of the small quantity of allergen introduced into the skin, prick testing is less likely to give false-positive results than intradermal tests (Table 9–2). Allergenic

Table 9–2   Advantages and Disadvantages of Prick and Intradermal Skin Tests for Immediate-Type Hypersensitivity

	PRICK TEST	INTRADERMAL TEST
Advantages	Lower false-positive rate Allergenic extracts are more stable May be more accurate for food sensitivities	More sensitive More reproducible
Disadvantages	Less reproducible Less sensitive	Higher false-positive rate

extract solutions for prick tests are more stable and have a longer shelf life. However, prick tests are also less reproducible than intradermal tests. Prick testing is an excellent screen to be used in conjunction with intradermal testing. Intradermal tests are more reproducible and are much more sensitive than prick tests. However, the sensitivity of intradermal testing is accompanied by an increased rate of false-positive results.

Single Dilution or Serial Dilution Skin Tests?

There is a legitimate controversy as to whether patients should be tested with a single concentration of allergenic extract or with a series of dilutions. The most accurate method is to test the patient with high dilutions and increase the concentration of allergen applied every 15 minutes until a reaction is seen. This technique certainly avoids a false-positive result caused by the use of too high a concentration of allergen and has great value in standardization of test reagents and in research studies in which one wants to stratify patients by the magnitude of their response. However, it is very impractical in a clinical setting. It limits the number of allergens that can be evaluated in one visit, it is difficult to apply reagents in an absolutely reproducible manner, and it is difficult to select skin sites that react in an identical fashion. By purchasing standardized allergenic reagents from a reliable source, gaining experience with the application and interpretation of tests using a known panel of reagents, including a reference histamine positive control, and interpreting the test results in the context of the clinical history, false-positive results are not likely to be a problem.

Some argue that testing with serial dilutions of allergenic extracts is helpful in the selection of appropriate allergen concentrations for immunotherapy. Proponents of the Rinkel method of immunotherapy use the results of dilution testing to calculate a treatment dose that is usually only modestly more concentrated than the test dose.[38] Patients treated under this protocol receive very low doses of allergen. Because clinical response to immunotherapy is directly correlated with the quantity of allergen administered, the Rinkel method often provides a less than optimal treatment.[39] Some clinicians favor the serial dilution method because it identifies the highest dose of allergen tolerated by the patient.[40] This information can be used to start immunotherapy with more concentrated solutions. If a patient can tolerate a 1:100 dilution of extract at the onset (typical starting doses are 1:100,000), one might question whether the level of sensitivity was an adequate indication for immunotherapy. Furthermore, with use of the typical dosing schedule for immunotherapy, even a 100-fold increase in the quantity of allergen delivered at the onset would move the patient's schedule up by only about 2 months. Given that immunotherapy must be administered for between 4 and 6 months before it is effective, this advantage seems minor compared with the considerable increase in time and expense involved with skin testing in serial dilutions.

Skin Tests or In Vitro Tests?

Both in vivo and in vitro tests have merits (Table 9–3). In vitro tests may have a specificity >90%, but the sensitivity is only to 60% to 70%.[3–7,41–43] Thus, skin tests are

Table 9–3 Advantages and Disadvantages of In Vitro and Skin Tests for Immediate-Type Hypersensitivity

	IN VITRO TEST	SKIN TEST
Advantages	Does not require skilled personnel in physician's office	More sensitive
	Minimal patient discomfort (venipuncture only)	Results available on same visit
	Not influenced by antihistamines	Allergenic extracts are identical to those used in immunotherapy
Disadvantages	Less sensitive	Requires trained personnel in physician's office
	More expensive	Potentially more discomfort
	Delay in obtaining results requires second office visit	Must stop use of antihistamines beforehand
	IgG antibodies from immunotherapy may interfere	Interference by dermatographism

more sensitive than in vitro tests. One might question the extent to which this increased sensitivity is clinically useful. Skin test results and in vitro tests tend to correlate well when the response to a specific allergen is strong. When in vitro results and skin test results are weak, there is often marked discordance. Thus, in vitro tests are not useful to evaluate weak or negative skin tests. If the goal of the physician is just to identify clinically relevant allergens in order to guide the patient in environmental modification, then either test, taken in conjunction with the clinical history, may be more than adequate.

In vitro testing entails minimal discomfort, is not influenced by concurrent administration of antihistamines, and may be particularly appropriate in patients with dermatographism or in small children who cannot tolerate skin testing. In vitro tests may be more suitable for the physician who uses allergy testing only on a sporadic basis. The theoretical disadvantages of in vitro testing are that one is not testing the whole biologic response to the allergenic challenge and, in patients receiving immunotherapy, there may some interference from specific IgG antibodies. In practice, the major objection to in vitro testing has been cost. In vitro tests are proportionally more expensive, especially when testing more than a very few allergens. Third-party payers are increasingly reluctant to pay for this type of testing. Proponents of in vitro testing have countered this criticism by limiting the number of tests ordered and using mixtures.[44] Although this may limit cost, it also curtails the amount of useful diagnostic information that is collected. Because in vitro test results are not available for at least several days after the blood is drawn, the patient must schedule a second office visit to review the test results and receive recommendations.

For the physician who uses allergy testing frequently, skin testing is more desirable. Short of nasal provocation, this approach comes closest to measuring the whole biologic response of the patient to the allergen. There is no interference from ongoing immunotherapy, but patients do need to stop use of antihistamines in advance of the test date. Once the allergenic extracts are obtained and personnel are trained, the cost per patient is considerably less than in vitro testing. Patients can be tested and the results reviewed within the same office visit. Patients often forget important parts of their clinical history, and the test results may lead to additional questions that help to identify clinically relevant allergens. The post-test interview provides an unparalleled opportunity to educate the patient about the pertinent allergens and the means by which they can minimize their exposure. Major issues such as elimination of pets or removal of carpeting to eliminate dust mites may be reinforced by showing the patient the reactions that these factors are causing in the body. The decision to implement immunotherapy places a considerable onus on the physician to identify the critical allergens with as much precision as possible, and skin testing will be the method of choice.

Single Allergen Extracts or Mixtures?

There is a great temptation to use mixtures of similar allergens for testing. The hope is that the number of tests can be minimized, the costs can be reduced, and useful information can still be collected. There are drawbacks to this approach. Depending on the quantity of allergen and the diversity of the allergens in the mixture, both false-positive and false-negative results may occur. For example, there is considerable cross-reactivity among the fescue family of grasses (timothy, june, ryegrass, orchard, and fescue), the four major ragweed groups (short, giant, western, and false), the birch family (birch, alder, and hazel), the olive family (olive, ash, and privet), and the cypress family (cedar and juniper). Beeches cross-react with oak pollens, and walnut cross-reacts with pecan and hickory pollens. There are also individual antigens associated with each of these plants. Thus, if a patient is sensitive to an allergen that is cross-reactive within a family, the dose of that allergen in the mixture may be high and a positive result will occur. However, if the relevant allergen is unique to only one of the pollens in the mixture, its concentration may be too low to elicit a reaction even in a person who is sensitive. Screening tests that use pollens from a single plant to estimate reactivity to the whole family also may miss some sensitive persons.

Mixtures of specific allergenic extracts are definitely to be avoided if the allergy tests are designed to identify allergens to be used for immunotherapy. The goal of immunotherapy is to inject patients with a limited number of allergens to which they show especially prominent reactivity. There are two reasons why the number of allergens in an immunotherapy program would be limited: (1) antigenic competition in which the immune system may respond to only a limited number of antigens out of a mixture administered (if too many antigens are injected at one time, the response to all may be suboptimal), and (2) to reduce the number of injections per session and the total volume that is given at one time. In practical terms, it is preferable to limit the number of antigens to 10 and certainly no more than 20.

Is Patient Risk a Consideration?

Patient risk is often cited as drawback of skin testing. However, reports tend to consider skin testing and immunotherapy together. A close examination of the literature shows that virtually all of the morbidity and mortality is associated with immunotherapy.[45] In a survey by the American Academy of Allergy and Immunology covering the years 1985 to 1989, all 117 fatalities were associated with immunotherapy. Of the persons who died of anaphylaxis, 77% had asthma. Only one of the patients who died had allergic rhinitis alone; this patient had cardiovascular disease and was receiving β-adrenergic blocker therapy.[45] There have been no fatalities associated with skin testing in the United States for 7 years. Previous fatalities involved patients who received intradermal testing without a screening percutaneous test and patients being tested with penicillin, venoms, or nut extracts. There were no adverse reactions to prick testing in a survey of approximately 16,000 patients as part of the National Health and Nutritional Examination Survey 1976–80.[46] Bousquet and Michel[47] reported only one generalized urticarial reaction among approximately 10,000 patients who had skin testing with 25 to 35 allergens in their clinic.

THE QUANDARY OF FOOD SENSITIVITY

Food Sensitivities

Although food allergies are believed to be frequent, the best objective evaluations indicate that the prevalence is low, occurring in only 1% of the population.[48,49] The incidence of food allergy is much higher in children than in adults. Milk, eggs, soybeans, and peanuts or other nuts are by far the most commonly implicated foods for IgE-mediated reactions.[50] However, not all adverse reactions involve type I hypersensitivity. Some foods contain vasoactive amines, and hot or spicy foods may trigger rhinorrhea through non-IgE-mediated mechanisms. Symptoms, particularly in the gastrointestinal tract, may occur in persons deficient in enzymes such as lactase. All of these issues have been extensively reviewed.[51]

Diagnostic Options

Allergy tests

Both cutaneous and in vitro allergy tests are less than satisfactory for the diagnosis of food allergies. When oral food challenges are used to evaluate the validity of in vitro or cutaneous tests, the false-positive rate has been as high as 60% to 65%.[50] Many foodstuffs contain substances that trigger histamine release in the absence of specific IgE, and this may account for the high false-positive rate, particularly with intradermal tests. Prick tests seem to be more specific than intradermal testing for food allergies. In the study by Bock et al.,[50] all patients with positive results of intradermal testing, whose sensitivity was subsequently confirmed by oral food challenge, also had positive results of prick testing.

False-negative results also may occur. It is always uncertain whether specific food extracts actually contain the offending allergen. Some persons, for instance, may be sensitive to foods when cooked but not to the same product when uncooked. Some allergens from fruits and vegetables are too unstable to be incorporated in test solutions.[52,53] Investigators have sought to compensate for this by doing "prick-prick" tests in which a needle is used first to prick the food and then the patient.

Food diaries and elimination diets

Food diaries, in which patients record everything they eat and their concurrent symptoms through the day, may help to identify suspicious foods. Food diaries are very tedious for the patient to keep. They may not always be aware when ingredients such as peanut products or eggs are present in prepared foods.[54] An elimination diet may be informative but also requires considerable dedication from the patient (and the family), depending on the stringency and number of products eliminated. After 2 weeks of avoidance, the food in question may be sampled to determine whether symptoms develop. Because of the potential for subjectivity and the non-blinded design of this approach, avoidance and re-challenge should be repeated on several occasions before a decision is made to eliminate a food from the diet. This type of deliberate challenge should not, of course, be attempted if a potentially life-threatening reaction such as anaphylaxis or asthma is suspected. It should be safe for patients who anticipate only symptoms of allergic rhinitis.

Oral challenges

Immunotherapy is not appropriate for food sensitivities; the only treatment is food avoidance in conjunction with medical therapy. It is difficult to comply with an exclusion diet, particularly if it includes common foodstuffs such as dairy products, wheat, or eggs. Therefore, the physician should make every effort to confirm the diagnosis before imposing draconian changes on a patient's lifestyle. The double-blind placebo-controlled food challenge protocol may be used to verify suspected sensitivities.[24]

REFERENCES

1. Havnen J, Amlie PA, Hvatum M, et al: IgE concentrations in allergic asthma in children. *Arch Dis Child* 1973; 48:850–855.
2. Kaliner M, Lemanske R: Rhinitis and asthma. *JAMA* 1992; 268:2807–2829.
3. Hamburger RN, Berger WE, Quiwa NB, et al: Skin testing compared with in vitro testing for screening allergic patients. *Ann Allergy* 1991; 67:133–137.
4. Kelso JM, Sodhi N, Gosselin VA, Yunginger JW: Diagnostic performance characteristics of the standard Phadebas RAST, modified RAST, and Pharmacia CAP system versus skin testing. *Ann Allergy* 1991; 67:511–514.
5. Eichler I, Gotz M, Jarisch R, et al: Reproducibility of skin prick testing with allergen extracts from different manufacturers. *Allergy* 1988; 43:458–463.
6. Seltzer JM, Halpern GM, Tsay Y-G: Correlation of allergy test results obtained by IgE FAST, RAST, and prick-puncture methods. *Ann Allergy* 1985; 54:25–30.
7. Williams PB, Dolen WK, Koepke JW, Selner JC: Comparison of skin testing and three in vitro assays for specific IgE in the clinical evaluation of immediate hypersensitivity. *Ann Allergy* 1992; 68:35–45.
8. Ogino S, Bessho K, Harada T, et al: Evaluation of allergen-specific IgE antibodies by MAST for the diagnosis of nasal allergy. *Rhinology* 1993; 31:27–31.
9. Homburger HA, Jacob GL: Initial results of the College of American Pathologists interlaboratory proficiency program for diagnostic allergy testing (abstract). *J Allergy Clin Immunol* 1988; 81:229.

10. Perelmutter L, Bergeron M, Mandy F: Assessment of the effect of IgG antibodies to ragweed and rye grass on the IgE antibody disc RAST. *Ann Allergy* 1983; 50:393–397.
11. Homburger HA, Jacob GL: Analytic accuracy of specific immunoglobulin E antibody results determined by a blind proficiency survey. *J Allergy Clin Immunol* 1982; 70:474–480.
12. Conroy MC, Adkinson NF Jr, Sobotka AK, Lichtenstein LM: "Releasability" of histamine from human basophils (abstract). *Fed Proc* 1977; 36:1216.
13. Gleich GJ, Hull WM: Measurement of histamine: a quality control study. *J Allergy Clin Immunol* 1980; 66:295–298.
14. Demoly P, Bousquet J, Manderscheid JC, et al: Precision of skin prick and puncture tests using nine methods. *J Allergy Clin Immunol* 1991; 88:758–762.
15. Lutz CT, Bell CE Jr, Wedner HJ, Krogstad DJ: Allergy testing of multiple patients should no longer be performed with a common syringe. *N Engl J Med* 1984; 310:1335–1337.
16. Nelson HS, Rosloniec DM, McCall LI, Ikle D: Comparative performances of five commercial prick skin test devices. *J Allergy Clin Immunol* 1993; 92:750–756.
17. Ghys L, Rihoux JP: Pharmacological modulation of cutaneous reactivity to histamine: a double-blind acute comparative study between cetirizine, terfenadine, and astemizole. *J Int Med Res* 1989; 17:24–27.
18. Almind M, Dirksen A, Nielsen NH, Svendsen UG: Duration of the inhibitory activity on histamine-induced skin weals of sedative and non-sedative antihistamines. *Allergy* 1988; 43:593–596.
19. Phillips MJ, Meyrick Thomas RH, Moodley I, Davies RJ: A comparison of the in vivo effects of ketotifen, clemastine, chlorpheniramine, and sodium cromoglycate on histamine and allergen induced weals in human skin. *Br J Clin Pharmacol* 1983; 15:277–286.
20. Galant S, Zippin C, Bullock J, Crisp J: Allergy skin tests. I. Antihistamine inhibition. *Ann Allergy* 1972; 30:53–63.
21. Long WF, Taylor RJ, Wagner CJ, et al: Skin test suppression by antihistamines and the development of subsensitivity. *J Allergy Clin Immunol* 1985; 76:113–117.
22. Jewett DL, Fein G, Greenberg MH: A double-blind study of symptom provocation to determine food sensitivity. *N Engl J Med* 1990; 323:429–433.
23. Naclerio RM, Baroody FM: Observations on the response of the nasal mucosa to allergens. *Otolaryngol Head Neck Surg* 1994; 111:355–363.
24. Bock SA, Sampson HA, Atkins FM, et al: Double-blind, placebo-controlled food challenge (DBPCFC) as an office procedure: a manual. *J Allergy Clin Immunol* 1988; 82:986–997.
25. Luczynska C, Li Y, Chapman MD, Platts-Mills TAE: Airborne concentrations and particle size distribution of allergen derived from domestic cats (*Felis domesticus*). Measurements using cascade impactor, liquid impinger, and a two-site monoclonal antibody assay for Fel d I. *Am Rev Respir Dis* 1990; 141:361–367.
26. Munir AKM, Einarsson R, Schou C, Dreborg SKG: Allergens in school dust. I. The amount of the major cat (*Fel d* I) and dog (*Can f* I) allergens in dust from Swedish schools is high enough to probably cause perennial symptoms in most children with asthma who are sensitized to cat and dog. *J Allergy Clin Immunol* 1993; 91:1067–1074.
27. McDonald LG, Tovey E: The role of water temperature and laundry procedures in reducing house dust mite populations and allergen content of bedding. *J Allergy Clin Immunol* 1992; 90:599–608.
28. Woodfolk JA, Luczynska CM, de Blay F, et al: The effect of vacuum cleaners on the concentration and particle size distribution of airborne cat allergen. *J Allergy Clin Immunol* 1993; 91:829–837.
29. Bentley AM, Jacobson MR, Cumberworth V, et al: Immunohistology of the nasal mucosa in seasonal allergic rhinitis: Increases in activated eosinophils and epithelial mast cells. *J Allergy Clin Immunol* 1992; 89:877–883.
30. Naclerio RM, Proud D, Togias AG, et al: Inflammatory mediators in later antigen-induced rhinitis. *N Engl J Med* 1985; 313:65–70.
31. Atkins PC, Schwartz LB, Adkinson NF, et al: In vivo antigen-induced cutaneous mediator release: simultaneous comparisons of histamine, tryptase, and prostaglandin D_2 release and the effect of corticosteroid administration. *J Allergy Clin Immunol* 1990; 86:360–370.
32. van Wijk RG, van Toorenenbergen AW, Zijlstra FJ, et al: Nasal hyperreactivity and its effect on early and late sequelae of nasal challenge with house-dust mite extract. *Allergy Proc* 1993; 14:273–281.
33. Andersson M, von Kogerer B, Andersson P, Pipkorn U: Allergen-induced nasal hyperreactivity appears unrelated to the size of the nasal and dermal immediate allergic reaction. *Allergy* 1987; 42:631–637.
34. Iliopoulos O, Proud D, Adkinson NF Jr, et al: Relationship between the early, late, and rechallenge reaction to nasal challenge with antigen: observations on the role of inflammatory mediators and cells. *J Allergy Clin Immunol* 1990; 86:851–861.
35. Stevens WJ, Vermeire PA, van Schil LA: Bronchial hyperreactivity in rhinitis. *Eur J Respir Dis Suppl* 1983; 128:72–80.

36. Ramsdale EH, Morris MM, Roberts RS, Hargreave FE: Asymptomatic bronchial hyper-responsiveness in rhinitis. *J Allergy Clin Immunol* 1985; 75:573–577.
37. Hagy GW, Settipane GA: Prognosis of positive allergy test in an asymptomatic population: a three-year follow-up of college students. *J Allergy* 1971; 48:200–211.
38. Willoughby JW: Serial dilution titration skin tests in inhalant allergy: a clinical quantitative assessment of biologic skin reactivity to allergenic extracts. *Otolaryngol Clin North Am* 1974; 7:579–615.
39. Van Metre TE Jr, Adkinson NF Jr, Lichtenstein LM, et al: A controlled study of the effectiveness of the Rinkel method of immunotherapy for ragweed pollen hay fever. *J Allergy Clin Immunol* 1980; 65:288–297.
40. Nalebuff DJ, Fadal RG, Ali M: Determination of initial immunotherapy dose for ragweed hypersensitivity with the modified RAST test. *Otolaryngol Head Neck Surg* 1981; 89:271–274.
41. Corey JP, Liudahl JJ, Young SA, Rodham SM: Diagnostic efficacy in in vitro methods versus skin testing in patients with inhalant allergies. *Otolaryngol Head Neck Surg* 1991; 104:299–302.
42. Finnerty JP, Summerell S, Holgate ST: Relationship between skin-prick tests, the multiple allergosorbent test and symptoms of allergic disease. *Clin Exp Allergy* 1989; 19:51–56.
43. Sogg AJ: Comparative skin and RAST test results—an update. *Laryngoscope* 1985; 95:1213–1215.
44. Nalebuff DJ: Use of RAST screening in clinical allergy: a cost-effective approach to patient care. *Ear Nose Throat J* 1985; 64:107–121.
45. Reid MJ, Lockey RF, Turkeltaub PC, Platts-Mills TAE: Survey of fatalities from skin testing and immunotherapy 1985–1989. *J Allergy Clin Immunol* 1993; 92:6–15.
46. Turkeltaub PC, Gergen PJ: The risk of adverse reactions from percutaneous prick-puncture allergen skin testing, venipuncture, and body measurements: Data from the second National Health and Nutritional Examination Survey 1976–80 (NHANES II). *J Allergy Clin Immunol* 1989; 84:886–890.
47. Bousquet J, Michel F-B: In vivo methods for study of allergy: skin tests, techniques, and interpretation, vol. 1, 4th ed., in Middleton E Jr, Reed CE, Ellis EF, et al (eds.): *Allergy: Principles and Practice*, St. Louis, Mosby, 1993, pp 573–594.
48. Bock SA: Prospective appraisal of complaints of adverse reaction to foods in children during the first three years of life. *Pediatrics* 1987; 79:683–688.
49. Host A, Halken S: A prospective study of cow milk allergy in Danish infants during the first 3 years of life. Clinical course in relation to clinical and immunological type of hypersensitivity reaction. *Allergy* 1990; 45:587–596.
50. Bock SA, Lee WY, Remigio L, et al: Appraisal of skin tests with food extracts for diagnosis of food hypersensitivity. *Clin Allergy* 1978; 8:559–564.
51. Anderson JA: A pediatrician's guide to food allergy. *Henry Ford Hosp Med J* 1988; 36:198–203.
52. Ortoloni C, Ispano M, Pastorello EA, et al: Comparison of results of skin prick tests (with fresh foods and commercial food extracts) and RAST in 100 patients with oral allergy syndrome. *J Allergy Clin Immunol* 1989; 83:683–690.
53. Rosen JP, Selcow JE, Mendelson LM, et al: Skin testing with natural foods in patients suspected of having food allergies. Is it a necessity? *J Allergy Clin Immunol* 1994; 93:1068–1070.
54. Sampson HA, Mendelson L, Rosen JP: Fatal and near-fatal anaphylactic reactions to food in children and adolescents. *N Engl J Med* 1992; 327:380–384.

10

Nasal Provocation Testing

MORGAN ANDERSSON, M.D., Ph.D.
LENNART GREIFF, M.D., Ph.D.
CHRISTER SVENSSON, M.D., Ph.D.
CARL PERSSON, Ph.D.

In recent years, understanding of the pathophysiology of allergic and nonallergic airway diseases has dramatically increased. Important contributions to the increased knowledge have been achieved by the development of new and better methods for provocation and monitoring of airway mucosal responses. The acquired results from nasal provocation experiments may in several respects also be true for processes in the tracheobronchial airways, because the nasal and tracheobronchial mucosal are similar, from both a structural and a functional point of view.

Nasal challenges with different kinds of agents and measurements of response have several advantages compared with studies of the lower airways. Nasal provocations can be performed easily and frequently over well-defined mucosal areas. Hence, several methods for provocation and measurement of nasal responses have been used in recent years. Each of the techniques has its advantages and restrictions. To correctly interpret the results, the investigator must be familiar with the methods used.

Choosing the most suitable technique for provocation and evaluation of the mucosal response requires that the intention be well defined. For clinical purposes it seems reasonable to choose techniques for qualitative measurements, but experimental research requires quantitative measurements with a high degree of reproducibility and standardization.

One of the most important factors in the diagnosis of allergic rhinitis is the history. Skin tests usually confirm allergens suggested by the history. If not, a further history must be taken with respect to the agents identified by positive skin tests. Other additional tests also may be used which can incorporate in vitro tests such as the radioallergosorbent test (RAST). Nasal allergen challenge is an additional in vivo test. For many otorhinolaryngologists, it is the most common form of provocation in the nose and it is an important tool that can be very helpful in routine clinical work.

For experimental research, many other agents and mediators have been used in nasal provocation experiments. This chapter addresses different techniques for nasal provocation and measurement of nasal responses. In the future, better diagnostic tools will likely be available, especially to investigate, classify, and understand the diverse group of diseases categorized as nonallergic (idiopathic) rhinitis.

DELIVERY SYSTEMS

Different techniques can be used to deliver solutions of challenging agents to the nose, including dripping,[1] and pipettes.[2] These methods, however, challenge only a selected area of the nose. In contrast several studies have shown that a nasal pump spray provides a fairly precise volume and achieves a widespread distribution of the aqueous solution in the nasal cavity.[3] The nasal pool is a newly invented method that may be appropriate for nasal provocation. It consists of a compressible plastic container. The solution can be kept in the nasal cavity as long as the pool device is compressed by the patient. The device can be loaded with different soluble agents and gives a widespread distribution over the mucosal surface for well-defined periods[4] (Fig. 10–1).

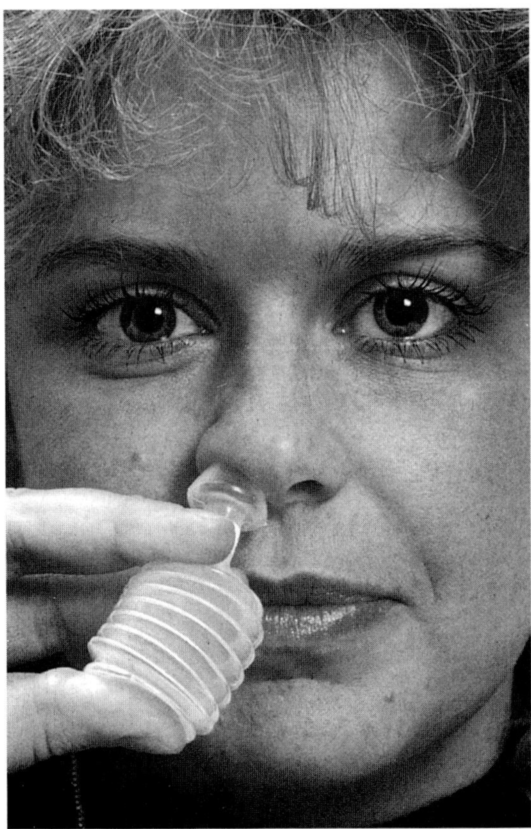

Figure 10–1. Nasal pool device. Nasal pool can be loaded with different kinds of agents and washes a well-defined mucosal area. The fluid can be kept in the nose for well defined periods.

As a means of imitating the natural exposure of pollens, dry powder in the form of whole pollen grains have been delivered to the nose over long periods.[5] The distribution of the pollens with this technique is imprecise, however. Paper disks soaked with pollens also have been used. They challenge a small and well-defined area of the mucosa.[6] This technique may be suitable for selected studies involving mechanisms of glandular secretion. Paper disks themselves, however, induce mucosal exudative inflammation and collect fluid from different compartments of the nasal tissue.[7] Pollens also can be delivered with nebulizers.[8]

Any system that delivers gases to the airways can be used to challenge the nose. Such methods have been used for both gases[9,10] and other physical stimuli, such as cold, dry air.[11] It is important that the amount and distribution of delivered gas or stimuli are known.

AGENTS

Many different substances have been used for nasal provocation. Especially for clinical work, allergens in dry or liquid soluble forms have been used. Provocations with putative inflammatory mediators, irritants, or physical stimuli are used for experimental challenge situations.

Allergens

Several types of allergens can be used. Most commonly used are pollen allergens such as grains or extracts. The stability, purity, and standardization of the extracts are crucial.[12] Fresh extracts should be kept cold between challenges, and stock solutions should be kept in a freezer. Allergen challenges can be performed during and outside the actual allergy season. There is a risk of an increased responsiveness when the provocation is performed during the actual allergy season.[5,13] Especially in the clinic and for safety reasons, this is an important consideration. Repeated challenges with allergen also can influence the reproducibility of the result. At least 1 week should elapse after termination of the pollen season before any nasal challenge is performed. In the asymptomatic state, at least 1 week should pass between each challenge done outside the pollen season.

Allergen provocation

Nasal challenges with allergen are probably the most common provocations and in vivo tests performed by the otorhinolaryngologist. There may be several reasons for performing this type of provocation (Table 10–1). The nasal response to a nasal provocation procedure may be affected by various factors, especially different anti-allergic drugs and other pharmacologic treatments that may have potential antihistamine-like properties. Some of these drugs are listed in Table 10–2. For clinical objectives in which merely a qualitative answer is needed (allergic or not allergic to a specific allergen), the following procedure is recommended. The patient should undergo routine allergologic tests. These tests (skin prick test or RAST) may

Table 10–1   Potential Indications for Nasal Allergen Provocations

1. Discrepancy between the history and result of skin prick test or radioallergosorbent test
2. Determination of a nasal sensitivity to allergens when history and other tests are not distinct
3. Producing allergic symptoms, when routine diagnosis is negative, but case history speaks for allergy
4. Confirmation of presence of local allergy before immunotherapy in patients sensitive to several allergens
5. Some special certified procedures
6. Means of convincing the patient of his or her allergy

Table 10–2   Factors Affecting Nasal Provocation: Suggested Time Between Medication and Provocation

DRUG	TIME
Sodium chromoglycates, nasal	3 days
Nasal corticosteroids	2 weeks
α-Agonists, nasal	1 day
Inhaled β-agonists	none
Oral corticosteroids	2 weeks
Antihistamines	
First-generation	2–4 days
Second-generation	
Astemizole	6–8 weeks
Others	1 week
Nonsteroidal analgesics	1 week
Central nervous system antihypertensive	3 weeks
Tricyclic anti-depressive drugs	3 weeks

indicate the intensity of the response. A rhinoscopic examination also should be performed before the challenge to disclose any structural abnormality that may influence the result. Any contraindications to the provocation also should be excluded (Table 10–3). The initial rhinoscopic examination can give the observer a "baseline" impression of the appearance of the nasal mucosa before the challenge. A diluent challenge is then given in one or both of the nasal cavities to exclude a nonspecific reactivity. Thereafter, increasing doses of standardized allergen extracts are sprayed into the nasal cavity with a mechanical pump spray. With a pump spray, which is easy to handle, a precise dose of allergen can be deposited in the nose. The allergen extracts should have been dissolved in the diluent solution previously given. After each of the increasing doses of allergens, the patient is told to count any sneezes and notify the examiner of any possible symptoms. At least 10 minutes should elapse between each challenge. This interval between challenge and clinical examination seems adequate from both a practical and a scientific point of view.[4,8,14]

**Table 10–3 Relative and Absolute Contraindications for Nasal
Allergen Provocation**

1. Acute mucosal inflammation of the nose or paranasal sinuses
2. Previous anaphylactic reactions in other shock organs
3. Suspicion of a high degree of sensitivity from case history or results of skin prick test or other in vitro tests
4. Not standardized extracts in which the adequate doses delivered are unknown
5. Pregnancy
6. Severe general diseases such as severe asthma, obstructive bronchial diseases, cardiopulmonary diseases with restricted capacity
7. Nasal operation, especially on the inferior turbinate, less than 6 to 8 weeks before provocation

Between each challenge, the nose is inspected to determine whether the appearance of the mucosa has changed. The procedure is continued until a positive response occurs. If after the highest allergen dose the patient still does not have any nasal symptoms, the result of provocation is interpreted as negative. Then it is less likely that the patient is allergic to the provocative agent, although allergy cannot be completely excluded. This kind of provocation procedure is used for clinical situations and is often sufficient when a qualitative answer is needed. To correctly interpret the result, the investigator must be familiar with the provocation technique used. The investigator also should be aware of any possible side effects and preventive measures should have been considered.

Mediators

Different kinds of mediators have been delivered topically to the nose to explore the pathophysiology of mucosal processes. For interpretation of the results, however, it is important to bear in mind that allergic and probably also nonallergic responses involve a cascade of different mediators and cytokines exerting their actions on many different inflammatory and structural cells in the nasal mucosa. Thus, a single mediator provocation cannot resemble the true nature of the complex pathophysiologic process in allergic or nonallergic process. For certain purposes, however, such as the investigation of different pharmacologic effects, single mediator provocations may be appropriate. Nevertheless, the limitations for provocation with mediators are the same as those for allergen extracts (standardization, deposition, etc.). Some of the biochemical mediators used for provocation also may interact with the delivery systems and thus reduce the actual quantity of delivered mediators.

Histamine is a potent exudative agent in the upper airways, and when topically applied to the nasal mucosa it mimics the full spectrum of symptoms associated with the acute allergic reaction in the nose. In contrast to allergen provocation, however, it cannot recruit inflammatory cells nor can it induce any late-phase reactions or hyperreactivity.[15]

Nasal histamine provocations have revealed small differences in nasal patency between a group of healthy controls and patients with nonallergic rhinitis (idiopathic rhinitis).[16] Also, a group of patients with nonallergic rhinitis who had rhinorrhea as the dominating symptom had an increased secretory response to histamine compared with healthy subjects.[17]

When other mediators are topically delivered to the nose, other response profiles are induced. Topical leukotriene D_4 and bradykinins induce microvascular exudative responses.[18] Prostaglandins,[19] serotonin,[20] and platelet-activating factor[21] may all display different responses in the nose. Therefore, when mediator provocations are performed, appropriate response measurements must be chosen, and these techniques must be related to the provocative stimulus.

Methacholine is a synthetic acetylcoline analogue. Topically administered to the nose, it induces glandular secretion.[22] Both methacholine and histamine have been used in the lower airways for assessing bronchial hyperreactivity.[23] In the nose, however, both methacholine and histamine have not been as successful for distinguishing between healthy subjects and patients with nonallergic nasal hyperreactivity. Some authors have found differences between groups of healthy subjects and unselected nonallergic patients.[24,25] When patients were selected according to their dominating symptom ("runners" or "blockers"), the group of runners showed increased secretory responsiveness to methacholine as compared with the group of blockers.[16]

Capsaicin releases neuropeptides from sensory nerve endings. When capsaicin was topically applied to the nose, it could not distinguish patients with nonallergic rhinitis from healthy subjects.[26] In animals, neurogenic mechanisms seem to have important pathophysiologic functions.[27] Alternatively, neurogenic stimulus seems to have many fewer important inflammatory properties in human airways. Thus, when neurogenic stimuli such as nicotine, substance P, or capsaicin are topically applied to the nose, only hyperalgesia and glandular secretion may occur.[28–30] Further, capsaicin provocations, with the potential risk of inhalation of the provocative agent, can induce severe bronchospasm. Hence, capsaicin provocations should be performed only by physicians who are familiar with the techniques and potential dangers of these kinds of provocations.

Irritants and Physical Stimuli

Different irritants such as cigarette smoke or ammonium gas have been applied to the nose. The major problem with these challenges is quantification of the doses given. Patients with nonallergic rhinitis often have nasal complaints when they are exposed to cold, dry air. In such circumstances, both nasal symptoms and release of mediators have been observed.[11] Whether this effect actually is related to the coldness or the dryness of the air is not known.

Temperature changes also have been used to investigate physiologic nasal reactions.[31,32] The studies have demonstrated that changes of temperature affecting one part of the body can induce vascular changes in the nose. Thus, when the nasal response to different kinds of provocations is measured, patients should first become acclimatized to the experimental environment before any measurements can be determined accurately. As a means to mimic possible mechanisms in exercise-induced asthma, fluids with different osmolarity[33,34] and hypertonic solutions[35] have been applied to the nose. In occupational medicine, other stimuli such as organic acid anhydrides have been shown to induce nasal symptoms in exposed workers.[36]

Acetylsalicylic Acid

In 1968, the clinical entity of intolerance against acetylsalicylic acid (ASA), nasal polyposis, and asthma was first described.[37] The diagnosis of intolerance against ASA has gained increased interest in recent years because of the observation that daily peroral aspirin provocations could promote tolerance to ASA.[38] Recently, both nasal and bronchial provocations with increasing doses of an acetylsalicylic acid analogue (lycine-ASA) have been performed.[39-41] After nasal provocations, the topically delivered lycine-ASA induced both increased nasal patency and nasal symptoms in aspirin-sensitive subjects.[39,40] The diagnosis of ASA intolerance has to be based on the provocation procedure, because there is no specific in vitro test for this type of diagnosis. Topical nasal challenges with aspirin analogues in ASA-intolerant subjects seem to be safer and easier than oral tests. The test, however, is less sensitive than oral provocations for confirming an intolerance, but it can be useful for determining whether an oral provocation test is indicated. Nasal challenges with ASA analogues are easy to perform, time-saving, and well tolerated. The test also can be performed in an outpatient setting.[40]

SAFETY OF NASAL PROVOCATIONS

Side effects in association with nasal provocations are few. Nevertheless, standard precautions and routine safety measures should always be considered.

MEASUREMENT OF THE NASAL RESPONSE

As mentioned, different provocative agents induce different kinds of nasal responses. Thus, the method for evaluation of the nasal response must depend on the provocative stimulus. The nose can respond to various stimuli in only a limited way. Changes in vascular tonus regulate nasal patency. Rhinorrhea is due to glandular secretion and microvascular exudation of plasma. Stimulation of sensory nerves provoke sneezes and itching.

Symptoms

As mentioned, symptom recording and rhinoscopy may be sufficient for clinical purposes when only a qualitative answer is needed. The primary method and the easiest to perform is assessment of symptoms by either the subject or the observer.[42] Symptoms of nasal congestion, rhinorrhea, and irritation can be rated, and the number of sneezes can be counted. A visual analogue scale may be more sensitive, however. A line is drawn with labels on both ends. The subjects mark the sensation of the different symptoms along the lines. Documentation of the symptoms is of most value for intrapersonnel evaluations. In addition to symptom scores, at least one objective measurement of the nasal response should be used.

A rhinoscopic investigation may itself affect the response and induce inflammatory changes; it is important to be aware of this effect when a clinical examination is performed before objective measurements of the nasal response. For more complicated research, more sophisticated methods of assessing nasal responses are needed.

Vascular Reactions

Different parts of the nasal vasculature can be monitored independently. Changes in the tonus of the capacitance vessels can be examined by measuring the volume of the nasal cavity and indirectly by changes in the airflow/pressure gradient. Different techniques for measuring vasculature reactions are listed in Table 10–4.

Nasal peak flow

Nasal peak flow measurement is the simplest technique. It is inexpensive, quick, and easy to perform. It may be useful for detecting changes in nasal patency for repeated measurements and compares well with rhinomanometry.[43] The reproducibility of peak flow measurements is less than that of rhinomanometry, however.[44]

Rhinomanometry

This technique attempts to measure nasal airway resistance by quantitatively measuring nasal flow and pressure.[44] It is based on the principle that air will flow through a tube only when there is a pressure gradient. When the nasal mucosa is decon-

Table 10–4   Different Techniques for Measuring of Nasal Vasculature Reactions

Capacitance vessels	
Rhinomanometry	
	Active (anterior/posterior)
	Passive (anterior/posterior)
Nasal peak flow	
	Inspiratory
	Expiratory
Acoustic rhinometry	
Rhinostereometry	
Resistance vessels	
^{133}Xe washout	
Hydrogen (^{3}H) clearance	
Laser-Doppler	

gested, the reproducibility of rhinomanometric results is good but time-consuming.[45] Active anterior rhinomanometry is recommended and most frequently used. Furthermore, it seems to be more sensitive than passive anterior rhinomanometry.[45]

Acoustic rhinometry

This is a fairly new technique for measurement of the geometrical cross-sectional area of the nasal cavity. It uses an audible sound pulse that is generated by a spark. The sound pulse is then propagated in a sound tube and passed into the nose, where it is altered by variations in the cross-sectional area. The reflected signal is picked up by a microphone and analyzed. From this measurement it is possible to determine the volume of the cavity.[46]

Rhinostereometry

This is an optical device. Variations of the distance of the nasal mucosal surface can be estimated through an eyepiece of a microscope.[47] The method measures changes in the mucosal swelling with a very high degree of accuracy, but the correlation to the patient's own subjective impression of nasal obstruction is poor.[48]

Resistance vessels

Blood flow in the resistance vessels can be measured with laser-Doppler flowmetry.[49] This method seems to measure blood flow changes in the superficial parts of the nasal mucosa, whereas another method of measuring blood flow in the resistance vessels, the $_{133}$Xe washout method, probably measures deeper parts of the mucosa.[50] Clearance of hydrogen ($_3$H) is another method and can be used for continuous measurement of blood flow. The technique, however, is both traumatic and technically difficult to perform.[51]

Nasal Discharge

Nasal discharge includes tear fluid, serous glands, seromucous glands, goblet cells, and plasma exudation. Various kinds of challenges generate different responses in the nose which then also influence the appearance and consistency of the nasal discharge.

Various methods have been used to collect nasal fluids: absorption,[52] suction,[53] blowing,[54] dripping,[24] washing,[55] and lavage.[8,56] Minimal mechanical and physical stimulation of the mucosa is, of course, important. Some investigators have inserted a catheter into the nasal cavity. With such a technique, the degree of mechanical stimulation may be considerable. Also, paper disks irritate the mucosal surface and may induce a selective absorption of different solutes from the surface.[57] Filter papers absorb not only surface liquid but also a considerable amount of subepithelial interstitial fluid.[7] When comparing results from different investigators, one must bear in mind the different techniques used.

Instillation of large volumes of saline (5 to 10 mL), with the head bent backward or forward, with the nasal pool device washes larger areas than the spraying technique[8] (Fig. 10–2). Nasal lavage causes minimal mechanical stimulation and no apparent alterations in the response to challenges, is well tolerated, and can be performed repeatedly.[4,5,8] It samples surface liquids from a large mucosal area, and multiple biochemical markers and mediators can be analyzed.[8,58] With the "nasal pool" device, patients themselves can lavage their noses and the fluid can be instilled into the nasal cavity for different time periods[4,5] (Fig. 10–1). The problem with total nasal congestion can be overcome by giving a nasal decongestant before the lavage.[8] The possible interaction between nasal decongestants and the measured parameters must, however, be considered.

Blown secretions can be quantified by volume measurements (that is, in a syringe)[59] (Fig. 10–3) or by weighing of handkerchiefs.[60] The nose also can be washed with tracers of known concentration. When an exogenous marker is added to the lavage fluid, the marker itself should not be absorbed or adsorbed to the mucosa. Exogenous albumin does not seem to be selectively retained in the nasal mucosa, and this marker molecule can be precisely measured by radioactive labeling.[57] The change in the concentration of the recovered lavage fluid permits calculations of the amount of discharge recovered. Lithium and radiolabeled albumin both have been used as tracers.[57,61] These techniques have provided useful information about the amount of discharge released, but they have not been able to define their sources, properties, or composition.

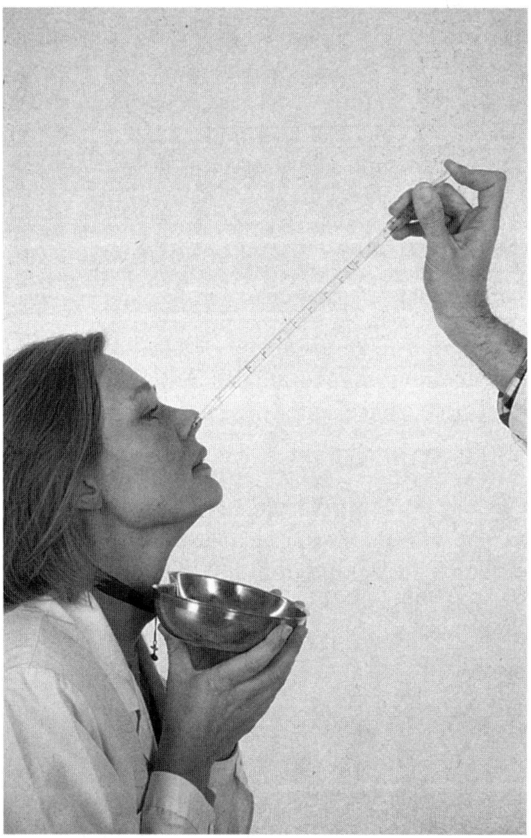

Figure 10–2. Nasal lavage technique. After nasal provocation with an agent, the nose can be washed by saline solution. In the lavage fluid, both the cellullar content and the levels of different mediators can be determined.

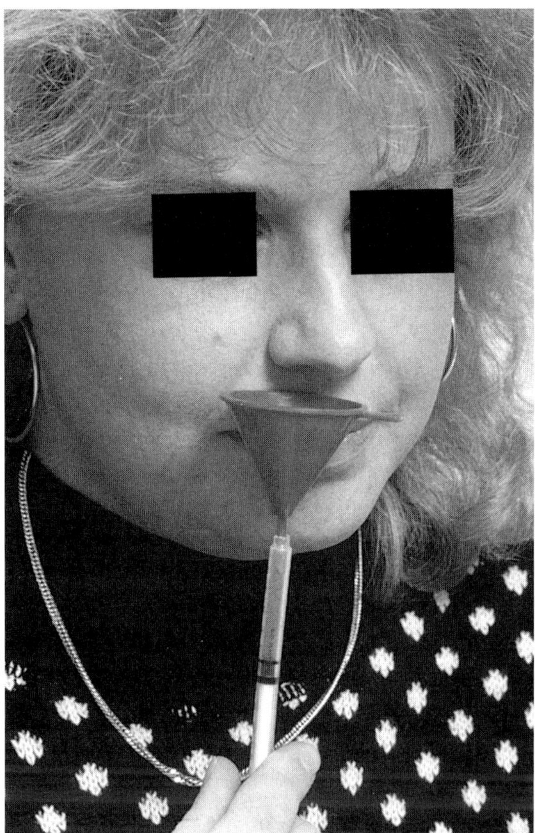

Figure 10–3. Volume of the glandular secretion can be measured by a funnel connected to a syringe.

Biochemical Markers

Several techniques and methods have been developed to measure mediators, plasma proteins, glandular secretory products, cytokines, and extracellular matrix molecules in response to various provocation factors. These methods reflect the amount of markers on the mucosal surface but also may mirror the amount in the mucosal tissue. Differences in the concentration may thus reflect not only the "true content on the mucosal surface" but also the ability of the substances to enter the lumen. Indeed, the measured levels of any possible product on the mucosal surface may not be the "true" amount of released substances but can very likely reflect different actions (such as exudative and secretory processes) that drive these factors from the mucosal and submucosal tissue out into the lumen. Not only the amount but also the physical properties of the discharge may vary as a result of different provocative factors. The viscosity and spinability of the discharge after allergen challenges differ from those after methacholine provocations.[62]

Cellular Responses

Various techniques have been used to obtain, process, evaluate, and interpret nasal cytologic specimens as well. The selection of the sampling method is dependent on the requirements of the specimen. The age of the patient, the need for repeated samplings, and the position or site of the mucosa of interest also must be considered.

Secretions can be blown onto paper or plastic wrap and thereafter placed onto a glass slide.[63,64] These methods for cell harvesting are collected from nasal secretions and may actually not reflect the true mucosal content of inflammatory cells. It can also be speculated whether the cells harvested from nasal secretions really reflect cells actively participating in a pathophysiologic process or are just cells maintained in the nasal cavity for an unknown period and are no longer fulfilling any operative role.

Cotton swabs can be used to collect cells. It is a simple procedure, but the reproducibility of this technique is low.[65] Imprints also can be used and utilize a thin plastic strip painted with 1% albumin to produce a sticky surface.[66] The swabs are pressed on the mucosal surface, normally the septum. The need for manual handling and the presence of a high quantity of secretions are disadvantages.[66] Nasal brushes also can be used for cell collection.[67] A small, plastic-coated steel-wire brush with nylon bristles is used. It is placed between the septum and inferior turbinate and is rotated while being removed (Fig. 10–4). The number of cells can be calculated because the volume of fluid in which the cells are dissolved is known.[67] The cells

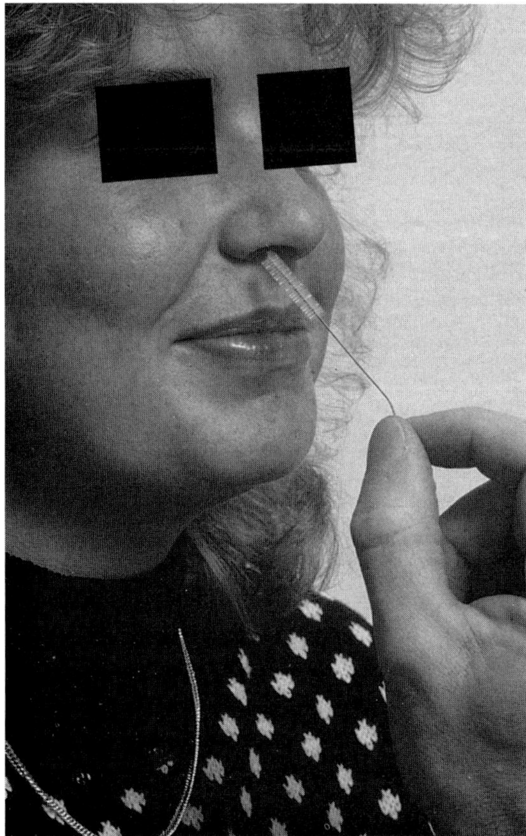

Figure 10–4. Nasal brush, a small, plastic-coated steel-wire brush with nylon bristles. It is introduced into the nasal cavity under direct visual guidance and rotated between the septum and inferior turbinate. Cells collected with this technique have a high morphologic quality.

obtained include those from secretions and the superficial layer of the mucosa. Cells collected with this method can be used for both biochemical analysis and morphologic studies. Unfortunately, the brush technique causes a slight irritation, which makes it unsuitable for use in children.

Nasal scrapings[68] and nasal lavages[69] are other methods of gathering cells. For the nasal scraping method, a plastic curette is introduced into the nasal cavity under direct visual guidance. In contrast to the nasal brush, this method seems to harvest cells from a more superficial layer of the nasal mucosa.[68] The cells collected by nasal brushes seem, however, to be better preserved than cells obtained by lavage techniques.[66,69] Cells also can be examined in biopsy specimens.[70] Disadvantages of the biopsy specimen are trauma and nasal bleeding, and biopsies are difficult to perform repeatedly. The biopsy specimen allows, however, analyses of the deeper layers of the mucosa, such as the basement membrane and the submucosal tissue. The Geritsma forceps is a newly developed forceps that collects specimens in which the morphology of both the epithelium and the cells is well preserved.[71] Anesthesia is needed before any biopsy can be taken, however. The anesthesia itself and the introduction of the anesthetic agent into the nasal cavity may affect the results. Furthermore, because the nasal mucosa is very abundant in vasculature, a vasoconstrictor usually is needed to reduce the risk of intraoperative or postoperative bleeding. Different techniques for the collecting of cells are listed in Table 10–5.

CONCLUSIONS

Several new techniques recently have been developed both for nasal provocation and for monitoring of responses. Each of these methods has its advantages and disadvantages. These need to be considered in order to select the proper provocative agent and to choose the correct method for observation of the nasal response in relation to the aim of the investigation and the question at issue.

Table 10–5   Cytologic Methods for Cell Collecting

METHOD	QUANTITATIVE	SECRETION	EM*	BIOCHEM†	EASE
Smear	No	Yes	No	No	+++
Blown secretion	No	Yes	No	No	++
Imprints	Yes	Yes	No	No	++
Nasal scraping	Yes	No	Yes	Yes	++
Lavage and cytocentrifuge	Yes	No	Yes	Yes	++
Brush and cytocentrifuge	Yes	No	Yes	Yes	+
Biopsy	Yes	No	Yes	Yes	++

*EM, electron microscopy.
†Biochem, possible to analyze biochemical markers and mediators with a high degree of precision.

REFERENCES

1. Karlsson G, Rundcrantz H: Peroral chromones. A new way to treat allergic rhinitis? *Acta Otolaryngol (Stockh) Suppl* 1979; 1360:27–29.
2. Kirkegaard J, Secher C, Borum P, Mygind N: Inhibition of histamine-induced nasal symptoms by the H_1 antihistamine chlorpheniramine maleate. Demonstration of topical effect. *Br J Dis Chest* 1983; 77:113–122.
3. Mygind N, Vesterhauge S: Aerosol distribution in the nose. *Rhinology* 1978; 16:79–88.
4. Greiff L, Pipkorn U, Alkner U, Persson CG: The "nasal pool" device applies controlled concentrations of solutes on human nasal airway mucosa and samples its surface exudations/secretions. *Clin Exp Allergy* 1990; 20:253–259.
5. Connell JT: Quantitative intranasal pollen challenge. II. Effect of daily pollen challenge, environmental pollen exposure, and placebo challenge on the nasal membrane. *J Allergy* 1968; 41:123–139.
6. Okuda M: Mechanisms in nasal allergy. *ORL Digest* 1977; 39:26–33.
7. Erjefält I, Persson CG: On the use of absorbing discs to sample mucosal surface liquids. *Clin Exp Allergy* 1990; 20:193–197.
8. Naclerio RM, Meier HL, Kagey-Sobotka A, et al: Mediator release after nasal airway challenge with allergen. *Am Rev Respir Dis* 1983; 128:597–602.
9. McLean JA, Mathews KP, Solomon WR, Brayton PR, Brayne NK: Effect of ammonia on nasal resistance in atopic and nonatopic subjects. *Ann Otol Rhinol Laryngo* 1979; 88:228–234.
10. Bacon JR, McLean JA, Mathews KP, Banas JM: Priming of the nasal mucosa by ragweed extract or by an irritant (ammonia). *J Allergy Clin Immunol* 1981; 67:111–116.
11. Togias AG, Naclerio RM, Proud D, et al: Nasal challenge with cold, dry air results in release of inflammatory mediators: possible mast cell involvement. *J Clin Invest* 1985; 76:1375–1381.
12. Aas K, Backman A, Belin L, Weeke B: Standardization of allergen extracts with appropriate methods. *Allergy* 1978; 33:130–137.
13. Andersson M: *Allergen-Induced Hyperreactivity*. Thesis, University of Lund, 1988.
14. Andersson M, von Kogerer B, Andersson P, Pipkorn U: Allergen-induced nasal hyperreactivity appears unrelated to the size of the nasal and dermal immediate allergic reaction. *Allergy* 1987; 42:631–637.
15. Svensson C, Pipkorn U, Alkner U, et al: Topical vasoconstrictor (oxymetazoline) does not affect histamine-induced mucosal exudation of plasma in human nasal airways. *Clin Exp Allergy* 1992; 22:411–416.
16. Clement PAR, Stoop AP, Kaufman L: Histamine threshold and nasal hyperreactivity in nonspecific allergic rhinopathy. *Rhinology* 1985; 23:35–42.
17. Gerth Van Wijk RG: *Nasal Hyperreactivity*. Thesis, Erasmus University, Rotterdam, 1991.
18. Svensson C, Greiff L, Andersson M, Persson CGA: Bradykinin-, leukotriene D_4-, and histamine-induced mucosal exudation of plasma in human airways in vivo (abstract). *Allergy Clin Immunol News* 1994; 2:85.
19. Jackson R: Prostaglandin E, as a nasal constrictor in normal human volunteers. *Curr Ther Res* 1970; 50:165.
20. Tönnesen P, Mygind N: Nasal challenge with serotonin and histamine in normal persons. *Allergy* 1985; 40:350–353.
21. Klementsson H, Andersson M: Eosinophil chemotactic activity of topical PAF on the human nasal mucosa. *Eur J Clin Pharmacol* 1992; 42:295–299.
22. Raphael GD, Druce HM, Baraniuk JN, Kaliner MA: Pathophysiology of rhinitis. I. Assessment of the sources of protein in methacholine-induced nasal secretions. *Am Rev Respir Dis* 1988; 138:413–420.
23. Hargreave FE, Ryan G, Thomson NC, et al: Bronchial responsiveness to histamine or methacholine in asthma: measurement and clinical significance. *J Allergy Clin Immunol* 1981; 68:347–355.
24. Borum P: Nasal methacholine challenge. A test for the measurement of nasal reactivity. *J Allergy Clin Immunol* 1979; 63:253–257.
25. Filiaci F, Zambetti G: Aspecific nasal reactivity in allergic and non-allergic rhinopathy. *Rhinology* 1983; 21:329–334.
26. Stjärne P, Lundblad L, Lundberg JM, Änggård A: Capsaicin and nicotine-sensitive afferent neurones and nasal secretion in healthy human volunteers and in patients with vasomotor rhinitis. *Br J Pharmacol* 1989; 96:693–701.
27. Lundblad L: *Protective Reflexes and Vascular Effects in the Nasal Mucosa Elicited by Activation of Capsaicin-Sensitive Nerve Fibers*. Thesis, University of Stockholm, 1984.
28. Karlsson G, Pipkorn U: Substance P and human nasal mucociliary activity. *Eur J Clin Pharmacol* 1986; 30:355–357.

29. Greiff L, Svensson C, Andersson M, Persson CGA: Effects of topical capsaicin in seasonal allergic rhinitis. *Thorax* 1995; 50:225–229.
30. Greiff L, Wollmer P, Erjefält I, Andersson M, Pipkorn U, Persson CGA: Effects of nicotine on the human nasal mucosa. *Thorax* 1993; 48:651–655.
31. Drettner B: Vascular reactions of the human nasal mucosa on exposure to cold. *Acta Otolaryngol (Stockh)* Suppl 1961; 166:1–109.
32. Flisberg K, Ingelstedt S: Vascular reactions to feet cooling in normal and allergic nose: an analysis of some physical and physiologic variables. *Acta Otolaryngol (Stockh)* 1962; 55:457–466.
33. Anderson SD: Recent advances in the understanding of exercise-induced asthma. *Eur Respir Dis* 1983; Suppl 128:225–236.
34. Silber G, Naclerio R, Eggleston P, et al: In vivo release of histamine by hyperosmolar stimuli (abstract). *J Allergy Clin Immunol* 1985; 75:176.
35. Greiff L, Wollmer P, Svensson C, Andersson M, Persson CGA: Effects of hypertonic saline on mucosal exudation of plasma in human airways (abstract). *Allergy Clin Immunol News* 1994; 2:76.
36. Nielsen J, Welinder H, Ottosson H, Bensryd I, Venge P, Skerfving S: Nasal challenge shows pathogenetic relevance of specific IgE serum antibodies for nasal symptoms caused by hexahydrophthalic anhydride. *Clin Exp Allergy* 1994; 24:440–449.
37. Samter M, Beers RF Jr: Intolerance to aspirin. Clinical studies and consideration of its pathogenesis. *Ann Intern Med* 1968; 68:975–983.
38. Stevenson DD, Simon RA, Mathison DA: Aspirin-sensitive asthma: tolerance to aspirin after positive oral aspirin challenges. *J Allergy Clin Immunol* 1980; 66:82–88.
39. Patriarca G, Nucera E, DiRienzo V, et al: Nasal provocation test with lysine acetylsalicylate in aspirin-sensitive patients. *Ann Allergy* 1991; 67:60–62.
40. Wellbrock M, Mertens J, Cornelius M, Brasch J: Intranasal provocation with lysine acetylsalicylic acid [German]. *HNO* 1993; 41:577–581.
41. Dahlén B, Zëtterström O: Comparison of bronchial and peroral provocation with aspirin in aspirin-sensitive asthmatics. *Eur Respir J* 1990; 3:527–534.
42. Weeke B, Davies RJ, Okuda M: Allergy Diagnosis In Vivo, in Mygind N, Weeke B (eds.): *Allergic and Vasomotor Rhinitis: Clinical aspects.* Copenhagen, Munksgaard, 1985, pp 97–107.
43. Holmström M, Scadding GK, Lund VJ, Darby YC: Assessment of nasal obstruction. A comparison between rhinomanometry and and nasal inspiratory peak flow. *Rhinology* 1990; 28:191–196.
44. Clement PAR, Hirsch C: Rhinomanometry—a review. *ORL* 1984; 46:173–191.
45. Clement PAR: Committee report on standardization of rhinomanometry. *Rhinology* 1984; 22:151–155.
46. Hilberg O, Jackson AC, Swift DL, Pedersen OF: Acoustic rhinometry: evaluation of nasal cavity geometry by acoustic reflection. *J Appl Physiol* 1989; 66:295–303.
47. Juto J-E, Lundberg C: An optical method for determining changes in mucosal congestion in the nose in man. *Acta Otolaryngol (Stockh)* 1982; 94:149–156.
48. Graf P, Juto J-E: Correlation between objective nasal mucosal swelling and estimated stuffiness during long-term use of vasoconstrictors. *ORL* 1994; 56:334–339.
49. Bende M: *Blood Flow in Human Nasal Mucosa.* Thesis, University of Lund, 1983.
50. Olsson P: *Studies of Blood Flow in Human Nasal Mucosa With ^{133}Xe Washout Technique and Laser Doppler Flowmetry.* Thesis, University of Lund, 1986.
51. Konno A, Togawa K, Nishihira S: Participation of vascular reflex in mucosal swelling in nasal allergy. *Acta Otolaryngol (Stockh)* 1982; 94:131–140.
52. Ingelstedt S, Ivstam B: The source of nasal secretion in the normal condition: fluorescein tests. *Acta Otolaryngol (Stockh)* 1949; 37:446–450.
53. Rawlins AG: Method of obtaining secretions from nasopharynx for diagnosis of nasal allergy. *Laryngoscope* 1947; 57:95–96.
54. Secher C, Kirkegaard J, Borum P, et al: Significance of H_1 and H_2 receptors in the human nose: rationale for topical use of combined antihistamine preparations. *J Allergy Clin Immunol* 1982; 7:211–218.
55. Johansson SGO, Deuschl H: Immunoglobulin in nasal secretion with special reference to IgE. I. Methodological studies. *Int Arch Allergy Appl Immunol* 1976; 52:364–375.
56. Remington JS, Vosti KL, Lietze A, Zimmerman AL: Serum proteins and antibody activity in human nasal secretions. *J Clin Invest* 1964; 43:1613–1624.
57. Bisgaard H, Krogsgaard OW, Mygind N: Measurement of secretion in nasal lavage. *Clin Sci* 1987; 73:217–222.
58. Greiff L, Persson CGA, Svensson C, et al: Loratadine reduces allergen-induced mucosal output of α_2-macroglobulin and tryptase in allergic rhinitis. *J Allergy Clin Imunol* 1995; 96:97–103.
59. Klementsson H, Andersson M, Baumgarten CR, et al: Changes in non-specific nasal reactivity and eosinophil influx and activation after allergen challenge. *Clin Exp Allergy* 1990; 20:539–547.

60. Mygind N, Borum P: Effect of a cholino-receptor antagonist in the nose. *Eur J Respir Dis* 1983; Suppl 128:167–174.
61. Linder A, Strandberg K, Deuschl H: Histamine concentrations in nasal secretion and secretory activity in allergic rhinitis. *Allergy* 1987; 42:126–134.
62. Brofeldt S, Mygind N, Sörensen CH, et al: Biochemical analysis of nasal secretion by methacholine, histamine, and allergen provocations. *Am Rev Respir Dis* 1986; 133:1138–1143.
63. Hansel FK: Observations on the cytology of the secretions in allergy of the nose and paranasal sinuses. *J Allergy* 1934; 5:357–366.
64. Hastie R, Heroy JH III, Levy DA: Basophil leukocytes and mast cells in human nasal secretions and scrapings studied by light microscopy. *Lab Invest* 1979; 40:554–561.
65. Whelan CFA: Problems in the examination of nasal smears in allergic rhinitis. *J Laryngol Otol* 1980; 94:399–404.
66. Pipkorn U, Karlsson G: Methods for obtaining specimens from the nasal mucosa for morphological and biochemical analysis. *Eur Respir J* 1988; 1:856–862.
67. Pipkorn U, Karlsson G, Enerbäck L: A brush method to harvest cells from the nasal mucosa for microscopic and biochemical analysis. *J Immunol Methods* 1988; 112:37–42.
68. Meltzer EO, Jalowayski AA: Nasal cytology in clinical practice. *Am J Rhinol* 1988; 2:47–54.
69. Klementsson H, Venge P, Andersson M, Pipkorn U: Allergen-induced changes in nasal secretory responsiveness and eosinophil granulocytes. *Acta Otolaryngol (Stockh)* 1991; 111:776–784.
70. Enerbäck L, Pipkorn U, Granerus G: Intraepithelial migration of mast cells in hay fever. *Int Arch Allergy Appl Immunol* 1986; 80:44–51.
71. Fokkens WJ, Bruijnzeel-Koomen CA, Vroom T, et al: The Langerhans cell. An underestimated cell in atopic disease. *Clin Exp Allergy* 1990; 20:627–638.

11

Obstructive Sleep Apnea

WOLFGANG PIRSIG, M.D.

Obstructive sleep apnea (OSA) is a relatively common and potentially life-threatening disorder characterized by recurrent partial or complete obstructions of the pharyngeal airway which lead to snoring, hypopneas, and apneas during sleep and cause mental or physical deficits.[1-3] This dynamic phenomenon occurs whenever the collapsing force of negative inspiratory pressure exceeds the dilating force of pharyngeal airway-maintaining muscular contraction. The precise region of the collapse within the three-segmented pharynx and the mechanism of collapse vary from patient to patient and even individually during the different stages of sleep. The site of collapse may occur at one or more segments of the unsupported muscular pharyngeal airway between the soft palate and the epiglottis.[4-7]

The OSA syndrome involves the basic sequence of cyclic events briefly summarized by Wiegand et al.[8] With the initial onset of sleep, the pharyngeal airway collapses as a result of the decreased pharyngeal muscle activity. Airflow ceases despite ongoing ventilatory effort. Airflow cessation leads to progressive hypoxia and hypercapnia, which increasingly stimulate ventilatory efforts against the occluded airway until arousal occurs. With arousal, the upper airway opens, and is associated with loud snoring, and airflow is restored. Arousal coincides with an increase of upper airway inspiratory muscle activity, in particular the genioglossus, as demonstrated in the classic article by Remmers et al.[5] Hyperventilation in response to the accumulated chemical ventilatory stimuli (hypercapnia and hypoxia) initially follows deocclusion of the upper airway. The subsequent decrease in carbon dioxide tension and increase in oxygen tension result in a decreasing ventilatory effort, which in connection with return to the sleeping state is followed by recurrent pharyngeal collapse. The cycle begins anew and may be repeated hundreds of times each night, resulting in significant sleep disruption and exposure to hypoxemia.

Many factors are known contributors to these sleep-related breathing disorders. Negative upper airway pressure is thought to play a key role in the destabilization of the pharyngeal walls leading to their obstruction. Because an increasing nasal resistance contributes to the increase of the transpharyngeal pressure gradient, increased nasal resistance may be a factor in the pathophysiology of OSA and snoring.

229

This chapter focuses on the significance of the nose for sleep-disordered breathing. However, the role of the nose in the pathogenesis of OSA remains unclear. In particular, the relevance of chronically increased nasal resistance in OSA is controversial. There is evidence that nasal obstruction may interfere with breathing during sleep.[9–12] For instance, bilateral choanal atresia or a teratoma of the nasopharynx in the newborn may be associated with OSA, which is resolved by a nasal operation. Experimentally induced acute nasal occlusion may lead to increased snoring and apneic events during sleep, and successful nasal operation with relief of the nasal airflow impediment may be partially effective for reducing the loudness of snoring, the number of apneic episodes, and daytime hypersomnolence.

However, no direct correlation has been demonstrated between the severity of nasal obstruction and the severity of OSA.[13–19]

One reason for this controversy is that most measurements of nasal functions were obtained in the awake patient in an upright position. Thus, these nasal measurements cannot be correlated with those obtained during sleep. To my knowledge, there is no publication about noninvasive tests of nasal function during sleep.

Furthermore, comparison of data is difficult or impossible because of several limitations of most studies of OSA. The terminology is imprecise for sleep-related criteria and variables such as apnea, hypopnea, oxygen saturation, hypersomnolence, and snoring loudness, and standard methods of recording are lacking. Often the subjects investigated are selected and there are no matched control groups in regard to age, sex, state of health, body mass index, body position, and sleep stage. Furthermore, in retrospective epidemiologic studies, confounding factors are not always adequately controlled.[20] Because the differentiation of abnormal from normal breathing is often difficult, the definition of "pathologic" or "success of treatment" is arbitrary or often depends on a sole criterion. Furthermore, many studies are retrospective and present data gained from unvalidated questionnaires, self-assessed symptoms, and short-term result.[21] Because of these shortcomings in many basic and clinical studies on OSA, validated and reliable data on sleep-disordered breathing, in particular information related to the nose, have remained rare and limited.

DEFINITIONS

There is no general agreement on the definition of OSA, a syndrome with an unknown natural history until today. Because the overlap between normal and pathologic breathing in sleep is wide and age-dependent, it is not possible even to define "pathological apnea." Arbitrarily and as a practical working definition, apnea is defined as cessation of airflow at the nose or mouth for at least 10 seconds. This minimal duration of an apnea is the most frequently accepted definition for adults. The apnea index (AI) is the number of apneas lasting 10 seconds or longer per hour of sleep. No agreement can be found on the operational definition of "hypopnea," but a broader consensus exists for a 4% or more decrease from baseline for the definition of an event of oxygen desaturation. Apneas are termed "central" when respiratory effort ceases, "obstructive" when there is no airflow at the mouth or nose despite respiratory effort, and "mixed," which is a combination of the other two, in which an obstructive apnea follows a central apnea.

Detailed comments on the dilemma of definitions and terminology associated with sleep-disordered breathing, in particular in finding cutoff points for "pathologic" and "benign," have been published by Berry and Phillips[21] and George and Kryger.[22] For the age group between 20 and 60 years, cutoff points of an apnea-hypopnea index (AHI) of 5, 8, 10, 15, and 20 or more have been considered pathologic levels of OSA by different investigators. Evaluation becomes more complex when the various operational definitions of the criteria of sleep-disordered breathing in the elderly or in children are compared. Thus, Rosen et al.[23] showed that the adult criteria for OSA did not identify children with serious obstruction of the upper airway. Utilizing the AHI $\geq$5 threshold, Berry and Phillips[21] found a high prevalence (mean, 41%) of sleep-disordered breathing in the elderly after having reviewed nine articles on this topic encompassing a total of 247 mainly healthy elderly men.

It is evident that the use of AI or AHI as the sole or primary criterion for OSA is insufficient. Therefore, Lugaresi et al.[24,25] proposed a classification of severity of OSA which involves some sleep variables and daytime sleepiness. The presence of functional impairment is also included in minimal criteria (both AHI $\geq$5 and daytime hypersomnolence) for the diagnosis of sleep apnea syndrome in the recently published international classification of sleep disorders by the American Sleep Disorders Association. As a harmless form of sleep-disordered breathing, "primary snoring" is defined as snoring without sleep disruption and the absence of the complaint of insomnia or excessive daytime sleepiness (EDS).[26]

The Stanford group[27] recently identified a subgroup of heavy snorers suffering from EDS who did not satisfy the criteria for OSA. This male subgroup was characterized by a relatively low BMI, an AHI less than 5, an increased respiratory-related arousal index, and a low score on the multiple sleep latency test. This condition, which has also been observed in children,[28] has been termed the "upper airway resistance syndrome" (UARS) and can be significantly improved by application of nasal continuous positive airway pressure.[29,30]

EPIDEMIOLOGY

Symptoms and signs of OSA are defined differently in different studies. Therefore, it is difficult to establish prevalence data on conditions that are not well defined.

Furthermore, there are no simple and validated instruments for measuring sleep-disordered breathing in large, unselected populations. Accepting certain limitations, several working groups have tried to outline the problem by collecting some data on the morbidity, mortality, and risk factors of sleep apnea. Most subjects have been selected from a large population on the basis of questionnaires and were studied by overnight polysomnography or screening procedures.

On the basis of the minimal criteria for OSA,[26] it is suspected that *ca* 2% of the middle-aged population have OSA. Several studies have shown that sleep-disordered breathing events markedly increase with age.[21] Concerning the male: female ratio, more recent studies have demonstrated that OSA seems to be more prevalent among women than was assumed from earlier studies.[31–33] In the study by Young et al.[33] of a random sample of 3,513 state employees (30 to 60 years), 2% of women and 4% of men met the minimal criteria for OSA,[26] that is, both a AHI ≥5 and daytime sleepiness. These authors also found that women are not so severely affected because their AHI is proportionally lower.

Obesity is one of the main risk factors associated with OSA, and epidemiologic studies showed a large increase in reported daytime sleepiness and habitual snoring with increasing weight.[34]

What is the pathologic significance of sleep-related breathing disorders detected in "healthy" persons? Heavy snoring and OSA have been linked to higher cardiovascular morbidity (in particular, cardiac arrhythmias, pulmonary and systemic hypertension, stroke, cognitive deficits, myocardial infarction, and cardiac failure) and thus to an increased mortality rate. Concerning cardiovascular complications, no prospective studies are available on mortality rate in patients with OSA. Data from retrospective studies[35–37] are certainly suggestive of an increased cardiovascular morbidity and mortality in patients with OSA. Although many data have been collected concerning cardiovascular diseases and neuropsychologic deficits in OSA, we still do not know what severity of sleep-disordered breathing is potentially harmful.[38–40]

As to the natural history of OSA, Lugaresi et al.[25] described, in a retrospective analysis, the hypothesis that the passage from primary snoring to heavy snorer's disease, or OSA, is a gradual process.[24] However, they admitted that only prospective studies will better clarify the relationships among snoring, obstructive apneas, cardiovascular risk, and risk of death.

THE NOSE AND SLEEP-DISORDERED BREATHING

The nasal passages can theoretically influence upper airway collapse by contributing to inspiratory airway resistance or by control of pharyngeal muscles via supposed nasal airflow receptors. Several studies have investigated both hypotheses. The pathophysiology of OSA involves the development of pharyngeal airway narrowing.[41] There are convincing arguments that this pharyngeal airway may behave like a Starling resistor in healthy and diseased persons because of the decreased upper airway muscle tone and phasic inspiratory activity during sleep.[42–45] The subatmospheric pressure generated within the collapsible segment of the pharynx contributes to the limitation of inspiratory flow.[42] Increased nasal resistance results in the generation of a more subatmospheric pharyngeal pressure during inspiration, because the force of diaphragmatic contraction is increased to move air through the narrowed nasal cavities. This might increase the pressure decrease across the smallest cross-sectional area in the pharynx, contributing to collapse. The contribution of nasal resistance toward this mechanism remains unclear.[13]

Several investigators[3,13–17,46,47] have searched for correlations between awake nasal resistance and sleep-related breathing factors. In all these studies, the awake nasal resistance was determined by rhinomanometry or by head-out body plethysmography. Most authors could not find correlations between awake nasal resistance and AI or AHI, whereas the relationship between snoring and awake nasal resistance has been controversial. Hoffstein et al.[15] briefly explained these differing results: "Neither the site of obstruction during apneas nor the site of generation of snoring is in the nose."

The measurement of nasal resistance during sleep presents several technical difficulties. No noninvasive method is available to measure nasal resistance during sleep. Olsen et al.[10] concluded from a comparison of esophageal pressures with the nose open then occluded that oral breathing appeared to be a high-resistance pathway during sleep in comparison with nasal breathing. This conclusion was drawn from very few data from some middle-aged healthy persons. Hudgel and Robertson[48] used small, multiply perforated nasopharyngeal catheters to measure nasal resistance of middle-aged healthy men during wakefulness, stage 2, and rapid eye movement (REM) sleep periods in both lateral positions. They found that total nasal resistance did not change significantly during sleep and did not differ significantly from that during wakefulness. Resistance on one side of the nose was considerably higher than on the other side and changed alternately during sleep. This spontaneously fluctuating resistance appeared to be independent of gravity. In another study, Hudgel and Hendricks[49] used three transnasally placed catheters and a face mask to measure upper airway resistance in healthy, nonsnoring men during wakefulness and stage 2 sleep. In these subjects, the increase in inspiratory supralaryngeal airflow resistance from wakefulness to sleep occurred at the level of the palate or hypopharynx and not within the nose. During sleep, nasal resistance increased minimally, whereas at 0.01 l/s inspiratory flow, transpalatal and hypopharyngeal resistances increased 200% and 400%, respectively. The limitation of all three studies is that they changed the natural conditions of the nasal cavities by the measuring methods. Because there are no adequate instruments to measure nasal function and particularly nasal resistance during sleep noninvasively, it is impossible to define criteria for selection of predisposed individuals for whom an increased nasal resistance may be an important factor in the pathogenesis of nonapneic snoring or OSA.

The alae nasi muscles dilate the nostrils, reducing nasal resistance. Therefore, several groups have been interested in studying the activity of these muscles in healthy individuals and patients with OSA. In normal subjects, activation of upper airway muscles seems to be precisely synchronized. Strohl et al.[50] measured the electromyography (EMG) activity of the alae nasi during wakefulness, quiet sleep, and CO_2-induced hyperapnea and compared the time from onset of EMG activity to the onset of inspiratory airflow in eight healthy women and men. They found a rhythmic increase in tone in the dilator naris muscles just preceding the onset of inspiration. During stages 2 and 3 of sleep, the interval between alae nasi EMG and airflow significantly increased when compared with wakefulness. During CO_2-induced hyperapnea, the alae nasi EMG to airflow interval and alae nasi EMG magnitude increased in direct proportion to CO_2 levels and minute ventilation. These data suggest that in humans, activation of upper airway muscles occurs before the onset of inspiratory flow and this sequence is more clearly evident during sleep or hyperapnea than during quiet breathing.

Suratt et al.[51] measured the alae nasi EMG and the contraction of the rib cage and diaphragm during apneas in nine male subjects with various degrees of OSA during sleep. They observed that during non-REM sleep, both alae nasi EMG activity and change in esophageal pressure decrease at the onset of obstructive apnea and increase as apnea progresses. As apnea progresses, alae nasi EMG activation occurs earlier relative to change in esophageal pressure. Alae nasi preactivation was thus greater at the end of an apneic episode than at the beginning of the episode. The same EMG activity pattern was found for the genioglossus. The authors concluded that earlier activation of upper airway muscles relative to the diaphragm and rib cage musculature during apneic episodes appears to be a compensatory attempt to open the airway before airway pressure is lowered by contraction of the diaphragm and rib cage muscles.

This decrease in EMG activity of upper airway muscles at the onset of apneas has been described by previous investigators.[5,52] In addition, Suratt et al.[53] observed that patients with OSA and high upper airway resistance had considerable phasic activation of the alae nasi and genioglossal muscles during inspiration. This phasic activity was found during wakefulness and during sleep. Phasic activity of alae nasi EMG signals during sleep was greater in patients with OSA than in young, normal-weight control subjects with low upper airway resistances. It was not significantly different, however, between patients and the older, normal-weight and the older, obese control subjects. The authors interpreted the increased phasic activity of these muscles in patients with OSA as representing a compensatory mechanism when upper airway patency becomes threatened during sleep.

To determine the relationship of hypothetical nasal receptors to respiratory rhythmicity during sleep, White et al.[54] and McNicholas et al.[55] monitored breathing in sleeping normal subjects after nasal anesthesia. Both working groups showed that topical nasal anesthesia resulted in a statistically but not clinically significant increase in the frequency of obstructive apneas and hypopneas during sleep. These results suggest that nasal receptors sensitive to airflow may play a role in maintaining breathing rhythmicity during sleep.

Several studies indicate an association between nasal obstruction and sleep-disordered breathing.[10,12,15,45,56] These obstructive breathing events occur both during natural nasal obstruction due to nasal allergy[12,57,58] and during severe nasal occlusion in association with nasal congenital anomalies, infections, trauma, and tumors. Some investigators have demonstrated that therapy of causative conditions eliminated or reduced obstructive symptoms (Table 11–1). Obstructive breathing events during sleep have also been observed during artificially induced total nasal occlusion in adult volunteers[9–11,64–66] and in patients with nasal packs for treatment of epistaxis or after nasal operation.[62–64] In some of the patients with the temporary nasal packs, the degree of sleep-related breathing disorders appeared to be more pronounced than in the healthy individuals. However, these studies did not control for other associated factors known to cause OSA; thus, their results cannot be compared with findings in healthy volunteers.

To find out whether nasal occlusion produces OSA by decreasing upper airway muscle activation via nasal reflexes or by increasing upper airway resistance, Wilhoit and Suratt[70] studied the effect of artificial intranasal occlusion on the activity of the alae nasi and genioglossal muscles in healthy men. Nasal occlusion produced OSA in all subjects and increased the phasic EMG activity of both muscles throughout sleep. Apneas tended to occur at the nadirs of EMG activity. This finding suggests that nasal occlusion generally increases respiratory drive to upper airway muscles

Table 11–1   Reported Effects of Nasal Surgery on Obstructive Sleep Apnea

REFERENCE	NO. OF PATIENTS	FOLLOW-UP TIME, MONTHS	PREOPERATIVE AHI	POSTOPERATIVE AHI	NO. OF RESPONDERS	POSTOPERATIVE SUBJECTIVE BENEFIT
59	2	2–3	AI: 29 resp. 66	AI: 25 resp. 72	0	yes (2)
60	23	no data	44.2	41.5	8/23* (35%)	no data
61	6	4–44	47 (12–85)	28 (15–53)	3/6* (50%)	yes (6)
62	3	2–12	290–350 apneas/night	40–106 apneas/night	3* (100%)	yes (3)
63	9	2–6	38.8	26.8	5/9* (55.5%)	yes (9)
3	20	2–3	39.8	36.8	4 normalized 4 improved 7 unchanged 5 worsened	yes

AHI: apnea-hypopnea index.
Responders are patients whose postoperative apnea-hypopnea index or apnea index decreased by more than 50% of the preoperative value.

during sleep. "The findings are consistent with the hypothesis that nasal occlusion forces subjects to breathe through a high resistance pathway—the mouth—during sleep. Breathing through a high resistance pathway would make the pressure in the pharynx more negative and thus requires more upper airway muscle activation to maintain airway patency. Apneas would occur when there is insufficient muscle activation to offset the more negative pharyngeal airway pressures."

Another pathogenetic aspect was discussed by Lavie and Rubin[65] who compared the effect of acute nasal occlusion in five healthy apneic-free sons of patients with fullblown sleep apnea with four age-matched normals without a familial history of OSA. Nasal occlusion caused a significant increase in the number of sleep apneas in the sons of patients with OSA as compared with controls, a finding that suggests the inheritability of sleep apnea proneness.

All these different nasal occlusion studies show that severe nasal obstruction leads to disordered breathing in sleep, but the relative importance of less severe degrees of nasal obstruction remains unclear. Some results suggest that the obstructive events observed are a consequence of nasal obstruction rather than elicited by specific nasal reflexes. Further research is required to clarify the role of the "resistor nose" for sleep-disordered breathing.

DIAGNOSTICS OF SLEEP-DISORDERED BREATHING

History

Symptoms of OSA are not specific. They may include snoring, disturbed sleep, nocturnal enuresis, excessive daytime somnolence, intellectual deterioration, personality change, hallucinations, automatic behavior, morning headaches, sexual impotence, accident proneness, and, particularly in children, hyperactivity and anti-social behavior.

OSA may be associated with symptoms caused by cardiovascular disorders or neuropsychological dysfunction. These sequelae are often treated as isolated diseases such as depression, impotence, systemic hypertension, or cardiac arrhythmias without being recognized as symptoms of sleep-related breathing disorders.

The history may be a help to diagnose OSA, particularly when patients complain about EDS or drowsiness when driving or when a partner reports or "stops breathing during sleep." In regard to the two complaints by a partner, Kapuniai et al.[71] found a predictive accuracy of 88% for AI more than 10. However, even detailed questionnaires cannot help to detect patients of risks from that obscure area between "still normal" and "mild apneic."[72,73] Viner et al.[73] performed a blinded comparison of history and physical examination with results of nocturnal polysomnography in 410 patients. They found a prevalence of OSA in 46% of their patients (AHI >10). Subjective impression alone identified correctly only 52% of patients with OSA, and it had a specifity of 70%. Bliwise et al.[74] could not achieve a high diagnostic accuracy with three questions about snoring after analyzing data on self-reported snoring and related behavior in 1,409 patients before nocturnal polysomnography. The value of a patient's history is also limited after treatment, when improvement of EDS leads to overestimation of the therapeutic efficacy (Table 11–1).

Physical examination

Although no physical findings are pathognomonic for OSA, a careful general, otorhinolaryngologic, and orthodontic examination is necessary to evaluate the anatomy of the upper airway. Depending on the history and findings, the diagnostic approach is completed by referring the patient to other specialists (internal medicine, pneumology, allergy, neurology, psychiatry, pediatrics, gerontology, radiology, orthodontics, maxillofacial surgery).

There is no need to repeat the list of potential pathologic conditions of the upper airway associated with OSA, such as bulky tongue, elongated and thick uvula, and retrognathia. They may present as a single anatomical or functional problem or may include several segments of the upper airway, sometimes being part of a craniofacial anomaly (such as Pierre Robin syndrome, Apert's syndrome), of a neuromuscular disorder (such as myasthenia gravis, Chiari malformation type 2), or of a general medical problem (such as Hodgkin's disease, Prader-Willi syndrome).[75] According to Schuller,[76] the combination of several anatomical alterations of the upper airway in OSA is considerably more common than OSA due to a single anatomical problem. He found that only 3 of approximately 200 patients with OSA had a single anatomical obstruction that could be sufficiently surgically corrected. Several attempts have been made to demonstrate that some findings are very characteristic for OSA, such as an excessively long soft palate, a retrognathic mandible, or kissing tonsils in children. For instance, in a prospective study of 150 patients with symptoms suggesting sleep apnea, Davies et al.[72] showed that neck circumference corrected for height is more useful as a predictor of OSA than general obesity. However, for most of these OSA-suspicious signs, no control studies are available. Furthermore, a large group of patients with OSA have no identifiable abnormality of the upper airway, and thus their condition is termed "idiopathic."[77]

Although the diagnostic value of some tests for OSA is doubtful or irrelevant, some of the following investigations in awake patients are performed according to the interests of the investigators: nasal resistance tests, acoustic rhinometry, pharyngeal acoustic reflection, upper airway pressures, pulmonary function tests, nasopharyngeal fiberoptic visualization, radiocephalometry, cinefluoroscopy, computed tomography, and magnetic resonance imaging.

Polysomnography

PSG is crucial for the diagnosis of sleep-disordered breathing, either by investigation in sleep laboratories or by home monitoring equipment. Several factors in the sleeping patient are registered by a polygraph strip chart recorder, and the patient might be videotaped throughout the night. The standard overnight polysomnographic study may include the following:

Electroencephalography (EEG)
Electro-oculography (EOG)
Nasal airflow
Oral airflow
Thoracic movement
Abdominal movement
Electrocardiography (ECG)
Skin-surface oximetry (ear or finger)
Electromyography (EMG of genioglossus)
Measurement of sleep-dependent breath sounds
Measurement of body position

In addition, registration of esophageal pressure, measurements of upper airway pressures and resistances, somnofluoroscopy, fiberoptic nasopharyngoscopy, and anterior tibial EMG may be performed in sleeping patients.

Many individuals need a sleep investigation because of suspected OSA or follow-up after treatment, but the number of sleep laboratories is limited. Therefore, several investigators, in particular in Europe, have tried to reduce the number of expensive and time-consuming conventional PSGs and to find cheaper screening tests suited also for home recordings. With the technical improvement of pulse oximeters, this method in combination with the history and clinical features is effective for diagnosing advanced cases of OSA; however, its sensitivity is low for mild to moderate disease.[78,80] One main question of all screening tests is how to measure factors by which sleep is documented and staged, with minimal sensors. The recording of movements allows an estimation of the sleeping time with good accuracy, as was shown by Svanborg et al.[81] These authors combined a static charge-sensitive bed with oximetry and found 34% of the patients as borderline cases who needed more extensive examinations. The German MESAM IV system combines oximetry, body position monitoring, and recording of intermittent snoring sounds. This system has been validated by Stoohs and Guilleminault[82] who found an acceptable correspondence only between oximeter findings and AHI. Douglas et al.[83] reported results in 200 consecutive patients with possible OSA. They combined oximetry with overnight recording of respiratory pattern and leg movements and found that the diagnosis could be made in most of the patients. Bradley[84] considered nocturnal monitoring of SaO_2 and of respiratory effort (such as by esophageal balloon, Respitrace) a reasonable alternative to full PSG.

It is very difficult to compare the various studies on screening for sleep apnea because different criteria for pathologic oximetry were used and validation was performed with different cutoff points of AHI. Nevertheless, there are some practical arguments to support the concept of screening for OSA by registration of the following factors: pulse oximetry, nasal and oral airflows, thoracic and abdominal movements, and breath sounds (recording the frequency range between 50 Hz and 1,500 Hz). To date, these screening methods have not been accepted for routine diagnostic purposes by either the American Thoracic Society or the American Sleep Disorders Association, which consider an all-night polysomnographic study mandatory for "the characterization and documentation of the presence and severity of sleep apnea."[26]

Multiple Sleep Latency Test

Chronic daytime sleepiness, from mild to excessive (EDS) degree, is one of the dominant symptoms of OSA. It is reported in 8% to 10% of middle-aged people. It impairs tasks that require sustained vigilance, especially when driving or working. Thus, EDS is the main reason why OSA is positively correlated with traffic and work accidents.[58,85] The patient's level of daytime sleepiness is measured by the multiple sleep latency test (MSLT)[29,86] or the multiple maintenance of wakefulness test.[87] These tests are not necessary to diagnose OSA, but they may help to find an objective document for an important complaint which also defines the degree of the morbidity. Roehrs et al.[88] analyzed the polysomnographic and MSLT data from 466 patients with suspected sleep-related breathing disorders and found that the respiratory-related arousal index was the best correlate of the degree of EDS as measured by the MSLT.

Evaluation of the Upper Airway

Knowledge of the precise location of the obstructive segment(s) of the upper airway is of special importance to establish criteria for the various surgical procedures for

Table 11–2   Techniques Used to Evaluate the Upper Airway

TECHNIQUE	SLEEP	QUANTITATION	RESEARCH TOOL	CLINICAL ROUTINE	DIS-ADVANTAGES
Measurement of upper airway pressure	+	+	+	(+)	SE
Fiberoptic pharyngoscopy	+	−	+	+	SE, RM
Breath sounds analysis	+	+	+	(+)	SE
Cinefluoro-scopy	+	−	+	−	IRE, RM
Fast computed tomography	+	+	+	−	IRE, EE, RM
Radio-cephalometry	−	+	+	+	IRE, RM
Acoustic reflection	−	+	+	AR+	SE, RM
Fast magnetic resonance imaging	−	+	+	−	EE, RM

AR: acoustic rhinometry; IRE: ionizing radiation exposure; EE: expensive equipment; SE: special experience; RM: representing a moment.

treating OSA. These additional techniques (Table 11–2) to evaluate the upper airway were reviewed by Shepard et al.[89] The disadvantage of many of these techniques is that they represent only a short moment of the dynamic changes of the upper airway and do not allow conclusions for the whole night. Some techniques cannot be performed during sleep, and most diagnostic procedures have not been established in clinical routine.

Measurements of upper airway pressure

Upper airway closing pressures: New insight into the pathophysiology of OSA could be gained by studying the pressure to produce upper airway collapse during sleep in nonsnorers, asymptomatic snorers, and patients with OSA. Yet, even these sophisticated studies hardly helped to elucidate the importance of the nose in OSA. Issa and Sullivan[90] used nasal continuous positive airway pressure (NCPAP) to identify the airway suction pressure that caused upper airway closure during sleep. In patients with moderate to severe OSA, they occluded the nasal airway and simultaneously recorded nasal cavity and esophageal pressures in the supine and lateral positions. During active inspiratory efforts, the upper airway closing pressures during NREM stages 3 and 4 ranged from -0.5 to -8.9 cm H_2O. In all three sleep stages, the upper airway closing pressure in the supine position was significantly lower than that recorded in the lateral position. Furthermore, that study documented that the upper airway was more collapsible in NREM stages 1 and 2 and REM sleep than during NREM stages 3 and 4. That study and other studies[44,91] have shown that the application of NCPAP can eliminate periodic upper airway occlusion in patients with OSA when the level of nasal pressure exceeds a given critical pressure.[44,90] This critical pressure was defined as the level of nasal pressure below which maximal inspiratory airflow ceases. Smith et al.[44] demonstrated positive critical closing pressures of 3.3 ± 3.3 cm H_2O in six patients with OSA, whereas Schwartz et al.[45] determined negative critical closing pressures of -13.3 ± 3.2 cm H_2O in normal subjects. These results of the pressure-flow relationship in the upper airway support the hypothesis that the upper airway behaves like a Starling resistor during sleep in normal persons, and patients with OSA.

Airflow pressures have been measured at different sites in the upper airway by means of different catheter systems to document the site(s) of upper airway collapse during sleep in patients with OSA.[4,92–97] The various catheters, including open catheters, balloon catheters, and transducer-tipped catheters (Millar type), are inserted transnasally. A face mask with pneumotachograph, a fiberendoscope, and NCPAP can be added to study other features (resistance, cross-sectional areas, modulation of intrapharyngeal pressure) of the upper airway.

Hudgel[4] measured pressure at four sites within the pharyngeal airway. He found a collapse of the velopharyngeal segment in nine patients (46%) with OSA and a collapse more caudally in the retroglossal region in 56%, which he defined as hypopharyngeal collapse.

Shepard et al.[95] constructed a multiport catheter to monitor pressures in the upper airway and esophagus during apneas. During NREM sleep, collapse was confined to the velopharyngeal segment in 10 (56%) of the 18 grossly obese patients with OSA. In the remaining eight patients, collapse extended into the retroglossal segment of the oropharynx.

Metes et al.[94] measured the airway pressure during several apneas at multiple sites along the airway by using a movable Millar catheter, the initial position of which was controlled by a lateral soft tissue radiograph of the head and neck. Among 51 patients, the obstruction was retropalatal in 30, retrolingual in 7, and undetermined in 14. Chaban et al.,[92] who validated this technique, documented that collapse was confined to the velopharynx in 50% of 10 patients with OSA.

Tvinnereim and Miljeteig,[97] using a Millar catheter, obtained continuous pressure recordings from the pharynx and esophagus during sleep from 12 patients with OSA. They identified the obstructive segments at the velopharyngeal level in six patients (50%), at the oropharyngeal level in two, and at the hypopharyngeal level in four.

Although different catheter systems were used, these studies have reported similar findings: approximately 50% of the patients had collapse confined to the velopharyngeal segment, whereas in the remaining patients collapse extended to the oropharyngeal and hypopharyngeal segments of the upper airway.

Launois et al.[93] developed an endoscopic method to identify regions of the passive pharyngeal airway most susceptible to narrowing or complete closure. Two pressure transducer catheters (Millar) and a fiberoptic endoscope were placed in the pharynx via the nose. The transducer tips of these catheters were positioned just above the glottis and at the rostral end of the nasopharynx to measure nasal and endopharyngeal pressures. By applying NCPAP pharyngeal resistances could be manipulated during sleep and genioglossal muscle activity removed. These investigators found a complex pattern of primary and secondary sites of narrowing in 18 overweight patients with severe OSA. The nasopharynx was a site of primary narrowing in 16 patients, but in 8 of these patients other sites of primary narrowing were also observed. Because different conditions for creating the collapse were used in the study, the results are not comparable with the data from the above-mentioned studies. In addition, comparison of data of all these studies is somewhat difficult because different definitions were used for the three pharyngeal segments.

From their review of different methods to evaluate the upper airway, Shepard et al.[89] concluded that the measurement of pressures within the upper airway during sleep is promising. Use of a movable pressure-sensitive catheter in combination with the monitoring of esophageal pressure is a relatively easy procedure. Although monitoring of upper airway pressures may be associated with some discomfort for the patients this technique can define the site(s) of pharyngeal collapse, which is a prerequisite to select patients for operation.

Fiberoptic nasopharyngoscopy

Since 1978, fiberoptic nasopharyngoscopy has been used to visualize the entire upper airway and to evaluate its anatomy undistorted with the mouth closed.[98,99] With topical anesthesia, this subjective technique can be performed during sleep[6,76,98,100,101] and wakefulness. Concomitant video recording documents the pharyngeal muscle activity during ventilation with performance of voluntary Mueller maneuver and simulated snoring. Thus, Borowiecki et al.[98] demonstrated that the dominant site of airway closure during apneic episodes in patients with OSA was confined to the velopharyngeal level. Other investigators have found for some apneic snorers that the airway collapse also extends into the tongue base level.[6,102,103]

The predictive value of a positive Mueller maneuver to select optimal candidates for uvulopalatopharyngoplasty (UPPP) has not been confirmed by subsequent studies.[104,105] Skatvedt,[96] comparing continuous, nocturnal pressure measurements in the upper aerodigestive tract and fiberoptic nasopharyngoscopy with the Mueller maneuver, even found the latter method not sufficiently accurate and recommended that it not be used in the diagnostic workup. Pringle and Croft[100] confirmed this opinion on the basis of their results. On the contrary, the use of fiberoptic nasopharyngoscopy in combination with a very thin pressure probe to measure pharyngeal pressures during sleep was found to be a reliable method to select patients as suitable candidates for UPPP.[93,106] This thin catheter alongside the fiberscope may also provide a calibration standard for measuring dimensions of the cross-sectional areas of the upper airway recorded on the video images. Thus, this combined method may partially overcome the main disadvantage of fiberoptic nasopharyngoscopy, namely, the difficulty of quantitating the fiberoptic examination findings. Furthermore, fiberoptic pharyngoscopic findings are lacking age- and weight-matched controls in whom polysomnography was performed to exclude asymptomatic OSA.

Analysis of sleep-dependent breath sounds

Anatomical properties and mechanical characteristics of the upper airway are reflected in snoring noise. This has been demonstrated for its intensity[46] and also for its spectral properties, as Schäfer found in adults[107] and children.[108] In 1988, Hoffstein et al.[46] showed that patients with OSA snore significantly louder and more frequently than nonapneic snorers. Schäfer[107,109] analyzed sleep-dependent breath sounds of the whole night by fast Fourier transformation for apneic and nonapneic snorers. He recorded a large variation in the frequency spectrum of the single snoring events in one individual depending on body posture, phase of respiration, and sleep stage. In nonapneic snorers, the frequency range of snoring sounds is from 25 to 500 Hz, whereas in patients with OSA substantial amplitudes at frequencies up to 2 kHz are found. After UPPP Schäfer found a shift of the fundamental note to higher frequencies and a reduction of low-frequency amplitude. Patients not responding to UPPP also showed a reduction in low-frequency amplitude but had large amplitudes in the range from 1,100 to 1,600 Hz before and after operation. This peak of amplitudes around 1,500 Hz is due to airway obstruction at the tongue base level, and the peak of low-frequency amplitudes is mainly produced by the velopharyngeal segment.

In unselected male apneic and nonapneic patients who underwent UPPP, Schäfer[109] analyzed snoring sounds before and at least 6 months after operation in the sleep laboratory. Frequency spectra of 24 nonresponders showed the large peak of amplitudes between 1,100 to 1,500 Hz, whereas 25 responders (AHI $\leq$ 10) did not. On the basis of these criteria, the positive predictive value of the frequency spectrum was 76% and the negative predictive value was 78%. Thus, that frequency analysis of snoring sounds is a useful predictor of suitable candidates for UPPP.

In a recent article, Perez-Padilla et al.[110] analyzed the characteristics of snoring noise in 10 nonapneic snorers and nine patients with OSA. They found that the ratio of power above 800 Hz to power below 800 Hz could be used to separate snorers from patients with OSA. The main disadvantage of sleep-dependent breath sound analysis is the lacking consensus as to standardized methods for measuring snoring noises.

Cinefluoroscopy (somnofluoroscopy)

Thick barium can be used to coat the mucosa surfaces and render the pharyngeal contours more visible radiographically. The images from the anteroposterior and lateral dimensions are documented with video recording. Some investigators[7,99,111,112] were able to study sleeping nonapneic and apneic snorers by fluoroscopy (somnofluoroscopy). In a few subjects they recorded the dynamic changes of the pharyngeal walls during ventilation, snoring, and collapse and analyzed the movements of the mandible and hyoid bone. Essential disadvantages of fluoroscopy are load of the subjects by ionizing radiation and the recording of only a short moment of the pharyngeal lumina during sleep.

Computed tomography

Although conventional computed tomography (CT) has been used since 1983[7,113] to evaluate the dynamic changes of the upper airway of awake patients with OSA, the results are far from clear. Launois et al.[93] demonstrated a lack of congruence between CT-identified sites of pharyngeal narrowing in awake patients and sites of narrowing of the passive pharynx during sleep evaluated by pressure measurements. Even the introduction of fast CT scanning to image the upper airway of patients with sleep-disordered breathing during wakefulness did not result in practically usable data.[114,115] For determining the site of upper airway collapse during sleep in patients with OSA, both conventional and fast CT have provided more consistent information.[103,116] According to these observations, airway closure during apneic episodes begins in the velopharyngeal segment and extends caudally into the tongue base level. Some patients showed changing levels of closure ("seesaw" closure pattern according to Crumley et al.[103]) and some also demonstrated an airway closure at the tongue base level. As expected, in most patients with airway collapse at the velopharyngeal and tongue base level, UPPP enlarged the airway diameters of the velopharyngeal level but did not change airway diameters in the tongue base level.[103]

Radiocephalometry

Lateral radiocephalometric examination is used to evaluate the skeletal and soft tissue anatomy to determine some dimensions of the upper airway. Under standardized conditions, cephalometry is performed in awake, seated subjects with the head fixed. Thus, this method delivers a two-dimensional static image of the lateral head and neck. In 1983, Riley et al.[117] described that patients with OSA demonstrated retrognathia, an elongated soft palate, a narrowed space between the base of the tongue and the posterior soft tissue, and an inferiorly positioned hyoid bone relative to the mandibular plane. Normative cephalometric databases for children and adolescents have been established by orthodontists; however, age- and set-matched control data with specific parameters for patients with sleep-disordered breathing are available for only relatively small cohorts.

Although a plethora of data have been collected by several investigators[37,77,118–122] concerning apneic and nonapneic snorers, consensus is lacking on the significance of the single cephalometric parameters for the pathogenesis of OSA and for selection of patients for certain therapies. Radiocephalometric values are generally necessary for the application of oral appliances and for planning maxillofacial surgery in patients with OSA.

Acoustic reflection techniques

The acoustic reflection technique was described by Jackson et al.[123] to evaluate airway geometry by analysis of acoustic pulse response measurements. The quick and noninvasive technique has been used with some success to make cross-sectional area measurements of the trachea, the pharynx,[124,125] and the supraglottal oral cavity. These measurements are performed via the oral cavity in wakefulness and quiet ventilation and have provided some new data about the dynamic picture of the oral cavity and the airway distal to the velopharyngeal segment. This technique has demonstrated that awake patients with OSA have both smaller and more compliant orohypopharyngeal airway segments than do normal subjects.[126] However, conclusions concerning the geometry of the upper airway during sleep cannot be drawn.

In 1989, Hilberg et al.[127] introduced the acoustic reflection technique to evaluate the geometry of the nasal cavity. Cross-sectional areas of the nose are obtained as a function of distance from the nostril. This new method, termed "acoustic rhinometry," is increasingly being used in various situations to measure cross-sectional areas in the nasal cavities. Lenders and Pirsig[128] used acoustic rhinometry to evaluate the dynamic variations of cross-sectional areas of the naso-pharynx in awake nonapneic and apneic subjects. The intraindividual variability of cross-sectional areas in the velopharyngeal segment of snorers was significantly greater than that in nonsnoring controls; 94% of all the patients showed values of standard deviation greater than 31% of mean values in this segment. In 46 patients, 3 to 6 months after UPPP, a striking change in the intraindividual variability of the nasopharyngeal cross-sectional areas was measured: all 46 patients who had operations showed the same degree of variability as normal controls. The mean values of cross-sectional areas in the velopharyngeal segment of the same awake individual remained unchanged before and after UPPP. The acoustic reflection technique is quantitated, but the disadvantage is that the area beyond a severe constriction may not be accurately estimated. This does not concern the airway measurements via the wide oral cavity, but it may be of importance in acoustic rhinometry, in which the smallest cross-sectional area is in the anterior part of the nasal cavity.[129,130] Furthermore, because there is no standard procedure for the use of acoustic rhinometry, it is difficult to compare results between laboratories.

Magnetic resonance imaging

Magnetic resonance imaging (MRI) is a noninvasive technique and gives an excellent insight, especially into the soft tissue anatomy that defines the walls of the upper airway in multiple planes. Unfortunately, it can be used only in awake subjects because monitoring of sleep parameters is impossible with electrodes in the magnetic field. Furthermore, probably only patients with very severe OSA will fall asleep with the noise of the scanner. Since 1988, several groups[131–134] have used MRI to study volume changes and wall displacements occurring in the pharynx in different body positions and under NCPAP therapy. More insight into the deposition of fat tissue in patients with OSA has been gained by MRI.[132] Shellock et al.,[135] using ultrafast spoiled GRASS MRI, determined the presence of occlusions and narrowings of the pharyngeal airway in 10 awake patients with OSA.

TREATMENTS IN SLEEP-RELATED BREATHING DISORDERS

Depending on the findings and the severity of the breathing disorder, several therapeutic options are available, which are applied as a single treatment or in combination. The goal is to achieve long-term effectiveness with a minimum of side effects. The therapy should also be well accepted by the patient and the social surrounding. Few reports in the literature meet all of these criteria. Furthermore, consensus is lacking on how to define criteria to evaluate therapeutic success. Some studies use only the patients' subjective assessments of the effect of treatment on snoring and other symptoms, and others combine self-assessments with one or more sleep parameters evaluated in the sleep laboratory. But even for the most frequently used parameter, the AI or AHI, criteria of success differ. Some investigators consider a decrease of more than 50% in AHI a success, and others use cutoff points of 5, 10, 15, or 20 AHI to indicate a good treatment response. The most common treatments are briefly presented below; the focus is on those that involve more rhinologic aspects.

Nonsurgical Approaches

Weight loss

Nonsurgical weight reduction, as the only measure or in combination with other therapies, has been demonstrated to be very effective for treating even the severest degrees of OSA.[59,136–141] However, patient compliance is a limiting factor for this therapy which is accepted by only a few percent of patients in the long run.[142]

Limitation of alcohol and sedatives

Alcohol adversely influences breathing during sleep. Snoring, apneas, and oxygen desaturations after alcohol ingestion mainly occur during the first hours of sleep in normal individuals and in patients with OSA.[143] Alcohol selectively decreases neural input and electromyographic activity of the pharyngeal dilator muscles, whereas diaphragmatic activity is preserved.[144] This disturbs the forces for maintaining pharyngeal balance during sleep. Because of its vasodilatory effect, alcohol causes nasal obstruction. Robinson et al.[145] found that moderate alcohol ingestion significantly increased nasal and pharyngeal resistance in normal subjects in a sitting posture.

This increase of nasal resistance after alcohol ingestion was supported by Eccles and Tolley[146] in normal subjects when they adopted a supine posture. Using NCPAP in sleeping asymptomatic snorers, Mitler et al.[147] demonstrated a higher resistance of the upper airway, in particular during the first 2 hours after alcohol ingestion. Although the advice to "Avoid alcoholic beverages within 3 hours before bedtime" is always recommended to nonapneic and apneic patients, no long-term studies have been done to evaluate patients' acceptance. The same restriction applies to tranquilizers, sleeping pills, antihistamines, and other sedatives.

Body position

Marked changes in nasal resistance result from changes in posture. Resistance increases when lying down[148] and on the dependent side when lying on one side.[149] The supine position also increases the pharyngeal resistance, especially in patients with OSA.[150] Therefore, sleeping in a lateral posture with the head elevated about 30° from horizontal may help to lessen the resistance of the upper airway. Sleeping in a lateral posture dramatically decreased apnea and snoring in four patients with mild to moderate OSA.[151] However, that report and others are limited by small patient numbers and lack of long-term follow-up and matched controls. Different devices have been developed during the past hundred years to train the nonapneic or apneic snorer to change from the supine to the lateral position during sleep. Tennis balls sewn into pajamas and sound-sensitive devices placed under the pillow which vibrate when snoring surmounts a certain loudness level may have a conditioning effect but, at the same time, they disrupt sleep, as does each type of apparatus based on the alarm-clock principle. Therefore, sleep position training is appropriate only as an interim treatment for patients with mild OSA who have position-related obstruction.[152]

Nasal dilators

Nonsurgical trials have been undertaken to reduce the upstream resistance to inspiratory airflow and thus lessen compliant obstructive narrowing of the pharynx. Topical application of an α-agonist results in a short-term decrease of nasal resistance; however, long-term use of local vasoconstrictors may induce rhinitis medicamentosa. Because the anterior nose is the most resistive segment of the normal nasal cavity,[129,130] attempts have been undertaken to dilate the nasal vestibule. Petruson[153] developed a nasal dilator (Nozovent) that significantly decreases nasal resistance in the awake patient. His group[154] and other investigators[15,18,155] studied the effect of Nozovent on sleep-disordered breathing. The findings, listed in Table 11–3, allow some statements. The groups investigated are rather small and are not comparable because of their inhomogeneity in regard to anthropomorphic data and degree of nasal pathology. Nozovent was used in different modalities during the night(s) of polysomnographic investigation. There is no standardized definition and method to measure snoring noises. All investigators measured nasal resistance by posterior rhinomanometry in the awake, seated subject, except for Kerr et al.[18] who measured subjects in recumbency. All investigators found a significant decrease in nasal resistance with Nozovent. The effects of Nozovent on sleep and snoring differed from "none" to "significant." Most investigators did not find a change in

Table 11–3   Reported Effects of Nozovent

REFERENCE	NO. OF PATIENTS	NASAL RESISTANCE	NOZOVENT	PSG	EFFECT ON NASAL RESISTANCE	EFFECTS ON SLEEP AND SNORING	EFFECTS ON AHI
153	16; normal noses	active post-RM awake, sitting	awake sitting	∅	Airflow increase of 24%	∅	∅
154	10 (6M, 4F) normal noses; AI > 5	active post-RM awake, sitting	overnight	2 nights + snoring noise	Airflow increase of 18% (P < 0.002)	snoring noise decrease min. SO_2 increase 78% to 84% (P < 0.03)	AI decrease 47% (P < 0.008)
155	10 heavy snorers; AHI > 15	computed-assisted post-RM awake, sitting	first or second half of sleep	1 night + snoring noise	Drop of 60% in 72 snorers	none	no change
15	15 (6F; 9M); normal noses; 8: AHI > 10 7: AHI < 10	RM in 7 patients awake	during second half of sleep	1 night + snoring noise	Drop from 1.62 to 0.94 H_2O/l/sec (P < 0.02)	all snoring parameters reduced in SWS sleep	no change
18	10 males; AHI > 15; 6 had chronic nasal obstruction	post-RM in recumbency before and after sleep	+ 0.05% oxymeta-zaline	3 nights	Drop of 73% (P < 0.001)	decrease in arousal index	no change

AHI: apnea-hypopnea index; AI: apnea index; PSG: polysomnography; RM: rhinomanometry.

AHI, except for Höijer et al.[154] who measured a significant decrease in AI with use of Nozovent.

Nasopharyngeal tube

Remmers et al.[151] used the nasopharyngeal tube to diagnose the site of occlusion in the upper airway by bypassing the obstructing tongue. In pediatric otorhinolaryngology, the nasopharyngeal tube has been successfully used to select children with OSA due to adenotonsillar hyperplasia for adenotonsillectomy and to improve insufficient preoperative cardiopulmonary conditions.[156] Since the first report by Afzelius et al.[157] on the elimination of all apneic events in two patients with OSA, by means of overnight insertion of a rubber nasopharyngeal tube, only a few studies have reported the effect of this simple and inexpensive device. Nahmias and Karetzky[158] documented a 62% decrease in the AI and a 39% decrease in disordered breathing events in 44 patients with OSA. The nasopharyngeal tube was successful in 16 of the 24 patients, and the overall tolerance (for at least 4 months) of the tube was 44%. The authors recommended the tube as a useful alternative treatment for selected patients with OSA and as an immediate therapy while the patient tries to lose weight.

Nasal continuous positive airway pressure (NCPAP)

NCPAP is currently the most effective nonsurgical method available for reversing upper airway obstruction during sleep in patients with OSA. There are different theories to explain the action of NCPAP. One hypothesis is that nasally administered continuous positive airway pressure provides a pneumatic splint and thus prevents collapse of the pharynx.[91,159–162] According to another theory, NCPAP acts by increasing functional residual capacity, which in turn reflexly dilates the pharynx.[125,163,164] This method was first described by Sullivan et al.[91] in 1981. They were able to eliminate obstructive apneas and snoring in patients with OSA by administering air under 4.5 to 10 cm H_2O pressure via nasal prongs sealed with the nares. A self-sealing nasal mask to deliver air under pressure was described by Rapoport et al.[165] and Sanders et al.[166] Rapoport et al. demonstrated the effectiveness of NCPAP in patients with "pickwickian syndrome," and in the following years NCPAP more and more replaced tracheotomy for treating these severe degrees of OSA. In 1984, Sanders[167] found NCPAP to be helpful for reducing central apneas, a use confirmed by Issa and Sullivan.[168] The NCPAP therapy is immediately effective. With titration of the increasing pressure to the optimal value, first apneas, then hypopneas, and finally snoring are reduced to normal limits on the first night of treatment. Sleep returns to normal after an initial rebound of REM sleep or slow-wave sleep or both.[169] The pressure necessary to alleviate apnea ranges from 2.5 to 15 cm H_2O. Recently, Hoffstein and Mateika[170] published a study done in 26 patients with sleep apnea to show the predictive value of an equation that helps to find the starting pressure for NCPAP treatment. The prediction equation involves body mass index, neck circumference, and AHI. Sanders and Kerl[171] published data supporting the hypotheses that expiratory-phase events are important in the pathogenesis of OSA and that there are differences in the magnitude of the forces destabilizing the upper airway during inspiration and expiration. They developed an NCPAP device, nasal

BiPAP, that permits independent adjustment of inspiratory and expiratory positive airway pressure. Using BiPAP in 13 patients with OSA, they showed that obstructive sleep-disordered breathing could be eliminated at lower levels of expiratory airway pressure than with conventional NCPAP therapy.

A plethora of studies deals with the physiologic and therapeutic effects of NCPAP, and these are not reviewed here. A practical overview of NCPAP was published by Sullivan and Grunstein.[162] All authors agree that the two most common complaints of patients with OSA, snoring and EDS, are to a large extent eliminated by NCPAP. NCPAP improves sleep quality, in particular by reestablishing slow-wave sleep, mental and neuropsychological deficits except for planning abilities, and manual dexterity.[172] Concerning EDS, there is a discrepancy between incomplete normalization of the mean sleep latency and the patients' self-evaluation that they no longer feel sleepy.[87] NCPAP also reduces morning headache, depression, fatigue, impotence, and gastroesophageal reflux. Cardiac function is positively influenced in many respects: normalization of nocturnal cardiac arrhythmias, disappearance of pulsus paradoxus,[173] elimination of the negative esophageal pressure, and improvement of heart failure, which also is reflected in reduced nocturia. A normalizing effect of NCPAP on blood pressure in hypertensive patients with OSA has also been demonstrated, although the exact mechanism of this effect is not clear. In patients with pickwickian syndrome, NCPAP has been shown to prevent daytime hypoxia and hypercapnia, to decrease hematocrit, and to improve diurnal lung functions.[174,175] NCPAP could also eliminate OSA during pregnancy[176] and reduce sleep-related breathing disorders in children with lingual or maxillofacial anomalies.[177] However, several investigators have shown that the effectiveness of NCPAP depends on regular use throughout the whole night and every night, which leads to problems of compliance.

Despite all these abilities of NCPAP to influence and change the pathogenetic mechanisms of OSA, initial tolerance and poor long-term compliance appear to be essential shortcomings for this therapy, although technical modifications of the devices have made NCPAP more convenient for patients. A universally accepted definition of therapeutic compliance has not been devised. Three studies of recent working groups have been selected, which try to measure compliance with objective criteria in a prospective study. They clearly point to the problems of defining and measuring compliance.

To evaluate whether continuous home use of NCPAP is associated with the maintenance of therapeutic pressures, Reeves-Hoche et al.[178] covertly installed an elapsed timer and mask pressure transducer recorder in NCPAP units of 47 patients with OSA. They defined compliance as the amount of time the machine was running divided by the reported hours of sleep. In addition, they wanted to document the percentage of time that the effective pressure (shown to eliminate 95% of the obstructive apneas and hypopneas) was maintained. There is no knowledge of the compliance in three subjects, and nine subjects discontinued NCPAP treatment within 3 months. In the remaining patients, a group mean compliance was 68% for the 6 months of observation. The AHI did not correlate with compliance, but it did correlate with effective use. Subjective initial complaints of EDS correlated with compliance only during the first visit. The authors did not find any predictor for compliance.

Kribbs et al.[179] calculated the objective NCPAP use by a sophisticated stratification of three duration criteria (use defined as ≥20 min, as ≥4 h, as ≥7 h), which provided information about the number of patients who were receiving acceptable treatment. The criterion used as an acceptable level for frequency was an average of 5 to 7 days or ≥ 70% of all days monitored. Thus, 35 patients with OSA were stratified into those who used NCPAP at least 4 h a day on at least 70% of all days ("regular users") and those who failed to meet these frequency and duration criteria ("irregular users"). When NCPAP was used, the mean duration of use was 4.88 ± 1.97 h. However, patients' reports of the duration of NCPAP use overestimated actual use by 69 ± 110 min. Both frequency and duration of NCPAP use in the first month reliably predicted use in the third month. Although most (60%) of patients claimed to use NCPAP nightly, only 16 of 35 (46%) met criteria for regular use. "Surprisingly, only 2 of the 35 patients studied used NCPAP for at least 7 h on ≥ 70% of days, suggesting that frequent, long-duration, quality sleep is a relatively rare occurrence in OSA patients treated with NCPAP."

Meurice et al.[138] defined compliance as a function of subjective (patient's statement concerning the use of the apparatus per night) and objective (time counter data) criteria. Patients had to use the apparatus throughout the night, for an average of 5 h or more per night. With application of these criteria, compliance was 68% among their patients (30 of 44). The authors based the choice of such strict criteria on the necessity of preventing oxygen desaturation during sleep.

Considering these three different definitions of compliance and the various definitions of other studies, it is impossible to compare data of patients' compliance. For practical purposes (Table 11–4), one should differentiate between primary (immediate refusers and after the first NCPAP trials) and secondary (in the long run) NCPAP failures.

Rauscher et al.[192] studied the frequency of and reasons for primary NCPAP failures in 95 unselected patients with an AHI of more than 15. Thirty patients refused the treatment and decided to undergo UPPP, to reduce body weight, or to have no treatment at all. Eighteen patients refused NCPAP after 1 to 3 nights of trial NCPAP. Thus, the acceptance rate of NCPAP treatment was only 49% in patients with an AHI of more than 15. Furthermore, the authors found, similar to other studies,[138,191] that the rate of acceptance increased with AHI and with the degree that the subject felt impaired by EDS. Other investigations, however, could not support this correlation between NCPAP acceptance and severity of OSA.[178,179,188]

McEvoy and Thornton[189] offered long-term home-based NCPAP to 11 patients with all severities of OSA and followed seven patients for periods ranging from 1 to 18 months. They had 36% primary NCPAP failures. The rate of primary failures is rarely reported in the literature. Anand et al.[181] reported failure in 104 of 299 (35%), Katsantonis et al.[193] 33 of 138 (24%), Krieger[188] 19 of 233 (8%), and Meurice et al.[138] 5 of 54 (9%).

Causes for early discontinuation of NCPAP therapy include choice of other treatments, the cost of the NCPAP equipment, claustrophobia, mental retardation, chronic alcoholism, insomnia, noise from the machine, and poorly fitting mask. Only a few studies point to the significance of an unobstructed nasal passage for better acceptance of NCPAP.[181,189,194,195] Successful nasal operation not only enhanced the acceptance of NCPAP but also reduced the optimal titration pressure.[194,195]

Table 11–4   Reported Data (Prospective and Retrospective) on Use of Nasal Continuous Positive Airway Pressure

REFERENCE	NO. OF PATIENTS	MEAN FOLLOW-UP, MO (RANGE)	PRIMARY NONCOMPLIANCE	COMPLIANCE NO. (%)	METHODS OF FOLLOW-UP
180	23	15		19 of 23 (83%)	sleep lab
181	50	10.9 (1–38)	104/299 = 35%	28 of 50 (56%)	sleep lab
182	115	12	18/116	60 of 115 (52%)	home care agency
183	11	36 ± 19.7	6	4 of 11 (36%)	sleep lab
184	138	18	33	42%	sleep lab (N = 44)
185	7	10.2 (3–22)		5 of 7 (71%)	sleep lab
186	138	17 ± 11		AHI < 10 105 of 138 (76%)	quest. N = 96 teleph. N = 42
187	117	1–48		105 of 117 (90%)	6 of 117; sleep lab
188	233 OSA	29 ± 1.5	19 = 8.2%	181 of 214 (77%–89%)	time counter questionnaire
	36 snorers	22 ± 3.0		26 of 36 (58%–78%)	
189	11	9.7 (1–18)	4	6 of 7 (86%)	sleep lab
138	54	6	5	30 of 44 (68%)	sleep lab
190	19	14.2		16 of 19 (84%)	sleep lab
178	47	6	3	35 of 44 (68%)	monitoring device; sleep lab
183	50	18 (9–42)		46 of 50 (92%)	sleep lab
191	S = 168	(1.5–78)		107 of 168 (64%)	interview; sleep lab
	21 Snorers	10.3		29%	
	71 EDS	22		55%	
	30 Hypoxemia	15.5		70%	
	45 EDS + Hypoxemia	25		89%	

OSA: obstructive sleep apnea; EDS: excessive daytime sleepiness.

Table 11–4 provides data about primary NCPAP failures and long-term compliance with NCPAP therapy. Some studies described results in selected cohorts without concern about primary NCPAP failures. Only a few studies were prospective and used criteria other than the answers of the patients. Only three groups reported a mean follow-up of more than 20 months, although NCPAP has been in wide use for more than 10 years. The rate of therapeutic compliance derived from all studies ranges from 36% to 92% (mean, 70%). If only the studies that include numbers about primary noncompliance are considered, the mean percentage of long-term compliance is 60%. Adverse effects associated with nocturnal NCPAP have been reported by several authors.[179,180,183,186,189,191–193,195–198] These effects include dry mouth, swallowing air, nasal mucosal irritation (dryness, congestion, secretion), lesions on facial regions pressed by the equipment, disturbance from the noise of the blower, and poorly fitting mask with leakage, which induces eye irritation and tends to wake the patient. In addition, respiratory infection is a frequent cause of temporary disruption in therapy. Some patients complain about chest wall discomfort, which is presumably due to NCPAP-related increase in lung volume.[198] Periodic leg movements in sleep leading to sleep disruption may become evident or increase in severity after treatment of OSA with NCPAP, particularly in elderly patients.[199] Rarely, problems with traveling or acceptance by the family or the bed partner also lead to withdrawal of the treatment. Complications linked to NCPAP therapy are rare. Prolonged rebound REM sleep can result in low levels of arousal and thus lead to dangerous levels of hypoxemia.[189,200] The initial NCPAP trial should, therefore, always take place in the laboratory.[181] There is one report of cerebrospinal fluid leak and pneumatocephalus after using NCPAP[201] and another in which OSA worsened because of an extremely lax epiglottis.[202] Other case reports have included massive epistaxis, sleepwalking, and atrial arrhythmia, but all the patients were able to continue with the NCPAP treatment.

The conclusion reached from all these partially intricate data is that long-term therapeutic compliance with NCPAP does not involve more than 60% of patients who start after successful trials. Consequently, other therapies for OSA need to be considered, particularly for mild and moderate OSA. Consensus has to be reached about the criteria that should be used to define therapeutic compliance. Criteria for a better selection of patients are also necessary as well as improved facilities to help the patients with their NCPAP machines at home.

Oral appliances

Oral appliances (oral devices, dental orthoses) have been used in nonapneic snorers and patients with mild to moderate OSA. They are worn in the mouth during sleep and modify the mandibular position or prevent the velar tissues and base of the tongue from obstructing the airway. The evolution and experience with different oral appliances were reviewed by Clark[203] and Hultcrantz.[204] There are four types of oral appliances: mandibular positioning devices, tongue-retaining device, soft palate lifters, and tongue posture training devices.

The most frequently used device is a mandibular positioner, which advances the mandible and thus pulls the tongue forward. The effectiveness of such a mandibular protracting device was prospectively demonstrated in 100 patients with OSA (mean AI, 61) by Meier-Ewert and Deutsch.[205] After a mean follow-up of 4 months, an AI less than 10 was recorded in 39% of the patients. Two-year compliance was 37%. There are several hypotheses about the mechanism by which these devices reduce sleep-related breathing disorders. It has been demonstrated, for instance, that the posterior airway space, visible on the lateral radiocephalogram, is enlarged by the device. Schmidt-Nowara et al.,[206] however, found other patients who had improvement with the device but did not have a significant change in the posterior airway space. All investigations of these devices are prospective, nonrandomized studies or case reports. No matched controls have been used, and all comparisons have been drawn between sleep studies before and during use of the special device. Edentulous patients and persons with poor dental or periodontic status have not been included.[204] Each oral appliance has to be fitted to the anatomy of the patient by an orthodontist. The ability to breathe through the nose has also been a prerequisite for use of the devices, which keep the mouth partially shut. Thus, there are some shortcomings, which explain why patient tolerance limits the value of certain oral appliances. Dental damage and injury of the temporomandibular joint are concerns with some dental devices, but the long-term risk of such complications has not yet been comprehensively studied. There is no doubt that some of the recently introduced oral devices, as a sole therapeutic measure or in combination with others, may significantly improve sleep-related breathing disorders if they are permanently used. One can expect further development and improvement in the design of the oral appliances.

Pharmacologic approaches

Several drugs have been suggested for the therapy of OSA, but most long-term results have been disappointing.[142,161,198,207] Medroxyprogesterone has been used because it increases respiratory drive during sleep. It may improve air exchange in obese patients without complete airway obstruction, but this hormone does not help in patients with severe OSA and is associated with side effects.[75]

Tricyclic antidepressants may enhance the activity of the genioglossal muscles and alter the pattern of sleep-disordered breathing. In particular, protriptyline has been used in some studies, which also revealed the cholinergic side effects of this drug.[75,193] Tricyclic antidepressants without cholinergic side effects may be helpful in mild to moderate REM-related OSA,[142] but they have not been tested in a large cohort.

The initial enthusiasm for theophylline and aminophylline to treat the wide range of severity of OSA has not continued.[75] It is difficult to establish an individual dosage with a minimum of adverse effects. Currently, a trial with theophylline is recommended as initial treatment in patients with mild OSA presenting with fewer than 100 episodes of apnea and hypopnea per night.[208] Acetazolamide, which impedes carbon dioxide transport, was shown to increase oxygen saturation during sleep. It reduces the number of apneas in patients with symptomatic central sleep apnea. There is no clear indication for this drug in patients with OSA. Several authors[12,57,58] demonstrated the deteriorating influence of allergic rhinitis on the course of OSA, and Freed[209] reported that milk allergy caused OSA in his son. Therefore, antiallergy treatment, depending on the test findings, is used to relieve symptoms in allergic patients with OSA.

Surgical Approaches

It is now generally accepted that the site of obstruction in OSA may involve one or multiple segments of the upper airway. Surgical treatment of OSA bypasses the site(s) of obstruction or modifies the anatomy of the collapsible or obstructive segments. Because of insufficient diagnostic methods and difficulties in evaluating the occluding sites during sleep, these different segments have often been treated independently, and some crucial segments have probably been neglected. This possibility is reflected in the unsatisfying and often confounding short- and long-term results of the various surgical procedures reported in the literature. To improve the clinical outcomes from operation, a protocol was formulated by the surgical group at the Stanford Sleep Disorders Center, presenting a concept of comprehensive upper airway reconstruction.[210] A combination of soft tissue and skeletal reconstruction in the potentially obstructive sites can enhance the surgical effectiveness and lead to successful rates that are comparable to those of NCPAP. This result has been documented[210,211] in 306 consecutively treated surgical patients with OSA and is discussed below.

The surgical therapies described are mainly applied as separate procedures or in various combinations.

Adenectomy or tonsillectomy

There is well-documented evidence that OSA in children is mainly caused by adenoidal or tonsillar hypertrophy and that complete resolution of symptoms is observed in most cases after adenectomy or tonsillectomy.[212–217] It is, however, important to follow children whose adenoids or tonsils have been successfully removed because OSA may reappear in puberty in some. In a prospective investigation with a minimum of 7.5 years follow-up, Guilleminault[142] was the first to point to the problems of children who were affected by OSA again in puberty.

In adults, the value of tonsillectomy for the resolution of OSA is still contentious.[59,62,63,218,219] There is no doubt that tonsillectomy in patients with OSA and huge tonsils will reduce symptoms of sleep-disordered breathing. For many surgeons, tonsillectomy is a part of the UPPP operation when tonsils are present. Stevenson et al.[220] evaluated the long-term significance of tonsillectomy in combination with UPPP or nasal airway operation in 84 selected adult patients with OSA. They found that patients who had tonsillectomy as a part of their surgical procedures showed significant improvement over those in whom tonsillectomy was not performed.

Surgery of the nose and sinuses

In 1974, Simmons and Hill[221] brought the sleep apnea syndrome to the attention of otorhinolaryngologists by describing a "new syndrome" that they found by polysomnographic studies: "intermittent upper airway obstruction which is usually hypopharyngeal but can also be nasal in origin." In a 44-year-old white man with a history of diurnal sleep attacks, loud snoring, and apneic events during the night, polysomnography revealed apneas lasting up to 2 minutes and lacking stage 3 or 4. Two months after submucous nasal resection, the patient noted a marked decrease in daytime sleepiness and a reduction of his nightly respiratory disturbances. However, data from a postoperative sleep study were not provided. Since then, several investigators have shown that surgical correction of nasal flow impediment may be partially effective in the treatment of OSA. However, interpretation of these surgical results is difficult because: (1) anthropologic parameters were incomplete for the mostly few patients; (2) associated pharyngeal abnormalities were not quantified; (3) tests for nasal patency in sleep or wakefulness were not performed; (4) sleep studies were lacking or incomplete; (5) AI or AHI was the sole or primary criterion to define the degree of severity of the sleep-related breathing disorders; (6) nasal operation was often combined with other surgical procedures (i.e., UPPP, adenoidectomy, tonsillectomy) and the results were presented as a total; (7) no comparable criteria to define the success of treatment were given; and (8) follow-up times were too short.

Table 11–1 presents data from six selected investigations, from which some indeterminate conclusions may be drawn concerning the beneficial effect of nasal operation in patients with sleep-related breathing disorders. Except for the study by Dayal and Phillipson,[61] the follow-up of these investigations is very short. The subjective benefit after operation in almost all patients was the reduction of excessive daytime sleepiness and an improvement of sleep quality. With AI or AHI as a criterion, no correlation could be found between the severity of the sleep-related breathing disorder and the severity of nasal obstruction.

However, except for the study by Series et al.[3] no data on nasal patency tests were described. Even Series et al.[3] measured nasal resistance in the supine position at the baseline and postsurgical visits in only 14 of their 20 awake patients. These authors concluded that radiocephalometry may be helpful in identifying patients with mild sleep apnea-hypopnea syndrome and chronic nasal obstruction who will benefit from nasal operation. They found that the presence of craniomandibular abnormalities makes it unlikely that nasal operation will improve sleep-related breathing disorders.[222]

None of the six selected studies presented data on the preoperative and postoperative measurement of snoring. Other studies, often cited in the literature, were discarded because they contained even fewer data to interpret the relationship between nasal obstruction and breathing disorders in sleep. An interesting study by Papsidero[223] evaluated seven patients with EDS and intranasal abnormalities, they were treated by septoplasty and turbinate cautery and outfracture. As a means to eliminate other factors known to cause EDS, the seven patients met the following criteria: (1) EDS as measured by MSLT, (2) normal AHI (range, 2.2 to 19), (3) positive subjective and rhinomanometric evidence for nasal obstruction, (4) normal spirometry, (5) absence of nocturnal myoclonus, and (6) normal psychometric battery. All seven patients experienced significant improvements in subjective and objective measures of nasal breathing. Six of the seven patients had a significant improvement in snoring. All had a marked reduction in EDS as measured by MSLT. Although there are no data on duration of follow-up, postoperative AHI, or the method used for measuring snoring, the study showed that many more factors have to be included in studies that intend to investigate the role of nasal obstruction in OSA. Results of the studies on the efficacy of nasal operations in snorers and patients with apnea show that there is no criterion for predicting the success of nasal operations, except in a few severe cases such as bilateral choanal atresia, massive polyposis, or other obstructing nasal tumors.

Uvulopalatopharyngoplasty

Since Ikematsu[224] introduced palatopharyngoplasty and partial uvulectomy for treating snorers, UPPP is frequently performed for sleep-related breathing disorders in adults but rarely in children. Surgical techniques, modifications, complications, and pitfalls were recently summarized.[225] UPPP can stabilize the airway at the velopharyngeal level but is unable to increase its cross-sectional area.[128,226]

Although several retrospective and prospective studies have been published, randomized controlled trials are lacking. In particular, there are no clear criteria predicting the outcome of UPPP. In the 1980s, each degree of severity of OSA had been operated on, even many patients with a high body mass index (BMI) and high AHI. Most authors did not perform a preoperative evaluation of the site(s) of obstruction during sleep. This is, however, necessary because it has been proved by different methods that only approximately 50% of patients with sleep-related breathing disorders have the site of obstruction solely confined to the velopharyngeal segment, whereas in the remaining patients more or other obstructive sites of the upper airway can be demonstrated. Larsson,[227] comparing the outcome of UPPP in the literature, found the responder rate to vary between 9%[228] and 83%.[229] The reported data are difficult to compare because of great variation between the different studies in the selection of patients, the methods of preoperative evaluation of occlusive sites of the upper airway, differences in surgical techniques, follow-up time and criteria for success. Many investigations are retrospective case-control studies with a high percentage loss of follow-up. Factors predicting the success of UPPP have not been analyzed in all studies, and when this has been done the results are sometimes controversial.[227] A new approach to analyze the outcome of UPPP was described by Schwartz et al.[230] They measured the upper airway critical pressure before and after UPPP in 13 patients with OSA to determine the relationship between changes in collapsibility and the response to UPPP. They concluded that the response to UPPP in OSA is determined by the magnitude of the decrease in the upper airway critical pressure and that it is not influenced by the initial degree of obesity, the severity of sleep apnea, or the initial preoperative level of critical pressure. Launois et al.[93] in a well-documented prospective study, outlined the complexity of predicting the outcome of UPPP. The upper airway of 18 selected overweight patients with OSA (mean BMI, 33.3 kg/m^2) was evaluated with a sophisticated endoscopic method during sleep to identify regions of the passive pharyngeal airway most susceptible to collapse. Four months after UPPP, the improvement rate for the patients who had narrowing only in the nasopharynx (86%) exceeded that for the patients who had at least one site of narrowing outside the nasopharynx (18%). However, another follow-up 14 months after UPPP showed that the predicted improvement rate declined from 86% to 29%. Their patients did not lose weight.

Because UPPP is done to change the resistance of only one obstructive region, namely, the velopharyngeal segment, the outcome of UPPP cannot be compared with that of NCPAP or tracheotomy, which eliminate or bypass all obstructive levels of the upper airway.[36,181,193] On the basis of the conflicting impressions from the literature and including some of the author's own operative experience in about 300 patients in 7 years, the success of UPPP (AHI < 10, reduced EDS) can be predicted in about 80% of patients, with the following exclusion criteria: AHI > 30; overweight with BMI > 29; marked malocclusion, in particular retrognathia; narrow hypopharyngeal segment diagnosed during sleep; chronic alcoholism; chronic lung diseases; and high anesthesia risk. The success rate probably increases if upper airway evaluation during sleep shows that the site of pharyngeal occlusion is confined exclusively to the velopharyngeal segment.[93,94,112,231] However, these endoscopic examinations to define the pharyngeal lumen during sleep are associated with some discomfort and arousal and are usually not tolerated by patients who have less severe OSA. Launois et al.[93] needed 2 to 4 h to visualize the pharynx during sleep in their severely diseased patients.

Reduction glossoplasty

The surgical goal is to enlarge the narrow retroglossal airway space by reduction of the tongue base. This can be achieved by laser midline glossectomy and lingualplasty, developed by Fujita and Woodson.[232,233] A different approach of lingualplasty was described by Djupesland et al.[234] As a rule, the procedure is performed in combination with a permanent or temporary tracheotomy. After removal of the midline segment of the tongue, redundant midline tissue including lingual tonsils, free part of the floppy epiglottis, and supraglottic mucosa are excised. Initial results in 22 selected patients with severe OSA (mean AHI, 58.8), 14 of whom had failed prior UPPP, showed 77% as responders with a postoperative AHI < 20 (mean AHI, 8.1). The complication rate was 27%. The long-term results reported by Djupesland et al.[234] after 8.7 months (postoperative AHI < 20) were less satisfying: only 35% of 20 unselected patients could be considered cured.

Maxillofacial surgery

In 1979, Kuo et al.[235] reported successful advancement osteotomies of the mandible in three patients with OSA. Maxillofacial surgery in OSA is directed at alleviating obstruction at the hypopharyngeal level. This type of procedure has mainly been developed at the Stanford Sleep Disorders Center.[236] Depending on the findings, procedures to advance the mandible and maxilla are combined with hyoid myotomy and suspension.[237] A stepwise approach is proposed. In phase I, patients with an obstruction in the soft palate segment receive UPPP and patients with an obstruction at the base of the tongue receive mandibular osteotomy/genioglossus advancement with hyoid myotomy/suspension. In patients with obstructions in the velopharyngeal and hypopharyngeal segments, UPPP and genioglossus advancement and hyoid myotomy/suspension are performed at the same setting. If patients have nasal deformities, the nose is corrected during phase I. If the postoperative recording after a minimum of 6 months shows an insufficient improvement, the patient is offered phase II reconstruction with maxillomandibular advancement. In

1993, the surgical group at Stanford[210] published a review of 306 of 415 treated patients (mean follow-up, 9.3 months). Operation was considered a success if the result was equivalent to NCPAP or the postoperative AHI was less than 20 with normal oxygenation. Of the 239 patients entered into phase I, 61% were responders. The nonresponders were more severely affected (AHI > 75; BMI > $33\,kg/m^2$; severe mandibular deficiency). Of the 91 patients who underwent phase II operation, 97% were successfully treated. The authors concluded that a comprehensive presurgical evaluation allows a logical approach to reconstruction of the upper airway, and patients who complete the surgical protocol have a long-term success rate of more than 95%.

Tracheostomy

Kuhlo et al.[238] demonstrated that tracheostomy was the only therapy that was 100% successful for even the severest degrees of OSA before NCPAP had been developed. Because it bypasses all sites of potential obstructions of the upper airway, it eliminates all obstructive episodes. In long-term follow-up studies, only some central apneas are registered by polysomnography in patients with OSA who have tracheostomy.[237] Tracheostomy is still indicated for patients with severe OSA who are unsuitable for NCPAP or other operation. It is used relatively often in pediatric otorhinolaryngology for treating children with craniofacial syndromes associated with obstructive events, such as in Pierre Robin sequence, and Apert, Treacher Collins, and Klippel-Feil syndromes.

Special surgery

Various types of benign and malignant tumors may cause OSA by obstructing segments of the upper airway.[59,240–242] Surgical removal of these relatively rare tumors usually eliminates OSA. Growth hormone-secreting tumors of the pituitary gland may lead to acromegaly and OSA.[243] The excessive soft tissues of the pharynx and the hypertrophy of the tongue usually have a tendency to regress after successful hypophysectomy, followed by a reduction of OSA symptoms. Gastroplasty is another type of operation used to treat OSA due to excessive weight.[244] Sugerman[245] reviewed the three different gastric operations used for morbid obesity associated with OSA.

Anesthesia

Severe complications and fatality in association with operation for OSA have been mainly reported to occur in the perioperative phases.[246–248] Craddock and Lees[249] and Esclamado et al.[246] summarized the sparse literature concerning the anesthetic aspects of patients with OSA who need operation. Many patients with OSA present with typical anatomical features, including receding chin, limited *possibility* to open the mouth, hypoplastic mandible, a bulky tongue, a short, stocky neck, and obesity. All these features may result in "difficult intubation." Other risk factors include cor pulmonale, hypertension, and cardiac arrhythmias. A special anesthetic risk in patients with OSA is sedative drugs, which enhance collapsibility of the pharyngeal and oral soft tissue and may lead to additional airway obstruction in the

Table 11–5 Algorithm and Treatment for Obstructive Sleep Apnea

History and Physical Examination

4 to 6 Channel Sleep Screening
or Polysomnography (and MSLT)

Consultation of Other Specialists

Candidate for Nonsurgical Treatment

Candidate for Surgery

Evaluation of Upper
Airways during Sleep

NONSURGICAL TREATMENT	SEVERITY OF DISEASE	SEGMENT-RELATED OPERATION	SEVERITY OF DISEASE
Weight loss	Mild to severe	Nose and sinuses	Mild to moderate
Limitation of alcohol	Mild to severe	Andenoidectomy	Mild to severe
Restriction of sedative	Mild to severe	Tonsillectomy	Mild to moderate
Body position	Mild	Uvulopalatopharyngoplasty	Mild
Exercise	Mild to severe	Base of tongue	Moderate to severe
Medication	Mild	Hyoidplasty	Moderate to severe
Nasal dilator	Mild	Mandibular advancement	Severe
Nasopharyngeal tube	Mild	Maxillomandibular correction	Severe
Oral appliances	Mild to moderate	Special surgery (i.e., gastroplasty)	Severe
Nasal continuous positive airway pressure	Moderate to severe	Tracheostomy	Severe

perioperative phase. Therefore, avoidance of sedative and narcotic premedication and postoperative observation in intensive care units of patients at risk are mandatory. In addition, experience by the anesthetist in "difficult intubation" is another prerequisite to care for patients with OSA. The use of nasal packs for the management of severe epistaxis[69] and in connection with nasal operation results in sleep-related obstructive breathing in most patients, in particular the middle-aged and elderly. Therefore, both groups of patients need careful monitoring and a limitation of sedatives.

SUMMARY

The role of the nose in the pathogenesis of OSA remains unclear. The lack of reliable data and methods of examination complicate rational diagnosis and management of sleep-related breathing disorders. Therefore, it is difficult to recommend a convincing algorithm for the physician (Table 11–5). Particularly, tools to diagnose mild to moderate degrees of sleep-related breathing disorders and to evaluate their impact on health are insufficient. Although only all-night polysomnography and MSLT can detect most variations of sleep-disordered breathing, a screening for OSA by four-channel registration can be recommended for daily routine. If awake nasal resistance is increased or cross-sectional areas of the nasal cavities are diminished to moderate or severe degrees, medical or surgical nasal treatment should be used before other options of therapy are proposed. Until now, only about half of patients have benefited from therapy.

Acknowledgment—The author thanks Thomas V. McCaffrey, M.D., Ph.D., Mayo Clinic, for reviewing this chapter, and Mrs. Astrid Heinrich for her careful help with preparation of the manuscript.

REFERENCES

1. Guilleminault C, van den Hoed J, Mitler MM: Clinical Overview of Sleep Apnea Syndromes, in Guilleminault C, Dement WC (eds.): *Sleep Apnea Syndromes.* New York, Alan R. Liss, 1978, pp 1–12.
2. Guilleminault C, Partinen M (eds.): *Obstructive Sleep Apnea Syndrome: Clinical Research and Treatment.* New York, Raven Press, 1990.
3. Series F, St. Pierre S, Carrier G: Effects of surgical correction of nasal obstruction in the treatment of obstructive sleep apnea. *Am Rev Respir Dis* 1992; 146:1261–1265.
4. Hudgel DW: Variable site of airway narrowing among obstructive sleep apnea patients. *J Appl Physiol* 1986; 61:1403–1409.
5. Remmers JE, de Groot WJ, Sauerland EK, Anch AM: Pathogenesis of upper airway occlusion during sleep. *J Appl Physiol* 1978; 44:931–938.
6. Rojewski TE, Schuller DE, Clark RW, Schmidt HS, Potts RE: Synchronous video recording of the pharyngeal airway and polysomnograph in patients with obstructive sleep apnea. *Laryngoscope* 1982; 92:246–250.
7. Suratt PM, Dee P, Atkinson RL, Armstrong P, Wilhoit SC: Fluorosopic and computed tomographic features of the pharyngeal airway in obstructive sleep apnea. *Am Rev Respir Dis* 1983; 127:487–492.
8. Wiegand L, Zwillich CW: Pathogenesis of obstructive sleep apnea: role of the pharynx. *Semin Respir Med* 1988; 9:540–546.

9. Zwillich CW, Pickett C, Hanson FN, Weil JV: Disturbed sleep and prolonged apnea during nasal obstruction in normal men. *Am Rev Respir Dis* 1981; 124:158–160.

10. Olsen KD, Kern EB, Westbrook PR: Sleep and breathing disturbance secondary to nasal obstruction. *Otolaryngol Head Neck Surg* 1981; 89:804–810.

11. Suratt PM, Turner BL, Wilhoit SC: Effect of intranasal obstruction on breathing during sleep. *Chest* 1986; 90:324–329.

12. McNicholas WT, Tarlo S, Cole P, et al: Obstructive apneas during sleep in patients with seasonal allergic rhinitis. *Am Rev Respir Dis* 1982; 126:625–628.

13. Atkins M, Taskar V, Clayton N, Stone P, Woodcock A: Nasal resistance in obstructive sleep apnea. *Chest* 1994; 105:1133–1135.

14. Blakley BW, Mahowald MW: Nasal resistance and sleep apnea. *Laryngoscope* 1987; 97:752–754.

15. Hoffstein V, Mateika S, Metes A: Effect of nasal dilation on snoring and apneas during different stages of sleep. *Sleep* 1993; 16:360–365.

16. Miljeteig H, Hoffstein V, Cole P: The effect of unilateral and bilateral nasal obstruction on snoring and sleep apnea. *Laryngoscope* 1992; 102:1150–1152.

17. Lenders H, Schäfer J, Pirsig W: Turbinate hypertrophy in habitual snorers and patients with obstructive sleep apnea: findings of acoustic rhinometry. *Laryngoscope* 1991; 101:614–618.

18. Kerr P, Millar T, Buckle P, Kryger M: The importance of nasal resistance in obstructive sleep apnea syndome. *J Otolaryngol* 1992; 21:189–195.

19. Olsen KD, Kern EB: Nasal influences on snoring and obstructive sleep apnea. Snoring. *Mayo Clin Proc* 1990; 65:1095–1105.

20. Waller PC, Bhopal RS: Is snoring a cause of vascular disease? An epidemiological review. *Lancet* 1989; 1:143–146.

21. Berry DTR, Phillips BA: Sleep disordered breathing in the elderly: review and methodological comment. *Clin Psych Rev* 1988; 8:101–120.

22. George CF, Kryger MH: When is an apnea not an apnea? *Am Rev Respir Dis* 1985; 131:485–486.

23. Rosen CL, D'Andrea L, Haddad GG: Adult criteria for obstructive sleep apnea do not identify children with serious obstruction. *Am Rev Respir Dis* 1992; 146:1231–1234.

24. Lugaresi E, Mondini S, Zucooni M, Montagna P, Cirignotta F: Staging of heavy snorers' disease. A proposal. *Bull Eur Physiopathol Respir* 1983; 19:590–594.

25. Lugaresi E, Cirignotta F, Gerardi R, Montagna P: Snoring and sleep apnea: Natural history of heavy snorers disease. In Guilleminault C, Partinen M (eds.): *Obstructive Sleep Apnea Syndrome: Clinical Research and Treatment.* New York, Raven Press, 1990, pp 25–36.

26. Thorpy MJ (ed.): *International Classification of Sleep Disorders. Diagnostic and Coding Manual.* Lawrence, Kansas, Allan Press, 1990.

27. Guilleminault C, Stoohs R: Upper airway resistance syndrome (UARS) (abstract). *Am Rev Respir Dis* 1991; 143 Abstracts:A589.

28. Downey R, Perkin RM, MacQuarrie J: Upper airway resistance syndrome: sick, symptomatic but underrecognized. *Sleep* 1993; 16:620–623.

29. Guilleminault C, Stoohs R, Duncan S: Snoring (1) daytime sleepiness in regular heavy snorers. *Chest* 1991; 99:40–48.

30. Strollo PJ Jr, Sanders MH: Significance and treatment of nonapneic snorers. *Sleep* 1993; 16:403–408.

31. Gislason T, Benediktsdóttir B, Björnsson JK, Kjartansson G, Kjeld M, Kristbjarnarson H: Snoring, hypertension, and the sleep apnea syndome. An epidemiologic survey of middle-aged women. *Chest* 1993; 103:1147–1151.

32. Schmidt-Nowara WW, Jennum P: Epidemiology of Sleep Apnea, in Guilleminault C, Partinen M (eds.): *Obstructive Sleep Apnea Syndrome: Clinical Research and Treatment.* New York, Raven Press, 1990, pp 1–8.

33. Young T, Palta M, Dempsey J, Skatrud J, Weber S, Bader S: The occurrence of sleep-disordered breathing among middle-aged adults. *N Engl J Med* 1993; 328:1230–1235.

34. Gislason T, Almqvist M, Eriksson G, Taube A, Boman G: Prevalence of sleep apnea syndrome among Swedish men—an epidemiological study. *J Clin Epidemiol* 1988; 41:571–576.

35. Burack B, Thorpy M, Rozycki DL, Ledereich P, McGregor P: The lethal combination of cardiovascular disease (CDV) and obstructive sleep apnea (OSA) (abstract). *Sleep Res* 1991; 20:295.

36. He J, Kryger MH, Zorick FJ, Conway W, Roth T: Mortality and apnea index in obstructive sleep apnea: experience in 385 male patients. *Chest* 1988; 94:9–14.

37. Partinen M, Jamieson A, Guilleminault C: Long-term outcome for obstructive sleep apnea syndrome patients; mortality. *Chest* 1988; 94:1200–1204.

38. Durieux P, Neukirch F: Epidémiologie du syndrome d'apnées du sommeil de l'adulte. *Rev Mal Resp* 1990; 7:441–449.

39. Hedner J: Outline of Cardiovascular Complications in OSA, in *Diagnosis and Management of Obstructive Sleep Apnea Syndrome*. Stockholm, Medicinska Forskningsradet, October 1993, pp 43–52.

40. Strohl KP, Roth T, Redline S: Cardiopulmonary and neurological consequences of obstructive sleep apnea. In Fairbanks DNF, Fujita S (eds.): *Snoring and obstrucive sleep apnea*. ed. 2. New York, Raven Press, 1994, pp 31–43.

41. Kuna ST, Sant' Ambrogio G: Pathophysiology of upper airway closure during sleep. *JAMA* 1991; 266:1384–1389.

42. Sauerland EK, Orr WC, Hairston LE: EMG patterns of oropharyngeal muscles during respiration in wakefulness and sleep. *Electomyogr Clin Neurophysiol* 1981; 21:307–316.

43. Park SS: Flow-regulatory function of upper airway in health and disease: A unified pathogenetic view of sleep-disordered breathing. *Lung* 1993; 171:311–333.

44. Smith PL, Wise RA, Gold AR, Schwartz AR, Permutt S: Upper airway pressure-flow relationships in obstructive sleep apnea. *J Appl Physiol* 1988; 64:789–795.

45. Schwartz AR, Smith PL, Wise RA, Gold AR, Perlmutt S: Induction of upper airway occlusion in sleeping individuals with subatmospheric nasal pressure. *J Appl Physiol* 1988; 64:535–542.

46. Hoffstein V, Chaban R, Cole P, Rubinstein I: Snoring and upper airway properties. *Chest* 1988; 94:87–89.

47. Jessen M, Fryksmark U: Is there a relationship between the degree of nasal obstruction and snoring? *Clin Otolaryngol* 1993; 18:485–487.

48. Hudgel DW, Robertson DW: Nasal resistance during wakefulness and sleep in normal man. *Acta Otolaryngol (Stockh)* 1984; 98:130–135.

49. Hudgel DW, Hendricks C: Palate and hypopharynx: Sites of inspiratory narrowing of the upper airway during sleep. *Am Rev Respir Dis* 1988; 138:1542–1547.

50. Strohl KP, Hensley MJ, Hallett M, Saunders NA, Ingram RH Jr.: Activation of upper airway muscles before onset of inspiration in normal humans. *J Appl Physiol* 1980; 49:638–642.

51. Suratt PM, McTier R, Wilhoit SC: Alae nasi electromyographic activity and timing in obstructive sleep apnea. *J Appl Physiol* 1985; 58:1252–1256.

52. Önal E, Lopata M, O'Connor T: Pathogenesis of apneas in hypersomnia-sleep apnea syndrome. *Am Rev Respir Dis* 1982; 125:167–174.

53. Suratt PM, McTier RF, Wilhoit SC: Upper airway muscle activation is augmented in patients with obstructive sleep apnea compared with that in normal subjects. *Am Rev Respir Dis* 1988; 137:889–894.

54. White DP, Cadeux RJ, Lombard RM, Bixler EO, Kales A, Zwillich CW: The effects of nasal anesthesia on breathing during sleep. *Am Rev Respir Dis* 1985; 132:972–975.

55. McNicholas WT, Coffey M, McDonnell T, O'Regan R, Fitzgerald MX: Upper airway obstruction during sleep in normal subjects after selective topical oropharyngeal anesthesia. *Am Rev Respir Dis* 1987; 135:1316–1319.

56. Fairbanks DNF: Effect of nasal surgery on snoring. *South Med J* 1985; 78:268–270.

57. Leznoff A, Haight JS, Hoffstein V: Reversible obstructive sleep apnea caused by occupational exposure to guar gum dust. *Am Rev Respir Dis* 1986; 133:935–936.

58. Lavie P, Gertner R, Zomer J, Podoshin L: Breathing disorders in sleep associated with "microarousals" in patients with allergic rhinitis. *Acta Otolaryngol (Stockh)* 1981; 92:529–533.

59. Auber-Tulkens G, Hamoir M, Van den Eeckhaut J, Rodenstein DO: Failure of tonsil and nose surgery in adults with long-standing severe sleep apnea syndrome. *Arch Intern Med* 1989; 149:2118–2121.

60. Caldarelli DD, Cartwright RD, Lilie JK: Obstructive sleep apnea: variations in surgical management. *Laryngoscope* 1985; 95:1070–1073.

61. Dayal VS, Phillipson EA: Nasal surgery in the management of sleep apnea. *Ann Otol Rhinol Laryngol* 1985; 94:550–554.

62. Heimer D, Scharf SM, Leiberman A, Lavie P: Sleep apnea syndrome treated by repair of deviated nasal septum. *Chest* 1983; 84:184–185.

63. Rubin AHE, Ehaschar I, Joachim Z, Alroy G, Lavie P: Effects of nasal surgery and tonsillectomy on sleep apnea. *Bull Eur Physiopathol Respir* 1983; 19:612–615.

64. Lavie P, Fischel N, Zomer J, Eliaschar I: The effects of partial and complete mechanical occlusion of the nasal passages on sleep structure and breathing in sleep. *Acta Otolaryngol (Stockh)* 1983; 95:161–166.

65. Lavie P, Rubin AE: Effects of nasal occlusion on respiration in sleep. Evidence of inheritability of sleep apnea proneness. *Acta Otolaryngol (Stockh)* 1984; 97:127–130.

66. Tanaka Y, Honda Y: Nasal obstruction as a cause of reduced PCO_2 and disordered breathing during sleep. *J Appl Physiol* 1989; 67:970–972.

67. Taasan V, Wynne JW, Cassisi N, Block AJ: The effect of nasal packing on sleep-disordered breathing and nocturnal oxygen desaturation. *Laryngoscope* 1981; 91:1163–1172.

68. Johannessen N, Jensen PF, Kristensen S, Juul A: Nasal packing and nocturnal oxygen desaturation. *Acta Otolaryngol (Stockh)* 1992: Suppl 492:6–8.
69. Wetmore SJ, Scrima L, Hiller FC: Sleep apnea in epistaxis patients treated with nasal packs. *Otolaryngol Head Neck Surg* 1988; 98:596–599.
70. Wilhoit SC, Suratt PM: Effect of nasal obstruction on upper airway muscle activation in normal subjects. *Chest* 1987; 92:1053–1055.
71. Kapuniai LE, Andrew DJ, Cromwell DH, Pearce JW: Identifying sleep apnea from self-reports. *Sleep* 1988; 11:430–436.
72. Davies RJ, Ali NJ, Stradling JR: Neck circumference and other clinical features in the diagnosis of the obstructive sleep apnea syndrome. *Thorax* 1992; 47:101–105.
73. Viner S, Szalai JP, Hoffstein V: Are history and physical examination a good screening test for sleep apnea? *Ann Int Med* 1991; 115:356–359.
74. Bliwise DL, Nekich JC, Dement WC: Relative validity of self-reported snoring as a symptom of sleep apnea in a sleep clinic population. *Chest* 1991; 99:600–608.
75. Guilleminault C: Diagnosis, pathogenesis, and treatment of the sleep apnea syndromes. *Ergeb Inn Med Kinderheilk* 1984; 52:1–57.
76. Rojewski TE, Schuller DE, Clark RW, Schmidt HS, Potts RE: Videoendoscopic determination of the mechanism in obstructive sleep apnea. *Otolaryngol Head Neck Surg* 1984; 92:127–131.
77. Rivlin J, Hoffstein V, Kalbfleisch J, McNicholas W, Zamel N, Bryan AC: Upper airway morphology in patients with idiopathic obstructive sleep apnea. *Am Rev Respir Dis* 1984; 129:355–360.
78. Cooper BG, Veale D, Griffiths CJ, Gibson GJ: Value of nocturnal oxygen saturation as a screening test for sleep apnea. *Thorax* 1991; 46:586–588.
79. Rauscher H, Popp W, Zwick H: Model for investigating snorers with suspected sleep apnoea. *Thorax* 1993; 48:275–279.
80. Williams AJ, Yu G, Santiago S, Stein M: Screening for sleep apnea using pulse oximetry and a clinical score. *Chest* 1991; 100:631–635.
81. Svanburg E, Larsson H, Carlsson-Nordlander B, Pirskanen R: A limited diagnostic investigation for obstructive sleep apnea syndrome: oximetry and static charge sensitive bed. *Chest* 1990; 98:1341–1345.
82. Stoohs R, Guilleminault C: MESAM 4: an ambulatory device for the detection of patients at risk for obstructive sleep apnea syndrome (OSAS). *Chest* 1992; 101:1221–1227.
83. Douglas NJ, Thomas S, Jan MA: Clinical value of polysomnography. *Lancet* 1992; 339:347–350.
84. Bradley D: Sleep Apnea in Patients With Cardiac Failure: Implications for Investigation and Management, in *Diagnosis and Management of Obstructive Sleep Apnea Syndrome*. Stockholm, Medicinska Forskningsradet, October 1993, pp 53–58.
85. Haraldsson PO, Carenfelt C, Tingvall C: Sleep apnea syndrome symptoms and automobile driving in a general population. *J Clin Epidemiol* 1992; 45:821–825.
86. Carskadin MA (ed.): Current perspectives on daytime sleepiness. *Sleep* 1982; 5. Suppl 2:S55–S202.
87. Sforza E, Krieger J: Daytime sleepiness after long-term continuous positive airway pressure (CPAP) treatment in obstructive sleep apnea syndrome. *J Neurol Sci* 1992; 110:21–26.
88. Roehrs T, Zorick F, Wittig R, Conway W, Roth T: Predictors of objective level of daytime sleepiness in patients with sleep-related breathing disorders. *Chest* 1989; 95:1202–1206.
89. Shepard JW Jr, Gefter WB, Guilleminault C, et al: Evaluation of the upper airway in patients with obstructive sleep apnea. *Sleep* 1991; 14:361–371.
90. Issa FG, Sullivan CE: Upper airway closing pressures in obstructive sleep apnea. *J Appl Physiol* 1984; 57:520–527.
91. Sullivan CE, Issa FG, Berthon-Jones M, Eves L: Reversal of obstructive sleep apnoea by continuous positive airway pressure applied through the nares. *Lancet* 1981; 1:862–865.
92. Chaban R, Cole P, Hoffstein V: Site of upper airway obstruction in patients with idiopathic obstructive sleep apnea. *Laryngoscope* 1988; 98:641–647.
93. Launois SH, Feroah TR, Campbell WN, et al: Site of pharyngeal narrowing predicts outcome of surgery for obstructive sleep apnea. *Am Rev Respir Dis* 1993; 147:182–189.
94. Metes A, Hoffstein V, Mateika S, Cole P, Haight JSJ: Site of airway obstruction in patients with obstructive sleep apnea before and after uvulopalatopharyngoplasty. *Laryngoscope* 1991; 101:1102–1108.
95. Shepard JW Jr, Thawley SE: Localization of upper airway collapse during sleep in patients with obstructive sleep apnea. *Am Rev Respir Dis* 1990; 141:1350–1355.
96. Skatvedt O: Localization of site of obstruction in snorers and patients with obstructive sleep apnea syndrome: A comparison of fiberoptic nasopharyngoscopy and pressure measurements. *Acta Otolaryngol (Stockh)* 1993; 113:206–209.
97. Tvinnereim M, Miljeteig H: Pressure recordings: a method for detecting site of upper airway obstruction in obstructive sleep apnea syndrome. *Acta Otolaryngol (Stockh)* 1992; Suppl 492:132–140.

98. Borowiecki B, Pollak CP, Weitzman ED, Rakoff S, Imperato J: Fibro-optic study of pharyngeal airway during sleep in patients with hypersomnia obstructive sleep-apnea syndrome. *Laryngoscope* 1978; 88:1310–1313.

99. Weitzman ED, Pollak CP, Borowiecki B, Burack B, Shprintzen R, Rakoff S: The hypersomnia-sleep apnea syndrome: site and mechanism of upper airway obstruction, in Guilleminault C, Dement WC (eds.). *Sleep Apnea Syndromes.* New York, Alan R. Liss, 1978, pp 235–248.

100. Pringle MB, Croft CB: A comparison of sleep nasendoscopy and the Muller manoeuvre. *Clin Otolaryngol* 1991; 16:559–562.

101. Rybak LP, Maisel RH: Endoscopic findings in sleep apnea syndrome. *J Otolaryngol* 1979; 8:487–493.

102. Sher AE, Thorpy MJ, Shprintzen RJ, Spielman AJ, Burack B, McGregor PA: Predictive value of Müller maneuver in selection of patients for uvulopalatopharyngoplasty. *Laryngoscope* 1985; 95:1483–1487.

103. Crumley R, Stein M, Gamsu G, Golden J, Dermon S: Determination of obstructive site in obstructive sleep apnea. *Laryngoscope* 1987; 97:301–308.

104. Katsantonis GP, Maas CS, Walsh JK: The predictive efficacy of the Müller maneuver in uvulopalatopharnygoplasty. *Laryngoscope* 1989; 99:677–680.

105. Wittig R, Fujita S, Fortier J, Zorick F, Potts G, Roth T: Results of uvulopalatopharyngoplasty (UPPP) in patients with both oropharyngeal and hypopharyngeal collapse on Mueller maneuver (abstract). *Sleep Res* 1988; 17:269.

106. Launois SH, Feroah TR, Campbell WN, Whitelaw WA, Remmers JE: Site of obstruction in obstructive sleep apnea: influence on the outcome of uvulopalatopharyngoplasty (abstract). *Am Rev Respir Dis* 1990; 141 Abstracts:A861.

107. Schäfer J: Spektralanalyse schlafabhängiger Atemgeräusche: Ihre Aussagekraft bei der Entscheidung über die operative Behandlung von Patienten mit obstruktiver Schlaf-Apnoe. *Eur Arch Otorhionlaryngol* 1992; Suppl II:69–71.

108. Schäfer J, Pirsig W: Digital signal analysis of snoring sounds in children. *Int J Pediatr Otorhinolaryngol* 1990; 20:193–202.

109. Schäfer J: Surgery of the upper airway—can surgical outcome be predicted? *Sleep* 1993; 16 (Suppl):S98–S99.

110. Perez-Padilla JR, Slawinski E, Difrancesco LM, Feige RR, Remmers JE, Whitelaw WA: Characteristics of the snoring noise in patients with and without occlusive sleep apnea. *Am Rev Respir Dis* 1993; 147:635–644.

111. Cirignotta F, Lugaresi E: Some cineradiographic aspects of snoring and obstructive apneas. *Sleep* 1980; 3:225–226.

112. Katsantonis GP, Walsh JK: Somnofluoroscopy: its role in the selection of candidates for uvulopalatopharyngoplasty. *Otolaryngol Head Neck Surg* 1986; 94:56–60,

113. Haponik EF, Smith PL, Bohlman ME, Allen RP, Goldman SM, Bleecker ER: Computerized tomography in obstructive sleep apnea. Correlation of airway size with physiology during sleep and wakefulness. *Am Rev Respir Dis* 1983; 127:221–226.

114. Shepard JW Jr, Stanson AW, Sheedy PF, Westbrook PR: Fast-CT evaluation of the upper airway during wakefulness in patients with obstructive sleep apnea. *Prog Clin Biol Res* 1990; 345:273–279.

115. Burger CD, Stanson AW, Sheedy PF II, Daniels BK, Shepard JW Jr: Fast-computed tomography evaluation of age-related changes in upper airway structure and function in normal men. *Am Rev Respir Dis* 1992; 145:846–852.

116. Horner RL, Shea SA, McIvor J, Guz A: Pharyngeal size and shape during wakefulness and sleep in patients with obstructive sleep apnoea. *QJ Med* 1989; 72:719–735.

117. Riley R, Guilleminault C, Herran J, Powell N: Cephalometric analyses and flow-volume loops in obstructive sleep apnea patients. *Sleep* 1983; 6:303–311.

118. DeBerry-Borowiecki B, Kukwa A, Blanks RH: Cephalometric analysis for diagnosis and treatment of obstructive sleep apnea. *Laryngoscope* 1988; 98:226–234.

119. Lyberg T, Krogstad O, Djupesland G: Cephalometric analysis in patients with obstructive sleep apnoea syndrome. I. Skeletal morphology. *J Laryngol Otol* 1989; 103:287–292.

120. Maltais F, Carrier G, Cormier Y, Series F: Cephalometric measurements in snorers, non-snorers, and patients with sleep apnea. *Thorax* 1991; 46:419–423.

121. Ryan CF, Dickson RI, Lowe AA, Blokmanis A, Fleetham JA: Upper airway measurements predict response to uvulopalatopharyngoplasty in obstructive sleep apnea. *Laryngoscope* 1990; 100:248–253.

122. Strelzow VV, Blanks RHI, Basile A, Strelzow AE: Cephalometric airway analysis in obstructive sleep apnea syndrome. *Laryngoscope* 1988; 98:1149–1158.

123. Jackson AC, Butler JP, Millett EJ, Hoppin FG Jr, Dawson SV: Airway geometry by analysis of acoustic pulse response measurements. *J Appl Physiol* 1977; 43:523–536.

124. Brown IG, Zamel N, Hoffstein V: Pharyngeal cross-sectional area in normal men and women. *J Appl Physiol* 1986; 61:890–895.
125. Hoffstein V, Zamel N, Phillipson EA: Lung volume dependence of pharyngeal cross-sectional area in patients with obstructive sleep apnea. *Am Rev Respir Dis* 1984; 130:175–178.
126. Bradley TD, Brown IG, Grossman RF, et al: Pharyngeal size in snorers, nonsnorers, and patients with obstructive sleep apnea. *N Engl J Med* 1986; 315:1327–1331.
127. Hilberg O, Jackson AC, Swift DL, Pedersen OF: Acoustic rhinometry: evaluation of nasal cavity by acoustic reflection. *J Appl Physiol* 1989; 66:295–303.
128. Lenders H, Pirsig W: Acoustic rhinometry: a diagnostic tool for patients with chronic rhonchopathies. *Rhinology* 1992; Suppl 14:101–105.
129. Bachmann W, Legler U: Studies on the structure and function of the anterior section of the nose by means of luminal impressions. *Acta Otolaryngol (Stockh)* 1972; 73:433–442.
130. Haight JS, Cole P: The site and function of the nasal valve. *Laryngoscope* 1983; 93:49–55.
131. Collop NA, Block AJ, Hellard D: The effect of nightly nasal CPAP treatment on underlying obstructive sleep apnea and pharyngeal size. *Chest* 1991; 99:855–860.
132. Horner RL, Mohiaddin RH, Lowell DG, et al: Sites and sizes of fat deposits around the pharynx in obese patients with obstructive sleep apnoea and weight matched controls. *Eur Respir J* 1989; 2:613–622.
133. Ryan CF, Lowe AA, Li D, Fleetham JA: Magnetic resonance imaging of the upper airway in obstructive sleep apnea before and after chronic nasal continuous positive airway pressure therapy. *Am Rev Respir Dis* 1991; 144:939–944.
134. Strohl KP, Hockje PL, Haacke EM, Brooks LJ: Localized variations in the response of the human upper airway to applied positive pressure (abstract). *Physiologist* 1988; 31 Suppl:A37.
135. Shellock FG, Schatz CJ, Julien P, et al: Occlusion and narrowing of the pharyngeal airway in obstructive sleep apnea: evaluation by ultrafast spoiled Grass MR imaging. *Am J Roentgenol* 1992; 158:1019–1024.
136. Browman CP, Sampson MG, Yolles SF, et al: Obstructive sleep apnea and body weight. *Chest* 1984; 85:435–438.
137. Fairbanks DN: Snoring: surgical vs. nonsurgical management. *Laryngoscope* 1984; 94:1188–1192.
138. Meurice JC, Dore P, Paguereau J, et al: Predictive factors of long-term compliance with nasal continuous positive airway pressure treatment in sleep apnea syndrome. *Chest* 1994; 105:429–433.
139. Rubinstein I, Colapinto N, Rotstein LE, Brown IG, Hoffstein V: Improvement in upper airway function after weight loss in patients with obstructive sleep apnea. *Am Rev Respir Dis* 1988; 138:1192–1195.
140. Schwartz AR, Gold AR, Schubert N, et al: Effect of weight loss on upper airway collapsibility in obstructive sleep apnea. *Am Rev Respir Dis* 1991; 144:494–498.
141. Smith PL, Gold AR, Meyers DA, Haponik EF, Bleecker ER: Weight loss in mildly to moderately obese patients with obstructive sleep apnea. *Ann Intern Med* 1985; 103:850–855.
142. Guilleminault C: Treatments in Obstructive Sleep Apnea, in Guilleminault C, Partinen M (eds.): *Obstructive Sleep Apnea Syndrome: Clinical Research and Treatment*. New York, Raven Press, 1990, pp 99–118.
143. Issa FG, Sullivan CE: Alcohol, snoring and sleep apnea. *J Neurol Neurosurg Psychiatry* 1982; 45:353–359.
144. Krol RC, Knuth SL, Bartlett D Jr: Selective reduction of genioglossal muscle activity by alcohol in normal human subjects. *Am Rev Respir Dis* 1984; 129:247–250.
145. Robinson RW, White DP, Zwillich CW: Moderate alcohol ingestion increases upper airway resistance in normal subjects. *Am Rev Respir Dis* 1985; 132:1238–1241.
146. Eccles R, Tolley NS: The effect of alcohol ingestion upon nasal airway resistance. *Rhinology* 1987; 25:245–248.
147. Mitler MM, Dawson A, Henriksen SJ, Sobers M, Bloom FE: Bedtime ethanol increases resistance of upper airways and produces sleep apneas in asymptomatic snorers. *Alcohol Clin Exp Res* 1988; 12:801–805.
148. Rundcrantz H: Postural variations of nasal patency. *Acta Otolaryngol (Stockh)* 1969; 68:435–443.
149. Cole P, Haight JS: Mechanisms of nasal obstruction in sleep. *Laryngoscope* 1984; 94:1557–1559.
150. Brown IB, McClean PA, Boucher R, Zamel N, Hoffstein V: Changes in pharyngeal cross-sectional area with posture and application of continuous positive airway pressure in patients with obstructive sleep apnea. *Am Rev Respir Dis* 1987; 136:628–632.
151. Chaudnary BA, Chaudnary TK, Kolbeck RC, Harmon JD, Speir WA Jr: Therapeutic effect of posture in sleep apnea. *South Med J* 1986; 79:1061–1063.
152. Cartwright RD, Lloyd S, Lilie J, Kravitz H: Sleep position training as treatment for sleep apnea syndrome: a preliminary study. *Sleep* 1985; 8:87–94.

153. Petruson B: Improvement of the nasal airflow by the nasal dilator Nozovent. *Rhinology* 1988; 26:289–292.
154. Höijer U, Ejnell H, Hedner J, Petruson B, Eng LB: The effects of nasal dilation on snoring and obstructive sleep apnea. *Arch Otolaryngol Head Neck Surg* 1992; 118:281–284.
155. Metes, A, Cole P, Hoffstein V, Miljeteig H: Nasal airway dilation and obstructed breathing in sleep. *Laryngoscope* 1992; 102:1053–1055.
156. Kravath RE, Pollak CP, Borowiecki B: Hypoventilation during sleep in children who have lymphoid airway obstruction treated by nasopharyngeal tube and T and A. *Pediatrics* 1977; 59:865–871.
157. Afzelius LE, Elmqvist D, Hougaard K, Laurin S, Nilsson B, Risberg AM: Sleep apnea syndrome: an alternative treatment to tracheostomy. *Laryngoscope* 1981; 91:285–291.
158. Nahmias JS, Karetzky MS: Treatment of the obstructive sleep apnea syndrome using a nasopharyngeal tube. *Chest* 1988; 94:1142–1147.
159. Popper RA, Leidingcr MJ, Williams AJ: Endoscopic observations of the pharyngeal airway during treatment of obstructive sleep apnea with nasal continuous airway pressure—a pneumatic splint. *West J Med* 1986; 144:83–85.
160. Rapoport DM, Garay SM, Goldring RM: Nasal CPAP in obstructive sleep apnea: mechanisms of action. *Bull Eur Physiopath Respir* 1983; 19:161–620.
161. Strohl KP, Cherniack NS, Gothe B: Physiologic basis of therapy for sleep apnea. *Am Rev Respir Dis* 1986; 134:791–802.
162. Sullivan CE, Grunstein RR: Continuous Positive Airways Pressure in Sleep-Disordered Breathing, in Kryger MH, Roth T, Dement WC (eds.): *Principles and Practice of Sleep Medicine.* Philadelphia, W.B. Saunders Campary, 1989, pp 559–570.
163. Brown I, Taylor R, Hoffstein V: Obstructive sleep apnea reversed by increased lung volume? *Eur J Respir Dis* 1986; 68:375–380.
164. Series F, Cormier Y, Lampron N, La Forge J: Increasing the functional residual capacity may reverse obstructive sleep apnea. *Sleep* 1988; 11:349–353.
165. Rapoport DM, Sorkin B, Garay SM, Goldring RM: Reversal of the "Pickwickian syndrome" by long-term use of nocturnal nasal-airway pressure. *N Engl J Med* 1982; 307:931–933.
166. Sanders MH, Moore SE, Eveslage J: CPAP via nasal mask: a treatment for occlusive sleep apnea. *Chest* 1983; 83:144–145.
167. Sanders MH: Nasal CPAP effect on patterns of sleep apnea. *Chest* 1984; 86:839–844.
168. Issa PG, Sullivan CE: Reversal of central sleep apnea using nasal CPAP. *Chest* 1986; 90:165–171.
169. Holzer BC, Pressman MR, Fry JM: REM sleep and slow wave sleep (SWS) rebound with nasal CPAP treatment of sleep apnea (abstract). *Sleep Res* 1985; 14:165.
170. Hoffstein V, Mateika J: Predicting nasal continuous positive airway pressure. *Am J Respir Crit Care Med* 1994; 150:486–488.
171. Sanders MH, Kern N: Obstructive sleep apnea treated by independently adjusted inspiratory and expiratory positive airway pressures via nasal mask: physiologic and clinical implications. *Chest* 1990; 98:317–324.
172. Bedard MA, Montplaisir J, Malo J, Richer F, Rouleau I: Persistent neuropsyhological deficits and vigilance impairment in sleep apnea syndrome after treatment with continuous positive airways pressure (CPAP). *J Clin Exp Neuropsychol* 1993; 15:330–341.
173. Shiomi T, Guilleminault C, Stoohs R, Schnittger I: Leftward shift of the interventricular septum and pulsus paradoxus in obstructive sleep apnea syndrome. *Chest* 1991; 100:894–902.
174. Leech JA, Önal E, Lopata M: Nasal CPAP continues to improve sleep-disordered breathing and daytime oxygenation over long-term follow-up of occlusive sleep apnea syndrome. *Chest* 1992; 102:1651–1655.
175. Sforza E, Krieger J, Weitzenblum E, Apprill M, Lampert E, Ratamaharo J: Long-term effects of treatment with nasal continuous positive airway pressure on daytime lung function and pulmonary hemodynamics in patients with obstructive sleep apnea *Am Rev Respir Dis* 1990; 141:866–870.
176. Feinsilver SH, Hertz G: Respiration during sleep in pregnancy. *Clin Chest Med* 1992; 13:637–644.
177. Guilleminault C, Nino-Murcia G, Heldt G, Baldwin R, Hutchinson D: Alternative treatment to tracheostomy in obstructive sleep apnea syndrome: nasal continuous positive airway pressure in young children. *Pediatrics* 1986; 78:797–802.
178. Reeves-Hoche MK, Meck R, Zwillich CW: Nasal CPAP: an objective evaluation of patient compliance. *Am J Respir Crit Care Med* 1994; 149:149–154.
179. Kribbs NB, Pack AI, Kline LR, et al: Objective measurement of patterns of nasal CPAP use by patients with obstructive sleep apnea. *Am Rev Respir Dis* 1993; 147:887–895.
180. Akashiba T, Kurashina K, Sasaki I, et al: Long-term effects and complications of home nasal CPAP therapy for obstructive sleep apnea patients. *Nippon Kyobu Shikkan Gakkai Zasshi* 1992; 30:604–608.

181. Anand VK, Ferguson PW, Schoen LS: Obstructive sleep apnea: a comparison of continuous positive airway pressure and surgical treatment. *Otolaryngol Head Neck Surg* 1991; 105:382–390.
182. Browman CP, Newman JC, Winslow DH: Nasal CPAP therapy for obstructive sleep apnea syndrome: determinants of long-term compliance (abstract). *Sleep Res* 1989; 18:206.
183. Chin K, Ohi M, Fukui M, Kuriyama T, Hirai M, Kuno K: Therapy and clinical symptoms in patients with obstructive sleep apnea in Japan. *Nippon Kyobu Shikkan Gakkai Zasshi* 1992; 30:270–277.
184. Dickins QS, Jenkins NA, Chambers GW, Schweitzer PK, Walsh JK: Long-term nasal CPAP use (abstract). *Sleep Res* 1989; 18:223.
185. Frith RW, Cant BR: Severe obstructive sleep apnoea treated with long term nasal continuous positive airway pressure. *Thorax* 1985; 40:45–50.
186. Hoffstein V, Viner S, Mateika S, Conway J: Treatment of obstructive sleep apnea with nasal continuous airway pressure. Patient compliance, perception of benefits, and side effects. *Am Rev Respir Dis* 1992; 145:841–845.
187. Issa FG, Costas LV, Berthon-Jones M, McCauley VJ, Bruderer J, Sullivan CE: Nasal CPAP treatment for obstructive sleep apnea (OSA): long-term experience with 117 patients (abstract). *Am Rev Respir Dis* 1985; 131:Suppl:A108.
188. Krieger J: Long-term compliance with nasal continuous positive airway pressure (CPAP) in obstructive sleep apnea patients and nonapneic snorers. *Sleep* 1992; 15: (Suppl 6):S42–46.
189. McEvoy RD, Thornton AT: Treatment of obstructive sleep apnea syndrome with nasal continuous positive airway pressure. *Sleep* 1984; 7:313–325.
190. Narui K, Kazuma K, Tsuboi E: Effect of Nasal Continuous Positive Airway Pressure on Obstructive Sleep Apnea Long-Term Therapy and Its Patient Compliance, in Togawa K, Katayama S, Horie T (eds.): *Sleep Apnea and Rhonchopathy*. Basel, Karger, 1993, pp 28–32.
191. Rolfe I, Olson LG, Saunders NA: Long-term acceptance of continous positive airway pressure in obstructive sleep apnea. *Am Rev Respir Dis* 1991; 144:1130–1133.
192. Rauscher H, Popp W, Wanke T, Zwick H: Acceptance of CPAP therapy for sleep apnea. *Chest* 1991; 100:1019–1023.
193. Katsantonis GP, Schweitzer PK, Branham GH, Chambers G, Walsh JK: Management of obstructive sleep apnea: comparison of various treatment modalities. *Laryngoscope* 1988; 98:304–309.
194. Mayer-Brix J, Becker H, Peter JH: Nasal high pressure ventilation in obstructive sleep apnea syndrome. Theoretical and practical otorhinolaryngology. *Laryngo-Rhino-Otol* 1989; 68:295–298.
195. Ripberger R, Pirsig W: Die nasale Überdruckbeatmung (nCPAP) zur Therapie der obstruktiven Schlafapnoe: Akzeptanz bei 50 Patienten. Laryngorhinootologie 1994; 73:581-585.
196. Meurice JC, Mergy J, Rostykus C, Dore P, Paquereau J, Patte F: Atrial arrhythmia as a complication of nasal CPAP. *Chest* 1992 102:640–642.
197. Sanders MH, Gruendl CA, Rogers RM: Patient compliance with nasal CPAP therapy for sleep apnea. *Chest* 1986; 90:330–333.
198. Sanders MH: Nonsurgical management of snoring and obstructive sleep apnea. In Fairbanks DNF, Fujita S (eds.): *Snoring and Obstructive Sleep Apnea*, ed. 2. New York, Raven Press, 1994; pp 57–75.
199. Fry JM, DiPhillipo MA, Pressman MR: Periodic leg movements in sleep following treatment of obstructive sleep apnea with nasal continuous positive airway pressure. *Chest* 1989; 96:89–91.
200. Krieger J, Weitzenblum E, Monassier JP, Stoeckel C, Kurtz D: Dangerous hypoxaemia during continuous positive airway pressure treatment of obstructive sleep apnoea (letter). *Lancet* 1983; 2:1429–1430.
201. Jarjour NN, Wilson P: Pneumocephalus associated with nasal continuous positive airway pressure in a patient with sleep apnea syndrome. *Chest* 1989; 96:1425–1426.
202. Anderson A, Alving J, Lildholdt T, Wulff CH: Obstructive sleep apnea initiated by a lax epiglottis: a contraindication for continuous positive airway pressure. *Chest* 1987; 91:621–623.
203. Clark GT: Obstructive sleep apnea and dental devices. *Calif Dental Assoc J* 1988; 16:26–33.
204. Hultcrantz E: Are Orthodontic- or Tongue Retaining Devices and "Low-Tech" Methods of Value in the Treatment of Obstructive Sleep Apnea? in *Diagnosis and Management of Obstructive Sleep Apnea Syndrome*. Stockholm, October 1993; pp 117–123.
205. Meier-Ewert K, Deutsch N: Prothetische-Behandlung des Obstruktiven Schlaf-Apnoe-Syndroms, in Meier-Ewert K, Rüther E (eds.): *Schlafmedizin*. Stuttgart-Jena, Fischer, 1993, pp 321–328.
206. Schmidt-Nowara WW, Meade TE, Hays MB: Treatment of snoring and obstructive sleep apnea with a dental orthosis. *Chest* 1991; 99:1378–1385.
207. George C, Kryger M: Management of sleep apnea. *Semin Respir Med* 1988; 9:569–576.
208. Thalhofer S, Dorow P, Kaufmann U: Langzeitbeobachtungen einer Therapie der Schlafapnoe mit abendlich eingenommenem retardierten Theophyllin. *Pneumologie* 1991; 45 (Suppl 1):290–292.

209. Freed D: Pulmonary hypertension in children who snore (letter). *Br Med J* 1981; 283:231.
210. Riley RW, Powell NB, Guilleminault C: Obstructive sleep apnea syndrome: a review of 306 consecutively treated Surgical patients. *Otolaryngol Head Neck Surg* 1993; 108:117–125.
211. Powell NB, Riley RW, Guilleminault C: The Hypopharynx: Upper Airway Reconstruction in Obstructive Sleep Apnea Syndrome, in Fairbanks DNF, Fujita S (eds.): *Snoring and Obstructive Sleep Apnea.* ed. 2. New York, Raven Press, 1994; pp 193–209.
212. Brouillette RT, Ferrbach SK, Hunt CE: Obstructive sleep apnea in infants and children. *J Pediatr* 1982; 100:131–140.
213. Brown OE, Manning SC, Ridenour B: Cor pulmonale secondary to tonsillar and adenoidal hypertrophy: management considerations. *Int J Pediatr Otorhinolaryngol* 1988; 16:131–139.
214. Guilleminault C, Korobkin R, Winkle R: A review of 50 children with obstructive sleep apnea syndrome. *Lung* 1981; 159:275–287.
215. Mauer KW, Staats BA, Olsen KD: Upper airway obstruction and disordered nocturnal breathing in children. *Mayo Clin Proc* 1983; 58:349–353.
216. Maw AR, Jeans WD, Cable HR: Adenoidectomy. A prospective study to show clinical and radiological changes two years after operation. *J Laryngol Otol* 1983; 97:511–518.
217. Stradling JR, Thomas G, Warley ARH, Williams P, Freel A: Effect of adenotonsillectomy on nocturnal hypoxaemia, sleep disturbance and symptoms in snoring children. *Lancet* 1990; 335:249–253.
218. Orr WC, Martin RJ: Obstructive sleep apnea associated with tonsillar hypertrophy in adults. *Arch Intern Med* 1981; 141:990–992.
219. Simmons FB, Guilleminault C, Dement WC, Tilkian AG, Hill M: Surgical management of airway obstructions during sleep. *Laryngoscope* 1977; 87:326–338.
220. Stevenson EW, Turner GT, Sutton FD, Doekel RC, Pegram V, Hernandez J: Prognostic significance of age and tonsillectomy in uvulopalatopharyngoplasty. *Laryngoscope* 1990; 100:820–823.
221. Simmons FB, Hill MW: Hypersomnia caused by upper airway obstructions: a new syndrome in otolaryngology. *Ann Otol Rhinol Laryngol* 1974; 83:670–673.
222. Series F, St. Pierre S, Carrier G: Surgical correction of nasal obstruction in the treatment of mild sleep apnoea: importanoe of cephalometry in predicting outcome. *Thorax* 1993; 48:360–363.
223. Papsidero MJ: The nose and its impact on snoring and obstructive sleep apnea, in Fairbanks DNF, Fujita S (eds.): *Snoring and Obstructive Sleep Apnea*, ed. 2., New York, Raven Press, 1994, pp 179–192.
224. Ikematsu T: Study of snoring. Therapy (in Japanese). *J Jpn Otol Rhinol Laryngol Soc* 1964; 64:434–435.
225. Fairbanks DNF, Fujita S (eds.): *Snoring and Obstructive Sleep Apnea*, ed. 2. New York, Raven Press, 1994.
226. Polo O, Brissaud L, Fraga J, Dejean Y, Billiard M: Partial upper airway obstruction in sleep after uvulopalatopharyngoplasty. *Arch Otolaryngol Head Neck Surg* 1989; 115:1350–1354.
227. Larsson H: Results of Surgical Treatment of Obstructive Sleep Apnea Syndrome, in *Diagnosis and Management of Obstructive Sleep Apnea Syndrome*, Stockholm, October 1993; pp 85–89.
228. Walker EB, Frith RW, Harding DA, Cant BR: Uvulopalatopharyngoplasty in severe idiopathic obstructive sleap apnea syndrome. *Thorax* 1989; 44:205–208.
229. Ryan CF, Lowe AA, Li D, Fleetham JA: Three-dimensional upper airway computed tomography in obstructive sleep apnea: a prospective study in patients treated by uvulopalatopharyngoplasty. *Am Rev Respir Dis* 1991; 144:428–432.
230. Schwartz AR, Schubert N, Rothman W, et al: Effect of uvulopalatopharyngoplasty on upper airway collapsibility in obstructive sleep apnea. *Am Rev Respir Dis* 1992; 145:527–532.
231. Hudgel DW, Harasick T, Katz RL, Witt WJ, Abelson TI: Uvulopalatopharyngoplasty in obstructive apnea: Value of preoperative localization of site of upper airway narrowing during sleep. *Am Rev Respir Dis* 1991; 143:942–946.
232. Fujita S, Woodson BT, Clark JL, Wittig R: Laser midline glossectomy as a treatment for obstructive sleep apnea. *Laryngocope* 1991; 101:805–809.
233. Woodson BT, Fujita S: Clinical experience with lingualplasty as part of the treatment of severe obstructive sleep apnea. *Otolaryngol Head Neck Surg* 1992; 107:40–48.
234. Djupesland G, Schrader H, Lyberg T, Refsum H, Lilleas F, Godtlibsen OB: Palato-pharyngoglossoplasty in the treatment of patients with obstructive sleep apnea syndrome. *Acta Otolaryngol (Stockh)* 1992; Suppl 492:50–54.
235. Kuo PC, West RA, Bloomquist DS, MacNeil RW: The effect of mandibular osteotomy in three patients with hypersomnia sleep apnea. *Oral Surg* 1979; 48:385–392.

236. Powell NB, Riley RW, Guilleminault C: Maxillofacial Surgery for Obstructive Sleep Apnea, in Guilleminault C, Partinen M (eds.): *Obstructive Sleep Apnea Syndrome: Clinical Research and Treatment*. New York, Raven Press, 1990, pp 153–182.

237. Riley RW, Powell NB, Guilleminault C: Inferior mandibular osteotomy and hyoid myotomy suspension for obstructive sleep apnea: a review of 55 patients. *J Oral Maxillofac Surg* 1989; 47:159–164.

238. Kuhlo W, Doll E, Franck MC: Erfolgreiche Behandlung eines Pickwick-Syndroms durch eine Dauertrachealkanüle. *Dtsch Med Wochenschr* 1969; 94:1286–1290.

239. Ledereich PS, Thorpy MJ, Glovinsky PK, et al: Five Year Follow-Up of Daytime Sleepiness and Snoring After Tracheostomy in Patients With Obstructive Sleep Apneas, in Chouard CH (ed.): *Chronic Rhonchopathy*. London, John Libbey Eurotext Ltd, 1988, pp 354–357.

240. Goldman JM, Barnes DJ, Pohl DV: Obstructive sleep apnoea due to a dermoid cyst of the floor of the mouth. *Thorax* 1990; 45:76.

241. Kenna MA: Transsphenoidal encephalocele. *Ann Otol Rhinol Laryngol* 1985; 94:520–522.

242. Pirsig W, Schäfer J: Obstruktives Schlaf-Apnoe-Syndrom im Alter aus der Sicht des Hals-Nasen-Ohren-Arztes, in Platt D (ed.): *Handbuch der Gerontologie*. Vol 6: Stuttgart, Hals-Nasen-Ohrenheilkunde, 1993, pp 208–235.

243. Pekkarinen T, Partinen M, Pelkonen R, Iivanainen M: Sleep apnoea and daytime sleepiness in acromegaly: relationship to endocrinological factors. *Clin Endocrinol* 1987; 27:649–654.

244. Rajala R, Partinen M, Sane T, Pelkonen R, Huikuri K, Seppalainen AM: Obstructive sleep apnoea syndrome in morbidly obese patients. *J Intern Med* 1991; 230:125–129.

245. Sugerman HJ: Gastric surgery for morbid obesity. *Prob Gen Surg* 1987; 4:258–269.

246. Esclamado RM, Glenn MG, McCulloch TM, Cummings CW: Perioperative complications and risk factors in the surgical treatment of obstructive sleep apnea syndrome. *Laryngoscope* 1989; 99:1125–1129.

247. Gabridczyk MR: Acute airway obstruction after uvulopalatopharyngoplasty for obstructive sleep apnea syndrome. *Anesthesiology* 1988; 69:941–943.

248. Katsantonis GP, Walsh JK, Schweitzer PK, Friedman W: Further evaluation of uvulopalatopharyngoplasty in the treatment of obstructive sleep apnea syndrome. *Otolaryngol Head Neck Surg* 1985; 93:244–250.

249. Craddock MK, Lees DE: Anesthesia for Obstructive Sleep Apnea Patients: Risks, Precautions, and Management, in Fairbanks DNF, Fujita S (eds.): *Snoring and Obstructive Sleep Apnea*, ed. 2. New York, Raven Press, 1994, pp 211–217.

12

Cerebrospinal Fluid Rhinorrhea

JAMES A. STANKIEWICZ, M.D.
KATHELYNE G. DELSUPEHE, M.D.

A dural defect with leakage of cerebrospinal fluid (CSF) from the cisterns into the nasal cavity is a serious medical problem. The communication between the upper respiratory tract and the intracranial space has a significant risk for severe meningitis that can be fatal even in the era of modern antibiotic therapy.

The increasing numbers of severe craniofacial injuries and the more aggressive surgical approach to skull base and intracranial diseases have led to an increased number of patients presenting with CSF rhinorrhea.

Physicians and otolaryngologists, in particular, should be aware of how CSF leaks occur, how new sophisticated diagnostic tools should be used, and how rhinorrhea should be managed. Endoscopic nasal surgery brought us new fears about intracranial complications, but, more importantly, it provided us with the possibility of precisely diagnosing and confidently closing a CSF leak, avoiding the risks of craniotomy.

CLASSIFICATION

CSF leaks are generally classified according to their cause or pathogenesis (Table 12–1). Traumatic CSF rhinorrhea represents approximately 90% of cases and is a complication of 2% of all head traumas.[1] Both craniofacial injuries and operation (sinus or intracranial procedures) can cause a transient or permanent CSF fistula. In young children, rhinorrhea rarely occurs after trauma, probably because of the increased pliability of the skull and the underdevelopment of the sinuses.[2,3]

Much less frequently, rhinorrhea occurs in patients without a history of trauma. It has been argued, however, that use of the term "spontaneous" to describe CSF leaks is misleading because all CSF leaks must have an underlying cause. Therefore, we prefer the term "nontraumatic."

In almost half the cases of nontraumatic leak, a tumor or hydrocephalus causes an increase in CSF pressure. If not, the leak is called primary nontraumatic (spon-

270

**Table 12–1   Classification of
Cerebrospinal Fluid Leaks**

Traumatic leak (90%)*
  Craniofacial injury (80%)
  Iatrogenic: after (para)nasal operation (0.9%)
          after intracranial operation (8%–16%)
Nontraumatic (spontaneous) leak (10%)
  High-pressure flow (secondary spontaneous leaks) (5%)
    Intracranial tumor
    Hydrocephalus
  Normal-pressure flow (primary spontaneous leaks) (5%)
    Focal bony atrophy or dehiscences
    Bony erosions by small encephaloceles
    Other underlying congenital defects
    Empty sella syndrome
    Idiopathic

*Numbers in parentheses are approximate rates of occurrence.

taneous). In cases with normal or low CSF pressure, the pathogenesis is less well understood. Most likely, bony acquired or congenital defects cause a CSF leak. However, few cases have been documented.[4–6]

The onset of traumatic rhinorrhea can vary and is commonly referred to as immediate (within 48 hours) or delayed. In 95% of cases of delayed traumatic CSF leaks, they occur within 3 months after trauma. Most cases of accidental rhinorrhea have immediate onset, and only half of postsurgical CSF leaks present the first week after operation.[7,8]

PATHOPHYSIOLOGY

The factors responsible for traumatic and spontaneous CSF fistulas are essentially the same: a disruption of the arachnoid and dura coupled with an osseous defect and CSF pressure gradient that is either continuously or intermittently greater than the (healing) tensile strength of the disrupted tissue.[9] Hence, traumatic rhinorrhea occurs when CSF leaks through a dural tear and bony defect or fracture. The mechanisms of delayed traumatic rhinorrhea are less clearly understood but may result from herniation of the dura and eventually dural tear into a nonhealed osseous fracture site or from the dissolution of a hematoma at the fracture site.[10]

Spontaneous CSF rhinorrhea usually occurs in adults, coinciding with attainment of the highest levels of normal CSF pressures (increase from 40 mm H_2O in infants to 140 mm H_2O in adults).[11,12] The normal arterial and respiratory pulse waves affect CSF pressure, along with position changes of the head, and are therefore subject to recurrent fluctuations. Valsalva-like actions such as nose blowing can lead to dural rupture at sites of skull base dehiscences by increasing intracranial pressure.[11,12] Increased intracranial pressure, however, is not necessary for the development of spontaneous CSF rhinorrhea. Theories for primary nontraumatic leaks in the anterior cranial fossa include focal atrophy, rupture of the arachnoid sleeves passing through the cribriform plate with olfactory nerve filaments, and persistence of an embryonic olfactory lumen.[11,12]

ANATOMY

The most common anatomical sites of CSF leaks are due to congenital weaknesses in the anterior cranial fossa and the type of surgical procedure performed. The most common locations are depicted in Figure 12–1.

According to one series of 53 patients with rhinorrhea of different causes, 39% of fistulas occurred in the area of the cribriform plate and cells of the ethmoid sinus, in 15% the fistulas extended into the frontal sinus, and in 15% the fistulas extended from the sella turcica to the sphenoid sinus.[13] More rarely, the fistula can originate from the middle or posterior cranial fossa to the mastoid cells; in this case, CSF fluid enters the nasal vault via the middle ear and eustachian tube.

DIAGNOSIS

Both the presence and the anatomical site of the dural fistula need to be identified. The precise localization of the leak is most important. Accurate preoperative locali-

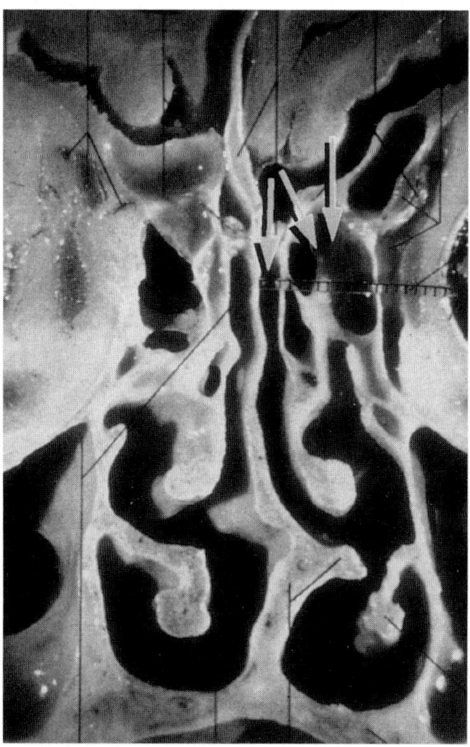

Figure 12–1. Most common sites of cerebrospinal fluid fistula.

zation allows planning for the most appropriate minimal procedure with a consequent reduction in complications and postoperative morbidity (Table 12–2).[19]

History and Clinical Signs

A thorough history is the first step toward arriving at the proper diagnosis. CSF leaks typically present with a history of clear, watery discharge, usually unilateral. Diagnosis is easier in a patient who has had recent trauma or operation. Delayed-onset fistulas can occur up to many years after trauma and, especially, after operation.[8] Some fistulas can therefore be unrecognized for years and ascribed to allergic or vasomotor rhinitis.

Sometimes the discharge will be accompanied by headaches relieved by CSF drainage. Drainage can be intermittent, because fluid may accumulate in one of the paranasal sinuses and empty with changes in head position ("reservoir sign"). A history of headaches and vision abnormalities can suggest increased intracranial pressure. Sometimes associated symptoms can point toward the localization of the leak. For instance, anosmia (present in 60% of posttraumatic rhinorrhea), especially when unilateral, indicates an injury near the olfactory area and anterior fossa. Interference with optic nerve function localizes the defect in the region of the tuberculum sellae, sphenoid sinus, or posterior ethmoid sinus.[15] In a patient with recurrent meningitis, especially pneumococcal, a dural defect with CSF leakage to the upper airway should be ruled out even if there is no demonstrable fluid drainage from the nose.

Physical examination should consist of complete rhinologic, otologic, head and neck, and neurologic studies, including a nasal endoscopy.[16] Nasal endoscopy can reveal abnormalities such as encephalocele or a meningocele (Fig. 12–2). Often the spinal fluid drainage can be initiated or increased by Valsalva maneuver or by compressing both jugular veins (Queckenstedt test) (Fig. 12–3). A change in head position can cause a gush of fluid ("reservoir sign") from CSF collected in an anatomical depression or an open sinus.

In patients with a head injury, blood may mix with CSF and mask the recognition of a CSF leak. CSF separates from blood when the mixture is placed on filter paper (or other media) and produces a clinically detectable sign, which has been called a "ring sign," "double-ring sign," or "halo sign" (Fig. 12–4). The appearance of the ring, however, is not exclusive for CSF and so the test can have false positive results.[17]

Table 12–2   Diagnosis of Cerebrospinal Fluid Leaks

History and clinical signs
Biochemical analysis of fluid
Anatomical localization
   Radiographic studies
   Nonradiographic dyes
   Nuclear studies

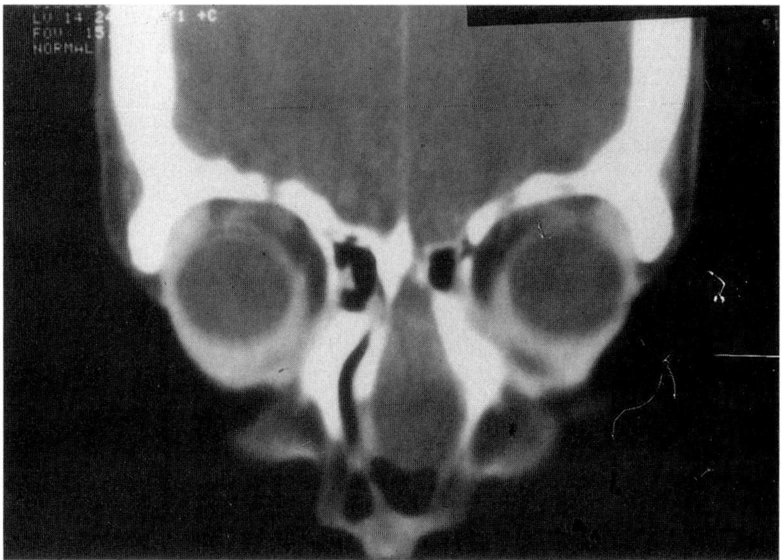

Figure 12–2. Endoscopic view of encephalocele in posterior cribriform plate (arrow). (Courtesy of Stankiewicz JA, *Advanced Endoscopic Sinus Surgery*. Philadelphia: Mosby, 1995, p 87.)

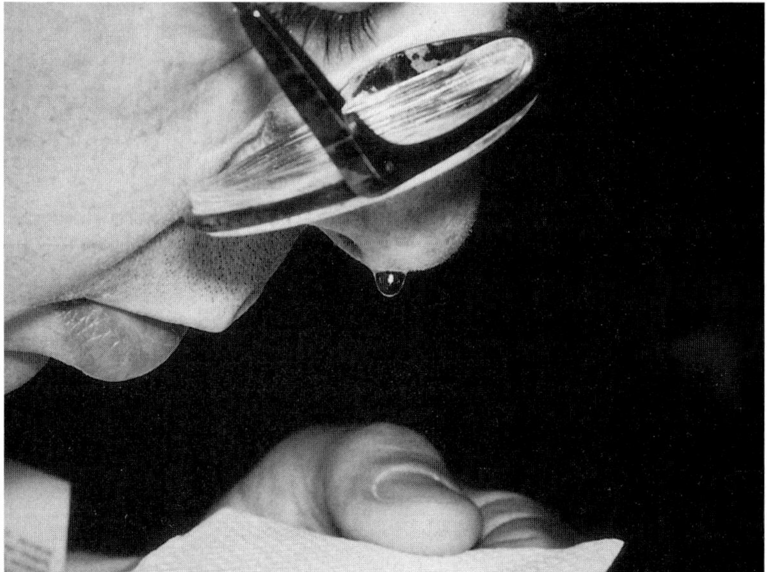

Figure 12–3. Spinal fluid slipping from patient's nose.

Bilateral rhinorrhea gives no clue about the site of the fistula, but when rhinorrhea is unilateral it seems logical that the defect of the skull base should be on the same site. Usually this is true. Paradoxical rhinorrhea does occur, however, when the midline structures (crista galli and vomer) are dislocated and CSF can flow through the nostril opposite to the defect.[12] The most frequently associated clinical findings of CSF rhinorrhea are meningitis (30%) or pneumocephalus (30%).[8]

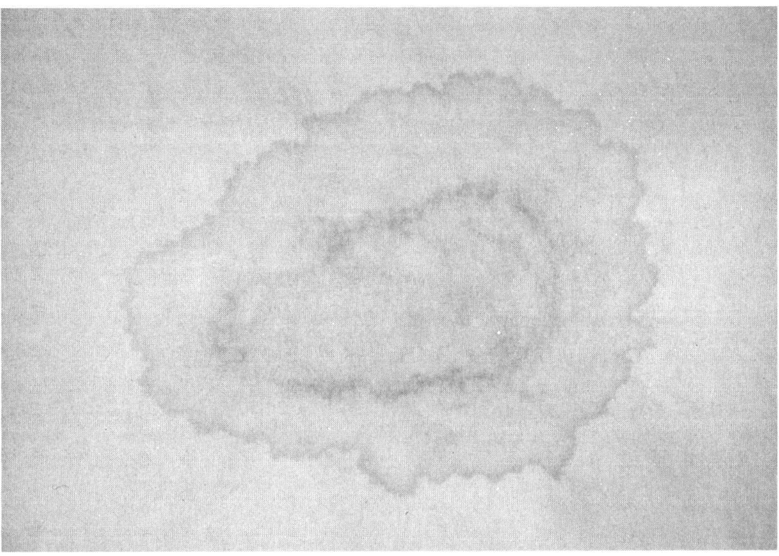

Figure 12–4. "Halo" sign, indicating cerebrospinal fluid leak.

Biochemical Tests

A quick but fairly unreliable test is a glucose content determination by *glucose oxidase papers*. False positive results can be caused by reducing substances present in the lacrimal gland secretions and nasal mucus; results can be positive with as little glucose as 5 mg/dL.[14] Active meningitis can lower glucose concentrations and therefore confound the results of quantitative glucose analysis. Glucose strip testing can be used as an inexpensive first-line diagnostic test in a patient with craniofacial injury. However, we think all positive test results should be confirmed by the more reliable β2 transferrin test.

Immunoelectrophoretic identification of CSF-specific marker proteins is the current standard for the identification of CSF fluid. β2 *transferrin assay* is the most widely used current test. It is a protein that is highly specific for human CSF. It may also be found in serum of newborns, vitreous humor, and patients with liver disease. The assay is a highly sensitive and selective, rapid, noninvasive test for the detection of CSF leakages. A minimum of 100 μL of fluid is usually necessary for electrophoresis.[18,19]

Total protein analysis, specific gravity analysis, and salt content test are not used any more because of the improved results obtained with other tests.

Anatomical Localization

Radiographic studies

Plain radiographs occasionally demonstrate a fracture or an air-fluid level in the sinus or an aerocele in the cranial cavity. The presence of air in the subarachnoid space on a plain radiograph is an almost pathognomonic sign of dural fistula. It is usually a consequence of a relatively large tear in the dural envelope. In the absence of a craniofacial injury, plain radiography is of little diagnostic value.

Computed tomography demonstrates not only the site of a fracture causing a traumatic leak but also underlying anatomical abnormalities causing a nontraumatic fistula (Fig. 12–5). It also provides valuable information about the condition of the brain and is the current standard in all craniofacial traumas. Sometimes a fluid level in the sphenoid sinus may indicate leakage; this finding does not necessarily mean that the site of leakage is located in this sinus, because fistulas in the posterior cribriform plate or posterior ethmoid roof can simply drain into the sphenoid sinus ostia. Pneumocephalus is diagnostic for a large dural tear (Fig. 12–6). A deviation of the crista galli has been reported as a radiologic sign in patients presenting with primary CSF rhinorrhea, a finding supporting congenital bony dehiscence as the etiologic basis for this condition.[20]

A modified technique with *digital subtraction cisternography* has been reported as useful if computed tomography cisternography does not identify the site of leakage.[21]

Magnetic resonance imaging is generally not recommended in the workup of CSF rhinorrhea because it does not demonstrate bony defects as effectively as computed tomography. However, heavily T2-weighted images have been reported to demonstrate severe CSF rhinorrhea.[22] Magnetic resonance imaging can also be helpful to evaluate exact extent when an encephalocele is present.

The diagnostic yield of computed tomography can be enhanced by injecting metrizamide (a water-soluble nonionic triiodinated contrast) or iohexol (Omnipaque) intrathecally. Metrizamide or Omnipaque computed tomographic cisternography (MCTC) documents precisely the presence of CSF leakage in most patients with an *active* leak (Fig. 12–7). This procedure has low morbidity and is best performed in the position of maximal leakage and provides high contrast against the

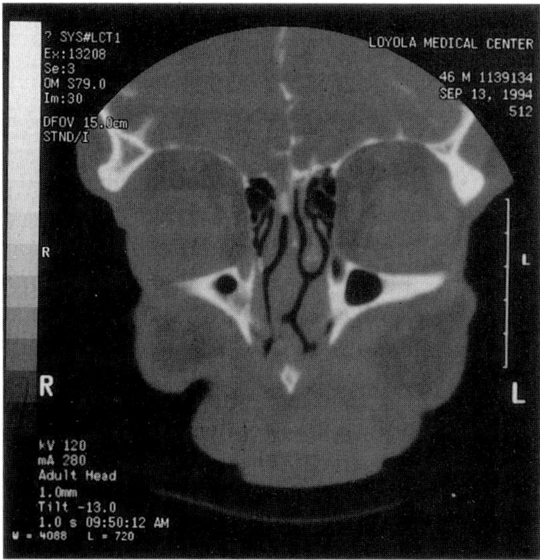

Figure 12–5. Computed tomography scan showing defect and mass coming through skull base from encephalocele.

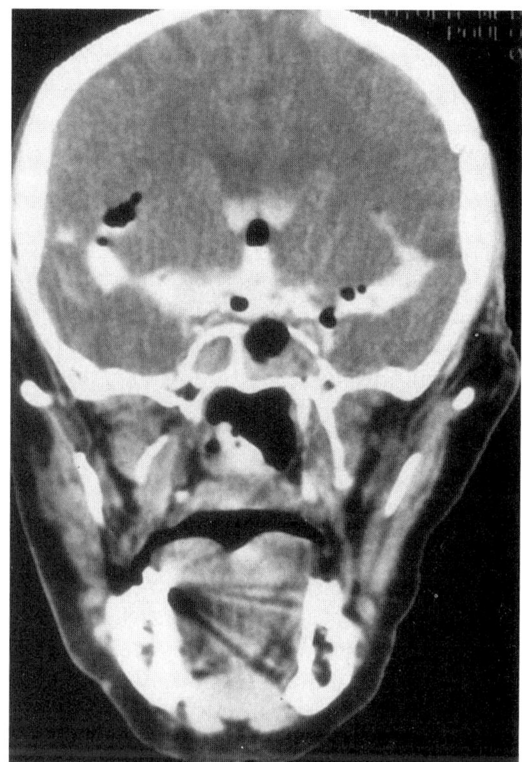

Figure 12–6. Computed tomography scan showing a pneumocephalus.

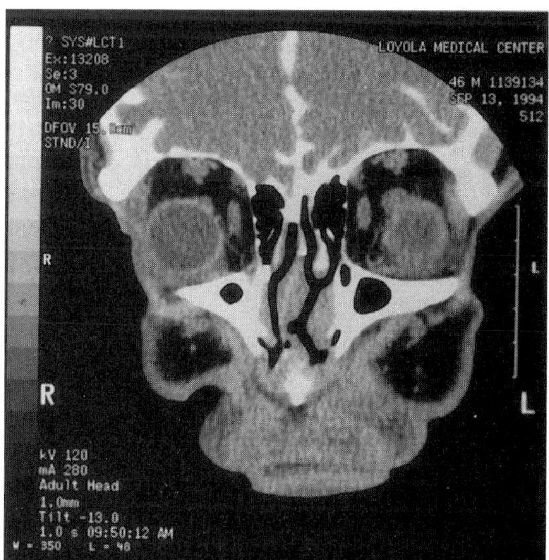

Figure 12–7. Positive computed tomography dye study (*arrow*) for a cribriform plate defect and active cerebrospinal fluid leak.

air within the paranasal sinuses.[23] However, neurotoxicity presenting as nausea, headaches, and acute organic psychosyndromes has been described. Severe toxicities have been reported only in patients undergoing myelography in which the dose of metrizamide is higher than that in routine MCTC.[24] There is some controversy as to whether MCTC can also precisely identify the site of CSF leakage. One study demonstrated positive localization by MCTC in 13 of 17 cases (76%). Of the 15 active fistulas, 13 (87%) were identified. None of the inactive fistulas could be demonstrated.[24]

Patients with slow or intermittent CSF leak in whom MCTC is unsuccessful can be restudied after electively increasing the intracranial pressure to activate the leak. This can be done by infusing saline intrathecally immediately before imaging.[23] Other authors have had good results using Valsalva maneuver or coughing to increase the intracranial pressure.[25] *Pneumocephalography* is an obsolete procedure that is uncomfortable (patient is in hanging-head position) and provides no contrast to the paranasal sinuses and nasal airway and has therefore been abandoned.[23]

Nonradiographic dyes

Dyes injected intrathecally and recovered on nasal pledges are of historic interest. The use of indigo carmine, methylene blue, and Evans blue has been abandoned because of neurologic toxicity (including paraplegia) and poor localization of the leak.[26] *Fluorescein* (0.2 mL 5% solution for injection mixed in 5 to 10 mL CSF) injected intrathecally is the most accurate method of localizing site of the leak, preoparatively and intraoperatively, to visually identify the fistula (Fig. 12–8). Transient neurologic complications have been reported.[26] Most accurate information can be obtained by direct nasal endoscopy 20 to 30 minutes after intrathecal injection to look for fluorescent CSF that is visible in the light of the endoscope. No additional ultraviolet light is necessary, but visualization may be enhanced by a blue light filter on the endoscope. A routine otologic examination can reveal fluorescein in the middle ear behind the eardrums, as can inspection of the posterior pharyngeal wall. Other methods include pledgets placed in key areas in the nasal cavities. The location of the stained cottonoid can then point toward the site of the leak.[27] We think that this technique can be useful if the precise location is not identified by MCTC and operation is considered. However, direct intranasal examination is preferred because the pledget technique is inaccurate as a result of possible saturation and contamination of neighboring pads.

Nuclear studies

Radioactive tracer isotopes are introduced into the CSF by lumbar or suboccipital puncture. Their distribution can be followed by serial scanning or scintiphotography of the head. Alternatively, pledgets can be inserted in the nasal cavity in all areas of potential leak. Different tracers have been used, including radioactive iodine (I^{131}), serum albumin (RISA), ytterbium (Yb^{169}) DTPA, indium (In^{111}) DTPA, technetium (^{99m}Tc) human serum albumin, and technetium (^{99m}Tc) pertechnetate.[11,25] Although isotope studies are considered relatively safe, several limitations undermine their clinical usefulness. Usually they cannot reveal the precise site of the leak. The isotope is absorbed by the bloodstream, causing extracranial contamination. Diffi-

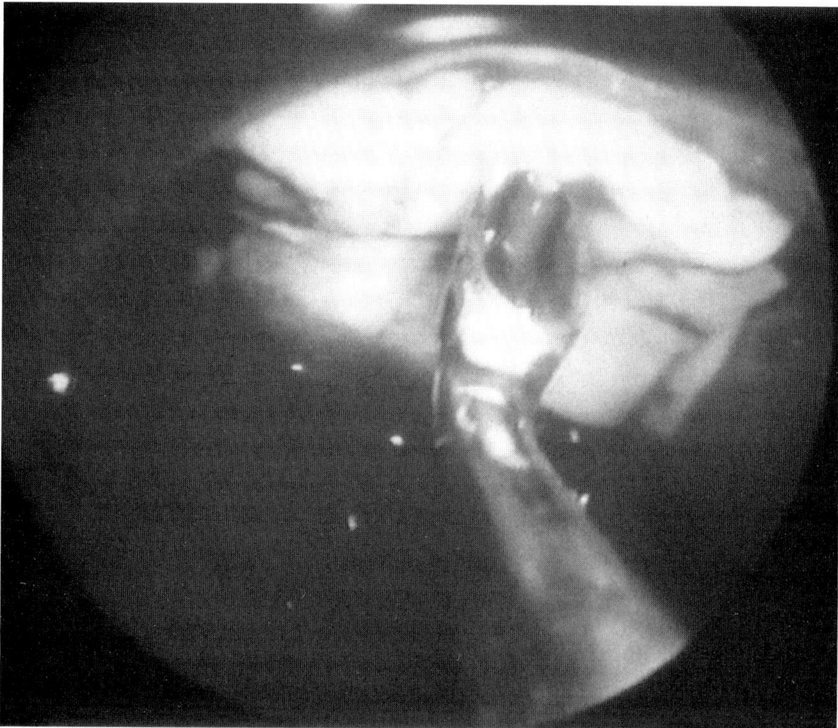

Figure 12–8. Fluorescein is noted coming from an active cerebrospinal fluid leak in sphenoid sinus. (Courtesy of Stankiewicz JA, *Advanced Endoscopic Sinus Surgery*. Philadelphia: Mosby, 1995, p 83.)

culties in positioning the patient may cause distal pledgets to saturate.[28] Finally and importantly, if the test is to be termed positive, the pledget readings should be impressively high. Borderline or slightly elevated readings are not reliable. Additionally, false positive results have been reported in up to 33% of patients.[6]

A silent fistula can be activated sometimes by increasing the intracranial pressure. One study compared "overpressure radionuclide cisternography" (ORNC) with MCTC in the detection of intermittent rhinorrhea in children. ORNC was more sensitive than MCTC for diagnosing the leak, but MCTC may be better for identifying the site of the leak[26] (Fig. 12–9).

MANAGEMENT

The treatment of CSF leaks depends mainly on the cause, location, and severity. In traumatic cases, the interval from trauma to manifestation, whether early or delayed rhinorrhea, is also important. The natural history of CSF leaks varies according to the underlying cause. Traumatic rhinorrhea often stops spontaneously. Leakage stops within 1 week in 70% of patients, within a few months in 20% to 30%, and within 6 months in most cases. Leakage rarely recurs. Conversely, only one-third of nontraumatic leaks cease spontaneously. Nontraumatic leaks typically persist for years with intermittent flow and recurrent leakage (Table 12–3).[30]

Table 12–3   Therapy of Cerebrospinal Fluid Leaks

Conservative therapy
    Bed rest (head-up position)
    Laxatives
    Serial lumbar punctures or continuous subarachnoidal
      catheter
    Antibiotics
Surgical therapy
    Intracranial approach
    Extracranial approach
      External sinus procedure
      Endoscopic sinus procedure

Conservative treatment consists of a 1- to 2-week trial of bed rest in a head-up position. Coughing, sneezing, nose blowing, and straining should be avoided. Laxatives are prescribed to minimize increased pressures during bowel movements. Closure of the defect can be facilitated by decreasing the intracranial pressure through repeated lumbar puncture or, better yet, an indwelling lumbar subarachnoid catheter.[31] The aim is to remove about 150 mL of CSF daily. There is some theoretical objection that such treatment could enhance the risk of meningitis. The decrease in CSF flow could theoretically allow bacteria to pass more easily through the fistula to the basal cisterns, but no evidence exists for this hypothesis. Lumbar drainage should obviously not be used in cases with marked brain edema and raised intracranial pressure.[12] The prophylactic use of antibiotics is controversial. Very few prospective, controlled studies are available, and no statistical, sound conclusions can be drawn. Most authors argue that routine use of antimicrobial agents cannot be advocated. The impression prevails that antibiotic prophylaxis is at least ineffective and may even be dangerous by selecting resistant organisms.[6,12] However, exceptions are conceivable in cases with a high risk of meningitis, including in patients with preexisting sinusitis/sinus operation or when another injury mandates their use. Restricting oral intake and the use of steroids, diuretics, or osmotically active medications can be considered, but they are probably minimally effective. The main disadvantage of the conservative approach is the risk for meningitis and brain abscess.

Therefore, *surgical repair* is generally advocated in patients with large fistulas (especially in the presence of pneumocephalus), nontraumatic leaks, acute and delayed-onset, prolonged traumatic leaks, or recurrent leaks. Immediate surgical exploration and simultaneous closure of dural fistula are also indicated in cases with open wounds that communicate with the dura, closed head injuries with intracranial complications, and fistula caused by and detected at operation, whether it is intracranial or nasal.[25,26]

No matter what surgical technique is used for closure, the above-mentioned conservative measures are generally used as an adjuvant the first days postoperatively.

Intracranial repair of CSF fistula was the standard therapy for many years, until recently. For fistulas in the frontal area of the cranial fossa, treatment usually consists of a frontal anterior fossa craniotomy. Rarely, temporal middle fossa craniotomy or occipital posterior fossa craniotomy is performed. Different techniques for repair have been described, including a pedicled or free periosteal or dural flap, a muscle plug for larger openings, mobilized portion of the falx, a fascia graft, or combined flaps and fibrin glue.[14] The sphenoid sinus is difficult to approach through an intracranial approach. The main benefits of the intracranial approach are direct access to the fistula with direct visualization of the dural tear, inspection and treatment of adjacent cortex, a better chance at tamponading a leak in the face of increased intracranial pressure, and the ability to treat coexisting intracranial abnormality. When preoperative maneuvers or operative exploration fails to demonstrate the site of fistula, an intracranial technique for a blind repair has been successful. In these cases, the cribriform areas (and sometimes the sphenoid sinuses) are covered with graft material.[14] Disadvantages of the intracranial closure techniques include considerable morbidity, a significant risk of permanent anosmia, brain retraction trauma (including edema, hematoma, hemorrhage, seizures, and cognitive impairment), and prolonged operative and hospitalization time.[13,26] The failure rate is surprisingly high, considering the extensive nature of the operation, ranging from 40% for the initial attempt to 10% overall, despite repeated craniotomies.[8,13]

Extracranial techniques are twofold: external approaches or endoscopic techniques. External approaches can consist of anterior osteoplastic flap through a coronal scalp or eyebrow incision, external ethmoidectomy, transethmoidal sphenoidotomy, transseptal sphenoidotomy, or transantral, depending on the site of leak. Similarly, grafts including fascia lata, temporal fascia, septal or turbinate mucosa, muscle or fat, and septal cartilage are used for both the external and the nasal endoscopic approaches.[1,26–28] The external approaches, although effective, are an alternative to the much more elegant and probably equally effective endoscopic closure. The endoscopic technique has been reported by several authors.[1,27,30–33]

For cribriform plate or fovea ethmoidalis fistula, a classic transnasal ethmoidectomy is performed (Fig. 12–10). For sphenoid sinus fistulas, an additional sphenoidotomy is performed, allowing a much more posterior repair (Fig. 12–11). The graft is placed over the fistula and gently positioned. When possible, the graft is "tucked in" above the bony skull base, ethmoid, or cribriform plate. The application of endoscopic techniques to intranasal closure of CSF leaks has several advantages over external ethmoidectomy or other intranasal methods, including excellent field of vision through enhanced illumination coupled with the ability to obtain angled magnified views, allowing exact localization of the leak; the ability to precisely clean mucosa from the bony defect without significantly increasing the size of the defect; and accurate position of the graft material over and into the defect.[1,27,32,33] Alternatively, Papay et al.[32] reported the use of endoscopic telescopes in a transseptal transsphenoidal approach to localize sphenoid CSF leaks.

Extracranial approaches have not been prospectively compared with the intracranial approaches, but several advantages are obvious: good visualization, far lower morbidity, and no anosmia. Success rates for the extracranial approaches vary from 86% to 100%, generally exceeding the outcome of the intracranial ap-

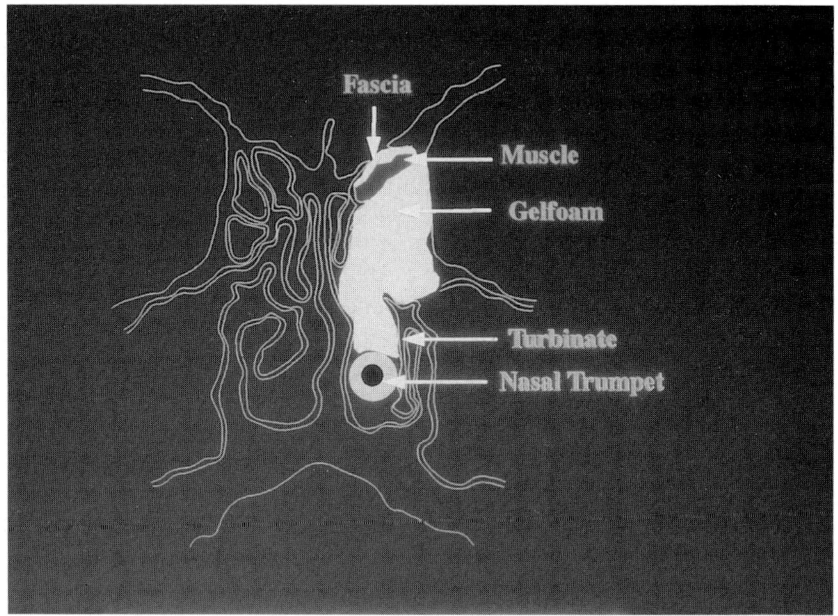

Figure 12–9. Layered repair of an endoscopically repaired ethmoid/cribriform cerebrospinal fluid fistula. (Courtesy of Stankiewicz JA, *Advanced Endoscopic Sinus Surgery*. Philadelphia: Mosby, 1995, p 84.)

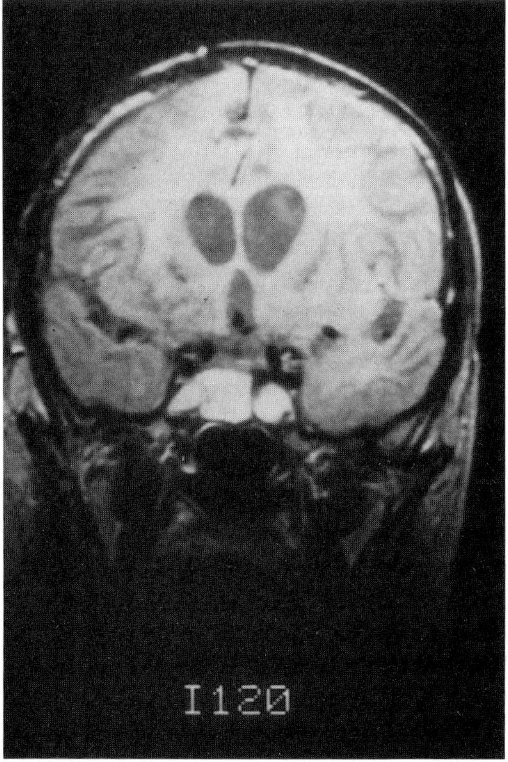

Figure 12–10. Wide sphenoidotomy in which cerebrospinal fluid leak is repaired with fibrin glue.

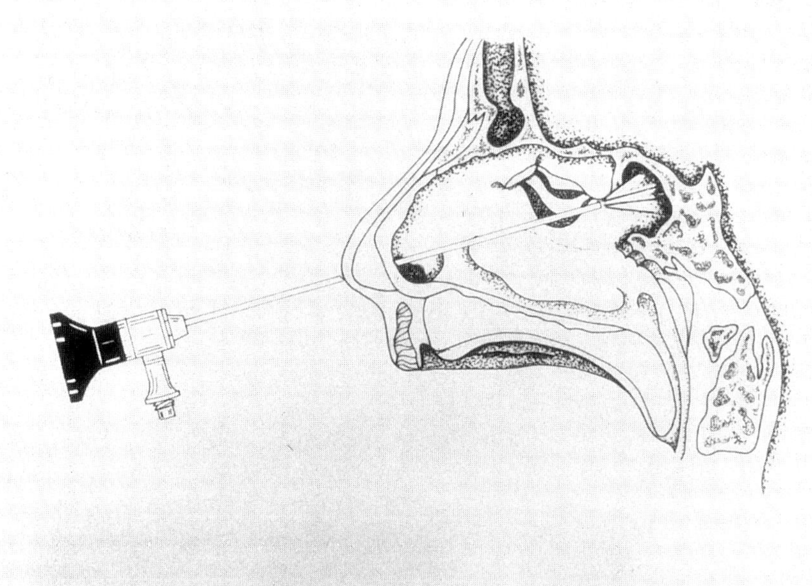

Figure 12–11.   Endoscopic repair through transnasal ethmoidectomy of sphenoid cerebrospinal fluid leak. (Courtesy of Stankiewicz JA, *Advanced Endoscopic Sinus Surgery*. Philadelphia: Mosby, 1995, p 82.)

proaches.[1,28,33,34] The main disadvantages include the inability to assess and treat concomitant intracranial abnormality, the difficulties encountered in treating frontal and sphenoid sinuses with prominent lateral extensions, and the undesirability of patching high-pressure leaks from the outside.[12–14] Consequently, because of the rarity of the latter two types of leaks, the most appropriate initial surgical management of CSF rhinorrhea is an extracranial rhinologic repair unless there is a coexisting indication for intracranial exploration.

OUTCOME AND COMPLICATIONS

Results and risks of operative treatment have to be compared with the results and risks of the natural, untreated course and of conservative treatment. Meningitis is the most frequent severe complication, with *Streptococcus pneumoniae* being the most common pathogen followed by *Haemophilus influenzae*.[2,35,36] The risk of meningitis during the first 3 weeks after trauma is estimated to be 10%.[12,35] In nontraumatic rhinorrhea, the rate of meningitis is much higher (40%).[12,35,36] According to the literature, meningitis caused by a persistent CSF fistula is associated with a very high mortality. Along with the lower rate of spontaneous closure, a conservative approach for these indications is discouraged.

Spontaneous closure rates of CSF fistula differ according to the cause of the fistula, and these are cited above. Recurrence rate after initial spontaneous closure was 7% in one large retrospective series.[11] Operative mortality ranges between 1% and 3% for intracranial procedures to negligible for external approaches. Morbidity

Suggested Diagnostic Work-Up of CSF Rhinorrhea

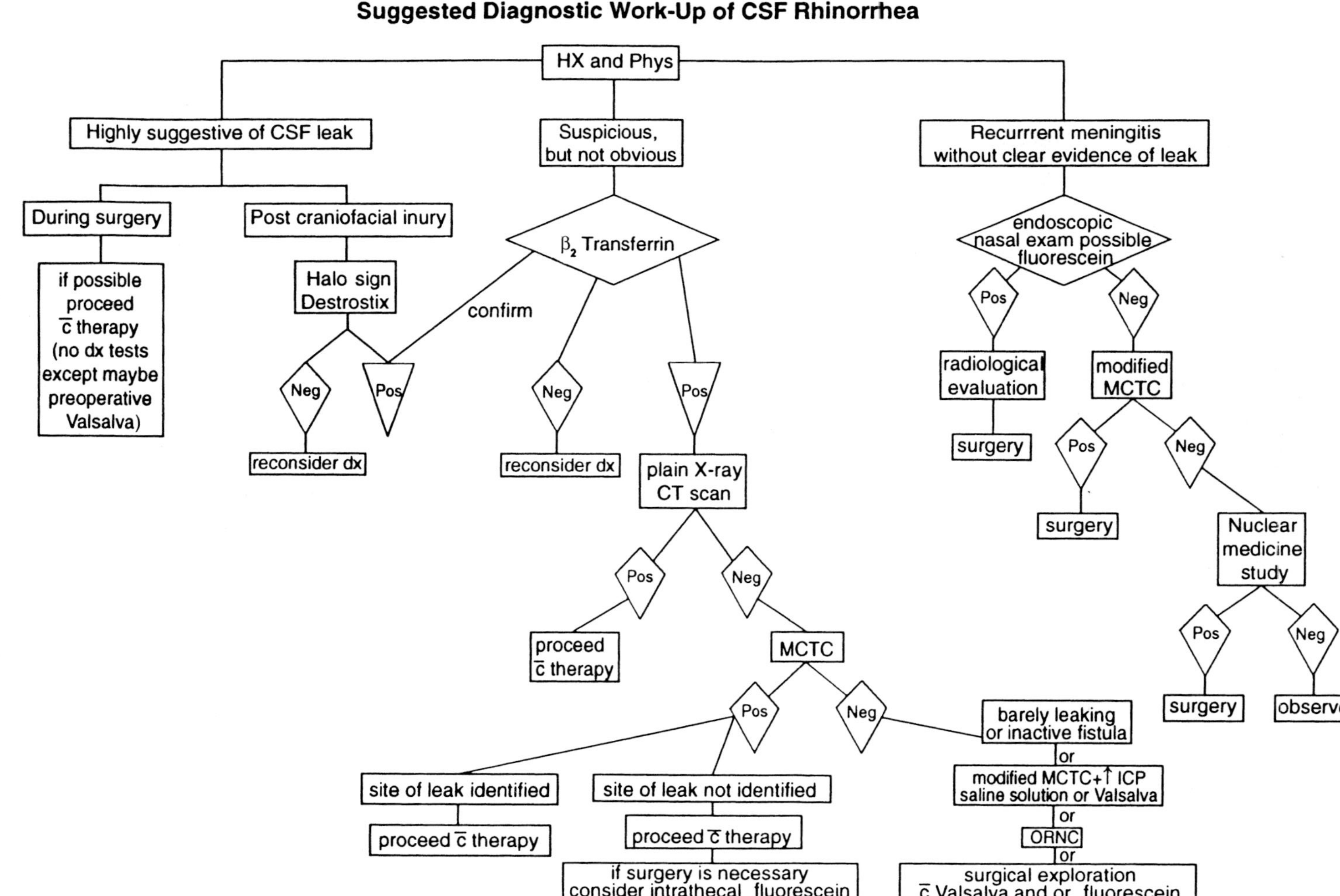

Suggested diagnostic workup in patients with cerebrospinal fluid rhinorrhea (CSF). Hx, history; Phys, Physical examination; dx, diagnostic, diagnosis; Neg, negative; Pos, positive; MCTC, metrigamide computed tomographic cisternography; ICP, intracranial pressure; ORNC, overpressure (stress) radionuclide cisternography.

with intracranial approaches can be significant (see above), and anosmia is the most often reported (10% to 25%).[11–13] Severe complications from external approaches are rarer and include all complications for ethmoidectomy and sphenoidotomy. Recurrent leaks are common, especially after intracranial approaches (the worst leaks), and serial operative procedures are often mandatory.[11–13]

CONCLUSION

CSF fistulas can occur after a trauma, whether iatrogenic surgical or a craniofacial injury, but also spontaneously. Several diagnostic tools are available to identify the site of leakage if a fistula is clinically suspected. In early-onset traumatic rhinorrhea, a conservative approach can be justified, but other fistulas will need immediate surgical intervention to avoid potentially fatal meningitis. A craniotomy can be avoided in most cases by using safer and successful external approaches.

The otolaryngologist head and neck surgeon now plays a primary role in the diagnostic and therapeutic management of patients with CSF rhinorrhea. Technology is now available for endoscopic nasal examination, diagnosis , and therapy of the anatomic site of the leak. Moreover, the extracranial, especially endoscopic, approach for repair of CSF leak for uncomplicated approachable fistula is quickly emerging as the treatment of choice. It has little attendant morbidity and is an excellent chance for permanent closure of the dural defect.

REFERENCES

1. Stankiewicz JA: Cerebrospinal fluid fistula and endoscopic sinus surgery. *Laryngoscope* 1991; 101:250–256.
2. Jones DT, McGill TJ, Healy GB: Cerebrospinal fistulas in children. *Laryngoscope* 1992; 102:443–446.
3. Park JI, Strelzow VV, Friedman WH: Current management of cerebrospinal fluid rhinorrhea. *Laryngoscope* 1983; 93:1294–1300.
4. Rontal M, Rontal E: Studying whole-mounted sections of the paranasal sinuses to understand the complications of endoscopic sinus surgery. *Laryngoscope* 1991; 101:361–366.
5. Ohnishi T: Bony defects and dehiscences of the roof of the ethmoid cell. *Rhinology* 1981; 19:195–202.
6. Beckhardt RN, Setzen M, Carras R: Primary spontaneous cerebrospinal fluid rhinorrhea. *Otolaryngol Head Neck Surg* 1991; 104:425–432.
7. Eljamel MS, Foy PM: Post-traumatic CSF fistulae: the case for surgical repair. *Br J Neurosurg* 1990; 4:479–483.
8. McCoy G: Cerebrospinal rhinorrhea: a comprehensive review. *Laryngoscope* 1963; 73:1125–1157.
9. Ommaya AK, DiChiro G, Baldwin M, Pennybacker JB: Non-traumatic cerebrospinal fluid rhinorrhoea. *J Neurol Neurosurg Psychiatry* 1968; 31:214–225.
10. Okada J, Tsuda T, Takasugi S, et al: Unusually late onset of cerebrospinal rhinorrhea after head trauma. *Surg Neurol* 1991; 35:213–217.
11. Hubbard JL, McDonald TJ, Pearson BW, Lewis ER Jr: Spontaneous cerebrospinal fluid rhinorrhea: evolving concepts in diagnosis and surgical management based on the Mayo Clinic experience from 1970 through 1981. *Neurosurgery* 1985; 16:314–321.
12. Loew F, Pertuiset B, Chaumier EE, Jaksche H: Traumatic, spontaneous and postoperative CSF rhinorrhea. *Adv Tech Stand Neurosurg* 1984; 11:169–207.
13. Ray BS, Bergland RM: Cerebrospinal fluid fistula: clinical aspects, techniques of localization, and methods of closure. *J Neurosurg* 1969; 30:399–405.
14. Calcaterra TC: Diagnosis and management of ethmoid cerebrospinal rhinorrhea. *Otolaryngol Clin North Am* 1985; 18:99–105.

15. Yerkes SA, Thompson DH, Fisher WS III: Spontaneous cerebrospinal fluid rhinorrhea. *Ear Nose Throat J* 1992; 71:318–320.
16. Bolger WE, Kennedy DW: Nasal endoscopy in the outpatient clinic. *Otolaryngol Clin North Am* 1992; 25:791–802.
17. Dula DJ, Fales W: The "ring sign." Is it a reliable indicator for cerebrospinal fluid? *Ann Emerg Med* 1993; 22:718–720.
18. Porter MJ, Brookes GB, Zeman AZ, Keir G: Use of protein electrophoresis in the diagnosis of cerebrospinal fluid rhinorrhoea. *J Laryngol Otol* 1992; 106:504–506.
19. Ryall RG, Peacock MK, Simpson DA: Usefulness of β_2-transferrin assay in the detection of cerebrospinal fluid leaks following head injury. *J Neurosurg* 1992; 77:737–739.
20. Tolley NS, Lloyd GA, Williams HO: Radiological study of primary spontaneous CSF rhinorrhoea. *J Laryngol Otol* 1991; 105:274–277.
21. Byrne JV, Ingram CE, MacVicar D, Sullivan FM, Uttley D: Digital subtraction cisternography: a new approach to fistula localisation in cerebrospinal fluid rhinorrhea. *J Neurol Neurosurg Psychiatry* 1990; 53:1072–1075.
22. Wakhloo AK, van Velthoven V, Schumacher M, Krauss JK: Evaluation of MR imaging, digital subtraction cisternography, and CT cisternography in diagnosing CSF fistula. *Acta Neurochir (Wien)* 1991; 111:119–127.
23. Naidich TP, Moran CJ: Precise anatomic localization of atraumatic sphenoethmoidal CSF rhinorrhea by metrizamide CT cisternography. *J Neurosurg* 1980; 53:227–228.
24. Chow JM, Goodman D, Mafee MF: Evaluation of CSF rhinorrhea by computerized tomography with metrizamide. *Otolaryngol Head Neck Surg* 1989; 100:99–105.
25. Nuss D, Costantino P: Diagnosis and management of cerebrospinal fluid leaks. In: *Otolaryngology-Head and Neck Surgery*. St. Louis: Mosby Yearbook, 1996, pp 79–95.
26. Zlab MK, Moore GF, Daly DT, Yonkers AJ: Cerebrospinal fluid rhinorrhea: a review of the literature. *Ear Nose Throat J* 1992; 71:314–317.
27. Mattox DE, Kennedy DW: Endoscopic management of cerebrospinal fluid leaks and cephaloceles. *Laryngoscope* 1990; 100:857–862.
28. Calcaterra TC: Extracranial surgical repair of cerebrospinal rhinorrhea. *Ann Otol Rhinol Laryngol* 1980; 89:108–116.
29. Yessenow RS, McCabe BF: The osteo-mucoperiosteal flap in repair of CSF rhinorrhea: a 20-year experience. *Otolaryngol Head Neck Surg* 1989; 101:555–558.
30. Wigand ME: Transnasal ethmoidectomy under endoscopic control. *Rhinology* 1981; 19:7–15.
31. Stankiewicz JA: Complications in endoscopic intranasal ethmoidectomy: an update. *Laryngoscope* 1989; 99:686–690.
32. Papay FA, Maggiano H, Dominguez S, et al: Rigid endoscopic repair of paranasal sinus cerebrospinal fluid fistulas. *Laryngoscope* 1989; 99:1195–1201.
33. Dodson EE, Gross CW, Swerdloff JL, Gustafson LM: Transnasal endoscopic repair of cerebrospinal fluid rhinorrhea and skull base defects: a review of 29 cases. *Otolaryngol Head Neck Surg* 1994; 111:600–605.
34. Persky MS, Rothstein SG, Breda SD, et al: Extracranial repair of cerebrospinal fluid otorhinorrhea. *Laryngoscope* 1991; 101:134–136.
35. Martinez E: Mixed bacterial meningitis associated with CSF leak. *Clin Infect Dis* 1992; 14:1263.
36. Tolley NS: A clinical study of spontaneous CSF rhinorrhea. *Rhinology* 1991; 29:223–230.

13

Use of Advanced Technology in Diagnosis of Bacterial Sinusitis and Associated Complications

DAVID H. SLAVIT, M.D.

Sinusitis is an extremely common chronic disease, affecting as many as 30 million Americans.[1] The disease is characterized by inflammation of the paranasal sinuses with associated obstruction of the sinus ostia, retention of secretions, and infection. The ciliated cell beat frequency is reduced, and ciliated cells convert to mucus-secreting goblet cells.[2,3] Mucous hypersecretion and impaired mucociliary transport can block drainage sites with symptoms of congestion, obstruction, pain, and pressure. If the sinus passageways remain blocked because of prolonged, recurrent, or inadequately treated infection, a chronic state may develop. Chronic sinusitis is generally used to describe the condition when symptoms exist for longer than 3 months.

DIAGNOSIS

The first firm diagnostic clues to sinusitis may come from the physical examination and history. The most common manifestations are combinations of facial tenderness or pain, nasal congestion, and purulent discharge. The posterior drainage of secretions into the throat often leads to the development of a cough. There may also be complaints of popping or clicking in the ears, muffled hearing, halitosis, and reduction in the senses of taste and smell.

Predisposing historical factors include nasal trauma, allergic rhinitis, viral upper respiratory tract infection, nasal polyps, foreign bodies, nasal intubation, dental abscess, and the prolonged use of nasal constrictor sprays. Other factors leading to sinusitis include defects of mucociliary clearance and abnormalities of the immune system. Factors that affect normal mucociliary function include structural deformities of cilia, altered mucous viscosity, Kartagener's syndrome, and cystic fibrosis.

Nasal Endoscopy

The diagnosis and management of sinus disease have been enhanced in recent years by technologically improved radiographic evaluation and methods for intranasal visualization.[4,5] Nasal endoscopy provides an in-depth display and evaluation of the nasal cavity and paranasal sinuses.[6] Decongestion of the nose with a topical α-adrenergic spray shrinks the mucosa to permit a more extensive view.

Physical findings in paranasal sinusitis can be variable, including nasal edema, erythema, purulent rhinitis, closure of the sinus ostia, posterior pharyngeal drainage, facial edema, orbital edema and cellulitis, facial cellulitis, and nasal polyps. Irritation of the nasal mucosa leads to inflammation with a bright red, irregular appearance. Prolonged nasal inflammation may lead to the formation of nasal polyps or polypoid degeneration of the nasal mucosa. During endoscopic assessment, careful attention should be given to the condition of the mucosa, including its color, size, and condition. The shape of the turbinates and septum should be assessed, with particular regard given to any anatomic narrowing of the osteomeatal complex.

The presence of pus or polyps should be determined. Use of the rigid or flexible fiberoptic endoscope permits viewing of the sphenoethmoid recess and osteomeatal complex to evaluate for areas of inflammation or pathologic drainage. In maxillary and anterior ethmoid infections, the pus is visible in the middle meatus. Pus is visible in the superior meatus or sphenoethmoidal recess when the posterior ethmoid cells are involved. The absence of visible pus does not rule out active infection, because drainage from the sinuses may be impeded or may be intermittent. Further inspection of the nasopharynx, oropharynx, and hypopharynx may reveal evidence of the purulent nasal discharge.

Sinus Culture Techniques

The reference standard for diagnosing infectious sinusitis is sinus aspiration and culture. The need for a sinus aspirate for culture is based on the poor correlation between nasal and nasopharyngeal cultures and bacteria isolated from sinus aspirates. Nasal cultures are unreliable unless one constricts the mucosa and aspirates directly from the ostium.[11] Culture specimens obtained in acute sinusitis frequently show mixed flora and are not usually of diagnostic importance in routine cases.[7,8] Cultures are particularly appropriate for guiding the choice of antibiotic in patients with complicated or refractory sinusitis, in which unusual organisms are often found.[9-11]

Puncture of the maxillary antrum is an office procedure that may be used for diagnostic aspiration or therapeutic lavage. Intranasal approaches may be made through the ostium of the maxillary antrum or through the inferior meatus. Sinus punctures can also be performed through the canine fossa.[12] Because the nasal vestibule is heavily colonized with aerobic and anaerobic bacterial species, there is a possibility of contamination with inferior meatal aspirations. This possibility of contamination can be compensated for by attempting to sterilize the nasal mucosa topically and by correlating the interpretation of the Gram stain with the results of bacterial culture.

Another limitation of maxillary sinus aspiration for culture is that the secretions are often too thick to be aspirated and thus require irrigation.[5] Irrigation complicates the quantification of bacteria. Irrigation also results in aeration of the specimen, which may impair the recovery of anaerobic organisms. Contaminated bacteria often have a low colony count on culture and are not seen on Gram stain. Furthermore, inadequate methods of obtaining a specimen can be suspected when the results of Gram stain are positive and those of culture are negative. Many institutions consider cultures positive only if a bacterial species is recovered in a colony count of at least 10^4 colony-forming units/mL.[7,8]

The preferred method of aspirating the maxillary sinus in children is by passing a large trocar beneath the inferior turbinate through the lateral nasal wall. The Caldwell-Luc approach to the maxillary sinus is not acceptable in children because of the developing dentition. Attempted cannulation of the natural ostium in the middle meatus is not advisable because of the possibility of inadvertent traumatization and subsequent scarring to this region.[4]

Bacteriology of Sinusitis

With antral culture techniques, there are consistent results regarding the aerobic bacterial contents of acute sinusitis in children and adults.[4,7,8,13] The predominant bacterial agents are *Streptococcus pneumoniae* and *Haemophilus influenzae* in adults[3,6,11] and *S. pneumoniae, H. influenzae*, and *Moraxella catarrhalis* in children.[7,14] In subacute sinusitis the bacterial flora was similar. However, in patients with subacute sinusitis and cystic fibrosis, the most common pathogens recovered were *Pseudomonas aeruginosa*, non-typeable *H. influenzae*, and α-hemolytic streptococci.[15]

In persistent and chronic sinusitis, bacterial invasion of the submucosa results in infiltration of the lamina propria by polymorphic neutrophils, mast cells, and lymphocytes.[16,17] Subsequent release of the chemical mediators histamine and prostaglandins causes vasodilation and edema of the submucosa. Persistent lymphatic and venous obstruction leads to edema of the mucosa, which can then become thick and edematous.[18] As secretions become trapped within the sinuses and the oxygen saturation is lowered, bacteria proliferate. Furthermore, the phagocytic function of the polymorphic neutrophils decreases, ciliary function ceases as adenosine triphosphate (ATP) levels decrease, and proteolytic enzmyes released from dying polymorphic neutrophils destroy the cilia.[7,8,18] The decreased oxygen content of the sinus cavity supports the growth of anaerobic organisms.

Studies of the bacterial findings on chronic maxillary sinusitis have reported consistent results regarding aerobic results.[9,17] The greatest controversy is the prevalence of anaerobic organisms in chronic sinusitis.[9,16,17,19–23] In adults, Erkan et al.[19] found anaerobic organism in 88% of culture-positive specimens. The predominant anaerobic organisms were cocci of *Bacteroides* species (*B. fragilis* and *B. melaninogenicus*) and *Peptostreptococcus*. The predominant aerobes were *Streptococcus* species and *Staphylococcus aureus*.

In children, anaerobes are rarely found in chronic sinusitis.[20,21] In a recent study of chronic sinusitis in children, culture specimens obtained from mucosa revealed that the most prevalent organisms were α-hemolytic streptococci and *Staphylococcus aureus* followed by *S. pneumoniae, H. influenzae,* and *M. catarrhalis.*[23] *M. catarrhalis* was more prevalent in children younger than 4 years, and *S. aureus* was more common in older children.[23] Children with symptoms for more than 1 year had an increased prevalence of *S. aureus* and anaerobic infections.[23] Of the 55 cultures in the study, only 12 anaerobic organisms and 4 fungi were isolated.[23] Because of the low incidence of anaerobes and fungi, their importance in pediatric chronic sinusitis is unclear.

In the critical care setting, sinusitis is often caused by gram-negative, anaerobic, and polymicrobial pathogens.[24–27] There is often inadequate ventilation, close-spaced bacterial overgrowth due to chronic mucosal inflammation, and growth of resistance organisms. The more common isolates include *Pseudomonas aeruginosa, Klebsiella pneumoniae, Enterobacteriaceae, Staphylococcus epidermidis, Escherichia coli, Enterococcus* species, *Serratia marcescens, Bacteroides* species, and other anaerobes.[24–27]

Immunologic Evaluation

Another cause of alteration in the microbial content of sinusitis is an abnormal immune status. Numerous reports have associated recurrent infections with IgG subclass deficiencies, particularly IgG2 in children and IgG3 in adults.[28–31] The clinical relevance of IgG subclass deficiency is controversial as measured by radioimmunodiffusion assays, because isolated deficiencies of each of the four IgG subclasses can be found in apparently healthy individuals.[32,33] Two newer methods, the immunoradiometric assay and the enzyme-linked immunosorbent assay (ELISA), appear to be more specific.[32] IgG3 deficiencies were reported in adults with recurrent upper and lower respiratory tract infections.[33,34] Also in adults, IgA deficiencies were observed in patients with chronic rhinitis and chronic sinusitis.

In children, IgG2 deficiencies have been most commonly associated with chronic or recurrent infections.[34,35] Antibodies to polysaccharide antigens are particularly associated with the IgG2 subclass. Patients with this deficiency have repeated infections with bacteria that have a polysaccharide capsule, such as *H. influenzae* and *Pneumococcus*. Partial deficiency of one or more IgG subclasses may be associated with an increased susceptibility to infections.[34]

The evaluation of immunologic status cannot be limited to determination of immunoglobulin class and subclass levels only. Evaluation for immunization hyporesponsiveness can detect patients who have normal immunoglobulin levels but fail to make appropriate specific immunoglobulin when challenged.[34,35] In a study of 61 patients with refractory sinusitis, 34 had abnormal results on immunologic studies when all these variables were evaluated.[35] If only immunoglobulin class and subclass levels were studied, immunologic abnormalities would have gone undetected in 17 of the 34 patients.[35] Patients, particularly children, with recurrent infections should be evaluated for their response to pneumococcal immunization, even if they have normal immunoglobulin levels.[36]

In acquired immunodeficiency syndrome (AIDS), the most common pathogens are those found in the general population; however, cases of opportunistic infections can exist.[37] Patients with AIDS have multiple immunologic deficits involving humoral and cell-mediated immunity. The humoral deficits place the patient at risk for recurrent bacterial infections. In patients with AIDS and sinusitis, the pathogens are commonly *S. pneumoniae*, *H. influenzae*, and, less commonly, *S. aureus*, *Salmonella enteritides*, *K. pneumoniae*, and *P. aeruginosa*.[39,40] Cytomegalovirus and *Pneumocystis carinii* have also been reported to cause sinusitis. The diagnosis of cytomegalovirus can be missed if surgical biopsy specimens or sinus aspirations for culture are not performed. The increasing use of cytotoxic drugs for human immunodeficiency virus (HIV) infections will put patients at higher risk for fungal complications. Currently, fungal sinusitis appears to be associated with late-stage AIDS when the CD4+ lymphocyte count is less than 150/mm.[38]

Fungal sinusitis due to *Aspergillus*, *Mucormycosis* and other agents has been increasingly recognized and reported in patients with and without immunologic compromise.[41,42] Fungal sinusitis has been classified as acute invasive disease and chronic disease of an invasive or noninvasive nature.[37,43] Extramucosal fungal infections may manifest as polypoid lesions due to saprophytic growth on retained secretions or appear as fungal balls. These are usually benign conditions related to *Aspergillus*. Infiltrating fungal sinusitis occurs in an immunocompetent host but is usually not as aggressive as the fulminant infections that occur in immunocompromised persons. The fulminant disease is the lethal form of infection and may be caused by *Mucormycosis* or *Aspergillus*. An additional type of sinusitis is allergic fungal sinusitis.[44]

RADIOGRAPHIC EVALUATION

Although the reference standard for diagnosing infectious sinusitis is sinus aspiration and culture, its use is generally limited to patients with complicated or refractory sinusitis. In general practice, sinus radiographs are readily obtained and can be considered a pragmatic reference standard. A standard four-view radiograph includes Caldwell (anteroposterior), Waters (occipital-mental), lateral, and submental vertex projections. Caldwell plain radiographs of the sinuses visualize the frontal and ethmoid sinuses. The Waters view is used for delineation of the maxillary sinuses. The submental vertex and lateral views are used for observation of the sphenoid sinuses. These films are considered diagnostic for sinusitis if they reveal mucosal thickening of more than 8 mm in adults, air-fluid level, or opacification.[45,46]

Plain Radiography

Plain radiography provides noninvasive and fast evaluation of the lower third of the nasal cavity and the maxillary, frontal, sphenoid, and posterior ethmoid sinus. However, it provides very limited information about the anterior ethmoid sinus and is not adequate for evaluation of chronic sinusitis when mucosal thickening alone may be present. Its drawback of overlapping structure makes evaluation of the osteomeatal complex, anterior ethmoid sinus, middle meatus, and sphenoid recess somewhat limited. Using air-fluid levels and opacification as criteria of disease and antroscopy as a standard of reference, Kuhn[47] found that the sensitivity of plain radiography was 54% and the specificity was 92%. When the criterion of mucosal thickening was used, the numbers reversed, and sensitivity was 99% and specificity only 46%. The accuracy of plain radiography diminishes when infections are limited to the osteomeatal complex region without involvement of the maxillary sinus.

Computed Tomography (CT) Imaging

Complex motion tomography, such as polytomography, has been replaced by CT scanning because of the better definition of images obtained and the decreased radiation exposure. The presence of air-fluid levels is typically associated with acute sinusitis, whereas the findings suggestive of chronic sinusitis include mucosal thickening, bone remodeling, polyposis, and bone thickening due to osteitis from adjacent chronic mucosal inflammation.[48] Hyperattenuated secretions on CT scans may be due to *inspissated* secretions, fungal sinusitis, or hemorrhage in the sinus.

CT scans can provide specific diagnoses and display the underlying causes of sinusitis in patients who have chronic or recurrent acute sinusitis. In recurrent sinusitis, CT examination is delayed until antibiotic therapy controls the acute exacerbation. At that point, CT scans can clarify anatomic relationships and variations that may play a role in sinusitis.

The early imaging manifestations of sinonasal fungal disease are usually nonspecific and cannot be distinguished from the imaging findings of the more common nonfungal infections.[66] Even with chronic fungal disease, distinction from chronic bacterial infection may not be possible on either CT or magnetic resonance imaging. Fungal disease of the sinonasal cavities is often first diagnosed because of the clinical failure to respond to routine antibiotic therapy implemented for an apparent bacterial infection.

There are circumstances in which a fungal infection or an aggressive infection can be suggested by the imaging study. Osteomyelitis is likely when the sinus cavity soft tissue is surrounded by a sinus bony wall, with variable areas of thickened reactive bone and localized areas of bone sequestration.[66] Another condition is the presence of maxillary sinus soft tissue disease continuous into the adjacent nasal fossa and extending into the soft tissues of the cheek.

Imaging Technique

To afford optimal demonstration of the anterior ethmoid sinuses and osteomeatal structures, CT imaging is performed in the coronal plane.[48] CT scanning enables the clinician to identify and evaluate systematically the frontal sinus, frontal recess, uncinate process, infundibulum, maxillary sinus, maxillary sinus ostia, ethmoid bulla, sinus lateralis, middle meatus, posterior ethmoid sinus cell, sphenoid sinus, and the sphenoid recess. Continuous 3-mm slices through the area of the osteomeatal complex show the specific components of the complex, and the actual coronal angle is not significant.[49-51] With 5-mm-thick images, only 45% of scans demonstrated good to excellent visualization of the osteomeatal complex. Because absolute coronal scan angle is not critical for 3-mm scan technique, imaging angle may be set to maximally avoid dental amalgam.[52] Even with artifacts from dental amalgam, direct coronal images are superior to reformatted coronal images obtained from axial data.[48] Full axial images with coronal reconstruction are used only in rare instances when patients are physically unable to assume a prone position.

In an attempt to decrease the radiation dose and the cost of the CT examination, "limited" CT examination of the nasal cavity and paranasal sinuses has been advocated. This examination may consist of coronal images performed with various gaps and thus provide a sampling of the extent of mucoperiosteal inflammation. The information gained through such an examination is incomplete with segmented display of regional morphology.[48] Furthermore, some radiologists believe that the setup time required to achieve individual coronal plains in such a scanning protocol may increase the time required for a study.

The radiation dose to the area as well as the time of the study can be decreased without sacrificing the complete display of regional anatomy. For a screening sinus CT scan, Babbel and Harnsberger[49] proposed the use of 3-mm continuous scan technique through the anterior half of the paranasal sinuses where the osteomeatal unit is found and the 5-mm continuous scan technique through the posterior half. This compromise allows optimal visualization of the osteomeatal unit with a decrease in the total number of required slices. The total amount of radiation used in this screening CT scan can be significantly reduced further by lowering the dose from the more standard brain and neck doses as a result of the use of bone algorithm technique.[51,53] The images are displayed and photographed with a wide window technique (2,500 HU/250 HU) using a high-resolution bone algorithm technique.[53] There is no significant decline in image quality or diagnostic usefulness of the scan until techniques less than 140 mA (70 mA at 2 seconds) are used. The advantages of reduced exposure techniques include decreased radiation exposure and decreased expense.

When initial images or clinical symptoms suggest tumor or complicated inflammatory sinus disease (i.e., intracranial or orbital extension), a full sinonasal CT protocol is indicated, including use of intravenous contrast agent, axial and coronal imaging of the sinuses and intracranial structures, and photography to emphasize both soft tissue and bone detail.[51] Axial images are useful for the evaluation of periorbital and intracranial complications of sinuses.

Interpretation and Diagnosis

Babbel et al.[50] categorized recurrent inflammatory sinonasal diseases into five patterns: infundibular, osteomeatal unit, sphenoidethmoidal recess, sinonasal polyposis, and sporadic or unclassifiable disease. The influndibular pattern is assigned when isolated maxillary sinusitis due to obstruction in the inferior aspect of the infundibulum is identified. The ostomeatal unit pattern is designated when the ipsilateral medial meatus is opacified, resulting in sinusitis within some or all of the ipsilateral frontal, maxillary, and anterior ethmoid sinuses. The sphenoidethmoidal recess pattern is applied when obstruction is present posteriorly within the region of the sphenoidethmoidal recess, resulting in sphenoid and posterior ethmoid sinusitis. Sinonasal polyposis describes a combination of polypoid soft tissue densities present throughout the nasal vault and paranasal sinuses in association with variable diffuse sinus opacification. There is often enlargement of the ostia, thinning of the adjacent bone, and air-fluid levels. Sporadic or unclassifiable patterns include sporadic inflammatory sinus findings such as retention cysts, mucoceles, and mild mucoperiosteal thickening without coexistent osteomeatal unit obstruction or sphenoidethmoidal recess obstruction.

Mucus retention cysts result from inflammatory obstruction of the seromucinous glands within the sinus lining and are included in the sporadic pattern of inflammatory sinonasal disease.[50] Mucus retention cysts are low-density, smooth, margined, homogeneous masses. These cysts are most commonly found in the maxillary sinus, although they can be found within any of the paranasal sinuses. Retention cysts are reported to be found in as many as 10% of CT scans. Although usually asymptomatic, they are indicative of prior inflammatory disease. A variation is the serous retention cyst. This cyst is a postinflammatory accumulation of fluid beneath the mucosal layer and is usually located in the dependent portion of the affected sinus.[54]

The more aggressive mucocele is a dilated mucus-filled sac lined by mucous membrane. Whereas a retention cyst occurs when an individual mucus gland is obstructed, the mucocele is formed by mucus secretions filling the sinus cavity as a result of obstruction of the sinus ostium. The cause of the obstruction may be inflammation, trauma, operation, or tumor. Mucoceles are more commonly found in the frontal sinus than within the ethmoid and sphenoid sinuses. They are least likely in the maxillary sinuses. Characteristic CT findings of mucoceles include a nonenhancing low-density mass that totally fills the affected sinus. If the secretions become inspissated, a high density count results. Often there is bony sinus expansion with bone remodeling due to pressure necrosis.[54] Contrast enhancement of the mucocele periphery is indicative of a pylomucocele.

Additional sinonasal CT abnormalities and anatomic variants are frequently encountered. These include septal deviation, septal spur, synechia or intranasal adhesions, and concha bullosa. Yousem et al.[55] found that the presence of a nasal septal deviation and a horizontally oriented uncinate process correlated with an increased prevalence of sinus inflammation. The presence of a concha bullosa did not increase the risk of sinusitis. Other studies have also shown a concha bullosa as well as paradoxical turbinates, Haller cells, and uncinate pneumatization occur as often in patients with chronic sinusitis as in patients without sinus symptoms.[56]

The size, not the presence, of these anatomic variations is probably the critical factor regarding the prevalence of sinusitis. A prominent concha bullosa with an enlarged, expanded, pneumatized middle turbinate can narrow the middle meatus and osteomeatal complex. Hypertrophied and paradoxical curvature of the middle turbinates in which the caudal portion of the turbinate curves medially rather than laterally can also narrow the middle meatus.[56] Haller cells are middle ethmoid air cells that are laterally placed extending along the inferior orbital floor, inferolateral to the ethmoid bulla. Haller cells can result in narrowing of the infundibulum, predisposing to maxillary sinusitis.

Magnetic Resonance Imaging

Magnetic resonance imaging (MRI) has many advantages in the evaluation of paranasal sinuses. It offers the best soft tissue contrast. This is especially valuable in the evaluation of neoplasms and complicated infections that extend beyond the sinuses. Furthermore, multiplanar sections may be obtained without disturbing the patient, and it is the only technique for obtaining direct sagittal scans. Images are obtained without the use of ionizing radiation, which is particularly desirable in children. However, MRI also has several limitations. These include high cost, long imaging times that makes sedation necessary in most children, and the inability to directly display bony landmarks.[54]

Sinus thickening is usually seen as high intensity on the T2-weighted image against the black background of air and cortical bone. On T1-weighted images, the mucosal thickening is low in intensity. One to two millimeters of ethmoid sinus mucosal thickening may not be due to inflammatory disease but rather reflect the normal intermittent congestion of the nasal cycle.[63] The sinuses are abnormal on MRI in 65% of patients in the presence of an upper respiratory tract viral infection and in 34% of patients with no history of a cold.[64]

Sinonasal secretions are not always bright on T2-weighted images and dark on T1-weighted images. Som et al.[65,66] described the changes in signal intensity and sinonasal secretions on the basis of protein concentration. Sinus secretions appear hypointense on T1-weighted images and hyperintense on T2-weighted images when the mucus is in its most liquid form (total protein concentration less than 19%). In the mildly to moderately protenacious form of mucus secretions (total protein concentration 20% to 25%), the mucus is hyperintense on T1- and T2-weighted images. In a highly proteinacious form (total protein concentration 25% to 28%), the mucus is hyperintense on T1-weighted images and hypointense on T2-weighted images. When the secretions are in a near solid form (total protein concentration more than 28%), the mucus is hypointense on T1- and T2-weighted images. There is thus the potential for misdiagnosing completely opacified sinuses when the concretions of very hyperproteinacious secretions show a signal void simulating aeration. Because chronically obstructed sinus secretions may have any combination of signal intensities, it may be difficult to distinguish inflammation from neoplasm solely on the basis of intensity patterns. However, the presence of rim enhancement is a reassuring finding that suggests inflammation rather than neoplasm, which tends to enhance centrally.[66]

MRI has the ability to demonstrate fungal spread of sinusitis into the intracranial cavity resulting in vascular abnormalities, including thrombosis or parenchymal infarcts.[66] Acute bacterial and fungal sinonasal disease are dominated physiologically be watery secretions and submucosal edema. As a result, the MRI findings are essentially those of water, which has a low T1-weighted signal intensity, high T2-weighted signal intensity, and low to intermediate proton density signal intensity.

MRI has a limited role in the evaluation of uncomplicated sinusitis, but it has great potential for evaluating intracranial and intraorbital complication of sinusitis. MRI is usually a secondary imaging examination for the small number of patients with sinus neoplasms or complex infectious disorders. It is the study of choice for the evaluation of possible intracranial extension of sinus disease. In this situation, its ability to obtain multiplane images and excellent soft tissue discrimination present unique and compelling advantages over even contrast-enhanced CT.[65]

CHILDREN

Nasal endoscopy and the clinical evaluation form the basis for diagnosis of chronic and recurrent sinusitis. Unfortunately, nasal endoscopy in the office setting is often limited in children. Therefore, CT examination is used to confirm clinical suspicion. Lazar et al.[45] reported that plain radiography was not specific or sensitive enough for the diagnosis of chronic sinusitis in children. Specifically, if the diagnosis is made on the basis of plain radiography only, 40% of patients with sinusitis would be missed and 36% would be treated for nonexistent disease. CT imaging is the most sensitive radiographic method available for the diagnosis of chronic sinusitis.[45,46] Despite the good results provided by CT scans, Lazar et al. often discovered more extensive disease intraoperatively than from the preoperative CT scan.[45]

Incidental maxillary and ethmoid sinus opacifications on axial CT scans have been observed in 18% to 50% of asymptomatic children undergoing cranial CT.[57,58] This rate emphasizes the need to interpret radiographic studies in their proper clinical context. The embryologic development of the paranasal sinuses is also important to consider when assessing a child with sinusitis. The maxillary and ethmoid sinuses are present and may be normally aerated at birth.[59] Pneumatization of the sphenoid is usually detectable at 3 years of age and progresses throughout childhood.[60] The frontal sinuses first expand above the roofs of the orbit at about 5 years but may remain hypoplastic or aplastic into adulthood.[59]

The incidence of bony anatomic abnormalities identified in children is similar to that reported in adults.[61,62] Specifically identified, in descending order of frequency, are concha bullosa, septal deformity, paradoxical curvature of turbinate, Haller cells, and large ethmoid bulla.

In a subgroup of children with cystic fibrosis, unique features were identified on CT scans.[61] Children with cystic fibrosis had medial displacement of the lateral nasal wall in the region of the middle meatus with uncinate process demineralization. These changes appeared to be related to mucocele formation of the maxillary sinus with secondary pressure causing medial displacement to the lateral nasal wall in the middle meatus and demineralization of the uncinate process.

COMPLICATIONS

Complications occur most frequently in children and patients with depressed immune function. In children, most sinus complications follow acute infection, and the particular sinus involved determines the type of complication. *Haemophilus influenzae*, *Streptococcus pneumoniae*, and *Staphylococcus aureus* are the most frequently cultured bacteria.

Complications of sinusitis can be divided into local, orbital, and intracranial problems. Local complications include mucocele and osteomyelitis. Mucoceles or mucopyoceles grow slowly and expand beyond the limits of the sinus by pressure and bone resorption. Mucoceles are diagnosed by radiography and may take years before they become symptomatic. Most mucoceles are located in the frontal sinus and can present as soft, painless tumors of the superior and medial aspects of the orbit. If the posterior wall of the sinus is eroded, infections of the central nervous system can result.

Osteomyelitis that results from sinusitis is an unusual finding.[67] It is most frequently found after trauma, radiation therapy, or debilitating disease. The frontal sinus is mostly frequently involved.[68] Osteomyelitis of the frontal sinus may involve the anterior wall, posterior wall, or the floor. This invasion may occur through direct invasion of venous channels. Anterior extension may form a subperiosteal pericranial abscess termed Pott's puffy tumor.[67,69] It is usually accompanied by high fever and requires surgical drainage with excision of the sequestered bone. The organisms recovered from patients with Pott's puffy tumor frequently are polymicrobial and predominantly include α- and β-hemolytic streptococci, anaerobic streptococci, *Bacteroides* species, and occasional *Staphylococcus* and *Enterococcus*. The anterior extension may also extend inferiorly, forming a periorbital abscess. Acute spread of osteomyelitis to the skull by septic thrombophlebitis via the valveless veins of Breschet can be life-threatening.[67,71] The development of osteomyelitis in the anterior wall of the frontal bone is often associated with osteomyelitis of the posterior wall of the frontal sinus. Posterior extension can lead to an intracranial infection. In frontal sinusitis associated with intracranial complications, anaerobes such as *Fusobacterium*, *Bacteroides* species, and anaerobic streptococci are the predominant pathogens.

The proximity of the orbit to the paranasal sinuses most likely accounts for the orbit being the most commonly involved structure in complications of sinusitis. The thin lamina papyracea is often dehiscent, allowing for direct extension of infection. The venous system in this area is valveless, which also allows for communication between the nose, ethmoid sinus, orbit, and cavernous sinus.[72] Direct spread from the paranasal sinus to the orbit is most likely to occur anteriorly through the thin lamina papyracea but also may occur posteriorly directly to the optic nerve from the sphenoid and the posterior ethmoid sinuses through their intimate anatomic relationship. Bansberg et al.[73] found that 88% of the sphenoid sinuses and 48% of the posterior ethmoid cells are intimately related to the ipsilateral optic canal.[73] The width of the optic canal wall that separated the optic nerve from the sinus cavity was no more than 1 mm. Dehiscenses of the sphenoid sinuses near the optic nerve and optic chiasm have been described along with dehiscenses of the ethmoid labyrinth near the optic nerve.[73,74]

In orbital complications of sinusitis, the bacteria found in children include *Haemophilus influenzae, Streptococcus* species, and *Staphylococcus* species.[75,76] In contrast, the most common pathogens in adults are both aerobic and anaerobic organisms.[77–79] CT scanning of the sinuses and orbits allows accurate localization of the sinus infection and usually enables an accurate grading of orbital inflammation.[72,80]

Orbital infection can range from mild cellulitis to abscess. The classification introduced by Hubert[81] and refined by Smith and Spencer[82] and later by Chandler and colleagues[84] divides inflammatory orbital involvement related to sinusitis into five groups. The first group, a preseptal infection, is the most common. Inflammatory edema of the upper eyelid causes a swollen appearance with no limitation of extraocular movement, no evidence of an orbital infection, and no loss of visual acuity. In the second group, orbital cellulitis, the orbital contents are diffusely invaded by inflammatory cells and bacteria without the formation of a discrete abscess. The edema results in proptosis of the globe, chemosis, and limitation of extraocular movement. The third group is subperiosteal abscess and is characterized by a collection of pus in the medial aspect of the orbit between the bone and the periorbita.[77,78] The extraocular movement is impaired and the globe is displaced downward and laterally. In later stages, visual acuity may be affected. In the fourth group, orbital abscess, there is usually severe proptosis and complete ophthalmoplegia. Visual acuity is usually impaired and may progress to irreversible blindness if not treated promptly. The final group is cavernous sinus thrombosis. Infection of the cavernous sinus is characterized by sepsis, orbital pain, chemosis, proptosis, and ophthalmoplegia. Cavernous sinus thrombosis results in paresis of cranial nerves III, IV, and VI and the ophthalmic and maxillary divisions of cranial nerve V. Both eyes are often involved because of the spread of infection throughout the cavernous sinuses. Vision is intact except in advanced cases, in which there is pressure and compression of the central retinal artery. With advanced disease there is often involvement of the contralateral eye through the cavernous sinus. *Staphylococcus aureus* is the most common organism, followed by *Streptococcus* and *Pneumococcus*. In immunocompromised patients, the bacteriology often differs, with *Mucormycosis, Cryptococcus* and necrotizing *Pseudomonas aeruginosa* sinusitis being reported.[84–86]

Acute visual loss can also result as a component of orbital apex syndrome.[80,89,90] Orbital apex syndrome is related to involvement of the vessels and nerves passing through the superior orbital fissure and the optic foramen. In the fully developed syndrome, the visual loss is accompanied by internal/external ophthalmoplegia due to paresis of the third, fourth, and sixth cranial nerves and by changes in the sensation due to involvement of the third branch of the ophthalmic nerve. Isolated visual loss diagnosed as optic neuritis has been attributed to sinusitis.[91,92]

Fortunately, the dreadful complication of visual loss can often be avoided if sinusitis is diagnosed and treated early and appropriately. Strict monitoring of visual acuity and evaluation by CT scanning are essential. The occurrence of visual loss in association with sinusitis is a rhinologic emergency requiring prompt use of intravenous antibiotics in combination with early surgical decompression and drainage of the sinus. In addition, any patient who shows progression of symptoms over 24 hours or who shows no improvement in 48 to 72 hours should undergo surgical exploration. CT scan evidence of abscess also requires immediate drainage.

Intracranial complications of sinusitis include meningitis, epidural abscess, subdural empyema, venous sinus thrombosis, and brain abscess. The frontal sinuses have the highest rates for intracranial complications.[68] Meningitis is generally regarded as the most common intracranial complication of sinusitis.[71] Affected patients often have mild headache, retro-orbital pain, or subtle changes in sensorium. Lumbar puncture is characteristic, revealing leukocytosis, elevated protein levels, and a decreased glucose level. A CT scan before lumbar puncture is important to rule out a space-occupying lesion.

Epidural abscess is usually caused by frontal sinusitis and is often associated with osteomyelitis of the posterior table.[93] Epidural abscess is an uncommon entity, occurring 5 times less often than subdural abscesses.[94] Most cases of epidural abscesses occur in male adolescents.[95] Intracranial spread most commonly occurs through the communicating diploic veins, which penetrate the posterior frontal sinus wall. The other pathway for intracranial spread is via direct erosion of the posterior wall of the sinus.[67,95,96] The initial symptoms are occasionally very subtle; headache and spiking fever are often the presenting findings. Neurologic deficits are usually absent from this neurologically relatively silent area.[71,93,96] Even if an abscess cannot be seen on CT scan, a bony defect adjacent to the dura should raise the suspicion of pachymeningitis.

Subdural empyema, a collection of pus between the dura and the leptomeninges, is a rare complication of sinusitis. The collection usually results from retrograde thrombophlebitis caused by an acute frontal sinusitis.[94,95,97] Patients present with fever, intense headaches, and meningeal signs. The clinic course is usually fulminant with progression of the disease to nuchal rigidity, altered level of consciousness, hemiparesis, hemiplegia, and seizures. *Staphylococcus* and *Streptococcus* are the most common causative organisms. *Escherichia coli, Pseudomonas, Proteus,* and many anaerobes have also been implicated.[71,98,99] In the areas of the ethmoid and sphenoid sinuses, the brain is so close to the floor of the skull that epidural and subdural spaces are virtually nonexistent. Consequently, the ethmoid and sphenoid sinuses do not give rise to epidural and subdural abscess.[100,101]

Sinusitis can lead to a brain abscess. Approximately 15% of brain abscesses are of sinus origin, and the frontal and ethmoid sinuses are the most common. The mortality rate approaches 20% to 30%, and seizures occur in 30% to 50% of survivors.[75,99]

Intracranial complications arising from infections in the ethmoid and sphenoid sinus include meningitis most frequently, as well as cavernous sinus thrombosis and brain abscess.

SUMMARY

The initial uncomplicated episode of sinusitis can probably be treated on the basis of the clinical findings. Radiographic studies can then be limited to patients who have recurrent or persistent problems after appropriate medical therapy. Nasal endoscopy in the clinical evaluation is the basis for the diagnosis of chronic and recurrent sinusitis. Nasal endoscopy should supplement clinical evaluation in all patients who have chronic or recurrent acute infections. CT should be used when endoscopy fails to explain symptoms of sinusitis. CT shows the extent of mucosal disease deep in the osteomeatal complex and optimally displays the regional anatomy. If clinical and radiographic abnormalities do not resolve with more intensive medical management, coronal CT should be considered. The value of this study is most informative if the patient receives the full benefit of antibiotic and decongestant therapy before the examination so the underlying obstructing lesions of the osteomeatal complex may be separated from surrounding mucosal edema and fluid.

In children younger than 6 years, only maxillary and ethmoid sinuses are clinically important. To assess maxillary and ethmoid sinuses, both Caldwell and Waters views are necessary. In older patients, the lateral view, allowing assessment of the frontal and sphenoid sinuses, should also be obtained. In complicated cases of acute sinusitis with either orbital or central nervous system complications, CT should be done. CT should also be reserved for patients with numerous recurrences or protracted and nonresponsive symptoms. Children who have periorbital swelling or proptosis should undergo immediate contrast-enhanced CT examinations of both axial and coronal planes. If symptoms or CT findings suggest intracranial extension, an MRI evaluation should then be performed, if this does not delay appropriate surgical management. The rare patients with malignancies or aggressive infections causing bone destruction may require both CT and MRI evaluation.

Bacteriologic evaluation of the infectious agent has been shown to be valuable in the diagnostic treatment protocol. The osteomeatal flora is often different from the flora found in the paranasal sinus. The middle meatus is the most frequent sign of initial pathology leading to the involvement of adjoining sinuses. This observation has led to the development of treatment protocols that differ in many ways from those in the past; specifically, cultures with sensitivity analyses from the osteomeatal unit under the middle turbinate with a mini-tip culture tube have been valuable in the choice of antibiotic in treatment protocol development.

REFERENCES

1. NIH Data Book 1990. Bethesda, MD, US Department of Health and Human Services, 1990, Table 44. (Publication 90–1261.)
2. Wilson R, Sykes DA, Currie D, Cole PJ: Beat frequency of cilia from sites of purulent infection. *Thorax* 1986; 41:453–458.
3. Carson JL, Collier AM, Hu SS: Acquired ciliary defects in nasal epithelium of children with acute viral upper respiratory infections. *N Engl J Med* 1985; 312:463–468.
4. Calhoun K: Diagnosis and management of sinusitis in the allergic patient. *Otolaryngol Head Neck Surg* 1992; 107:850–854.
5. Druce HM: Emerging techniques in the diagnosis of sinusitis. *Ann Allergy* 1991; 66:132–136.

6. Stammberger H: Nasal and paranasal sinus endoscopy: a diagnostic and surgical approach to recurrent sinusitis. *Endoscopy* 1986; 18:213–218.
7. Wald ER, Milmoe GJ, Bowen A, Ledesma-Medina J, Salamon N, Bluestone CD: Acute maxillary sinusitis in children. *N Engl J Med* 1981; 304:749–754.
8. Gwaltney JM Jr, Scheld WM, Sande MA, Sydnor A: The microbial etiology of antimicrobial therapy of adults with acute community-acquired sinusitis: a fifteen-year experience at the University of Virginia and review of other selected studies. *J Allergy Clin Immunol* 1992; 90:457–462.
9. Tinkelman DG, Silk HJ: Clinical and bacteriologic features of chronic sinusitis in children. *Am J Dis Child* 1989; 143:938–941.
10. Schlanger G, Lutwick LI, Kurzman M, Hoch B, Chandler FW: Sinusitis caused by Legionella pneumophila in a patient with acquired immune deficiency syndrome. *Am J Med* 1984; 77:957–960.
11. Jousimies-Somer HR, Savolainen S, Ylikoski JS: Macroscopic purulence, leukocyte counts, and bacterial morphotypes in relation to culture findings for sinus secretions in acute maxillary sinusitis. *J Clin Microbiol* 1988; 26:1926–1933.
12. McNeill RA: Comparison of findings on transillumination, X-ray and lavage of the maxillary sinus. *J Laryngol Otol* 1963; 77:1009–1013.
13. Evans FO Jr, Sydnor JB, Moore WEC, Moore GR, Manwaring JL, Brill AH, et al: Sinusitis of the maxillary antrum. *N Engl J Med* 1975; 293:735–739.
14. Wald ER, Reilly JS, Casselbrant M, Ledesma-Medina J, Milmoe GJ, Bluestone CD, et al: Treatment of acute maxillary sinusitis in childhood: a comparative study of amoxicillin and cefaclor. *J Pediatr* 1984; 104:297–302.
15. Gwaltney JM Jr, Sydnor A Jr, Sande MA: Etiology and antimicrobial treatment of acute sinusitis. *Ann Otol Rhinol Laryngol* 1981; 90 Suppl:68–71.
16. Frederick J, Braude AI: Anaerobic infection of the paranasal sinuses. *N Engl J Med* 1974; 290:135–137.
17. Brook I: Bacteriologic features of chronic sinusitis in children. *JAMA* 1981; 246:967–969.
18. Carenfelt C: Pathogenesis of sinus empyema. *Ann Otol Rhinol Laryngol* 1979; 88:16–20.
19. Erkan M, Aslan T, Ozcan M, Koc N: Bacteriology of antrum in adults with chronic maxillary sinusitis. *Laryngoscope* 1994; 104:321–324.
20. Goldenhersh MJ, Rachelefsky GS, Dudley J, Brill J, Katz RM, Rohr AS, et al: The microbiology of chronic sinusitis in children with respiratory allergy. *J Allergy Clin Immunol* 1990; 85:1030–1039.
21. Sturdivant T, Cannon CR: The bacteriology of chronic sinusitis in pediatrics. *J Miss State Med Assoc* 1993; 34:183–185.
22. Feigin RD, Cherry JD (eds.): *Textbook of Pediatric Infectious Diseases*, ed. 2. Philadelphia, Saunders, 1987, pp 161–168.
23. Muntz HR, Lusk RP: Bacteriology of the ethmoid bullae in children with chronic sinusitis. *Arch Otolaryngol Head Neck Surg* 1991; 117:179–181.
24. Pope TL Jr, Stelling CB, Leitner YB: Maxillary sinusitis after nasotracheal intubation. *South Med J* 1981; 74:610–612.
25. Caplan ES, Hoyt NJ: Nosocomial sinusitis. *JAMA* 1982; 247:639–641.
26. Perlman DM, Caplan ES: Nosocomial sinusitis: a new and complex threat. *J Crit Illness* 1987; 2:219–225.
27. Deutschman CS, Wilton PB, Sinow J, Thienprasit P, Konstantinides FN, Cerra FB: Paranasal sinusitis: a common complication of nasotracheal intubation in neurosurgical patients. *Neurosurgery* 1985; 17:296–299.
28. Soderstrom T, Soderstrom R, Hanson LA: Immunoglobulin G subclasses in immunodeficiency. *Ann Clin Res* 1987; 19:280–284.
29. Heiner DC: Recognition and management of IgG subclass deficiencies. *Pediatr Infect Dis J* 1987; 6:235–238.
30. Shackelford PG, Polmar SH, Mayus JL, Johnson WL, Corry JM, Nahm MH: Spectrum of IgG2 subclass deficiency in children with recurrent infections: prospective study. *J Pediatr* 1986; 108:647–653.
31. Diaz JD, Nelson RP, Lockey RF: IgG subclass deficiency and recurrent infections. *Ann Allergy* 1988; 61:333, 375–378.
32. Meissner C, Reimer CB, Black C, Broome C, Rabson A, Siber GR, et al: Interpretation of IgG subclass values: a comparison of two assays. *J Pediatr* 1990; 117:726–731.
33. Armenaka M, Grizzanti J, Rosenstreich DL: Serum immunoglobulins and IgG subclass levels in adults with chronic sinusitis: evidence for decreased IgG3 levels. *Ann Allergy* 1994; 72:507–514.
34. Scadding GK, Lund VJ, Darby YC, Navas-Romero J, Seymour N, Turner MW: IgG subclass levels is chronic rhinosinusitis. *Rhinology* 1994; 32:15–19.
35. Shapiro GG, Virant FS, Furukawa CT, Pierson WE, Bierman CW: Immunologic defects in patients with refractory sinusitis. *Pediatrics* 1991; 87:311–316.

36. Zora JA, Silk HJ, Tinkelman DG: Evaluation of postimmunization pneumococcal titers in children with recurrent infections and normal levels of immunoglobulin. *Ann Allergy* 1993; 70:283–288.

37. Meiteles LZ, Lucente FE: Sinus and nasal manifestations of the acquired immunodeficiency syndrome. *Ear Nose Throat J* 1990; 69:454–459.

38. Rubin JS, Honigberg R: Sinusitis in patients with the acquired immunodeficiency syndrome. *Ear Nose Throat J* 1990; 69:460–463.

39. Simberkoff MS, El Sadr W, Schiffman G, Rahal JJ Jr: Streptococcus pneumoniae infections and bacteremia in patients with acquired immune deficiency syndrome, with report of a pneumococcal vaccine failure. *Am Rev Resp Dis* 1984; 130:1174–1176.

40. Schrager LK: Bacterial infections in AIDS patients. *AIDS* 1988; 2 Suppl 1:S183–S189.

41. Washburn RG, Kennedy DW, Begley MG, Henderson DK, Bennett JE: Chronic fungal sinusitis in apparently normal hosts. *Medicine (Baltimore)* 1988; 67:231–247.

42. Morgan MA, Wilson WR, Neel HB III, Roberts GD: Fungal sinusitis in healthy and immunocompromised individuals. *Am J Clin Pathol* 1984; 82:597–601.

43. Viollier AF, Peterson DE, De Jongh CA, Newman KA, Gray WC, Sutherland JC, et al: Aspergillus sinusitis in cancer patients. *Cancer* 1986; 58:366–371.

44. Corey JP: Allergic fungal sinusitis. *Otolaryngol Clin North Am* 1992; 25:225–230.

45. Lazar RH, Younis RT, Parvey LS: Comparison of plain radiographs, coronal CT, and intraoperative findings in children with chronic sinusitis. *Otolaryngol Head Neck Surg* 1992; 107:29–34.

46. McAlister WH, Lusk R, Muntz HR: Comparison of plain radiographs and coronal scans in infants and children with recurrent sinusitis. *AJR* 1989; 153:1259–1264.

47. Kuhn JP: Imaging of the paranasal sinuses: current status. *J Allergy Clin Immunol* 1986; 77:6–8.

48. Zinreich SJ: Imaging of chronic sinusitis in adults: x-ray, computed tomography, and magnetic resonance imaging. *J Allergy Clin Immunol* 1992; 90:445–451.

49. Babbel RW, Harnsberger HR: A contemporary look at the imaging issues of sinusitis: sinonasal anatomy, physiology, and computed tomography techniques. *Semin Ultrasound CT MRI* 1991; 12:526–540.

50. Babbel RW, Harnsberger HR, Sonkens J, Hunt S: Recurring patterns of inflammatory sinonasal disease demonstrated on screening sinus CT. *AJNR* 1992; 13:903–912.

51. Babbel R, Harnsberger HR, Nelson B, Sonkens J, Hunt S: Optimization of techniques in screening CT of the sinuses. *AJNR* 1991; 12:849–854.

52. Chow JM, Mafee MF: Radiologic assessment preoperative to endoscopic sinus surgery. *Otolaryngol Clin North Am* 1989; 22:691–701.

53. Chakeres DW: Computed tomography of the ethmoid sinuses. *Otolaryngol Clin North Am* 1985; 18:29–42.

54. Som PM, Bergeron RT: *Head and Neck Imaging,* ed. 2. St Louis, Mosby Year Book, 1991.

55. Yousem DM, Kennedy DW, Rosenberg S: Ostiomeatal complex risk factors for sinusitis: CT evaluation. *J Otolaryngol* 1991; 20:419–424.

56. Bolger WE, Butzin CA, Parsons DS: Paranasal sinus bony anatomic variations and mucosal abnormalities: CT analysis for endoscopic sinus surgery. *Laryngoscope* 1991; 101:56–64.

57. Diament MJ, Senac MO Jr, Gilsanz V, Baker S, Gillespie T, Larsson S: Prevalence of incidental paranasal sinuses opacification in pediatric patients: a CT study. *J Comput Assist Tomogr* 1987: 11:426–431.

58. Glasier CM, Ascher DP, Williams KD: Incidental paranasal sinus abnormalities on CT of children: clinical correlation. *AJNR* 1986; 7:861–864.

59. Maresh MM: Paranasal sinuses from birth to late adolescence; size of the paranasal sinuses as observed in routine posteroanterior roentgenograms. *Am J Dis Child* 1940; 60:55–78.

60. Fujioka M, Young LW: The sphenoidal sinuses: radiographic patterns of normal development and abnormal findings in infants and children. *Radiology* 1978; 129:133.

61. April MM, Zinreich SJ, Baroody FM, Naclerio RM: Coronal CT scan abnormalities in children with chronic sinusitis. *Laryngoscope* 1993; 103:985–990.

62. Kennedy DW, Zinreich SJ: The functional endoscopic approach to inflammatory sinus disease: current perspectives and technique modifications. *Am J Rhinol* 1988; 2:89–96.

63. Zinreich SJ, Kennedy DW, Kumas AJ, Rosenbaum AE, Arrington JA, Johns ME: MR imaging of normal nasal cycle: comparison with sinus pathology. *J Comput Assist Tomogr* 1988; 12:1014–1019.

64. Cooke LD, Hadley DM: MRI of the paranasal sinuses: incidental abnormalities and their relationship to symptoms. *J Laryngol Otol* 1991; 105:278–281.

65. Som PM, Dillon WP, Fullerton GD, Zimmerman RA, Rajagopalan B, Marom Z: Chronically obstructed sinonasal secretions: observations on T_1 and T_2 shortening. *Radiology* 1989; 172:515–520.

66. Som PM: Imaging of paranasal sinus fungal disease. *Otolaryngol Clin North Am* 1993; 26:983–994.
67. Wenig BL, Goldstein MN, Abramson AL: Frontal sinusitis and its intracranial complications. *Int J Pediatr Otorhinolaryngol* 1983; 5:285–302.
68. Sable NS, Hengerer A, Powell KR: Acute frontal sinusitis with intracranial complications. *Pediatr Infect Dis* 1984; 3:58–61.
69. Feder HM Jr, Cates KL, Cementina AM: Pott puffy tumor: a serious occult infection. *Pediatrics* 1987; 79:625–629.
70. Pott P: *The Chirurgical Works of Percival Pott.* London, Clark & Collins, 1965.
71. Clayman GL, Adams GL, Paugh DR, Koopmann CF Jr: Intracranial complications of paranasal sinusitis: a combined institutional review. *Laryngoscope* 1991; 101:234–239.
72. Clary RA, Cunningham MJ, Eavey RD: Orbital complications of acute sinusitis: comparison of computed tomography scan and surgical findings. *Ann Otol Rhinol Laryngol* 1992; 101:598–600.
73. Bansberg SF, Harner SG, Forbes G: Relationship of the optic nerve to the paranasal sinuses as shown by computer tomography. *Otolaryngol Head Neck Surg* 1987; 96:331–335.
74. Weille FL, Vang RR: Sinusitis as focus of infection in uveitis, keratitis, and retrobulbar neuritis. *Arch Otolaryngol* 1953: 58:154–165.
75. Fairbanks, DNF, Milmoe GJ: The diagnosis and management of sinusitis in children. Complications and sequelae: an otolaryngologist's perspective. *Pediatr Infect Dis* 1985; 4 Suppl 6:75–79.
76. Bernstein L: Pediatric sinus problems. *Otolaryngol Clin North Am* 1971; 4:127–142.
77. Moloney JR, Badham NJ, McRae A: The acute orbit. Preseptal (periorbital) cellulitis, subperiosteal abscess and orbital cellulitis due to sinusitis. *J Laryngol Otol* 1987; 12 Suppl:1–18.
78. Harris GJ: Subperiosteal inflammation of the orbit. A bacteriological analysis of 17 cases. *Arch Ophthalmol* 1988; 106:947–952.
79. Baker AS: The role of anaerobic bacteria in sinusitis and its complications. *Ann Otol Rhinol Laryngol* 1991; 154 Suppl:17–22.
80. Holt H, de Rötth A: Orbital apex and sphenoid fissure syndrome. *Arch Ophthalmol* 1940: 24:731–741.
81. Hubert L: Orbital infections due to nasal sinusitis: Study of 114 cases. *NY State J Med* 1937; 37:1559–1564.
82. Smith AT, Spencer JT: Orbital complications resulting from lesions of the sinuses. *Ann Otol Rhinol Laryngol* 1948; 57:5–27.
83. Chandler JR, Langenbrunner DJ, Stevens ER: The pathogenesis of orbital complications in acute sinusitis. *Laryngoscope* 1970; 80:1414–1428.
84. O'Donnell JG, Sorbello AF, Condoluci DV, Barnish MJ: Sinusitis due to Pseudomonas aeruginosa in patients with human immunodeficiency virus infection. *Clin Infect Dis* 1993; 16:404–406.
85. Bodenstein NP, McIntosh WA, Vlantis AC, Urguhart AC: Clinical signs of orbital ischemia in rhino-orbitocerebral mucormycosis. *Laryngoscope* 1993; 103:1357–1361.
86. Cheung SW, Lee KC, Cha I: Orbitocerebral complications of pseudomonas sinusitis. *Laryngoscope* 1992; 102:1385–1389.
87. Koltai PJ, Maisel BO, Goldstein JC: Pseudomonas aeroginosa in chronic maxillary sinusitis. *Laryngoscope* 1985; 95:34–37.
88. Fried MP, Kelly JH, Strome M: Pseudomonas rhinosinusitis. *Laryngoscope* 1984; 94:192–196.
89. Kjoer I: A case of orbital apex syndrome in collateral pansinusitis. *Acta Ophthalmol (Copenh)* 1945; 23:357–366.
90. Abramovich S, Smelt GJC: Acute sphenoiditis, alone and in concert. *J Laryngol Otol* 1982; 96:751–757.
91. Rothstein J, Maisel RH, Berlinger NT, Wirtschafter J: Relationship of optic neuritis to disease of the paranasal sinuses. *Laryngoscope* 1984; 94:1501–1508.
92. Sanborn GE, Kivlin JD, Stevens M: Optic neuritis secondary to sinus disease. *Arch Otolaryngol* 1984; 110:816–819.
93. Remmler D, Boles R: Intracranial complications of frontal sinusitis. *Laryngoscope* 1980; 90:1814–1824.
94. Harris LF, Haws FP, Triplett JN Jr, Maccubbin DA: Subdural empyema and epidural abscess: recent experience in a community hospital. *South Med J* 1987; 80:1254–1258.
95. Smith HP, Hendrick EB: Subdural empyema and epidural abscess in children. *J Neurosurg* 1983; 58:392–397.
96. Bluestone CD, Steiner RE: Intracranial complications of acute frontal sinusitis. *South Med J* 1965; 58:1–9.
97. Farmer TW, Wise GR: Subdural empyema in infants, children and adults. *Neurology* 1973; 23:254–261.
98. Idriss ZH, Gutman LT, Kronfol NM: Brain abscesses in infants and children: current status of clinical findings, management and prognosis. *Clin Pediatr (Phila)* 1978; 17:738–740, 745–746.

99. Brewer NS, MacCarty CS, Wellman WE: Brain abscess: a review of recent experience. *Ann Intern Med* 1975; 82:571–576.
100. Hadley JA, Bakos R, Regenbogen V: Middle cranial fossa epidural abscess: an unusual complication of acute sinusitis. *Am J Rhinol* 1991; 5:181–186.
101. Maniglia AJ, Goodwin WJ, Arnold JE, Ganz E: Intracranial abscesses secondary to nasal, sinus, and orbital infections in adults and children. *Arch Otolaryngol Head Neck Surg* 1989; 115:1424–1429.

14

Diagnosis of Fungal Sinusitis

THOMAS V. McCAFFREY, M.D., Ph.D.

Fungi are ubiquitous in the environment. Their spores are present suspended in the atmosphere and are continuously deposited on the mucosal surfaces of the nasal airway. However, colonization and infection of the paranasal sinuses are relatively uncommon occurrences. Infection usually requires some predisposing condition that impairs normal defense mechanisms. These conditions include a compromised immune system as a result of intense chemotherapy,[1,2] acquired immunodeficiency syndrome (AIDS),[3] or diabetes mellitus. Occasionally fungi do infect non-immunocompromised healthy persons when the inoculum is large or when there is ostial obstruction.

The initial manifestations of fungal infections are often subtle and may be overlooked until the infection is life-threatening. This chapter discusses the pathogenesis and predisposing factors for fungal sinusitis and its diagnosis.

CLINICAL CHARACTERISTICS OF FUNGAL SINUSITIS

Many fungi that produce disease in humans are organisms that are normally saprophytic but become pathogenic under particular circumstances. Reduced host immune defense may lead to invasion of tissue. The neutrophil is especially important in the defense against fungi, and reduced neutrophil counts or impaired neutrophil function as in diabetes mellitus predisposes to opportunistic fungal infection.

In a discussion of fungal diseases of the paranasal sinus, two aspects of the problem of pathogenesis need to be considered: the characteristics of the fungi that permit invasion of the host, and host factors that predispose to invasion. The particular combination of fungal virulence and host susceptibility leads to characteristic clinical presentations. In immunocompromised patients, the presentation of fungal sinusitis is most likely to be aggressive and fulminant. The range of clinical presentations of fungal infection of the sinuses is shown in Table 14–1. The first

Table 14–1 Types of Fungal Sinusitis

CLINICAL CONDITION	HOST FACTORS	PROGRESSION	PATHOLOGY	ORGANISMS
Mycetoma	Sinus Obstruction	Chronic	Fungus Ball	*Aspergillus,* dematiaceous fungi
Chronic	Sinus Obstruction	Chronic	Granuloma	*Aspergillus*
Fulminant	Immunocompromised	Acute	Tissue Invasion	*Aspergillus, Mucor*
Allergic	Allergy	Chronic	Allergic Mucin	*Aspergillus,* dematiaceous fungi

three conditions are discussed in this chapter, and allergic fungal sinusitis is discussed in Chapter 15.

Mycetoma

Mycetoma, or "fungus ball," is a colonization of a sinus with a noninvasive confluent mass of hyphae (Fig. 14–1). This form of sinus involvement has been most often reported in infections of *Aspergillus*. In the United States, *Aspergillus niger* is the most common species identified. However, in the Sudan, where *Aspergillus* infection is very common, *Aspergillus flavus* is the usual causative organism. Eighty-seven percent of culture-confirmed cases of fungal sinusitis contain some *Aspergillus* species as a pathogen.[4]

Chronic Invasive Fungal Sinusitis

The chronic invasive form of fungal sinusitis occurs most commonly in endemic areas such as the Sudan or Saudi Arabia, but it may also occur in patients with diabetes. The histologic appearance includes features of mycetoma with an associated granulomatous inflammation and necrosis. Noncaseating granulomata with foreign body or Langerhans-type giant cell are seen.

The distinction between mycetoma and chronic invasive sinusitis is not sharp. The mere presence of bony erosion does not define the invasive form of the disease. It is necessary to confirm the presence of fungal hyphae within the tissue. This finding of invasion requires systemic antifungal therapy for effective treatment.

Fulminant Fungal Sinusitis

Acute fulminant fungal sinusitis occurs in immunocompromised patients, particularly in patients with hematologic malignancies and reduced granulocyte counts. In

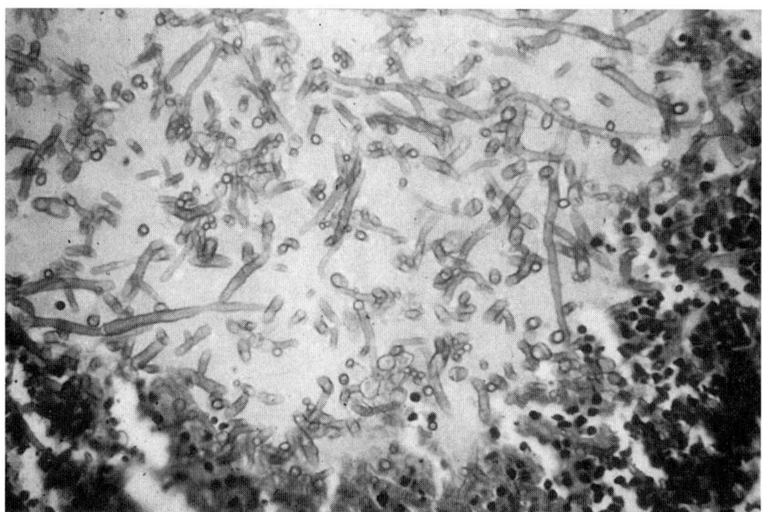

Figure 14–1.   Histologic appearance of a fungus ball. Large numbers of hyphal elements are present without evidence of tissue or vascular invasion.

these cases, the hyphae tend to grow diffusely with minimal inflammation. Vascular invasion produces mycotic thrombosis and tissue necrosis. Hyphae may grow in vessel lumens (Fig. 14–2). The proliferation of fungal hyphae around and through vascular spaces is the hallmark of fulminant invasive fungal disease. This growth pattern permits the infection to extend rapidly from the nasal sinuses into the soft tissue of the face or into the orbit and cranial cavity (Fig. 14–3).

Allergic Fungal Sinusitis

This form of fungal sinusitis occurs with an intense immunologic reactivity and is characterized by the formation of abundant quantities of allergic mucin. Charcot-Leyden crystals are seen as a result of eosinophil degranulation. Fungal hyphae are sparse and noninvasive. Because of its prevalence and increasing importance in rhinologic practice, this clinical presentation of fungal sinusitis is detailed in Chapter 15.

MYCOLOGY OF FUNGAL SINUSITIS

A wide variety of fungi are known to produce fungal infection of the sinuses. Essentially all of these organisms are widely present in the environment and are normally saprophytic. They produce infection of the sinuses when particular host factors permit them to proliferate. Alternatively, the pathogenic fungi, *Histoplasma capsulatum, Coccidioides immitis, Paracoccidioides braziliensis,* and *Blastomyces dermatitidis,* produce disseminated infection of the skin, lungs, brain, and other internal organs but rarely present as isolated sinus infections.

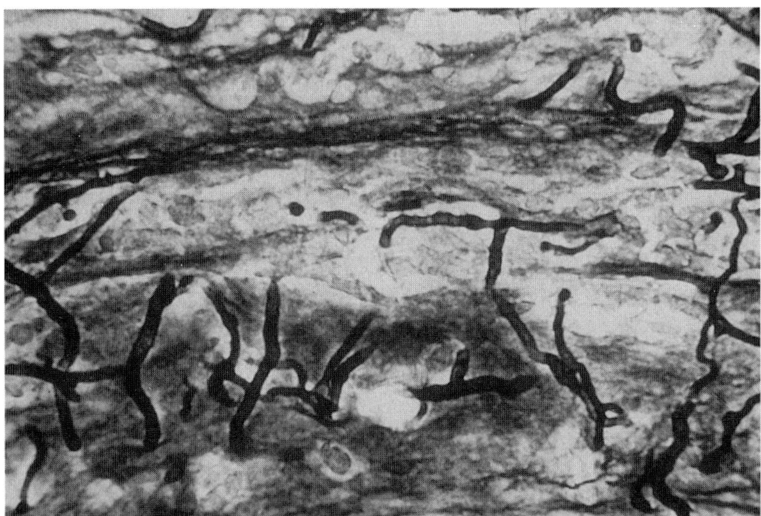

Figure 14–2. Vascular invasion in fulminant invasive fungal sinusitis. Vessel lumens are plugged with hyphae. This leads to infarction of tissue and further progression of the infection.

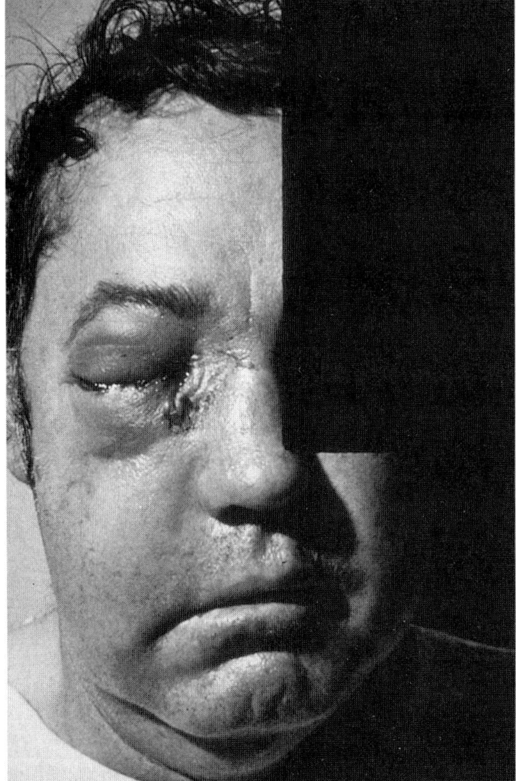

Figure 14–3. Clinical appearance of invasive fungal sinusitis. Invasion of the soft tissue of the face and orbit can be seen.

Most fungi that infect the paranasal sinuses can exist as yeast or hyphal forms, and the hyphal form is identifiable in histologic specimens. However, several species infect as yeast forms only. These include *Rhinosporidium seebri, Sporothrix schenkii, Cryptococcus neoformans*, and *Candida albicans*.

Yeast Form Fungi

Rhinosporidiosis

Rhinosporidum seebri produces specific nasal and sinus disease. Rhinosporidiosis is identified most commonly in India and Ceylon, but it is occasionally reported in other parts of the world.[5] The mode of transmission of the infection is not known with certainty but is thought to be by inhaling fungal spores, which are deposited on traumatized mucosal surfaces.

The pathogenic lesion of rhinosporidiosis is a pedunculated mass of granulation tissue with a "strawberry" appearance. The major symptom is nasal obstruction with an enlarging nasal mass that produces epistaxis and a mucopurulent nasal discharge. Histologically, the lesions consist of a fibromyxomatous stroma with cystic spaces with spores and sporangia along the margins of the tumor.

Hotchkin-Machman stain best defines the spores and sporangia. Diagnosis is based on the histopathologic appearance of the stained smears because it has not been possible to culture this organism.

Sporotrichosis

Sporothrix schenkii usually produces infections after trauma to the skin by thorns and splinters, insect bites, and insect stings, but sinus infection by *S. schenkii* has been reported.[6] *Sporothrix* occurs as a globose yeast form in the tissue with single budding. The inflammatory response is usually granulomatous.

Cryptococcosis

Cryptococcus neoformans is a yeast associated with pigeon excreta and pigeon nesting sites. Human infection occurs by inhalation of aerosolized droppings and can produce pulmonary granulomas or disseminated disease in the immuno-compromised patient. Frontal and maxillary sinusitis has been reported in a patient with AIDS and cryptococcal meningitis.[7]

A characteristic of *C. neoformans* is a thick polysaccharide capsule that can be stained with mucincarmine stain. This permits this organism to be definitively diag-nosed in histologic specimens.

Candidiasis

Candida albicans is a common fungus that can produce invasive sinonasal disease in patients with cancer and rarely in normal individuals.[8] The yeast form is prominent in the tissue. Pseudohyphae without true branching can also be seen in tissue specimens.

Hyphae-Forming Fungi

Most fungi producing fungal infection of the nose and paranasal sinuses are opportunistic invaders. They exist widely in the environment as saprophytes or plant pathogens and produce disease only under conditions of increased host susceptibility. *Aspergillus* is the most common organism producing infection of the nose and sinuses. Other organisms involved in paranasal sinus disease are listed in Table 14–2.

Aspergillus

Aspergillus is the most common cause of all forms of sinus fungal disease, and *Aspergillus fumigatus* is the most common pathogen. The spores of *A. fumigatus* are ubiquitous. They are present in soil, compost, and other decaying organic matter, and they form the majority of airborne fungi.

Although once thought to be a rare cause of human disease, it has become an increasingly important pathogen in immunocompromised patients. Depending on the immune status of the host and the size of the inoculum, this fungus can produce mycetoma, chronic invasive sinusitis, acute fulminant sinusitis, or allergic fungal sinusitis, as previously described.

Histologically, the fungus can be identified by its characteristic appearance. The hyphae are abundant with frequent acute branching. The hyphae have frequent septae. The characteristic appearance permits this organism to be identified even before definitive culture results are available (Fig. 14–4).

Mucor

The class Zygomycetes includes the orders Mucorales and Entomorphthorales, which are fungi found in decaying fruit, bread, vegetables, and soil. Zygomycetes are nonseptate fungi (Fig. 14–5). *Rhizopus* and *Mucor* are the most common species isolated from mucormycosis. Mucormycosis typically occurs in patients with uncontrolled diabetes or in immunosuppressed patients. The association of mucormycosis with diabetic ketoacidosis is related to the active ketone reductase system of

Table 14–2   Organisms Causing Fungal Sinusitis

ORGANISM	INCIDENCE
Aspergillus	Common
Mucor	Common
Dematiaceous fungi	Common
Fusarium	Rare
Sporothrix	Rare
Paecilomyces	Rare
Basidiomyces	Rare

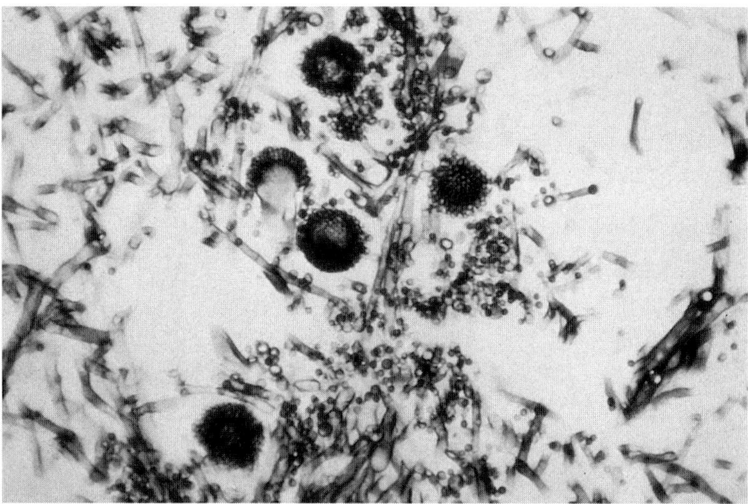

Figure 14–4. Histologic appearence of *Aspergillus fumigatus.* The hyphae are thin and branch at acute angles. Prominent septae are also present.

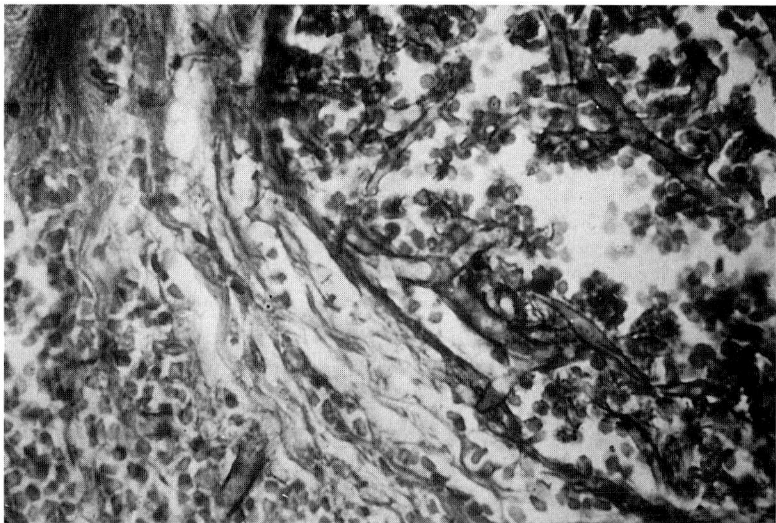

Figure 14–5. Histologic appearence of *Rhizopus.* The hyphae are broad and nonseptate. The branching is at right angles.

Rhizopus, which permits it to grow most favorably in acidic media with a high glucose content.

Once the organism enters tissue it becomes angioinvasive with a predilection for the elastic lamina of arteries. This invasion produces thrombosis and infarction, and the vascular lumina provide a route for further invasion and extension of the infection (Fig. 14–6).

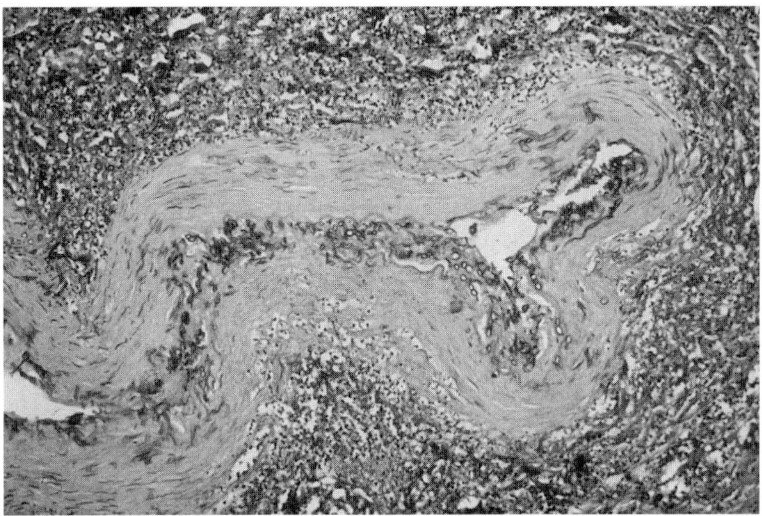

Figure 14–6. *Rhizopus* invading vascular lumen

Table 14–3 Characteristics of Dematiaceous Fungal Sinusitis

ORGANISM	INVASION	HOST IMMUNITY	SITE
Bipolaris	Rare	Normal	Multisinus
Curvularia	Rare	Normal	Multisinus
Exserohilum	Yes	Normal	Multisinus
Alternaria	Rare	Normal	Single sinus
Cladosporium	Yes	Normal	Brain

Dematiaceous fungi

The dematiaceous fungi are saprophytic fungi with septate hyphae that, unlike *Aspergillus*, contain melanin in their cell walls, giving them a dark color in tissue and in culture (Table 14–3). Phaeohyphomycosis is the term used to identify infection by the pigmented dematiaceous fungi. Multiple organisms in this group have been identified in human infections in normal and immunocompromized hosts.[9] While it was once believed that dematiaceous fungi were not pathogenic in humans, these organisms are now known to be not only pathogenic but capable of producing invasive disease in nonimmunocompromized individuals.[2,10,11]

DIAGNOSIS OF NASAL FUNGAL INFECTIONS

History

The onset of fungal sinusitis may be acute or insidious. The immune status of the host will determine the progression of the disease. Mycetomas may remain essentially asymptomatic for many years or present with symptoms of chronic nasal obstruction with nasal discharge. At the other end of the spectrum, fulminant invasive fungal sinusitis has rapidly progressing symptoms of pain, facial swelling, and often orbital symptoms and central nervous system symptoms as the disease extends to adjacent areas. Early recognition of the fulminant form of fungal sinusitis is important because death may occur within hours.

Predisposing Conditions

Fungi of the class Mucor have a propensity to grow in acidic media with high glucose. It is not surprising that this organism affects patients who have uncontrolled diabetes with ketoacidois. Also, the neutrophil is particularly important in host defense against fungal infections. Patients with absolute neutrophil counts less than 500 cells/µl are particularly susceptible to fungal infections. T-cell defects, such as occur in AIDS and hematologic malignancies, are also predisposing factors.[3] In particular, patients receiving chemotherapy for hematologic malignancies are affected.[12]

Sinus fungal disease must therefore be suspected in patients with even minimal changes on computed tomography of the sinus who are neutropenic or have uncontrolled diabetes. Repeated clinical examination with careful rhinoscopy and biopsy should be perfomed every 24 hours or as indicated in susceptible patients in whom developing fungal sinusitis is suspected. Biopsy specimens from high-risk patients should be sent for culture and microscopic examination. The Gomori methenamine silver stain is particularly effective for demonstrating fungal hyphae.

Radiographic Diagnosis

Fungal infections of the sinuses have a wide range of radiographic appearances, from nonspecific mucosal thickening without bony involvement to opacified sinus with areas of reactive osteitis and focal bone erosion. It is the combination of soft tissue and bone changes that may suggest the presence of fungal infection.[13]

On computed tomography or conventional sinus radiography, mycetoma is suggested by the presence of a high-attenuation region within the sinus surrounded by a region of mucous or soft tissue attenuation (Fig. 14–7). The high attenuation centrally is due to the dense desiccated mass of fungal hyphae surrounded by the mucous and inflammatory mucosa.[14] On magnetic resonance imaging, this appears as a central low T1-weighted and T2-weighted signal intensity as a result of the semisolid nature of the mycetoma.[15] Although these findings are characteristic of mycetoma, they are not necessarily specific for this condition. Other chronic sinus diseases producing inspissated secretions can produce similar findings.[16] However, fungal sinusitis produces greater attenuation than bacterial sinusitis.[17]

The radiographic characteristic of fulminant sinus fungal disease is an extension of the inflammatory changes into the surrounding tissue of the cheek, orbit, or brain.[16]

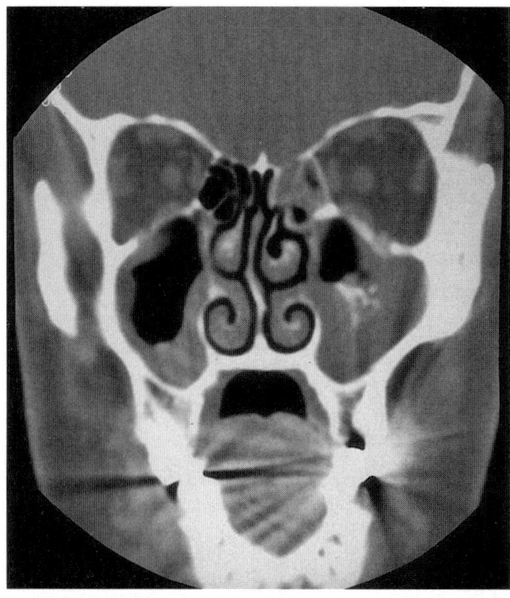

Figure 14–7. Computed tomographic scan of nasal sinuses showing high attenuation in maxillary sinus characteristic of a fungus ball. The finding of a fungus ball was confirmed by operation and biopsy.

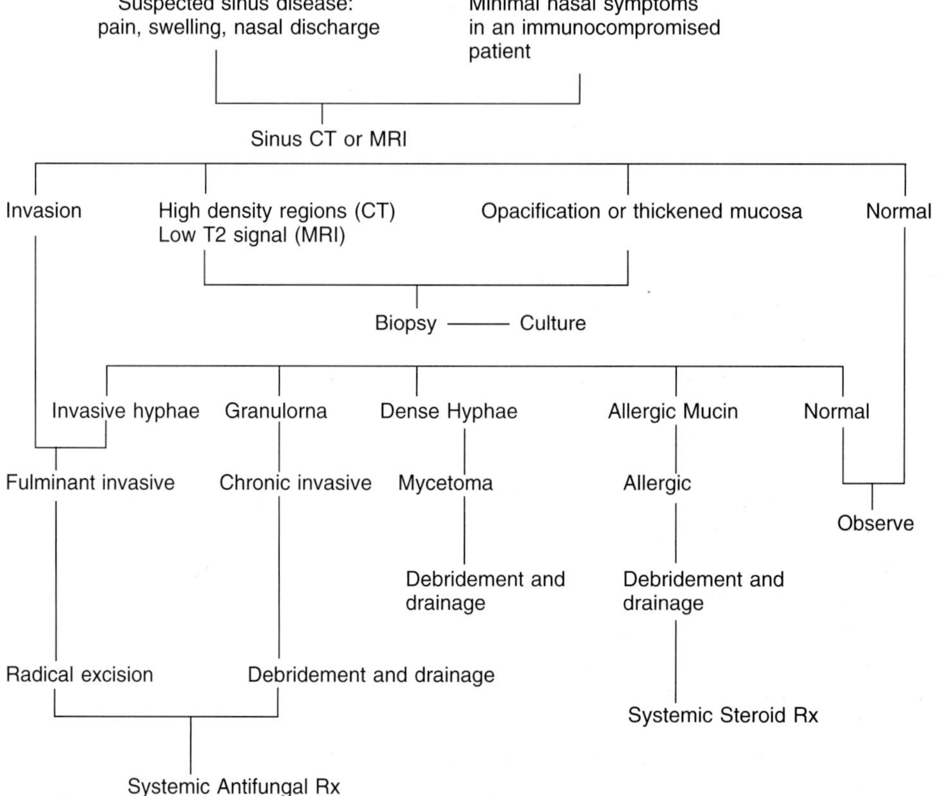

Figure 14–8. Diagnostic algorithm.

Histologic Identification

Direct examination of tissue specimens for fungal elements is a useful diagnostic test that can often provide a diagnosis before culture results are available. The simple preparation of specimens with 10% potassium hydroxide to clear the specimens provides much diagnostic information. Other useful stains include Gram stain, periodic acid-Schiff, and methenamine silver. Some species of fungi can be diagnosed on the basis of their histologic appearance.

The appearance of *Aspergillus* is characteristic: hyphae are abundant and there is frequent acute branching. The hyphae are thin and have frequent septae (Fig. 14–4). Mucorales produces broad hyphae with thin walls and lacks septations. Hyphal branching is perpendicular to the hyphal axis (Fig. 14–5). Other organisms that can be positively identified morphologically include *Candida, Pseudoallesheria, Rhinosporidium,* and *Cryptococcus.*[18]

Culture Identification

The definitive method for identifying fungi is in culture. The specimens for culture should be collected before antifungal therapy is initiated. There are many media for isolation of fungi, and no single medium is ideal for all fungi; thus, multiple media must be used. Because some fungi are slow-growing, at least 8 weeks should be allowed for growth of the fungi. Therefore, it is usually necessary to begin treatment before definitive identification of the infecting agent.

Once fungi are grown and recovered, multiple characteristics such as colony morphology and pigmentation, growth rate, biochemical reactions, and microscopic morphology can be used for exact identification.

Diagnostic Algorithm

A simplified diagnostic algorithm is presented in Figure 14–8.

REFERENCES

1. Kaczmarski R, Pagliuca A, Pullon H, Philpott-Howard J, Salisbury J, Mufti G: Fulminant fungal sinusitis following intensive chemotherapy. *Q J Med* 1990; 75:365–370.
2. Morrison VA, Weisdorf DJ: Alternaria: a sinonasal pathogen of immunocompromised hosts. *Clin Infect Dis* 1993; 16:265–270.
3. Meyer RD, Gaultier CR, Yamashita JT, et al: Fungal sinusitis in patients with AIDS: report of 4 cases and review of the literature. *Medicine (Baltimore)* 1994; 73:69–78.
4. Stammberger H, Jakse R, Beaufort F: Aspergillosis of the paranasal sinuses. X-ray diagnosis, histopathology, and clinical aspects. *Ann Otol Rhinol Laryngol* 1984; 93:251–256.
5. Lasser A, Smith HW: Rhinosporidiosis. *Arch Otolaryngol* 1976; 102:308–310.
6. Ogura S: Sporotrichosis of the maxillary antrum that simulated symptoms of a maxillary tumor. *Otol* 1955; 27:541–543.
7. Choi SS, Lawson W, Bottone EJ, Biller HF: Cryptococcal sinusitis: a case report and review of literature. *Otolaryngol Head Neck Surg* 1988; 99:414–418.
8. Ioannovich D: Odontogenous maxillary sinusitis due to Candida Albicans. Report of a case. *Arch Otolaryngol* 1961; 74:699–702.

9. Zieske LA, Kopke RD, Hamill R: Dematiaceous fungal sinusitis. *Otolaryngol Head Neck Surg* 1991; 105:567–577.

10. Killingsworth SM, Wetmore SJ: Curvularia/Drechslera sinusitis. *Laryngoscope* 1990; 100:932–937.

11. Pingree TF, Holt GR, Otto RA, Rinaldi MG: Bipolaris-caused fungal sinusitis. *Otolaryngol Head Neck Surg* 1992; 106:302–305.

12. Drakos PE, Nagler A, Or R, Naparstek E, et al: Invasive fungal sinusitis in patients undergoing bone marrow transplantation. *Bone Marrow Transplant* 1993; 12:203–208.

13. Centeno RS, Bentson JR, Mancuso AA: CT scanning in rhinocerebral mucormycosis and aspergillosis. *Radiology* 1981; 140:383–389.

14. Som PM: Imaging of paranasal sinus fungal disease. *Otolaryngol Clin North Am* 1993; 26:983–994.

15. Som PM, Dillon WP, Curtin HD, Fullerton GD, Lidov M: Hypointense paranasal sinus foci: differential diagnosis with MR imaging and relation to CT findings. *Radiology* 1990; 176:777–781.

16. Som PM, Curtin HD: Chronic inflammatory sinonasal diseases including fungal infections. The role of imaging. *Radiol Clin North Am* 1993; 31:33–44.

17. Zinreich SJ, Kennedy DW, Malat J, et al: Fungal sinusitis: diagnosis with CT and MR imaging. *Radiology* 1988; 169:439–444.

18. Brandwein M: Histopathology of sinonasal fungal disease. *Otolaryngol Clin North Am* 1993; 26:949–981.

15

Allergic Fungal Sinusitis (AFS) and AFS-Like Syndrome

D. THANE CODY II, M.D.
DAVID A. KHAN, M.D.
EUGENE B. KERN, M.D.

Allergic fungal sinusitis (AFS) is a misunderstood and misdiagnosed disease, and although we claim to understand it, the theories that have been proposed to explain the pathogenesis of this disease are not supported. We are attempting to correlate the histologic appearance of surgical specimens with clinical data. Slowly, we are beginning to understand this process, which affects up to 20% of patients operated on for chronic sinusitis. Our understanding, however, is still in its infancy.

Fungal sinus disease may be classified into four types based on histologic findings. Two types are saprophytic—mycetoma and AFS—and two are infectious—invasive and granulomatous fungal sinusitis.[1] Table 15–1 compares some of the features of these four diseases.

The mycetoma is an extramucosal fungus ball that grows in concentric rings, similar to fungal colonies in vitro. Little or no surrounding tissue reaction is present. AFS is the most recently described of the four forms of fungal sinusitis and is hypothesized to be a hypersensitivity reaction to fungal organisms present within the sinus. Invasive fungal sinusitis is characterized by tissue invasion, often with extensive necrosis. Clinically, invasive disease may be fulminant or indolent. Granulomatous fungal sinusitis shows a granulomatous reaction to fungal organisms. This is most often seen in endemic areas such as the Sudan.

To facilitate communication among physicians, the histopathologic diagnosis is used to describe patients with fungal sinus disease. However, the four diseases represent a spectrum of host responses to fungal organisms, and patients may show overlap between two or more of the four basic forms of fungal sinusitis. Patients with disease that overlaps two or more of these entities should be described as such, with a careful description of the histopathologic findings.

Once the diagnosis is established, modifiers describing the clinical course, type of organism, sinuses involved, and the duration of symptoms may be included.

Table 15–1   Four Forms of Fungal Sinus Disease

DISEASE	HOST IMMUNITY	PATHOLOGY	PATHOGENESIS
Allergic	Immunocompetent	Allergic mucin+ hyphae	Types I, III hypersensitivity
Mycetoma	Immunocompetent	Fungus ball Little tissue reaction	Unknown
Invasive	Immunocompromised	Tissue/vascular invasion Necrosis	Infection
Granuloma	Immunocompetent	Granuloma	Infection

Terms such as "aspergillosis" should be avoided because they describe so many different clinical entities that they have become meaningless.

BACKGROUND

In 1976, Safirstein[2] described a 24-year-old woman with allergic bronchopulmonary aspergillosis (ABPA) associated with nasal obstruction, nasal polyps, and nasal cast formation. This was the first case report of a patient with AFS. In 1981, Millar et al.[3] reported five other cases of chronic sinusitis in which the histologic features of the sinus contents were identical to these of ABPA. Millar suggested a relationship between allergic lung disease and sinus disease and coined the term "allergic aspergillosis of the paranasal sinuses."

After Millar's report, Katzenstein et al.[4] retrospectively reviewed specimens from 119 sinus operations. Nine cases demonstrated histologic features that were indistinguishable from those of mucoid impaction of the bronchi seen in patients with ABPA. The term "allergic mucin" was used to describe this mucus. Seven of the nine specimens also showed scattered fungal hyphae whose morphologic features resembled *Aspergillus*. The term "allergic *Aspergillus* sinusitis" was used to describe these seven cases. Robson et al.[5] later modified this description to "allergic fungal sinusitis" after it was recognized that fungi other than *Aspergillus* were being cultured from specimens from the sinuses of patients with AFS.

Since the first review by Katzenstein, there have been three retrospective studies and several case reports of patients with AFS, and to date there are 118 documented cases. As knowledge of this disease process increases among otorhinolaryngologists, allergists and pathologists, more cases are being identified, and consequently a better understanding of the disease process is developing.

DEFINITION AND PATHOLOGIC FEATURES

A patient has AFS if two criteria are met: first, the mucin must be of the allergic type[4]; second, fungi must be identified in the histologic sections or in cultures of the sinus contents or both. Patients with allergic mucin but without demonstrable fungal organisms in the sinus contents or in cultures represent a subpopulation of patients who are clinically indistinguishable from patients with AFS.[6] We describe these patients as having AFS-like syndrome.

The gross appearance of the sinus contents is thick, paste-like, green to brown mucus (Fig. 15–1).

Light microscopic examination of the mucus reveals allergic mucin (Fig. 15–2). Allergic mucin contains eosinophils and other debris within a background of eosinophilic to basophilic, amorphous mucin. The cellular debris is frequently arranged in multilayered rows or sheets giving rise to a laminated appearance. Individual cells within these sheets are often degenerating, with pyknotic nuclei. Charcot-Leyden crystals are small, hexagonal, bipyramidal crystals formed from the degranulation of eosinophils, and they are present in many specimens.

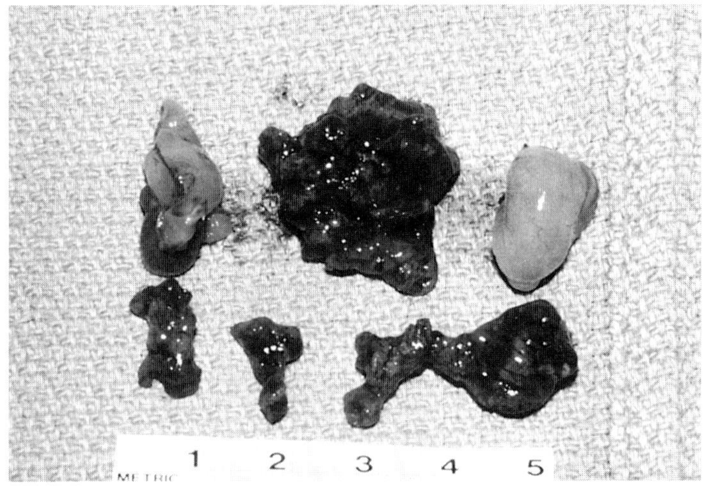

Figure 15–1.   Gross surgical specimen of sinus contents of a patient with allergic fungal sinusitis.

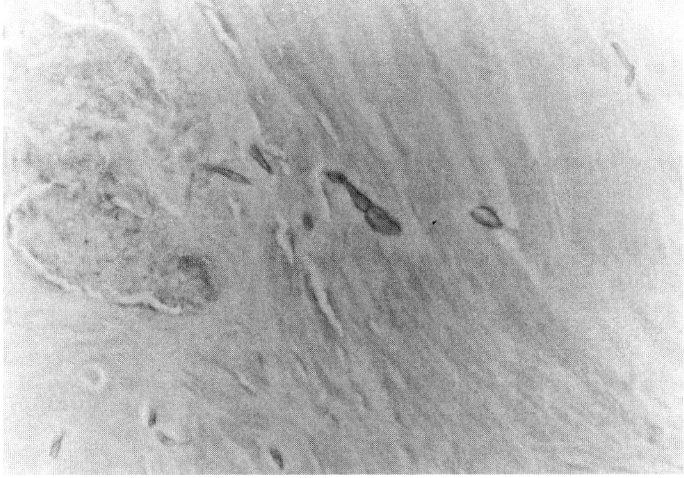

Figure 15–2.   Sinus contents of a patient with allergic fungal sinusitis. (Hematoxylin-eosin.)

Fungal hyphae are sparsely distributed in the mucus and often are not visible with routine hematoxylin eosin stains. Special stains may help demonstrate hyphae. These include Gomori's methenamine silver stain (Fig. 15–3), Grocott's silver stain, and the Fontana-Masson stain. The Fontana-Masson stain stains for the melanin pigment found in the cell walls of dematiaceous fungi, which is an advantage in differentiating dematiaceous fungi with most *Aspergillus* species in histologic sections. The key to identifying the disease is recognizing that microscopic examination of the mucus and debris in the sinuses is as important as examining the mucous membranes. The mucosa often shows mild to moderate nonspecific inflammation, and no fungal invasion into the mucous membranes is seen.

Species identification is done by culturing the organism and examining the morphologic features of the conidia under the microscope. Proper identification allows interpretation of laboratory data, such as results of skin testing and specific IgE, IgG, and IgM levels.

PROPOSED ETIOLOGY AND PATHOGENESIS

The pathogenesis of AFS is uncertain. Some possibilities are listed in Table 15–2. The hypothesis that is commonly accepted is that airborne spores or hyphae or both enter the sinus and elicit a type I or a type III Gell and Coombs hypersensitivity reaction or both.[4,5,7] This hypothesis has been extrapolated from patients with ABPA and from some preliminary immunologic evidence in patients with AFS.[7–11]

ABPA is a complex of asthma, transient pulmonary infiltrates, central bronchiectasis, and immediate cutaneous hypersensitivity and serum precipitins to *Aspergillus* antigens. Other features of ABPA include elevated total and specific IgE and IgG to *Aspergillus* and peripheral eosoinophilia. Mucoid impaction of the

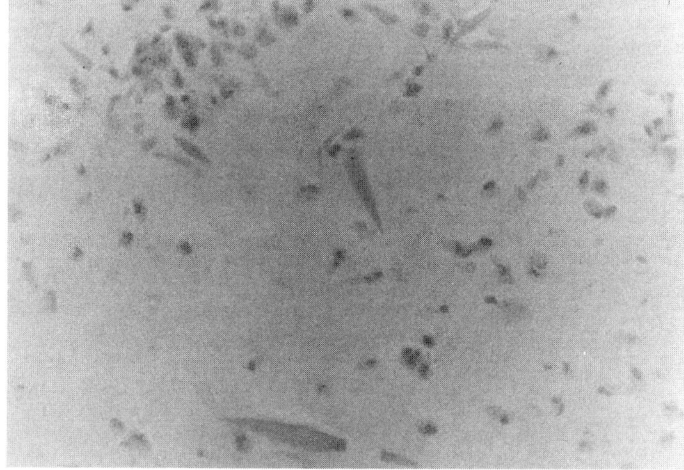

Figure 15–3. Sinus contents of a patient with allergic fungal sinusitis showing characteristic allergic mucin with sheets of eosinophils. (Gomori's methenamine silver stain.)

**Table 15–2   Possible Theories of the
Pathogenesis of Allergic Fungal Sinusitis**

Type I hypersensitivity reaction
Type III hypersensitivity reaction
Combination of types I and III hypersensitivity reactions
Obstruction to normal sinus drainage
Abnormal production of mucus or mucin
Impaired ciliary motility
Altered local or systemic host immunity
Other

bronchi in patients with ABPA is histologically identical to the allergic mucin in the sinuses of patients with AFS. Because of the histologic similarities, AFS has been suggested to be a sinus variant of ABPA. This hypothesis has not been supported by a prevalence of patients with concomitant AFS and ABPA that is greater than in the general population. To date, five cases have been reported. Therefore, it may not be appropriate to extrapolate theories regarding the pathogenesis of AFS from experience with ABPA. Further studies are needed to clarify the relationship between AFS and ABPA.

The pathogenesis of fungal sinus disease in general is unknown. The organism must contact the mucosal surface for a sufficient duration to initiate a host response. Additionally, the organism must overcome nasal defenses, enabling itself to grow on the mucosal surface more quickly than it is removed. Virulence factors such as the ability to bind to receptors on the mucosal surface, avoidance of detection by the immune system, or production of products that interfere with the mucociliary transport system may give an organism the ability to cause disease.

In the tracheobronchial tree, colonization can occur in patients with mucosal damage from diseases such as cancer, tuberculosis, sarcoidosis, or vasculitides. In contrast, patients who have AFS are a relatively young, disease-free population, with the exception of a 50% incidence of asthma.

Ostial obstruction from polyps is common in AFS, but whether this is a cause or sequela of the disease is unknown. We know from experience that patients with mycetomas frequently have patent ostia and aerated sinuses, and patients with AFS may have a large portion of the lateral nasal wall removed during operation. Despite an aerated sinus, these patients still have disease.

Preliminary evidence has shown that ciliostatic substances are released by *Aspergillus fumigatus* and *Alternaria alternata*. It is also known that some species produce exotoxins that can suppress lymphocyte function, inhibit complement, and impair macrophage phagocytosis and T-cell induction. *Aspergillus* can also produce elastase and protease, facilitating mucosal injury.

Because the predominant inflammatory cell in AFS is the eosinophil, this cell likely plays a role in the pathogenesis. The eosinophil granule contains several well-characterized cationic proteins, such as major basic protein (MBP), that have potent, toxic tissue effects.[12] In vitro, MBP can produce ciliostasis, bleb formation, and exfoliation of epithelial cells. Furthermore, MBP can induce histamine release in mast cells and basophils,[13] and Charcot-Leyden crystal protein (a lysophospholipase) also has inflammatory properties; however, its role in allergic diseases remains unclear.[14]

The toxicity of eosinophils also has been established in various human diseases, including chronic sinusitis, in which MBP has been localized to sites of tissue destruction and implicated in the pathogenesis of this disease.[15] Recently, Khan et al.[16] demonstrated striking extracellular MBP deposition (with lesser amounts of neutrophil elastase) in the periphery of allergic mucin in the absence of intact eosinophils, a finding suggesting that eosinophils have released the contents of their granules in AFS. Furthermore, a recent study demonstrated elevated levels of eosinophilic cationic protein in the serum and allergic mucin of patients with AFS.[17] Given the known toxicity of eosinophil granule proteins to the upper and lower airways, these toxic proteins possibly are contributing to the tissue destruction in AFS.

Interleukin-5 (IL-5) increases various eosinophil functions, including survival in vitro, adhesion to endothelium, and eosinophil activation. The predominant source of IL-5 in allergic diseases such as allergic rhinitis is thought to be T lymphocytes.[18] ABPA also is characterized by peripheral and tissue eosinophilia. In a murine model of ABPA, an anti-IL-5 antibody abrogated peripheral and tissue eosinophilia induced by *Aspergillus fumigatus* antigens.[19] The role of T lymphocytes and cytokines in the pathogenesis of AFS is currently unknown.

There is evidence to support an IgE-mediated (type I) reaction in AFS. In culture-proven cases of AFS, skin testing to the putative fungus has been positive in 100% of reported cases. In vitro testing for specific IgE also has demonstrated, almost uniformly, elevations in specific IgE to the cultured fungus. Manning et al.[20] studied 16 patients with AFS using modified radioallerapsorbent testing (RAST) to various fungi. Of this group, only four patients had cultured fungi in which species-specific RAST results were available, and all had positive results. A control group of five patients with chronic sinusitis and polyposis showed negative reactivity to all of the fungal RAST. Although the prevalence of mold allergy is unknown in chronic sinusitis, it is likely less than that in AFS.

As in ABPA, there are also data to suggest that an immune complex (type III) reaction may play a role in the pathogenesis of AFS. In more than 85% of culture-proven AFS cases, testing demonstrates serum precipitins and elevated fungi-specific IgG.

On the basis of this evidence, we propose the following immunopathogenesis of AFS. Fungal spores are inhaled and deposited in the upper airway mucosa. Persons with asthma, nasal polyposis, and rhinitis may have more viscid secretions, which could enhance trapping of the fungal organism. Ciliostasis produced by the fungus itself could further promote fungal growth. Fungal spores could cross-link specific IgE antifungal antibody present on mast cells, causing activation and degranulation. Mast cells through release of chemotactic factors and various cytokines would ultimately lead to tissue infiltration of eosinophils, T lymphocytes, and neutrophils. Cytokines such as IL-5 could activate eosinophils and increase their survival. Finally, eosinophil toxic granule proteins and neutrophil elastase could then contribute to tissue destruction and ultimate formation of allergic mucin.

ETIOLOGIC AGENTS

Many cases of AFS are culture-negative (37%). This rate reflects a combination of misinterpretation of positive cultures as contaminants, difficulty culturing fungi, the toxic effect of eosinophil degranulation, and inappropriate selection of specimens.

Table 15–3 shows culture results of reported cases. These include dematiaceous fungi (*Alternaria, Bipolaris, Curvularia, Exserohilum*), and *Aspergillus* species. *Bipolaris* is the most common species cultured in AFS.

Organisms in the family Dematiaceae are members of the class Hyphomycetes. These fungi are common soil saprophytes and are found on plants, soil, and other debris. They form melanin pigment in their cell walls in culture and often in host tissue. The Fontana-Masson stain can be used to stain for this pigment, assisting identification of the hyphae in the mucin.

Aspergillus species are ubiquitous. They are members of the class Hyphomycetes and the family Moniliaceae. They are also found in soil and decaying organic debris. There are well over 100 species and several varieties, 16 of which have been known to cause disease in humans. By far the most common are *Aspergillus fumigatus* and *Aspergillus flavus. Aspergillus* represents only 9.8% of culture-positive cases of AFS.

DIAGNOSIS

Patients with AFS are a homogeneous population whose features, when recognized, can suggest the diagnosis preoperatively.[20] If the disease is suspected, the pathologist can examine the mucous membranes, secretions and other debris in the sinus for allergic mucin and hyphae. Ultimately, it is the pathologist and the microbiologist who will confirm or confute the primary physician's initial clinical suspicions.

Table 15–3   Culture Results by Species (*n* = 102)

ORGANISM	NO.	%
Negative	38	37.3
Alternaria	11	10.8
Aspergillus	10	9.8
Bipolaris	21	20.6
Curvularia	13	12.8
Dreschslera	3	2.9
Exserohilum	2	2.0
Other*	4	3.8

*Includes Fusarium and Helminthosporium cultures that were positive but could not be identified.

Prevalence

The prevalence of AFS is reported to vary from 3.7% to 7.0%.[4,6,21,22] The prevalence increases to 17.1% if patients with allergic mucin but no hyphae or positive fungal cultures are included.[21]

Clinical Features

The age at presentation varies from 8[23] to 72 years old.[21] Patients are typically in their third or fourth decade, and the mean age at diagnosis is 31.4 years. The male: female ratio is approximately 1:1 (Table 15–4).

Patients present with chronic sinusitis, asthma, atopy, and nasal polyposis. A history of multiple operations and multiple, unsuccessful antibiotic trials is common. Many patients will have been treated with intravenous antibiotics without success.

No association with hobby or environmental or industrial exposures has been found; however, because many of the pathogens identified in AFS are soil or plant saprophytes, a history of gardening, farming, or composting should be determined.

Nasal obstruction is the most common complaint and occurs in two-thirds of patients (Table 15–5). Symptoms of local pain occur in one-third of patients, as does rhinorrhea. The character of the face pain is nonspecific and may include tenderness over the wall of an involved sinus, frontal, occipital, or vertex headaches of varying duration, and patterns with or without specific aggravating factors. In up to 60% of patients, pain is not a significant factor. The character of the nasal drainage is also nonspecific, although several authors have reported the presence of large nasal casts in patients with AFS.

**Table 15–4   Clinical Features of
Allergic Fungal Sinusitis**

| | PATIENTS | |
FEATURE	NO.	%
Age, yr (*n* = 113)		
0–19	34	30.1
20–39	44	38.9
40–59	29	25.7
>60	6	5.3
Sex (*n* = 101)		
Male	55	54.5
Female	46	45.5
Asthma (*n* = 95)	48	50.5
Polyps (*n* = 115)	111	96.5
ASA sensitivity (*n* = 70)	13	18.6

**Table 15–5   Presenting Symptoms in
Allergic Fungal Sinusitis (n = 42)**

	PATIENTS	
	NO.	%
Nasal obstruction	25	60
Rhinorrhea*	13	31
Pain†	14	33
Visual‡	7	17

* Anterior or posterior.
† Any type of face or head pain.
‡ Includes diplopia, blurred vision, and blindness.

Visual symptoms occur in 17% of patients. This finding reflects the local expansile potential for this disease. Symptoms include diplopia, blurring, and, rarely, blindness.

Other vegetative symptoms are frequently present as a result of the chronic nature of this disease. Many patients have undergone multiple surgical drainage procedures and have become frustrated with their illness.

Sinus disease should initiate a search for disease in the lower airway. Half of patients with AFS have asthma. This may be severe and steroid-dependent or mild. Other disorders such as ABPA, primary ciliary dyskinesias, cystic fibrosis, allergic angilitis, and granulomatosis should be considered.

Finally, the history should clearly delineate the patient's past and present immunologic status. Patients with AFS typically are immunocompetent, and this can be confirmed with the appropriate laboratory testing.

Physical Examination

All patients should have a thorough endoscopic endonasal examination. On examination, 97% of patients have nasal polyps. Many patients have expansile disease. This appears to be more common in the pediatric population[23] and is manifested by a periorbital or perinasal mass with or without associated visual symptoms. Because of these findings, the disease is often confused with malignancy.

The condition of the mucosa at endoscopy is dependent on prior instrumentation. In the unoperated nose, there are no specific mucosal findings. Evidence of bacterial superinfection may be present. Thick, green to brown nasal casts have occasionally been described. The turbinates may be red and edematous, and the lateral nasal wall may bow medially, similar to patients with cystic fibrosis. Patients who have undergone multiple and extensive operations often have mucosal atrophy. Thick scar formation and altered surgical landmarks can make the nasal examination difficult. The remainder of the head and neck examination is nonspecific, and other findings such as prominent cervical adenopathy point to a diagnosis other than AFS.

Differential Diagnosis

The goal of the evaluation is to differentiate chronic bacterial rhinosinusitis, abnormalities in mucociliary transport, and malignancy. A brief differential diagnosis is listed in Table 15–6.

**Table 15–6 Differential Diagnosis in
Allergic Fungal Sinusitis**

Congenital
  Cystic fibrosis
  Immunoglobulin deficiency
    IgG subclass
    IgA
  Complement deficiency
  Primary ciliary dyskinesia
Drug-induced
  Acquired immunodeficiency
Anatomic
  Foreign body
  Septal deformity
  Choanal atresia
  Adenoid hypertrophy
  Other
Infection
  Chronic bacterial
  Mycobacterial
  Fungal
Inflammatory
  Allergic angiitis and granulomatosis
  Wegener's granulomatosis
  Sarcoid
Nasal polyposis
Mucocele
Pyocele
Neoplasm
  Benign
    Inverting papilloma
    Meningocele
    Angiofibroma
    Other
  Malignant
    Squamous cell carcinoma
    Salivary gland
    Other

Laboratory Evaluation

Laboratory tests that may be helpful in the evaluation of the patient with signs and symptoms suggestive of AFS are shown in Table 15–7. These studies are aimed at ruling out disorders in the differential diagnosis of AFS while providing evidence for a type I or type III hypersensitivity reaction to fungal antigen. Specific antibodies to fungal antigens are limited in their usefulness because of cost, limited availability, and unknown sensitivity and specificity.

In the young atopic patient considered a candidate for operation on the basis of the history, physical examination, and failed medical management for chronic sinusitis, preoperative laboratory investigations should include a complete blood cell count with differential and determination of total IgE level. In certain persons with refractory sinusitis, testing of IgA and IgG with subclasses, determination of complement levels, sweat chloride test, determination of ciliary beat frequency, chest radiography, and serum electrolyte testing with fasting glucose may be of value. Skin tests can be done in patients who have a history suggestive of allergic rhinitis and who are not taking steroids. After operation, if the fungal species is identified, specific IgG and IgE levels can be determined for that organism. Serologic tests such as total IgE, specific IgE and IgG, and serum precipitins have not been adequately evaluated in regard to following disease remission or predicting recurrence. However, in reports of AFS in the literature, total IgE levels have decreased with treatment in 10 of 11 cases, and specific IgE has decreased in 4 of

Table 15–7   Laboratory Data in Evaluation of Allergic Fungal Sinusitis

TEST	USE
Complete blood cell count with differential	All patients in whom sinusitis is suspected
IgE	
IgG with subclasses	Patients with suspected
IgM	immunodeficiency
IgA	
Complement levels	
Specific IgE	To confirm host
Serum precipitins	response to known pathogen
Sweat chloride test	Suspected cystic fibrosis
Nasal cytology	Patients with suspected
Radioallergasorbent test	allergic rhinitis
Skin testing	
Ciliary beat frequency	Ciliary abnormality
Transmission electron microscopy of cilia	
Chest radiography	Patient with
Pulmonary function test	concomitant pulmonary process
Angiotensin converting enzyme	Suspected systemic disease
Anti-neutrophil cytoplasmic antibody	
Erythrocyte sedimentation rate	

5.[5,7,8,17,20,21,24,25] In recurrence of AFS after treatment, only one-third of patients had an increase in IgE, and in two patients in whom specific IgE was measured, neither had an increase. Furthermore, Bartynski et al.[7] described a patient who had symptomatic and radiographic improvement yet had a 24-fold increase in specific IgE to the cultured fungus. Clearly, further serologic data in AFS must be collected and analyzed before clinically meaningful information can be obtained.

Radiographic Evaluation

Computed tomography (CT) of the sinuses in the direct coronal plane is essential in the evaluation and treatment of AFS. With disease in the sphenoid, CT in the axial plane should also be done to delineate structures related to the lateral wall of the sphenoid sinus, such as the carotid artery. In general, patients with AFS have three

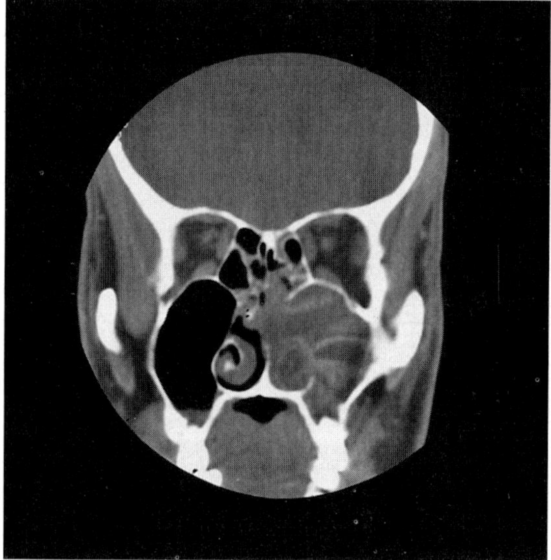

A

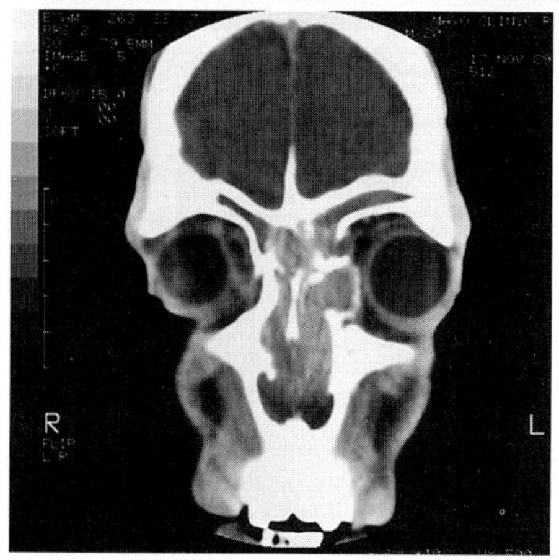

B

Figure 15–4. Computed tomogram in the direct coronal plane demonstrating pansinusitis with areas of increased attenuation in the maxillary sinuses without evidence of bony destruction (**A**) and with extensive bony destruction (**B**), representing the spectrum of disease.

or more sinuses involved with disease. Approximately 20% have bony erosion or expansion on the CT scan. Bony sclerosis is often not prominent. The CT appearance of the sinuses in AFS is heterogeneous, showing central areas of increased attenuation with surrounding areas of lower attenuation (Fig. 15–4). The degree of attenuation roughly correlates with the thickness of the secretions at the time of operation.

The CT findings in patients with AFS may be similar to those in patients with mycetomas or in patients with copious inspissated secretions from chronic bacterial sinusitis. Mycetomas, however, involve a single sinus, and the central areas are often metal-dense, making differentiation by CT straightforward.

Magnetic resonance imaging (MRI) scanning has not been used extensively in patients with AFS. Interpretation of MRI is more difficult than that of CT. As the density of the sinus contents increases, it becomes hard to differentiate air from solid mass, and objects as diverse as air and bone appear similar. MRI can be useful if invasion into the anterior or middle cranial fossa is suspected. It is also helpful for differentiating inspissated secretions from tumor mass. In general, the MRI in AFS shows low-signal intensity on T1-, T2-, and proton density-weighted images.

MANAGEMENT

Surgical Treatment

The mainstay of treatment in the patient suspected of having AFS is surgical drainage. The goal of operation is removal of all inspissated secretion, debris, and diseased tissue with preservation of normal nasal anatomy and tissue. The type of procedure needs to be individualized to the patient, the disease, and the preferences of the surgeon. Endoscopic sinus operation, conventional endonasal operation, Caldwell-Luc approach, or external ethmoidectomy can be considered. Limited operation on the ostiomeatal complex is not sufficient to treat AFS. Antrostomy should be large enough to allow complete examination of the sinus and removal of all diseased tissue. As previously mentioned, patients with AFS often have had prior operation, and the normal surgical landmarks may be absent. Care must be taken to

**Table 15–8   Laboratory Studies in
Allergic Fungal Sinusitis**

	PATIENTS	
	NO.*	%
Eosinophilia ($n = 39$)	24	61.5
Total IgE ($n = 39$)	30	77
Specific IgE† ($n = 10$)	10	100
Serum precipitins† ($n = 10$)	10	100

*No. is the number of reported cases with elevated or positive results.
†Positive test result to the organism cultured in the sinus contents.

avoid complications, such as injury to the orbit, optic nerve, or carotid artery or violation of the cribriform.

Medical Treatment

Treatment of the patient with AFS involves a multidisciplinary approach. Medical treatment options are available after surgical debridement. The more common treatment options are listed in Table 15–9. Postoperatively, patients should receive steroids orally and intranasally unless a contraindication exists. The ABPA treatment with oral prednisone is outlined in Table 15–9 and is the most commonly used regimen.

Careful postsurgical follow-up is the best way to identify recurrent disease. Follow-up evaluations should be done every other day for the first week, biweekly for the next 3 weeks, and once a month for 3 to 6 months. They should include nasal endoscopy on each visit. If polypoid change of the mucosa is noted on endoscopy or symptoms recur, more aggressive treatment is necessary.

Immunotherapy using specific extracts of the cultured fungus has not been evaluated in AFS. In ABPA, immunotherapy to *Aspergillus* is avoided because of concerns of increasing fungus-specific IgG and the theoretical risks associated with this phenomenon. However, in AFS, immunotherapy to other relevant antigens was advocated by Goldstein et al.[24] to reduce other sources of IgE-mediated inflammation. In one case report, a child with an orbital mass and AFS due to an unidentified fungus was treated with a "mold mixture" and other allergens after a recurrence of

**Table 15–9   Medical Treatment
Options in Allergic Fungal Sinusitis**

Treatments aimed at local reduction in antigen load
    Nasal saline irrigation
    Nasal antifungal washes*
Treatments aimed at decreasing the inflammatory response
    Inhaled nasal steroids
    Oral prednisone ABPA† regimen: 0.5 mg/kg per day for 2
      weeks, then every other day for 3 to 6 months, then
      taper
    Parenteral steroids
    Antihistamines
Antifungals‡
Avoidance of antigen
Immunotherapy§

*Sensitivities of the organism to the antifungal agent need to be known to begin therapy. No specific regimens are available for which we are aware.
†ABPA, Allergic bronchopulmonary aspergillosis.
‡Not recommended in the absence of tissue invasion.
§Theoretical risks to the development of specific IgG antibodies exist. Consultation with an allergist is recommended.

disease.[26] During immunotherapy, there was a reduction in the orbital mass and symptomatic improvement.

Recurrent disease refractory to treatment in a symptomatic patient is an indication to reoperate.

Complications of the Disease

The complications of AFS are related to local expansion. This can involve the orbit and anterior and middle cranial fossae. Patients may complain of blurred vision, diplopia, loss of vision, or other neurologic symptoms. Blindness, which occurs rarely, is a surgical emergency. Optimal treatment of AFS-induced blindness includes sinus decompression and parenteral steroids. However, steroids are contraindicated in patients with visual impairment from invasive fungal disease, a situation underlining the importance of accurate and timely histopathologic evaluation.

Expansion into the cranial cavity also presents a surgical dilemma. The diagnosis of AFS is often unknown, and malignancy or invasive infection is suspected. Even if AFS is diagnosed early in the surgical procedure, an intracranial abscess may have formed or concomitant invasive disease may be present. An attempt at complete surgical debridement, often with frontal craniotomy in combination with an intransasal operation, is required. Medical management postoperatively involves a collaborative effort among the otorhinolaryngologist, neurosurgeon, allergist, and infectious disease specialist.

Complications of Management

Complications of both the surgical and the medical management of AFS have been reported. One of the more common and least-recognized problems is the development of atrophic rhinitis after multiple, extensive procedures. It is prudent to recognize that patients with AFS often require more than one operation; therefore, surgical drainage should be conservative, sparing as much normal nasal architecture as possible. Maximizing medical therapy also may help decrease the number of operations.

Complications of nasal operation are well recognized, and revision procedure is best left to experienced hands.

Because steroid therapy is the focus of medical management, patients should be questioned regarding a history of tuberculosis, osteoporosis, gastric or duodenal ulcer, cataract, or other processes that may be exacerbated with steroid use.

PROGNOSIS

Patients with AFS appear to fall into three categories: those with rapid recurrence, those with delayed recurrence, and those with cure after a single operation. Predictors of recurrence other than a past history of multiple surgical procedures have not

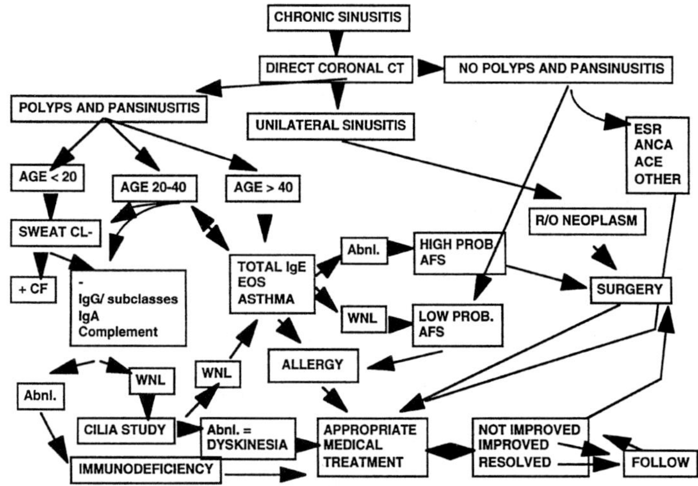

Figure 15–5.   Management algorithm for allergic fungal sinusitis.

been identified. Following serial total IgE levels may prove to be helpful in predicting recurrent disease or documenting remission,[8] but this approach is unproved. All patients should be counseled about the recurrent nature of AFS, and frequent and thorough endoscopic examinations should be done. In this way, the disease can be controlled in most patients.

CONCLUSION

AFS is becoming recognized as a significant cause of chronic sinusitis. As knowledge of the disease increases among otorhinolaryngologists, allergists, and pathologists, the number of documented cases will also increase. With this will come an improved understanding of the pathogenesis of AFS and improved treatment options.

AFS should be considered in the differential diagnosis of a young, atopic, immunocompetent patient with nasal polyps. An appropriate evaluation, including complete blood cell counts and peripheral differential, determination of total IgE levels, and radiographic examination that includes a direct coronal CT scan should be done. Other tests are dictated by the patient's clinical presentation. The definitive diagnosis will, however, be made by the pathologist after microscopic examination of the surgical specimen.

Currently, surgical sinus debridement and aeration is the mainstay of therapy, with aggressive postoperative medical management that can include oral steroids and frequent postoperative follow-up.

In the future, the physician may have several laboratory tests available to diagnose AFS preoperatively and follow the disease process postoperatively. However, until the efficacy of these tests is shown in controlled prospective clinical trials, their use is limited.

REFERENCES

1. Hartwick RW, Batsakis JG: Sinus aspergillosis and allergic fungal sinusitis. *Ann Otol Rhinol Laryngol* 1991; 100:427–430.
2. Safirstein BH: Allergic bronchopulmonary aspergillosis with obstruction of the upper respiratory tract. *Chest* 1976; 70:788–790.
3. Millar JW, Johnson A, Lamb D: Allergic aspergillosis of the maxillary sinuses. *Proc Scottish Torac Soc* 1981; 36:710.
4. Katzenstein AL, Sale SR, Greenberger PA: Allergic *Aspergillus* sinusitis: a newly recognized form of sinusitis. *J Allergy Clin Immunol* 1983; 72:89–93.
5. Robson JM, Hogan PG, Benn RA, Gatenby PA: Allergic fungal sinusitis presenting as a paranasal sinus tumour. *Aust NZ J Med* 1989; 19:351–353.
6. Cody DT II, Neel HB III, Ferreiro JA, Roberts GD: Allergic fungal sinusitis: the Mayo Clinic experience. *Laryngoscope* 1994; 104:1074–1079.
7. Bartynski JM, McCaffrey TV, Frigas E: Allergic fungal sinusitis secondary to dematiaceous fungi— *Curvularia lunata* and *Alternaria Otolaryngol Head Neck Surg* 1990; 103:32–39.
8. Brummund W, Kurup VP, Harris GJ, Duncavage JA, Arkins JA: Allergic sino-orbital mycosis. A clinical and immunologic study. *JAMA* 1986; 256:3249–3253.
9. Ence BK, Gourley DS, Jorgensen NL, Shagets FW, Parsons DS: Allergic fungal sinusitis. *Am J Rhinol* 1990; 4:169–178.
10. Travis WD, Kwon-Chung KJ, Kleiner DE, et al: Unusual aspects of allergic bronchopulmonary fungal disease: report of two cases due to *Curvularia* organisms associated with allergic fungal sinusitis. *Hum Pathol* 1991; 22:1240–1248.
11. Waxman JE, Spector JG, Sale SR, Katzenstein AL: Allergic *Aspergillus* sinusitis: concepts in diagnosis and treatment of a new clinical entity. *Laryngoscope* 1987; 97:261–266.
12. Gleich GJ, Adolphson CR: The eosinophilic leukocyte: structure and function. *Adv Immunol* 1986; 39:177–253.
13. O'Donnell MC, Ackerman SJ, Gleich GJ, Thomas LL: Activation of basophil and mast cell histamine release by eosinophil granule major basic protein. *J Exp Mol* 1983; 157:1981–1991.
14. Ackerman SJ, Zhou Z, Tenen DG, Clark MA, Tu Y-P, Irvin CG: Human Eosinophil Lysophospholipase (Charcot-Leyden Crystal Protein): Molecular Cloning, Expression, and Potential Functions in Asthma, in Gleich G, Kay A (eds.): *Eosinophils in Allergy and Inflammation.* New York, M Dekker, 1994, pp 21–54.
15. Harlin SL, Ansel DG, Lane SR, Myers J, Kephart GM, Gleich GJ: A clinical and pathologic study of chronic sinusitis: the role of the eosinophil. *J Allergy Clin Immunol* 1988; 81:867–875.
16. Khan DA, Gleich GJ, Leiferman KM: Immunohistologic analyses of allergic fungal sinusitis (abstract). *J Allergy Clin Immunol* 1994; 93:236.
17. Frazier TC, Rupp NT, Kuhn FA, Wray BB, Stafford CT, Dolen WK: Serum and allergic mucin levels of eosiniphil cationic protein in allergic fungal sinusitis (abstract). *J Allergy Clin Immunol* 1994; 93:234.
18. Ying S, Durham SR, Barkans J, et al: T cells are the principal source of interleukin-5 mRNA in allergen-induced rhinitis. *Am J Respir Cell Molec Biol* 1993; 9:356–360.
19. Murali P, Kumar A, Choi H, Banasal NK, Fink JN, Kurup VP: *Aspergillus fumigatus* antigen induced eosinophilia in mice is abrogated by anti-IL-5 antibody. *J Leukocyte Biol* 1993; 53:264–267.
20. Manning SC, Mabry RL, Schaefer SD, Close LG: Evidence of IgE-mediated hypersensitivity in allergic fungal sinusitis. *Laryngoscope* 1993; 103:717–721.
21. Allphin AL, Strauss M, Abdul-Karim FW: Allergic fungal sinusitis: problems in diagnosis and treatment. *Laryngoscope* 1991; 101:815–820.
22. Gourley DS, Whisman BA, Jorgensen NL, Martin ME, Reid MJ: Allergic *Bipolaris* sinusitis: clinical and immunopathologic characteristics. *J Allergy Clin Immunol* 1990; 85:583–591.
23. Manning SC, Vuitch F, Weinberg AG, Brown DE: Allergic aspergillosis: a newly recognized form of sinusitis in the pediatric population. *Laryngoscope* 1989; 99:681–685.
24. Goldstein MF, Atkins PC, Cogen FC, Kornstein MJ, Levine RS, Zweiman B: Allergic *Aspergillus* sinusitis (clinical conference). *J Allergy Clin Immunol* 1985; 76:515–524.
25. Holland C, Smith YE, Bielory L: Immunologic and CAT scan correlates of *Aspergillus* allergic fungal sinusitis treated with prednisone vs. no Rx (abstract). *J Allergy Clin Immunol* 1991; 93:144.
26. de Juan E Jr, Green WR, Iliff NT: Allergic periorbital mucopyocele in children. *Am J Opthalmol* 1983; 96:299–303.

16

Nose and Sinus Tumors

KERRY D. OLSEN, M.D.

Tumors of the nose and paranasal sinuses are not common. They are recognized late, and the prognosis is poor. Nose and sinus neoplasms are usually not found until results of imaging studies and biopsy are obtained. Unfortunately, the basic diagnostic components of medicine, the history and physical examination, are often overlooked.

The poor prognosis of malignant nose and sinus neoplasms is due to late diagnosis. Most nasal and sinus tumors initially cause symptoms such as nasal obstruction, rhinorrhea, or epistaxis. However, these symptoms are also common with multiple inflammatory disorders. Early symptoms often are ignored and diagnosis is not made until tumors are advanced with obvious findings of malignancy: facial deformity, orbital symptoms, loose teeth, or cranial nerve paralysis. Tumors can reach a considerable size before patients seek medical attention. We must stop equating the diagnosis of nose and sinus tumors with facial deformity, orbital symptoms, severe pain, and cranial nerve weakness. Improvement in survival will not occur until earlier diagnosis is made[1] (Fig. 16–1). It is important to teach family practitioners, internists, otolaryngologists, oral surgeons, dentists, and surgical residents how to identify these tumors sooner.

Physicians should be suspicious of a nose or sinus tumor when a patient has symptoms that are recurrent, are unilateral, or do not respond to normal medical therapy.[2] Early diagnosis of tumors is difficult when they are inaccessible to direct inspection. Therefore, it is important to know the characteristic behavior of the benign and malignant neoplasms found in the nose and paranasal sinus region. Appreciation of the anatomic basis for symptoms and physical findings also can lead to earlier diagnosis. The management goals of nasal and sinus tumors are not different from those of other head and neck neoplasms. Early diagnosis is preferable. Next, one obtains an accurate assessment of the tumor's extent and determines the pathologic diagnosis. Finally, an experienced head and neck oncology team plans and initiates appropriate treatment.

Because malignant tumors often mimic benign disorders initially, physicians must be suspicious and have the appropriate background knowledge to diagnose

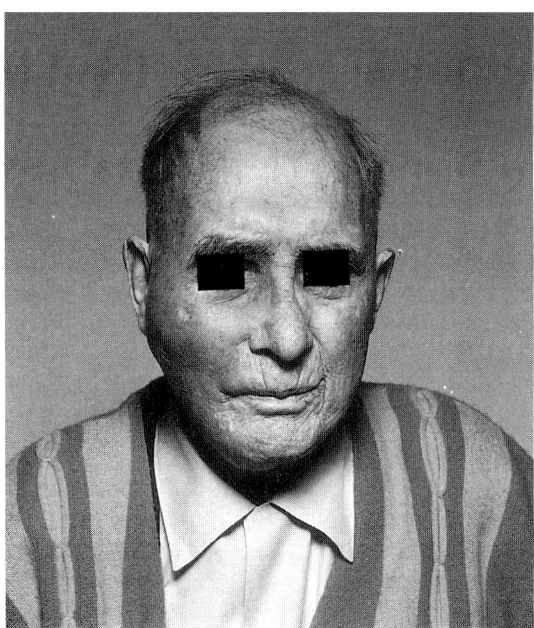

Figure 16–1. Advanced maxillary sinus carcinoma.

these tumors early. The cosmetic and functional changes that occur as a result of the tumor's growth and treatment cause tremendous emotional effects.[3]

TUMORS

The incidence of nasal tumors in the United States is less than 1 per 100,000. In Japan and Uganda, the incidence is two times greater.[3] Malignant tumors of the nose and paranasal sinuses account for only 0.2% to 0.8% of all malignancies.[2,4] Cancer of the nose and paranasal sinuses is more common in males. In the antrum, the male:female ratio is 2:1, and 95% of cases occur in persons older than 40 years.[2] In the ethmoid sinus, the male:female ratio is 1.4:1. Overall, 75% of all malignant tumors occur in persons older than 50 years.[2] The maxillary antrum is the site of 80% of sinus malignancies, and 95% of patients are older than 40 years and 75% are in the sixth, seventh, or eighth decade of life.[5] The incidence of maxillary sinus tumors is equal in blacks and whites.

For all nose and sinus tumors, the nose is the primary site in 25% and the sinuses in 75%.[2] Of all sinus neoplasms, 60% to 80% originate from the maxillary antrum.[5] With large tumors, it is often difficult to determine the exact site of origin. As a result, the tumor distributions noted in the literature are variable. One report found that 89% of sinonasal carcinomas developed in the maxillary sinus, 6% in the nasal cavities, 4% in the ethmoid sinuses, and less than 1% in the sphenoid or frontal sinuses.[6]

Tumors in the nasal cavity are evenly divided between benign and malignant neoplasms. Inverting papillomas predominate in the former, and squamous cell carcinoma in the latter.[7] Adenocarcinomas more commonly originate from the nasal fossa and ethmoids than from the maxilla. An adenocarcinoma is more likely nasal in origin because there are more mucous glands present in the nose than in the sinuses. Lymphomas arise equally from the nasal cavity and maxilla, and melanomas are equally found in the nasal cavity and ethmoids.[8]

Environmental factors are related to the cause of nasal and paranasal sinus tumors in approximately 80% of cases.[3] Woodworkers with exposure to hardwoods have a higher incidence of adenocarcinomas of the ethmoid and antrum[9] (Fig. 16–2), and exposure to nickel refining is a cause of squamous cell carcinoma of the ethmoids.[10] Smoking is associated with an elevated risk of nasal cancer, especially squamous cell carcinoma of the maxillary antrum.[11] Other occupations linked to the tumors include nuclear refinery work, boot and shoe manufacturing, chrome pigment work, textile work, flour milling, bakers, and radium painting, which are associated with an increased risk of squamous and anaplastic carcinomas.[5] Thorium dioxide (Thorotrast), when used as an imaging agent, causes antral squamous cell and mucoepidermoid carcinomas.[5] Children with prior radiation therapy for retinoblastoma also are at higher risk for the development of sinus tumors.[5]

Of all malignant tumors of the nose and paranasal sinuses, 75% to 80% are squamous cell carcinoma or its variants. The variants include anaplastic carcinoma, undifferentiated carcinoma, and transitional cell carcinoma. Other types of malignant tumors are salivary gland malignancies, 4% to 15% of tumors; sarcomas, 6%; and other tumors, including melanomas, lymphomas, and olfactory neuroblastomas.[7] The prognosis of malignant tumors seems to be more dependent on extent than on the degree of dedifferentiation. Anaplastic carcinomas, however, do behave worse.[2]

The maxillary antrum is the site for most malignant neoplasms of the nose and paranasal sinuses. In a review of 119 cases of maxillary sinus cancer, extension to the cheek, nose, palate, or orbit was found in all. One site was involved in 22%, two sites in 50%, three sites in 26%, and four sites in 1%.[12] Nodal metastasis was present initially in 10% to 18% of patients and eventually developed in 25% to 30%. Nodal metastasis was two times higher when cancer invaded the palate.[12]

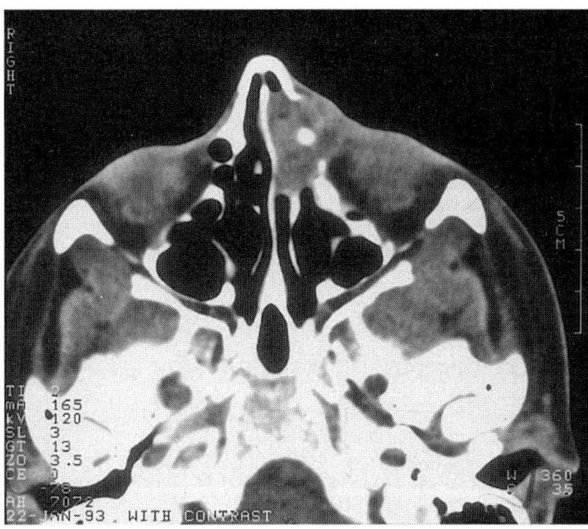

Figure 16–2.   Adenocarcinoma of superior nasal cavity.

Tumors spread easily from the nose to the sinus and vice versa. Tumors presented with bone destruction in 70% to 80% of cases.[2] They easily spread through surrounding foramina and fissures and into soft tissue. Cancer of the nasal cavity and paranasal sinuses often presents with regional disease. It is uncommon to have tumor confined to one location in the nose or sinus. Although the maxillary sinus is the site of origin for approximately 80% of all sinus neoplasms, tumors are isolated to the maxillary sinus alone in only 25% of cases.[13]

Delay in diagnosis of nose and paranasal sinus tumors is a major problem. The time from initial symptoms until diagnosis is 6 months or more.[2] During that time, 45% of tumors involve the orbit and 10% have extension to the pterygoid plates.[2] These tumors do have signs and physical findings that may allow for earlier diagnosis.

ANATOMIC BASIS OF DISEASE

An understanding of the anatomy of the nose and paranasal sinuses in necessary to diagnose tumors early. Because most nasal and paranasal sinus malignancies begin in the maxillary sinus, knowledge of antral anatomy is essential. The anatomy of the maxilla has been well described by Pearson.[1] The maxilla has four surfaces. The facial surface can easily be palpated through the skin of the face or beneath the upper lip in the labial gingival sulcus. The upper lip and cheek are innervated by the second division of the fifth cranial nerve. However, the labial surface of the gingiva of the incisor teeth is innervated by the anterior superior alveolar nerve. This nerve branches from V2 adjacent to the floor of the orbit before the nerve exits the infraorbital foramen. If the incisor teeth and upper lip are numb and there is no palpable mass on the facial surface of the maxilla, the tumor must involve the nerve before it exits the infraorbital foramen. The orbital surface of the maxilla cannot be palpated directly. However, it is important to appreciate that as a cancer involves more of the medial and posterior orbital surface, the tumor comes closer to the superior orbital fissure and optic canal. The nasal surface of the maxilla is largely dehiscent as a result of the large bony hiatus separating the maxilla from the nasal cavity. Anteriorly and superiorly to the hiatus is the nasolacrimal duct, and posterior to the hiatus are the greater palatine nerve and artery. Anterior and superior tumor involvement of the nasal surface can cause tearing due to obstruction of the nasolacrimal duct. The bony hiatus offers no barrier to tumor extension from the maxillary antrum to the nasal cavity. Posterior and inferior tumor involvement of the nasal surface can result in hemipalatal anesthesia of the hard and soft palate due to involvement of the greater palatine nerve.

Cancer high in the posteromedial portion of the antrum has the worst prognosis because of access to natural ostia to the brain and to the osteolymphatics. Early symptoms of tumor in this area, however, are only a stuffy nose and postnasal drainage. The final surface is the infratemporal fossa. This surface can be palpated as an early step in the performance of a maxillectomy. A fine groove on the infratemporal surface of the maxilla contains the posterosuperior alveolar nerve. This nerve supplies sensation to the buccal surface only of the gingiva of the posterior alveolus and molar and premolar teeth. Anesthesia of these areas implies tumor extension through the infratemporal fossa surface of the maxilla.

It is difficult to determine whether a cancer begins in the maxillary antrum or ethmoid sinus because tumors often involve both regions. The ethmoid labyrinth contains numerous small air cells separating the maxilla from the anterior cranial fossa. There are generally nine laminae in this region, four on each side: the uncinate, ethmoid bulla, middle turbinate, and superior turbinate.[1] The middle lamina is also called the ethmoid plate of the septum. This portion of the septum is extremely thin and offers a minimal barrier to the spread of cancer from one side of the upper nasal cavity to the other. The fovea ethmoidalis and cribriform areas of the nose also offer little barrier to intracranial spread of tumor.[6] The lateral border of the ethmoid cavity, the lamina papyracea, also is a very thin bone with little resistance to tumor spread. The anterior ethmoid artery marks the anterior extent of the cribriform.

The sphenoid sinus is situated in the sphenoid bone, which occupies the center of the skull. The sphenoid bone has three processes: the lesser wing, the greater wing, and the pterygoid process. The superior orbital fissure separates the greater and lesser wings of the sphenoid, and the roof of the greater wing is perforated by the foramen rotundum. With the exception of the anterior wall, it is not possible to adequately excise or resect a malignancy that invades the area outside the sphenoid sinus. Superiorly, one encounters the optic nerve and pituitary gland; laterally, the carotid artery and cavernous sinus. The bone laterally is generally thin and may be dehiscent. Inferior to the sphenoid sinus, one encounters the vidian nerve and nasopharynx. As with all the sinuses, there are venous communications with the intracranial veins that form a route for tumor spread.[6]

The cribriform plate is actually stronger than the ethmoidal roof even though it has numerous perforations. It lies slightly lower than the roof of the ethmoid, its external landmark being the medial canthal tendon. The anterior ethmoid nerve follows the anterior ethmoid artery and supplies sensation to the tip of the nose. This can be tested clinically.[1]

When tumor extends to the posterior nasal cavity, laterally through the sphenopalatine foramen or posteriorly from the maxillary antrum, it can involve the pterygopalatine fossa. When this occurs, the ipsilateral palate will be numb and the patient notes absence of tearing. Absence of tearing is due to involvement of the secretomotor fibers from the sphenoid ganglion which lead to the lacrimal gland. Further posteromedial spread from the maxilla can readily involve the middle cranial fossa via the foramen rotundum and the foramen lacerum via the pterygoid canal. Tumor extension from the sphenopalatine foramen or directly through the maxilla can involve the pterygomaxillary fissure, the pterygopalatine fossa, or the infratemporal fossa. The orbital apex can be involved via the infraorbital fissure or directly through the orbital floor. When the pterygopalatine fossa is involved with tumor, it also affects the sphenopalatine ganglion that lies at the upper medial portion of the fossa. This can be a cause for deep facial pain.[1]

The lymphatic flow from the nose and paranasal sinuses occurs in two directions. The anterior nasal cavity and vestibular lymphatics drain primarily to the submandibular nodes. Lymphatics from the nose also spread laterally to the buccal fat pad and to the submandibular nodes.[1] The remaining sinus and nasal mucosal lymphatics drain just anterior to the eustachian tube orifice on the lateral wall of the nasopharynx. This pretubal plexus is a posterior collecting channel that connects with the lateral pharyngeal lymph nodes near the base of the skull.[9] Metastasis to these nodes is one of the main reasons for use of radiation to treat paranasal sinus malignancies (Fig. 16–3). The lateral pharyngeal lymph nodes connect with the deep jugular nodes. Palpable cervical adenopathy due to paranasal sinus cancer, therefore, is a secondary and not a primary site of metastasis. These lymphatic pathways were first described by Ohngren in 1933.[14] When tumors spread to the retropharyngeal nodes, they also can cause unilateral Horner's syndrome and deep upper neck, eye, and frontotemporal pain.[1]

Nasal tumors spread easily throughout the nasal cavity. The nasal spine, septal cartilage, tissue of the upper lip, columella, nasal mucoperiosteum and perichondrium, premaxilla, and vomer are minimal barriers to tumor spread.[15] Tumors in the nasal vestibule spread by direct invasion into contiguous structures. These include the septal and alar cartilages. Tumors in this region are more likely to metastasize if they involve the upper lip, the skin on the nasal dorsum, or multiple sites or if they are poorly differentiated.[5]

Nasal cavity tumors are located, in decreasing order of frequency, on the turbinates, nasal septum, floor of the nose, and nasal vestibule.[16] Tumors have easy access to the septum and floor of the nose.[16] Once the septum is involved, tumor spread can occur submucosally. Septal invasion can extend to the anterior cranial

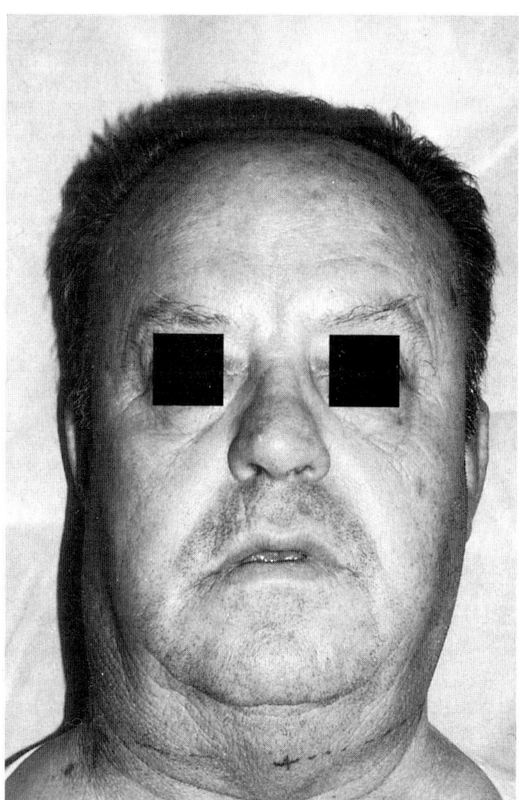

Figure 16–3. Bilateral cervical metastasis from advanced posterior nasal cavity carcinoma.

base and inferiorly to the premaxilla and floor of the nose with little resistance to periosteal invasion.

The antral mucosa also contacts the roots of the teeth posterior to the canine tooth. Dental symptoms can occur with involvement of the inferior antral mucosa. If the alveolar process is involved with tumor, pain can occur, and patients may note loose teeth or pain while wearing dentures.[1]

SYMPTOMS

No symptoms of nasal and sinus tumors are characteristic of early lesions. Benign and malignant neoplasms can present similarly and often have symptoms indistinguishable from those of nonneoplastic nasal and sinus disorders. Rice and Stanley[2] reported that 30 of 50 cases of nasal cavity cancer had chronic sinusitis and nasal polyps as initial symptoms. The diagnosis was delayed because the symptoms seemed subtle or trivial or even may have transiently responded to antibiotics and decongestants. Often, symptoms are so minimal that tumors are not suspected until a pathologist examines tissue that has been removed and erroneously thought to be benign inflammatory polyps.

Butlin,[17] in 1887, presented a classic description of the progression of symptoms of malignant nose and sinus neoplasms. He stated the following: "Sometimes the appearance of the tumor is preceded by pain, but in many instances, there is no pain until the disease is advanced. The first sign of serious disease is the appearance of a swelling of the face over the antrum or a fullness and obstruction of the corresponding side of the nose. With the fullness of the nostril, there may be a discharge of bloody fluid. Swelling gradually increases, not only in directions in which it first was noticed, but also up toward the orbit, down toward the mouth, and back into the sphenomaxillary fossa. The eye may be pushed up and the hard palate pushed down, but the swelling in the fossa is not so easily perceived. The nostril on the affected side often becomes completely obstructed. As the disease advances, the bony walls may be destroyed and the protrusion may take place, with effection of the soft parts around the bone. The skin of the face in this way becomes adherent to the tumor and immovable over it, and the result may be a vast ulcer with a thrusting forth of a fungus mass."

Rubin[18] described four phases of the natural history of nasal and sinus tumors. During the first phase, the tumor creates an inflammatory response. In the second phase, a dull ache becomes manifest as the surrounding bone is eroded. Phase three is accompanied by hypoesthesia and deep pain from nerve invasion. In phase four, there is major deformity with gross local and distant spread. Symptoms of nasal and sinus neoplasms can be divided into local, regional, and systemic. This classification and the description by Rubin are helpful for characterizing the symptoms of nasal and sinus neoplasms.

The examiner must also maintain a high index of suspicion for possible nose and sinus neoplasms when evaluating patients with nasal symptoms. This approach is especially important when symptoms are unilateral or when there has been failure to respond to the usual treatments. The surrounding inflammatory response to a tumor may transiently improve with antibiotics and decongestants. Rarely, however, does an inflammatory disorder cause nerve symptoms.

LOCAL SYMPTOMS

Nose and Nasal Cavity

One of the most frequent symptoms of nasal and sinus neoplasms is nasal obstruction. The nasal cavity is a minimal barrier to tumor spread, and unilateral nasal obstruction is a frequent presenting complaint. Unilateral obstruction rapidly becomes bilateral as the tumor grows into the nasopharynx or through the nasal septum. Extension through the septum is common in the thin bone of the superior nasal septum. Tumors also often cause epistaxis. Epistaxis can be minimal, or the patient may describe blood-tinged mucous drainage or brisk, profuse, and occasionally life-threatening epistaxis. Manipulation of friable, necrotic, or vascular neoplasms also can cause hemorrhage during examination. Another early symptom is rhinorrhea. Nasal discharge can be anterior or posterior and vary from watery, purulent, to occasionally clear. Cerebrospinal fluid rhinorrhea rarely occurs. The presence of unilateral rhinorrhea should help to distinguish possible neoplasm from vasomotor rhinitis or allergic rhinitis. Anytime a patient describes unilateral obstruction, bleeding, or rhinorrhea, a nasal or sinus tumor must be suspected.

The patient may be aware of a nasal mass that is visible or felt with a finger. The mass can be cancer, a benign tumor, or a polyp due to the tumor.[12] Vestibular cancers are not difficult to diagnose because they are readily visible. The patient complains of a persistent nodule or ulcerative lesion on one side of the nose anteriorly. Rarely, nasal vestibular cancers can be confused with an inflammatory process.[5] There may also be local soreness or burning.[8] As nasal cavity tumors progress in size, lesions originating on the lateral portion of the nose can infiltrate the overlying skin and lateral nasal bones. The nasal dorsum broadens, and an obvious nasal deformity occurs.

The nasal cavity also can be involved by tumors originating in the nasal skin. The most common malignancy of the nasal skin is basal cell carcinoma. According to Roenigk et al.,[9] the nose is involved in 25% of all basal cell carcinomas of the facial area (Fig. 16–4). These authors found that 87% of nasal skin tumors were basal cell carcinoma and 10.7% were squamous cell carcinoma. Nasal malignancies also may masquerade as inflammatory processes involving the skin of the overlying nose. These tumors may erroneously be thought to be infections, rosacea, or other inflammatory conditions[19] (Fig. 16–5). Additional nasal symptoms include pain, anosmia, or decreased sense of smell.

Sinus

Benign and malignant neoplasms can cause sinusitis as a result of blockage of the sinus ostia. Stasis of secretions and bacterial infections occur. Often, neoplasms originating in the sinus are misdiagnosed as mucoceles or pyoceles. As tumors

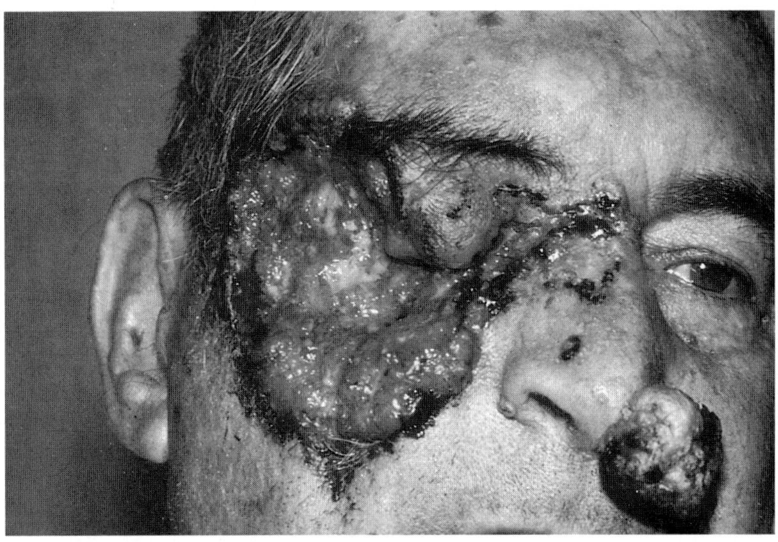

Figure 16–4. Extensive basal cell carcinoma involving maxillary antrum, nose, and nasal cavity.

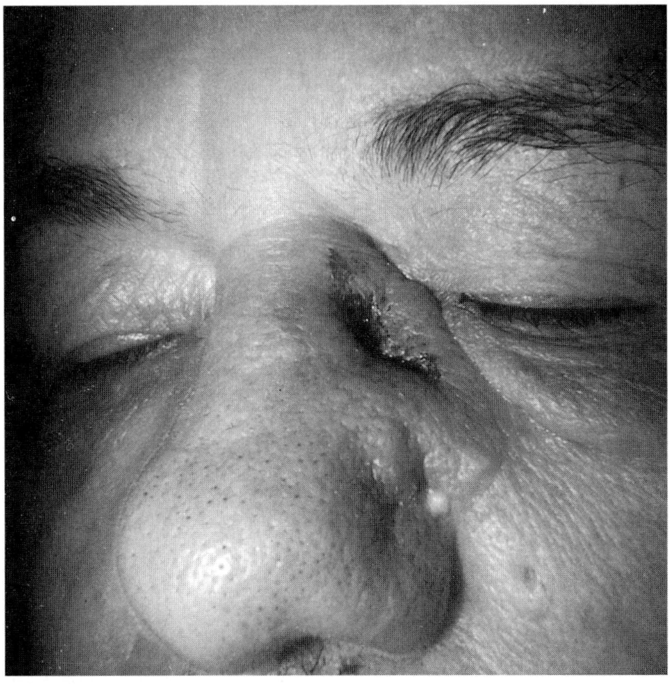

Figure 16–5. Squamous cell carcinoma of nasal cavity simulating nasal cutaneous infection.

extend beyond the bony walls of the sinus or have a secondary inflammatory reaction, facial swelling can occur. When the frontal sinus is involved, pain and swelling occur. Other symptoms in this area include ocular symptoms in 27% of cases, bloody rhinorrhea in 12%, and purulent nasal discharge in 9%.[20] Almost all patients have some forehead swelling with extension into the orbital area. A misdiagnosis of mucoceles, pyoceles, or osteomyelitis is common. Headache and facial pain are other symptoms due to sinus involvement.

Orbit

Unilateral tearing is a common symptom with nose and sinus neoplasms from obstruction anywhere along the course of the lacrimal duct or by tumor invasion of the lacrimal sac. Tumor obstruction of the inferior meatus also may cause occlusion of the lacrimal duct opening. The finding of a dry eye is worrisome for tumor extension into the pterygopalatine fossa. Tumor growth from the maxilla or laterally from the ethmoids through the lamina papyracea can cause proptosis, chemosis, or a palpable mass in the lower lid or medial canthal region. Diplopia occurs from direct muscle invasion, and decreased vision and blindness result from progressive orbital involvement or tumor extension to the orbital apex. When the orbital apex is involved, ocular muscle palsies, blindness, and forehead numbness from involvement of the ophthalmic branch of the trigeminal nerve occur.[13] One report reviewed the ophthalmic findings noted during the initial visit for maxillary sinus carcinoma[21] (Fig. 16–6). That study found epiphora, proptosis, upper displacement of the globe, diplopia, ocular motility disturbance, lid swelling, palpable orbital mass, and sudden visual loss. These findings occurred in 18 of 34 patients with malignant tumors of the nose and paranasal sinuses. These symptoms were similar to the initial symptoms of patients with paranasal sinus mucopyoceles.

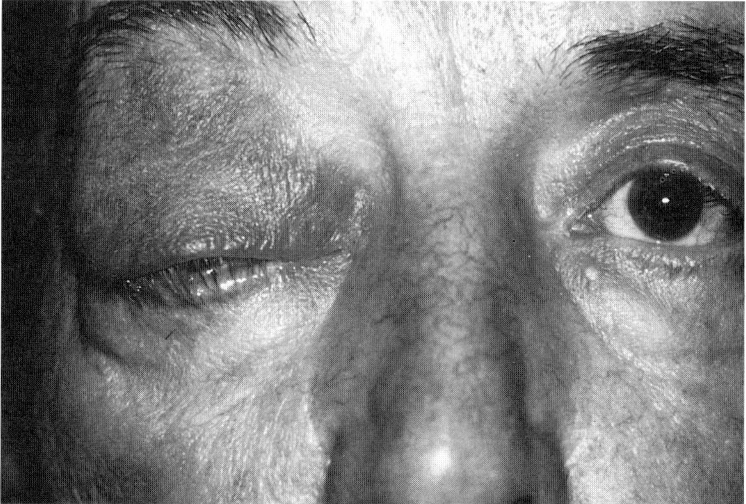

Figure 16–6.   Orbital involvement with maxillary sinus squamous cell carcinoma.

Dental Problems

Tumor involvement of the inferior portion of the maxilla or nasal cavity can involve the adjacent teeth. Pain, infection, or loosening of the teeth can occur. With maxillary tumors, the premolar and molar teeth are involved. Commonly, an extraction site will not heal or a persistent oroantral fistula can occur (Fig. 16–7). The alveolar arch can be altered such that significant malocclusion occurs. For edentulous patients, an early symptom may be pain while wearing the denture. Later, swelling or a mass on the palate or alveolar ridge may make wearing dentures impossible because of improper fit or discomfort. A mass visible on the roof of the mouth implies significant tumor spread and bony invasion.

Neurogenic Symptoms

Maxillary sinus neoplasms can involve the second division of the fifth cranial nerve and cause numbness of the cheek and upper lip. Involvement of the anterior alveolar superior nerve causes numbness of the gingiva on the labial surface of the incisor and canine teeth. Involvement of the posterior alveolar superior nerve causes numbness of the gingiva and alveolar ridge on the labial surface of the premolar and molar teeth. Tumors of the nasal cavity or maxillary sinus also can involve the descending palatine nerve and cause anesthesia of the hard and soft palates (Fig. 16–8). Vidian nerve involvement also can occur from tumor extension into the pterygopalatine fossa. Olfactory nerve involvement from tumor extension to the cribriform region and anterior cranial fossa can result in anosmia. Tumor extension to the orbital apex or through the superior orbital fissure also can involve cranial nerves II, III, IV, V(1), and VI. Tumor extension laterally from the sphenoid sinus

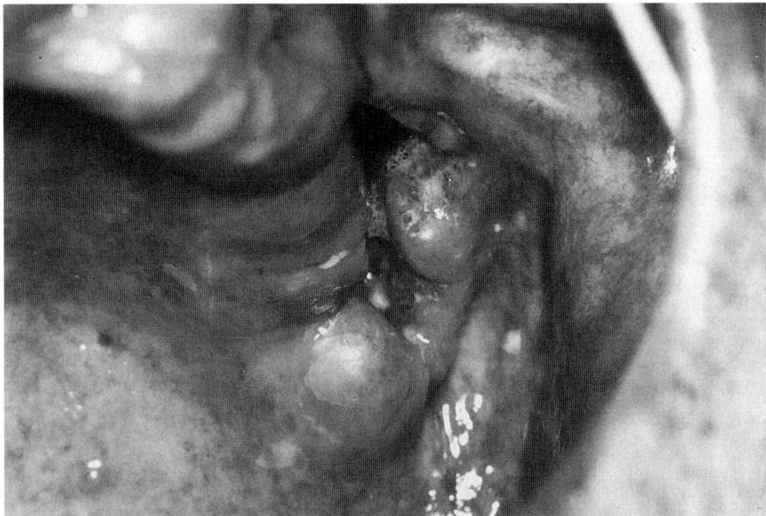

Figure 16–7. Oral antral fistula and involvement of alveolar arch from maxillary squamous cell carcinoma.

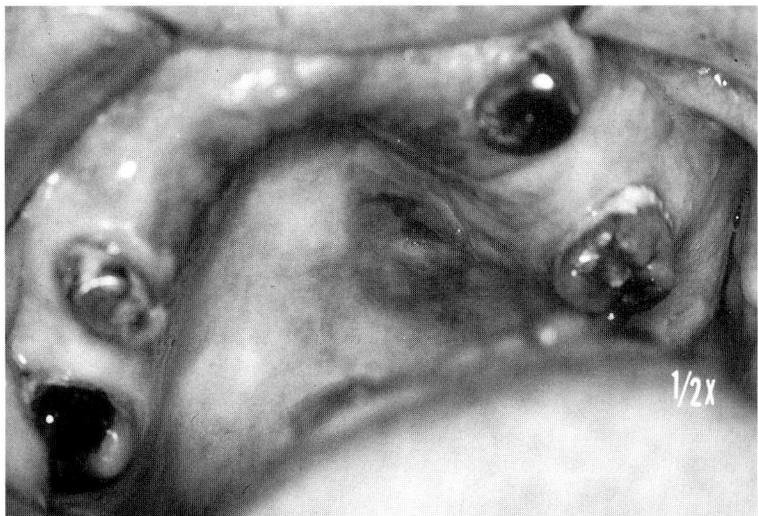

Figure 16–8. Adenoid cystic carcinoma of antrum involving descending palatine nerve and palate.

affects the abducens nerve first because of its lateral location in the cavernous sinus. This nerve has the longest course through the cavernous sinus. Tumor extension along the skull base to the petrous apex can involve cranial nerves VII, VIII, IX, X, and XI.

Cranial base tumors of long duration can cause severe headaches and neuropsychological changes. Patients may be disoriented and confused.[22] Meningitis also can occur. Intracranial and dural involvement, however, may cause no specific symptoms except for mild headache, even with massive intracranial tumor. When the sphenoid sinus is involved, pain is common. However, localization of sphenoid sinus pain can be variable. Pain may be felt at the occiput and mimic tension headaches or be noted at the vertex of the skull, the parietal bone, or retro-orbital areas. Many sites are possible for referred sphenoid sinus pain.[13]

Regional Symptoms

Patients may complain of decreased hearing as a result of serous otitis media from obstruction of the eustachian tube. Nasopharyngeal extension of nose and sinus tumors also can cause pain, skull base involvement, or bilateral nasal symptoms. As tumor extends into the infratemporal fossa, trismus may occur from invasion of the medial pterygoid muscle. Direct involvement of the cheek and temporal skin from tumor growth from the infratemporal or temporal fossa indicates advanced disease.

A mass in the neck may be metastatic spread of nose and sinus tumors. Involvement of the submandibular nodes, parotid nodes, or buccal nodes can occur with nasal cavity or vestibular tumors. Metastasis to the deep cervical nodes then can occur. Enlargement of the jugulodigastric nodes generally indicates secondary spread from the retropharyngeal nodes. The frequency of metastasis from cancer of the nose and sinus has been reported to range from 17.5% to 49.8%.[2] Metastatic disease is more common when there is tumor extension to the oral cavity, skin, orbit, or infratemporal fossa. Invasion of the cheek allows direct access to facial lymphatics and increases the risk for neck disease.[5]

Systemic Symptoms

Systemic symptoms occurs as a result of direct and indirect tumor effects. Indirect effects of tumor include infection, fever, fatigue, weakness, or generalized inanition. Systemic symptoms during the course of a nasal and sinus malignancy compound the direct tumor effects and often cause a painful, prolonged death. Distant metastasis occurs in approximately 12% of cases. The causes of death are hemorrhage (3%), intracranial extension (18%), systemic metastasis (8%), or bronchopneumonia (71%).[23]

Various studies have looked at the duration and frequency of symptoms present with nose and sinus tumors. Marchetta et al.[12] reported 119 patients with squamous cell carcinoma of the maxillary sinus. At the time of diagnosis, all patients had extension of the cancer outside the maxillary antrum to the orbit, nasal cavity, oral cavity, or skin of the cheek. The 5-year survival rate was only 25%. Another series[24] found the most common symptoms of nose and paranasal sinus tumors to be unilateral nasal obstruction (48%), facial or palatal swelling (41%), facial pain (41%), nasal discharge (37%), and epistaxis (35%). The time from the onset of symptoms until diagnosis was more than 8 months. The delay in diagnosis was greater for adenocarcinomas than for squamous cell carcinomas. Tumors that originated from the mucosal surface reached an advanced stage before causing many symptoms such as nasal stuffiness (40%), facial pain and swelling (29%) from bone destruction and infection, and epistaxis (29%) by erosion of small mucosal vessels. Symptoms often were treated conservatively because of an incorrect diagnosis of chronic sinusitis or nasal polyps. Delays in diagnosis ranged from 6 to 9 months.[5]

Chaudhry et al.,[25] in 1960, classified the signs and symptoms of nasal and sinus tumors into five groups. Group 1 (25% to 35%) were the oral signs and symptoms. These included dental-pulpal-type pain, loose teeth, malocclusion, trismus, or oroantral fistula after dental extraction. Group 2 were the findings from medial extension into the nasal cavity. These included unilateral nasal obstruction, unilateral watery or purulent rhinorrhea, epistaxis, pain, and awareness of a nasal mass. Group 3 were findings from orbital invasion. Ocular symptoms were found in 25% and included exophthalmos, diplopia, impaired vision, or fullness of the lower lid. Group 4 were facial symptoms from anterior tumor extension to the cheek. Loss of the nasolabial fold on the involved side was followed by obvious swelling and bulging. This was often painful, and signs of local inflammation were common. Other symptoms included cheek swelling, numbness, paresthesias, skin ulceration, and widening of the nasal dorsum. Group 5 were neurologic symptoms. When tumor extends into the base of the skull, meninges, and cranial nerves, headache, anosmia, meningitis, and cranial nerve deficits can occur.

Symptoms of nose and sinus tumors are listed in Table 16–1.

Table 16–1   Symptoms of Nose and Sinus Tumors

NASAL	SINUS	OPHTHALMOLOGIC	DENTAL	NEUROGENIC	OTHER SYMPTOMS
Nasal obstruction	Pain	Epiphora	Pain	Numbness of the cheek	Trismus
Rhinorrhea	Facial swelling	Proptosis	Loose teeth	Numbness of gingiva	Neck mass
Epistaxis		Chemosis	Oral antral fistula, extraction site, nonhealing	Numbness of palate	Decreased hearing
Pain		Diplopia		Dry eye	
Anosmia		Blindness	Inability to wear dentures	Diplopia	
Nasal mass		Palpable mass	Palatal mass	Forehead numbness	
Nasal deformity		Pain		Headache	
				Disorientation	
				Confusion	
				Numbness-V3	
				Involvement of cranial nerves VII–XII	

PHYSICAL EXAMINATION

Inspection of the nasal cavity provides the most information on physical examination. Before any examination, the nasal cavity must be decongested with a topical vasoconstrictor. Phenylephrine can be used as a spray, or cocaine and epinephrine solution can be applied on cotton pledgets. Concentrated lidocaine solution also can be used for topical anesthesia. During the waiting for the decongestant to work, the patient's head and neck area should be examined for external swelling, asymmetry, broadening or saddling of the external nasal dorsum, swelling of the cheek, proptosis, or neck swelling (Fig. 16–9).

The nasal cavity is then inspected with use of a nasal speculum and adequate illumination. Tumors in the nasal area may be necrotic, polypoid, or firm and smooth. Polypoid swollen mucosa from reaction to the tumor may obscure the lesion. Masses in the superior nasal cavity should be observed for pulsations, and the patient should be asked to perform a Valsalva maneuver so enlargement of the mass or a cerebrospinal fluid leak can be detected.

In one study, a fungating mass was found in 20% of cases and an ulcerative mass in 52% of cases of nasal cavity carcinoma.[5] Other tumor characteristics should be noted, including the shape, extent, degree of vascularity, color, friability to palpation, and possible site of origin. Tumors can be gently palpated with a cotton-tipped applicator to note their site of origin, their friability, and involvement of

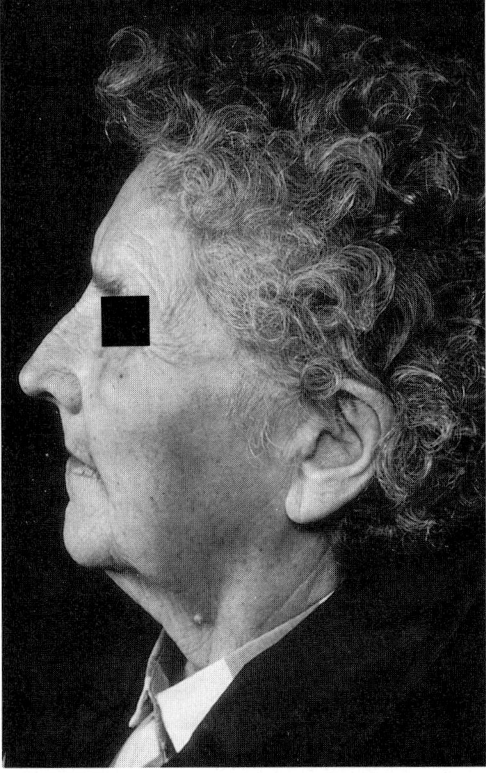

Figure 16–9. Swelling over zygoma from infratemporal fossa extension from squamous cell carcinoma of antrum.

adjacent structures. With use of a long-bladed nasal speculum and gentle palpation, it is often possible to determine whether the tumor is merely pushing or invading the septum, turbinates, lateral wall, or floor of the nose.

Palpation also plays an important role in the examination of nose and sinus tumors. Small tumors arising from the mucosal lining of the turbinates, septum, or sinus cavity cannot be palpated. However, vestibular lesions can be felt as a swelling, sore, or ulceration in the nasal vestibular skin. The nasal bones may show softening as a result of replacement of bone by tumor. The medial canthal region may reveal tumor extension from the ethmoids to the orbit with loss of the nasal bones and frontal process of the maxilla. Palpation should continue over the face of the maxilla to look for tumor extension into the soft tissues of the cheek. It is important to determine whether the skin is mobile or fixed to the tumor.[8] The inferior, medial, and superior orbital rims should be felt, and with a finger in the mouth the upper labial gingival sulcus and facial surface of the maxilla can be palpated. One can feel behind the maxillary tuberosity to assess the inferior infratemporal fossa. It is easy to directly inspect and palpate the teeth, alveolar ridge, and hard palate. The canine fossa and floor of the nose also can be easily assessed by finger palpation.

The neck should be examined for signs of cervical metastasis. The parotid glands, facial nodes, submandibular nodes, submental region, and the upper, middle, and lower jugular nodes must all be felt. Bimanual palpation of the neck is helpful for assessing the deeper nodes. Approximately 10% of cases have metastasis to the cervical nodes.[8]

Special nasal studies can be performed in the office and provide additional information about the tumor's characteristics and extent. Transillumination of the maxillary, ethmoid, and frontal sinuses may demonstrate sinus opacification. Endoscopic examination of the nose has become the most useful adjunct to the physical examination of the nose and sinus area. After the nose is adequately decongested and topically anesthetized, the nasal cavity, nasopharynx, inferior and middle meatus, sinus ostia, and superior nasal cavity all can be inspected with 0°, 30°, and 70° rigid scopes. A flexible fiberoptic scope also can be used and, in some cases, passed through the natural ostia into the maxillary sinus. Endoscopic examination of the nose should always be done whenever tumors are suspected.

A scratch-and-sniff smell test can be given to the patient to look for evidence of anosmia. This simple screening test can be followed by a more complete smell evaluation if hyposmia is noted. The presence of malingering can be detected by using ammonia because this will stimulate the fifth nerve and not the olfactory nerve. Olfaction should always be tested when a lesion involves the superior nasal cavity.

When a suspicious lesion is found on clinical examination, in most cases a biopsy should be performed. A contraindication to biopsy includes suspicion of angiofibroma, metastatic hypernephroma, or other vascular lesions. Another contraindication to biopsy is a known bleeding diathesis. In these cases, a biopsy should be done only in a hospital. In 99% of nasal and sinus tumors, when a mass is visible in the nasal cavity, biopsy can be safely done in the office. After the nose has been decongested, cocaine and epinephrine solution can be used to anesthetize the mass and surrounding area. Lidocaine and epinephrine then can be injected into the mass. After an appropriate time passes for vasoconstriction to occur, a biopsy specimen is taken with a small cups forceps and the specimen is sent for pathologic review. Cautery, if necessary, can be done with a silver nitrate stick or suction, or by placing a piece of absorbable gelatin sponge on the biopsy site. Packing is rarely necessary, but should be available. Biopsy of any suspicious lesions visualized during endoscopic examination should be done. This may result in an earlier diagnosis of nasal and sinus neoplasms.[6] A good light source, suction, and an assistant are helpful in performing a biopsy. Suction removes retained secretions, mucus, and blood to assist visualization. If the tumor is in the posterior nose or nasopharynx, a rigid or flexible scope can be placed into one side of the nose and a cups forceps placed through the opposite side of the nose for biopsy. For any lesion that is suspicious or not responding to medical management, biopsy should be done.[6]

Symptoms or physical findings may be suspicious for a neoplasm in the sinus region when a mass is not visible in the nose. This situation occurs most often with the maxillary sinus. In this case, the sinus can be inspected in the office after infiltrating the labial gingival sulcus with lidocaine and epinephrine. An incisive puncture is made into the antrum with a small trocar. The trocar is removed, and an endoscope is placed to examine the sinus. A separate opening can be used for a biopsy.

In the ethmoid region, when a tumor is suspected but no visible mass is seen in the nose, a swelling may be noted in the medial canthal area. Such lesions can undergo biopsy with a fine needle. For any palpable neck mass, biopsy can be done with a fine needle. Lesions in the pterygopalatine fossa, frontal or sphenoid sinus, or posterior ethmoids may require a surgical approach to the involved area in the operating room. For lesions not amenable to a safe endoscopic or direct biopsy in the office, biopsy should always be done in the operating room. The ethmoid sinus can be approached endoscopically or through a small external incision. The *frontal sinus* is inspected through a small external inferior frontal sinusotomy. The *sphenoid sinus* is opened endoscopically or through the transethmoidal or transeptal approach. The biopsy site should be located so subsequent operation would remove that area and sinus drainage provided if radiation therapy is planned.[26]

During examination of a nose and sinus tumor, the neck should be exposed completely. The neck is carefully palpated for any evidence of cervical adenopathy. The patient should remove dentures, and a complete head and neck examination is performed. The oral cavity is inspected closely to evaluate the hard palate and alveolar ridge (Fig. 16–10). One looks for loose teeth or other dental problems. The nasopharynx must be inspected with a mirror or a fiberoptic or rigid endoscope. The ears should be checked for evidence of serous otitis media or middle ear mass. A complete laryngeal and hypopharyngeal examination is done to complete the assessment of all cranial nerves.

V2 is evaluated by testing sensation of the cheek and upper lip. The anterior superior alveolar nerve is assessed by checking sensation on the facial surface of the gingiva of the incisor and canine teeth. The posterior superior alveolar nerve is tested by measuring sensation on the labial surface of the gingiva of the molar and premolar teeth and alveolar ridge. The descending palatine nerve is assessed by testing sensation of the hard and soft palate.

Ophthalmologic consultation may be necessary with nasal or sinus tumors to assess orbital involvement. At that time, the degree of proptosis, ocular mobility,

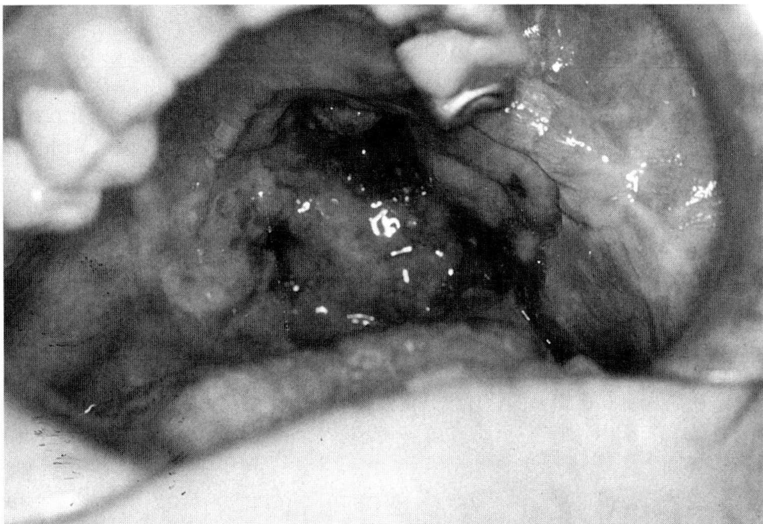

Figure 16–10. Invasive verrucous carcinoma of nasal cavity extending into palate.

visual field, and visual acuity can be tested. An accurate preoperative assessment of these factors is important. Schirmer's test is done to measure tearing by placing a filter paper in each lower conjunctiva for 5 minutes. The length of moistening of the paper is measured in millimeters. One side is compared with the other for asymmetry.

Some authors advocate initial exploration of nose and sinus tumors via a Caldwell-Luc approach to determine the tumor's extent, plan treatment, and perform a biopsy. The author does not agree. The tumor's extent should be adequately determined by a complete history, physical examination, and imaging studies. Exploratory operation for debulkment and assessment of the tumor's extent is not indicated given the ease of biopsy and advances in imaging.

Knowledge of nose and sinus anatomy, a thorough history, and a thorough head and neck examination should provide invaluable information about the extent of nose and sinus neoplasms. The involved area is complex, and an in-depth examination and history are necessary. Information gained from the examination should augment and enhance that obtained from additional studies.

OTHER STUDIES

Accurate determination of the tumor's location and histologic features is necessary to formulate treatment, predict prognosis, and report the results of therapy. Imaging studies are the most useful means to determine the tumor's extent. Plain films, tomograms, and ultrasound evaluations have no current role in the evaluation of nose and sinus neoplasms. Currently, computed tomography (CT) and magnetic resonance (MR) are the studies of choice. They complement one another, and often both are performed. High-resolution, fast, thin-section CT scans best determine bone erosion. CT is especially helpful to study the ethmoid sinus, cribriform plate, orbital walls, posterior maxillary fossa, pterygoid plates, and sphenoid walls (Fig. 16–11). The use of contrast is essential to identify intracranial spread. Direct axial and coronal CT images should be obtained if the patient can tolerate the positioning necessary for a coronal image. CT also has replaced linear and polypleural directional tomography, ultrasonography, and radioisotope scanning.[2]

With CT it is difficult to distinguish soft tissue tumor extension from inflammatory tissue or retained secretions from blockage of sinus ostia. MR does delineate tumor from surrounding soft tissue, inflammatory tissue, and retained secretions.[27] MR is performed with gadolinium enhancement and has the advantage of providing multiplanar information with no radiation exposure. MR is especially helpful for detecting neurogenic spread. In addition, MR has no loss of detail from dental amalgams.[4] For nose and sinus tumors, MR is not a superior imaging study to CT but is used in conjunction with CT to give additional information.[4]

Imaging studies are necessary to look for evidence of involvement of the middle fossa, cavernous sinus, lateral portion of the sphenoid wall or clivus, or evidence of distant metastasis. Reduced survival is noted with these findings. Prognosis is also poor when the pterygopalatine fossa, infratemporal fossa, cervical nodes, eustachian tube area, or nasopharynx is involved.[3]

With MR, the tumor's extent is best seen on T2-weighted images. Inflammatory tissue has a bright T2 image. Only 5% of tumors have a bright T2 image. These tumors include minor salivary gland neoplasms and neuromas. Most squamous cell carcinomas can be distinguished from adjacent inflammatory tissue with the use of MR.[27] One study compared CT and MR for nasal and sinus tumors. The correlation between histologic findings at operation and CT was only 85.2%. A positive correlation between MR and histologic findings was 94.1%. This rate increased to 98.4% with the use of gadolinium.[28]

It is not always possible to delineate a malignant from a benign neoplasm on the basis of imaging studies. Squamous cell carcinomas have aggressive bone destruc-

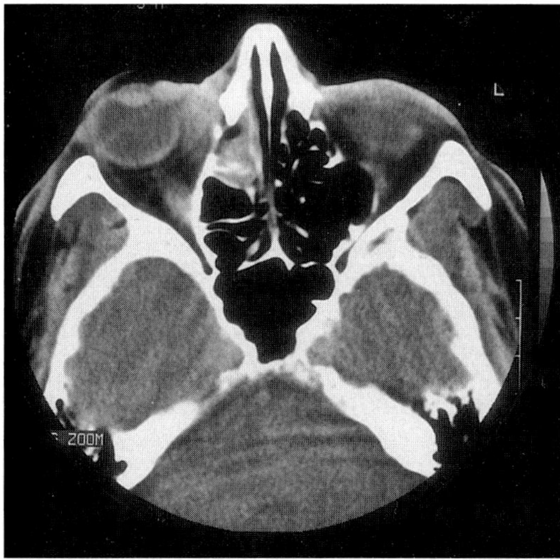

Figure 16–11. Squamous cell carcinoma of ethmoid sinus with invasion of orbit, well depicted with computed tomography.

tion without remodeling or reshaping in 80% of cases.[8] Opacification, expansion, or destruction of bone can occur in both benign and malignant neoplasms. Unfortunately, many of the signs, symptoms, and radiographic findings of benign and malignant neoplasms are similar. Bone destruction with a mass lesion can be seen with a mucocele or a cancer.[8] Slow-growing neoplasms can remodel the nasal vault and facial bones rather than destroying them. Once remodeling is seen, the radiographic impression is a nonaggressive lesion. When aggressive bone destruction is present, generally the radiographic interpretation is cancer.[29] However, if the involved bone is non-sinus, such as the floor of the anterior fossa, cavernous sinus, or floor of the middle fossa, bone destruction may be due to a benign process. The bones of the skull base may erode easier than the facial bones.[29]

Angiography may be indicated for certain nose and sinus tumors. When the history and physical examination suggest an angiofibroma, and if the tumor extends beyond the nasal cavity and maxillary sinus, angiography is always indicated. With enhancement on CT or when a tumor extends to the carotid artery, angiography may be helpful. Vascular tumors, such as hemangiomas, hemangiopericytomas, or metastatic hypernephromas, that involve the sphenoid and middle fossa often are studied by angiography. Other lesions, rhabdomyosarcomas and esthesioneuroblastomas, may show moderate enhancement on contrast CT but do not require angiography.

Patients with tumors that involve the nasopharynx or appear to have their origin from the nasopharynx should have Epstein-Barr virus titers determined to measure early antigen and viral capsid antigen titers. All patients should have chest radiography and liver function tests to rule out distant disease.

Accurate pathologic interpretation of biopsy specimens is essential. Standard microscopic hematoxylin-eosin examinations will diagnose most nasal and paranasal sinus tumors. The high-grade undifferentiated malignancies, however, may require special studies, especially lesions involving the cribriform plate region. Diagnostic dilemmas include undifferentiated carcinoma, anaplastic carcinoma, rhabdomyosarcoma, esthesioneuroblastoma, neuroendocrine carcinoma, lymphoma, and melanoma. For these tumors, paraffin section immunostains are helpful. The keratin stain looks for evidence of carcinoma. S-100 and HMB-45 staining are done for melanoma. A leukocyte common antigen stain will be positive in lymphoma. Synaptophism or neuron-specific enylase are two neuroendocrine markers positive in olfactory neuroblastoma or neuroendocrine carcinoma. Other markers such as actin, desmin, and myoglobin are positive in rhabdomyosarcoma. For lymphoma, it is often necessary to obtain fresh frozen tissue for immunostains or molecular genetic studies.

Tumor staging for nose and sinus tumors is not universally reported or accepted. The American Joint Committee on Cancer does have a staging system for maxillary antral carcinomas that makes use of Ohngren's line (a theoretical plane joining the medial canthus with the angle of the mandible). It recognizes four stages: T1, a tumor confined to the antral mucosa of the infrastructure with no bone erosion or destruction; T2, a tumor confined to the suprastructure mucosa without bone destruction or to the infrastructure with destruction of the medial or inferior bony walls only; T3, a more extensive tumor invading skin of the cheek, orbit, anterior ethmoid sinuses, or pterygoid muscles; and T4, massive tumor with invasion of the cribriform plate, posterior ethmoid, sphenoid, nasopharynx, pterygoid plates, or base of the skull. Numerous staging systems are used for olfactory neuroblastoma, angiofibroma, and other specific tumors of the nose and paranasal sinuses. No universal staging system exists for lesions of the nasal cavity or other sinus areas.

Table 16–2 lists some of the common benign and malignant neoplasms found in the nasal and sinus cavity. Select symptoms and physical findings for certain benign and malignant tumors follow.

SPECIFIC BENIGN NEOPLASMS

Inverting papillomas are common benign tumors usually found in the nasal cavity. Seventy-five percent of the patients are between 40 and 70 years old, and males are predominantly affected. The most common symptoms in one series were nasal obstruction (65%), awareness of a polyp in the nose (21%), sinusitis or pain (14%), nasal bleeding (12%), and postnasal drip (7%).[30] These tumors generally are found on the lateral wall of the nose. They rarely are found in the paranasal sinuses alone. These tumors are described as polypoid, irregular, papillomatous, or firm. Bone erosion or destruction of the lateral wall of the nose is not uncommon.[30]

Angiofibromas are unique, vascular, benign neoplasms occurring in male adolescents. The age range in one series was 7 to 29 years. The median age at diagnosis was 15 years.[31] Epistaxis (87%), nasal obstruction (80%), nasal drainage (3%), facial deformity (13%), otitis (3%), palatal bulging (3%), and proptosis (13%) all occurred. Patients may be misdiagnosed with sinusitis, rhinitis, or an antrochoanal polyp. The duration of symptoms has decreased from that in earlier series and is now 6 months. The gross appearance is a pale blue, smooth, often lobulated mass arising in the posterolateral nasopharynx.

Table 16–2 Nose and Sinus Tumors

BENIGN	MALIGNANT
Osteoma	Squamous cell carcinoma
Inverting papilloma	Adenocarcinoma: high-grade, low-grade, colonic type
Fungiform papilloma	Adenoid cystic carcinoma
Ossifying fibroma	Minor salivary gland malignancies
Hemangioma	Sarcomas
Lymphangioma	Chondrosarcoma
	Fibrosarcoma
	Osteogenic sarcoma
	Hemangiopericytoma
	Esthesioneuroblastoma
	Lymphoma
	Plasmacytoma
	Malignant melanoma
	Metastatic tumors

SPECIFIC MALIGNANT NEOPLASMS

A review of 1,297 patients with malignant tumors of the nasal and sinus cavity found 91% carcinomas, 7% sarcomas, 2% melanomas, and 0.3% esthesioneuroblastomas.[6] The most frequent symptoms at the time of onset were swelling of the cheek (29%), nasal obstruction (28%), epistaxis (20%), and nasal discharge (20%). At the time of initial examination, swelling of the cheek was present in 80%, nasal obstruction in 70%, discharge in 70%, dysesthesias in 60%, epistaxis in 52%, and lacrimation in 50%.[6]

Study of maxillary sinus carcinoma found that pain and nasal obstruction were the most common symptoms[32] (Fig. 16–12). A mass in the cheek was the most frequent physical finding. Eighty-two percent of all maxillary sinus tumors presented as advanced disease, stage III or IV. Palpable neck nodes at the time of diagnosis were present in 10%.

Rare sphenoid sinus tumors have been reported. Six isolated tumors of the sphenoid sinus were squamous cell carcinomas, lymphoepitheliomas, and adenocarcinomas.[33] Three patients had diplopia, two presented with pain, and one had nasal congestion, tinnitus, and unilateral sensorineural hearing loss. Before diagnosis and treatment, five of the six patients had visual alterations, and four had progressive retro-orbital, frontoparietal, or occipital pain or headache. All six had

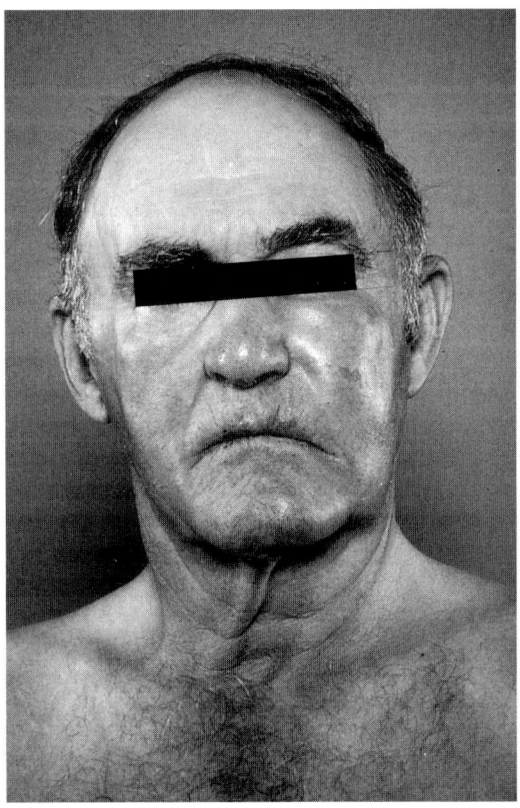

Figure 16–12. *A*, Facial deformity from extensive squamous cell carcinoma of antrum. *B*, Tumor extent well delineated on computed tomography. *C*, Surgical resection before free flap reconstruction.

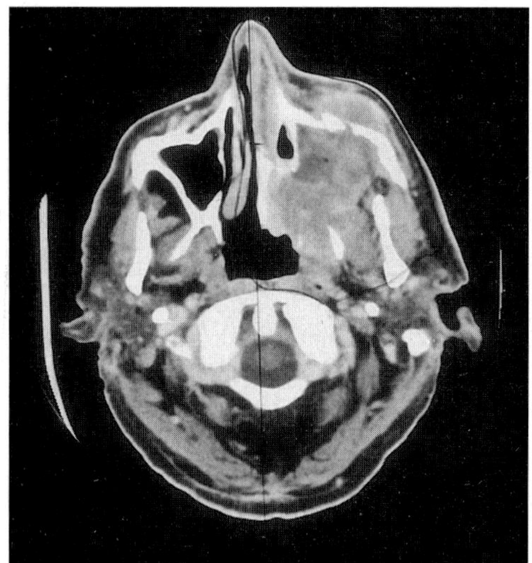

B

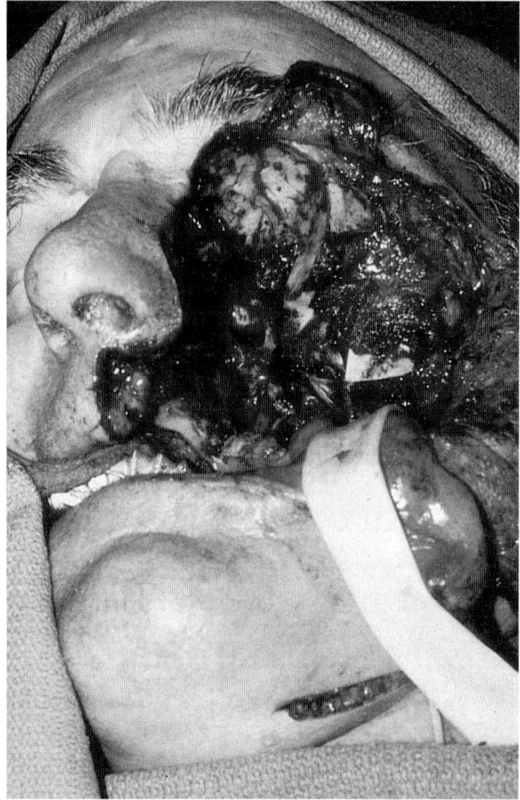

C

Figure 16–12. *Continued.*

evidence of proptosis and cranial nerve involvement. Cranial nerves II through VII were affected. Two patients had cervical lymphadenopathy. The tumors were all high-grade lesions treated with radiation therapy. There were no survivors beyond 33 months.[34]

Adenocarcinomas make up less than 10% of all malignant nose and sinus tumors. These include adenoid cystic carcinomas and low- and high-grade adenocarcinomas.[3] A small group of pure adenocarcinomas mimic adenocarcinoma of the colon histologically and are termed "colonic-type" adenocarcinoma. These are generally large, vascular-appearing, polypoid masses found in the nasal cavity. They often present with nasal obstruction and epistaxis. They are commonly found during the fifth through the seventh decades. The likely site is the superior nasal cavity or ethmoid region.[35] Adenocarcinomas have three patterns of growth: sessile, papillary, and alveolar. Invasion and destruction of adjacent soft tissue and bone occur, yet the low-grade tumors rarely metastasize.[3]

Chondrosarcomas are the most frequent sarcoma. The main symptoms are nasal obstruction, nasal discharge, and epistaxis. Facial pain, toothache, diplopia, and epiphora are less common. The male:female distribution was equal in one series.[31] On clinical examination, the lesions were a moderately firm to hard mass. Two patients presented with proptosis, and one had an external deformity of the cheek. The gross appearance is a pale, glistening, fleshy mass varying in consistency from soft to firm.[36]

Esthesioneuroblastomas (olfactory neuroblastomas) are rare neoplasms of neuroectodermal origin. They are commonly found in the cribriform region, in the upper third of the nasal septum, and along the superior and supreme nasal turbinates. Epistaxis and nasal obstruction are the most frequent symptoms, but other symptoms at the time of diagnosis can include tearing, pain, diplopia, proptosis, and anosmia. The time from onset of symptoms until diagnosis can be long, ranging from several months to 10 years. These tumors generally bleed easily on palpation and often are a red, granular, polypoid mass. They may appear to be a small polypoid area filling the cribriform area. Cervical metastasis at some time during the patient's illness can occur in up to 40% of cases. The tumors generally are found equally in males and females and are most commonly found in the sixth decade of life.[37]

Melanomas account for 1% of all nasal and paranasal sinus lesions. They are often multicentric, and early metastasis is common. They are generally gray, blue, or black. There is no sex predilection, and the lesions occur from the fifth to the eighth decade of life. In one series, 54 of 56 melanomas had an obvious nasal mass and 18% had cervical metastasis.[38] In 14% of cases a polypoid growth pattern was found. Epistaxis and nasal obstruction were present in 88% of patients, 16% complained of pain, and 5% to 9% noted swelling of the face, nose, palate, or neck. Patients with melanoma in the nose had a better prognosis than those whose lesions arose in the sinus.

Patients with spheno-occipital chordoma may present with nasal symptoms that include unilateral nasal obstruction, rhinorrhea, and hyponasal speech. One study found patients with nasal symptoms but no neurologic complaints.[35] These tumors are present at birth and, at some unspecified time, become aggressive. Unilateral nasal abnormality should always be viewed with suspicion. Clival chordomas are difficult to extirpate surgically.

Hemangiopericytomas of the nasal cavity are usually considered to be malignant. In a report of 10 patients from the Mayo Clinic, 8 were male and 2 were female.[37] The average age was 52 years (range, 44 to 72 years). Hemangiopericytomas can originate from the floor of the nasal vestibule, the posterior superior portion of the nasal septum, the choana, the nasopharynx, and the cribriform area and ethmoids. Signs and symptoms of hemangiopericytoma were nasal obstruction in five patients, epistaxis in two, and awareness of a mass in three. The duration of signs and symptoms ranged from several months to as long as 15 years. The tumors are nonencapsulated, firm, and often pink to tan. Only occasionally is the vascular nature suspected from gross examination.

Metastasis to the nose and paranasal sinuses occurs in 1% of cancers in this area. Renal cell carcinoma is the most frequent tumor and can be vascular. Other undifferentiated tumors from the breast, lung, prostate, and pancreas also can metastasize to the nasal area.

Unfortunately, there rarely are symptoms and physical findings that are unique to specific nasal or sinus tumors. Diagnosis, assessment of extent, and appropriate treatment still depend on an appropriate history, a complete physical examination, imaging studies, and accurate pathologic interpretation of biopsy specimens.

REFERENCES

1. Pearson BW: The surgical anatomy of maxillectomy. *Surg Clin North Am* 1977; 57:701–721.
2. Rice DH, Stanley RB Jr: Surgical Therapy of Nasal Cavity, Ethmoid Sinus, and Maxillary Sinus Tumors, vol. 1, in Thawley SE, Panje WR, Batsakis JG, Lindberg RD (eds): *Comprehensive Management of Head and Neck Tumors*. Philadelphia, Saunders, 1987, pp 368–390.
3. DeSanto LW: Neoplasms, vol. 1, in Cummings CW, Fredrickson JM, Harker LA, Krause CJ, Schuller DE (eds): *Otolaryngology–Head and Neck Surgery*. St. Louis, Mosby, 1986, pp 639–650.
4. Krespi YP, Levine TM: Tumors of the Nose and Paranasal Sinuses, in Paparella MM, Shumrick DA, Gluckman JL, Meyerhoff WL (eds): *Otolaryngology*, Vol 3: Head and Neck, ed. 3. Philadelphia, Saunders, 1991, pp 1935–1958.
5. Kramer TS: Nasal Vestibule, Nasal Cavity, and Paranasal Sinuses, in Larramore G (ed): *Radiation Therapy of Head and Neck Cancer*. New York, Springer-Verlag, 1989, pp 145–170.
6. Miyaguchi M, Sakai S, Mori N, Kitaoku S: Symptoms in patients with maxillary sinus carcinoma. *J Laryngol Otol* 1990; 104:557–559.
7. Osguthorpe JD: Sinus neoplasia. *Arch Otolaryngol Head Neck Surg* 1994; 120:19–25.
8. Sisson G, Becker S, Snyderman NL: Cancer of the Nasal Cavity and Paranasal Sinuses, in Suen JY, Myers EN (eds): *Cancer of the Head and Neck*, ed. 2. New York, Churchill Livingstone, 1981, pp 311–336.
9. Roenigk RK, Ratz JL, Bailin PL, Wheeland RG: Trends in the presentation and treatment of basal cell carcinomas. *J Derm Surg Oncol* 1986; 12:860–865.
10. Barton RT: Nickel carcinogenesis of the respiratory tract. *Otolaryngology* 1977; 6:412–422.
11. Zheng W, McLaughlin JK, Chow WH, et al: Risk factors for cancers of the nasal cavity and paranasal sinuses among white men in the United States. *Am J Epidemiol* 1993; 138:965–972.
12. Marchetta FC, Sako K, Mattick WL, Stinziano GD: Squamous cell carcinoma of the maxillary antrum. *Am J Surg* 1969; 118:805–807.
13. Donald PJ: Surgical Evaluation: Tumors of the Nasal Cavity and Paranasal Sinuses, vol. 1, in Thawley SE, Panje WR, Batsakis JG, Lindberg RD (eds): *Comprehensive Management of Head and Neck Tumors*. Philadelphia, Saunders, 1987, pp 304–326.
14. Ohngren LG: Cited by Pearson BW.[15]
15. Pearson BW: Surgical Therapy of the Nasal Cavity and Paranasal Sinuses: Surgical Anatomy, vol. 1, in Thawley SE, Panje WR, Batsakis JG, Lindberg RD (eds): *Comprehensive Management of Head and Neck Tumors*. Philadelphia, Saunders, 1987, pp 353–367.
16. Shockley WW: Special problems associated with carcinoma of the nose. *Otolaryngol Clin North Am* 1993; 26:247–264.
17. Butlin HT: *On the Operative Surgery of Malignant Disease*. London, J & A Churchill, 1887.
18. Rubin P: Cancer of the head and neck. *JAMA* 1972; 219:336–338.
19. Stanley RJ, Olsen KD, Muller SA, Roenigk RK: Aggressive intranasal carcinoma mimicking infection or inflammation. *Cutis* 1988; 42:288–293.

20. Brownson RJ, Ogurra JH: Primary carcinoma of the frontal sinus. *Laryngoscope* 1971; 81:71–89.
21. Hayasaka S, Sekimoto M, Shibasaki H, et al: Ophthalmologic complications in patients with malignant tumors of the nose and paranasal sinuses. *Ann Ophthalmol* 1992; 24:429–433.
22. Neubauer U, Fahlbusch R, Wigand ME, Weidenbecher M: Malignant tumors of the anterior cranial skull base. *Neurosurg Rev* 1992; 15:187–192.
23. Harrison DFN: The natural history of some cancers affecting the head and neck. *J Laryngol Otol* 1972; 86:1189–1202.
24. Tabb HG, Barranco SJ: Cancer of the maxillary sinus: An analysis of 108 cases. *Laryngoscope* 1971; 81:818–827.
25. Chaudhry AP, Gorlin RJ, Mosser DG: Carcinoma of the antrum: A clinical and histopathologic study. *Oral Surg Oral Med Oral Pathol* 1960; 13:269–281.
26. Weymuller EA Jr: Neoplasms, vol. 1, in Cummings CW, Fredrickson JM, Harker LA, Krause CJ, Schuller DE (eds): *Otolaryngology–Head and Neck Surgery*. St. Louis, Mosby, 1986, pp 923–926.
27. Som PM, Shapiro MD, Biller HF, et al: Sinonasal tumors and inflammatory tissues: differentiation with MR imaging. *Radiology* 1988; 167:803–808.
28. Lund VJ, Howard DJ, Lloyd GA, Cheesman AD: Magnetic resonance imaging of paranasal sinus tumors for craniofacial resection. *Head Neck* 1989; 11:279–283.
29. Som PM, Lawson W, Lidov MW: Simulated aggressive skull base erosion in response to benign sinonasal disease. *Radiology* 1991; 180:755–759.
30. Suh KW, Facer GW, Devine KD, et al: Inverting papilloma of the nose and paranasal sinuses. *Laryngoscope* 1977; 87:35–46.
31. Spiro JD, Soo KC, Spiro RH: Squamous carcinoma of the nasal cavity and paranasal sinuses. *Am J Surg* 1989; 158:328–332.
32. Wyllie JW III, Kern EB, Djalilian M: Isolated sphenoid sinus lesions. *Laryngoscope* 1973; 83:1252–1265.
33. Coates HL, Pearson BW, Devine KD, Unni KK: Chondrosarcoma of the nasal cavity, paranasal sinuses, and nasopharynx. *Trans Am Acad Ophthalmol Otolaryngol* 1977; 84:919–926.
34. Campbell WM, McDonald TJ, Unni KK, Laws ER Jr: Nasal and paranasal presentations of chordomas. *Laryngoscope* 1980; 90:612–618.
35. Salassa JR, McDonald TJ, Weiland LH: "Colonic type" adenocarcinoma of the nasal cavity and paranasal sinuses. *Otolaryngol Head Neck Surg* 1980; 88:133–135.
36. Freedman HM, DeSanto LW, Devine KD, Weiland LH: Malignant melanoma of the nasal cavity and paranasal sinuses. *Arch Otolaryngol* 1973; 97:322–325.
37. Olsen KD, DeSanto LW: Olfactory neuroblastoma: Biologic and clinical behavior. *Arch Otolaryngol* 1983; 109:797–802.
38. Gorenstein A, Facer GW, Weiland LH: Hemangiopericytoma of the nasal cavity. *Otolaryngology* 1978; 86:405–415.

17

Nasal Trauma

JAN L. KASPERBAUER, M.D.

The diagnosis of nasal trauma begins in various settings because the population of patients and the injuries involved are diverse. Otolaryngologists may have initial contact with a patient who has sustained nasal injuries in the outpatient setting, the emergency room, or the operating room. To diagnose nasal trauma accurately in each of these settings, the history, examination, and ancillary investigations performed vary accordingly. The flow diagram in this chapter presents the major activities and decisions required by a physician evaluating nasal trauma. Obviously, every decision made by a physician cannot be detailed. The goal of this chapter is to outline key points in history taking, examination, and ancillary studies to diagnose nasal injuries accurately (Fig. 17–1).

BACKGROUND INFORMATION

Scope of Nasal Injuries

Three structural elements of the nose must be assessed in cases of nasal injuries in order to plan treatment correctly: the skin and soft tissue covering of the nose, the bony and cartilaginous elements, and the mucosa.

The skin and soft tissues of the nose begin superiorly at the nasofrontal angle and in the midline extend to the base of the columella. The lateral margins of the nasal skin extend from the alar base inferolaterally to the medial border of the upper and lower eyelid skin superiorly. Skin injuries include abrasions, contusions, lacerations, degloving injuries, and tissue loss. The unique characteristics of the tissues at the alar margins, the alar base, and the soft tissue facets require close scrutiny. The soft tissue triangle at the apex of the nostril (bridging the columella and the ala) is *soft*, pliable, and thin in most persons. Accurate diagnosis and repair of cutaneous injuries in this area are mandatory to maintain the integrity of this structure. The alar base lacks any underlying cartilaginous or bony skeleton to maintain its unique shape, and very accurate closure of lacerations is required when cutaneous injuries involve the alar base. If injuries along the margin of the ala are lacking in tissue approximation, notching and resultant asymmetry are striking.

The bony and cartilaginous injuries of the nose include nondisplaced fractures, nondisplaced fractures with hematoma, fracture with displacement, and fractures associated with mucosal or skin disruption. For cosmetic and functional considerations, key areas to assess for fracture displacement include the nasal bones, pyriform aperture, frontal process of the maxilla, tip support structures, and septum.

Mucosal injuries are common in nasal trauma and are frequently signaled by epistaxis. Mucosal injuries may include the same spectrum as skin injuries. Close attention must be directed toward detecting hematoma formation in the potential space between the cartilage and perichondrium of the cartilages of the nose. Identification and treatment of hematomas are mandatory because fibrosis of a hematoma may subsequently cause displacement and malpositioning of a cartilage. More significantly, infection and abscess formation related to a hematoma may result in loss of the underlying cartilage.

Simple and complex nasal injuries have not been clearly differentiated. Factors that increase the potential for residual dorsal deformity, external scarring, and nasal obstruction contribute to complex nasal injuries. Many factors must be considered in determining which injuries are at high risk for cosmetic or functional sequellae and therefore yield a complex nasal injury. Features that contribute to complex nasal injuries include high-velocity injuries, multiple associated facial fractures, and tissue loss. Simple nasal injuries, however, typically are low-velocity injuries, lack other associated facial fractures, and have minimal tissue disruption.

Elements in Diagnosis of Nasal Injury

Key elements in diagnosing nasal injuries include the history, physical examination, and ancillary studies. During the evaluation, information may be gained in a disjunctive fashion, but key elements in each of these areas help a physician determine the presence and extent of the nasal injury.

Information regarding the energy and direction of impact are important elements in the diagnosis of nasal trauma because these variables influence the extent of injury and the potential for associated injuries involving the remaining facial skeleton, orbit, cervical spine, or other body cavities.[1] High-energy forces typically result in more extensive injuries and increase the likelihood of associated facial, orbital, and cervical spine injuries. Injuries sustained in a motor vehicle accident, falls, and other high-energy insults require investigation through either consultation with appropriate specialists or radiologic investigation of the cervicothoracic spine and potential injuries of the central nervous system. Further information regarding the setting of the injury may increase the likelihood of implantation of foreign bodies, necessitating close inspection of the wound for various particles. If a history of a penetrating injury rather than blunt injury is gained, more detailed investigation of deeper tissues is required.

Several general historical factors need to be considered. A history of a bleeding diathesis or use of anticoagulant medication is important to document. The potential for infectious disease must be assessed. Further, any medical allergies must be detected. Documentation of a patient's premorbid appearance (old photographs) and sense of smell are important to note. Further, the blood loss associated with the injury must be estimated.

The physical examination together with the history should provide an accurate assessment of the extent of injuries and allow formulation of a treatment plan.[1,2] The steps in the physical examination vary, depending on the extent of injury and the patient's condition. If epistaxis is ongoing, often the initial steps are examining the mucosal surfaces of the nose and controlling the epistaxis. Regardless of the initial efforts required related to the trauma and initial condition of the patient, a complete head and neck examination should be performed, and the orbits should also be assessed. Depending on the severity of the injury, assessment for other facial injuries, spinal cord injuries, or other bodily cavity injuries may need to be done. An intregal part of the physical examination includes the patient's vital signs. A focused nasal examination includes assessment of the skin, bony cartilaginous structures, and the mucosal surfaces of the nose. Marked swelling and edema may prevent accurate assessment of the degree of bony and cartilaginous injury and can be repeated in 5 to 10 days, once the swelling has significantly decreased. Evidence for a cerebrospinal fluid leak with high-energy injuries should also be sought in the physical examination.

Instrumentation, a key element in the diagnosis, required for accurate assessment of nasal injuries includes an indirect light source to allow both hands to be used for palpation. The recent addition of endoscopic examination, with both flexible and rigid telescopes, provides another avenue to investigate the middle and posterior intranasal structures with greater accuracy. Palpation is a key element in the assessment of nasal trauma because crepitus overlying the bony skeleton of the nose strongly suggests fracture and dislocation. Subcutaneous emphysema also can produce crepitus with a distinctly different tactile sensation. Lacerations should be closely inspected to determine depth and potential involvement for underlying cartilaginous structures and exposure of bone. Through and through incisions require identification also. If significant swelling has not occurred, or once the swelling has resolved, the symmetry and alignment of the bony and cartilaginous structures should be assessed and compared to the pre-morbid condition of the nose.

Several ancillary studies may be useful in evaluating nasal trauma. These include laboratory investigations, radiography, and photography. Laboratory studies are helpful if there is a history of a bleeding diathesis or significant blood loss in which transfusions may be required. Radiographic investigations are of limited use in simple nasal injuries unless there are radiopaque foreign bodies that require localization. With increasing severity of injuries, the utility of computed tomography increases to investigate the degree of comminution and potential for intracranial and other craniofacial injuries. Photographic documentation should be routinely done in nasal injuries, and the highest quality photographs available should be obtained. However, when patients with multiple injuries are rapidly transferred to the operating room, studio-quality photographic documentation is not possible. Such information, however, is useful for characterizing the initial extent of injury.

PATHWAY IN THE DIAGNOSIS OF NASAL TRAUMA

The information initially presented to an evaluating physician begins the process of characterizing the extent of nasal injury. This information may be relayed from the emergency room, another physician, the patient, or parent for describing the mecha-

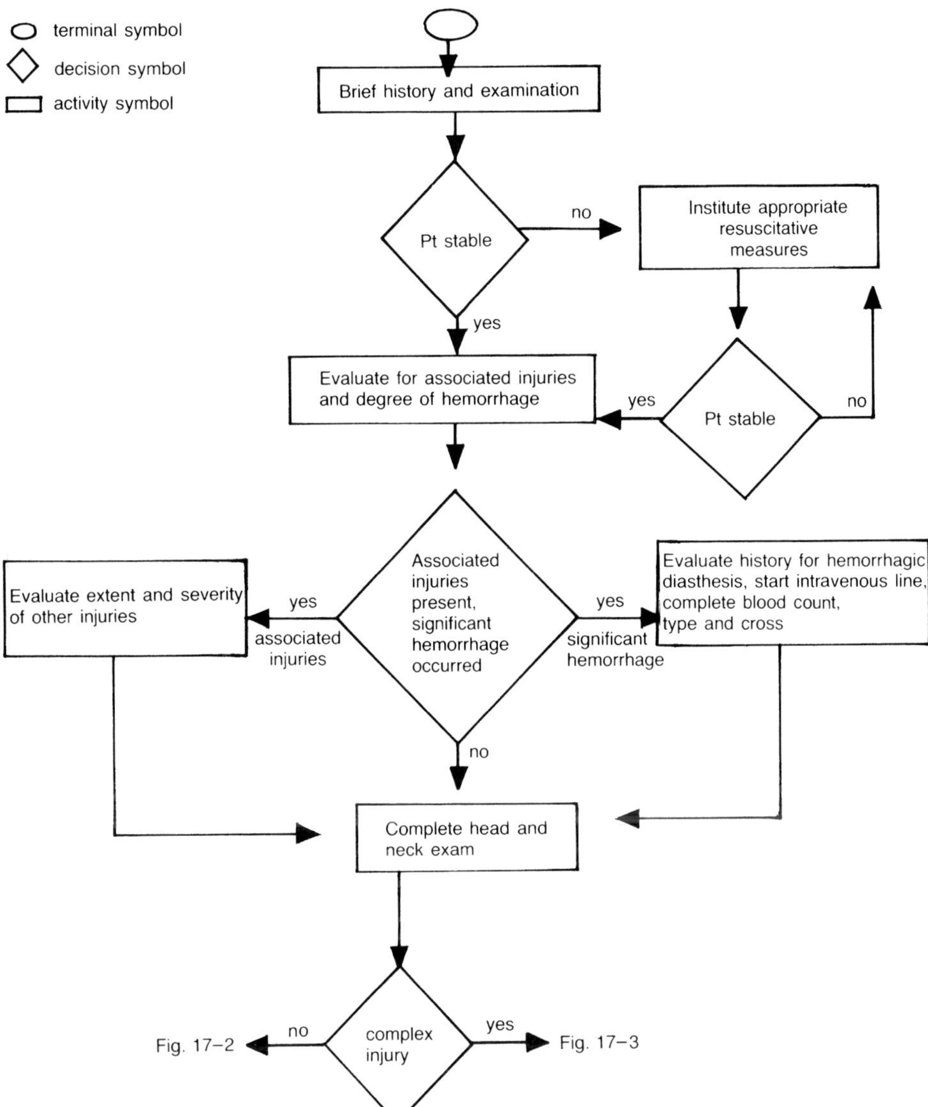

Figure 17–1. Initial evaluation of nasal trauma.

nism of injury. A brief visual examination of the patient in combination with data regarding the injury and vital signs enables a physician to establish whether a patient is stable.

Example 1: A patient presents in the office 5 days after an altercation in which he was struck in the nose with a fist. Brief epistaxis occurred, and he notes a nasal deformity and difficulty breathing through his nose. A brief examination reveals a C-shaped deformity of the dorsum, bony crepitus, minimal ecchymosis, and a septal deformity.

Example 2: A 25-year-old woman presents to the emergency room with a nasal injury and ongoing epistaxis after a blow to the nose and midface with a softball bat while catching at a softball game. The epistaxis has been profuse, and the patient is light-headed and tachycardic. Brief examination reveals bilateral epistaxis, ecchymosis, and edema of the nasal dorsum, left infraorbital region, and conjunctiva. The patient's blood pressure is 100/60 mm Hg.

Example 3: A patient involved in a motor vehicle accident sustained multiple orthopedic injuries and is en route to the operating room. The nasal injury, including a laceration, prompts an otolaryngology consultation. The patient is unconscious and intubated. Screening computed tomography of the head does not reveal any intracranial injuries. A brief examination before the onset of orthopedic surgery reveals a laceration of the right nose through the alar margin extending to the right nasal bone. The nasal bones are comminuted, and there is watery drainage intermixed with a slight hemorrhagic ooze from the right side of the nose.

If, based on this information, the patient is unstable, whether related to airway, breathing, or circulation, appropriate resuscitative measures should be instituted. Once the patient is stable, subsequent evaluation for associated injuries and assessment of the degree of hemorrhage can be done. If there has been significant hemorrhage, then type and cross-matching, intravenous fluid resuscitation, and complete blood cell count should be done. Historical information regarding a bleeding diathesis or use of anticoagulant medication should also be sought. The history of the injury and associated physical findings suggesting other associated injuries, whether orbital, intracranial, cervical, or thoracic spine, also may require further evaluation. If there is a question regarding the potential of intracranial or spinal injuries, then appropriate consultation with neurological/neurosurgical services is warranted, and these assessments should take priority over the nasal injury. A complete head and neck examination should be included when allowed by the patient's condition.

In example 1, there is no evidence to suggest that the patient is unstable. Therefore, evaluation can progress to assessing any associated injuries and degree of hemorrhage. Certainly, historical information regarding any loss of consciousness, any changes in vision, and any history of pain at other sites in the body is important. If the hemorrhage was brief, then evaluation proceeds to a more complete head and neck examination, including a more complete past medical history.

In example 2, the stability of the patient is not certain, and further evaluation of hypotension blood loss, and appropriate resuscitative measures are certainly indicated. Once this issue has been addressed, evaluation for associated injuries and the degree of hemorrhage can be completed. In this patient, injury to the region of the orbit and maxilla is certainly possible, and evaluations to determine the extent and severity of these potential injuries are indicated. The evidence for a potential orbital injury should prompt an ophthalmologic examination and an ophthalmologic consultation. Close attention to the dentition and maxilla during the complete head and neck examination influences subsequent decisions regarding radiographic examination. Because of the history of significant epistaxis in addition to resuscitative measures, which may include administration of blood products, evaluation of any bleeding diasthesis, both by history and with laboratory studies, is indicated.

In example 3, the patient is unstable and has already undergone resuscitative measures of a significant degree, and multiple other extensive injuries have relegated evaluation and treatment of the nasal injury to a low priority. Given the brief examination and history, however, one can suspect significant associated injuries to the anterior skull base or temporal bone and other facial bones. This patient has severe and potentially life-threatening injuries, and appropriate evaluation of these has likely been completed. It is, however, important for the otolaryngologist to ensure that the cervical spine is stable. In this patient, the possibility of a cerebrospinal fluid leak must be kept in mind also. It is obvious that a complete head and neck examination is not possible, but when it can be completed, a complete examination is necessary because patients with injuries related to a high-velocity impact frequently sustain multiple head and neck injuries.

Subsequent to stabilization of the patient, if necessary, evaluation for associated hemorrhage, establishing the extent of severity of other injuries, and completion of a head and neck examination, the physician must determine whether a radiographic evaluation is warranted. This decision-making process is aided by understanding that the purpose of radiographic evaluation in nasal trauma is not to determine whether a fracture is present or whether reduction is necessary. Rather, a radiographic evaluation should be aimed at establishing or detecting injuries to the adjacent facial skeleton or skull base. Therefore, the usefulness of a radiographic evaluation in nasal trauma increases as the complexity of the injury increases. Computed tomography and plain film evaluations may complement each other in establishing the extent of facial injuries. Routinely obtaining plain films is not cost-effective or necessary.[3,4]

The patient in example 1 does not require a radiographic evaluation. The injury was not a high-velocity injury, and neither the examination nor the history suggest injury to the adjacent bony skeleton. In example 2, however, the injury suggests a greater energy of impact and there is potential for an orbital injury. If significant edema precludes an adequate examination of the orbital rims, then computed tomography may be helpful in evaluating an associated bony orbital injury. In example 3, the patient has clearly had a very high-energy impact, and physical examination suggests a cerebrospinal fluid leak. Frequently, screening computed tomography of the head in patients with trauma inadequately evaluates the anterior skull base and orbital/maxillofacial region. Therefore, before reduction is attempted in this patient, a close radiographic evaluation is required.

The method of photographic documentation of a nasal injury varies, depending on the facilities available. When the patient is seen in the outpatient setting, otolaryngologists who also practice facial plastic surgery will have a mechanism available to accurately photograph nasal and facial structures. Poses similar to those used before rhinoplasty should serve adequately for most nasal injuries. In the emergency room setting or for cases in which severe injures have prompted rapid transport to the operating room, alternative methods are required. The goal of any photographic documentation is multiple views to provide accurate information regarding the extent of nasal injury. In settings that are less than optimum, multiple photographs taken in various wide settings may be useful.

The diagnosis and management of nasal trauma are aided by determining whether the nasal injury is simple or complex. Patients with complex nasal injuries require a greater involvement of physician time and have greater morbidity and mortality. Table 17–1 lists factors that potentially characterize a nasal injury as

**Table 17–1   Characteristics of a
Complex Nasal Injury**

Life-threatening injury or injury that prevents acute
  reduction
Tissue loss
Associated facial fractures
Cerebrospinal fluid leak
Bleeding diathesis
Infectious diseases

complex. Certainly, injuries with tissue loss have a significant potential for morbidity related to the injury. Blunt injuries likely produce tissue loss with jagged edges and irregular borders with the potential to follow superficial planes. Nasal injuries from sharp objects or penetrating wounds have tissue loss that may not follow planes of dissection. Large crush injuries are unlikely to produce tissue loss; however, with severe crush injuries, realignment of intranasal structures can be a challenge and results in disruption of the nasal septum. For evaluation of these wounds, it is important to identify whether the tissue loss is skin, skin and supporting structures, or a full-thickness defect including mucosa.

A second element that characterizes complex nasal injuries is life-threatening injuries or injuries that preclude acute reduction. With high-velocity, high-energy impacts, the facial skeleton and, in particular, the nose are frequently injured. In addition, intracranial, thoracic, abdominal, and orthopedic injuries can also occur and may preempt addressing the nose in a timely fashion. In these situations, and for situations in which it is uncertain whether the associated injuries will result in the patient's death, delayed treatment of the nasal injury is appropriate. The patient's general condition and other associated injuries determine complex management considerations.

Associated fractures of the facial skeleton increase the complexity and potential morbidity of nasal injuries. Zygomatic, naso-ethmoid, and Le Fort fractures increase the potential for a persistent external deformity and increase the time involved in reducing the bony fractures. The presence of a cerebrospinal fluid leak significantly increases the complexity of a nasal or head injury. Consideration must be given to the potential for meningitis, but a cerebrospinal fluid leak also indicates a fracture of sufficient magnitude to result in a dural injury. The presence of clear, watery drainage and hemorrhage increase the suspicion of a cerebrospinal fluid leak. β_2-Transferrin in this fluid supports the diagnosis of a leak. There are multiple potential sites for cerebrospinal fluid rhinorrhea in patients with significant head injuries, including the temporal bone.

A bleeding diathesis in the setting of nasal trauma results in a complex injury because of the potential need for initial management of the coagulopathy and the potential for intraoperative hemorrhage or postreduction hemorrhage. Finally, nasal trauma in a patient with known contagious infectious diseases increases the complexity because of the risk to the physician and may indeed require extra time and precaution in management.

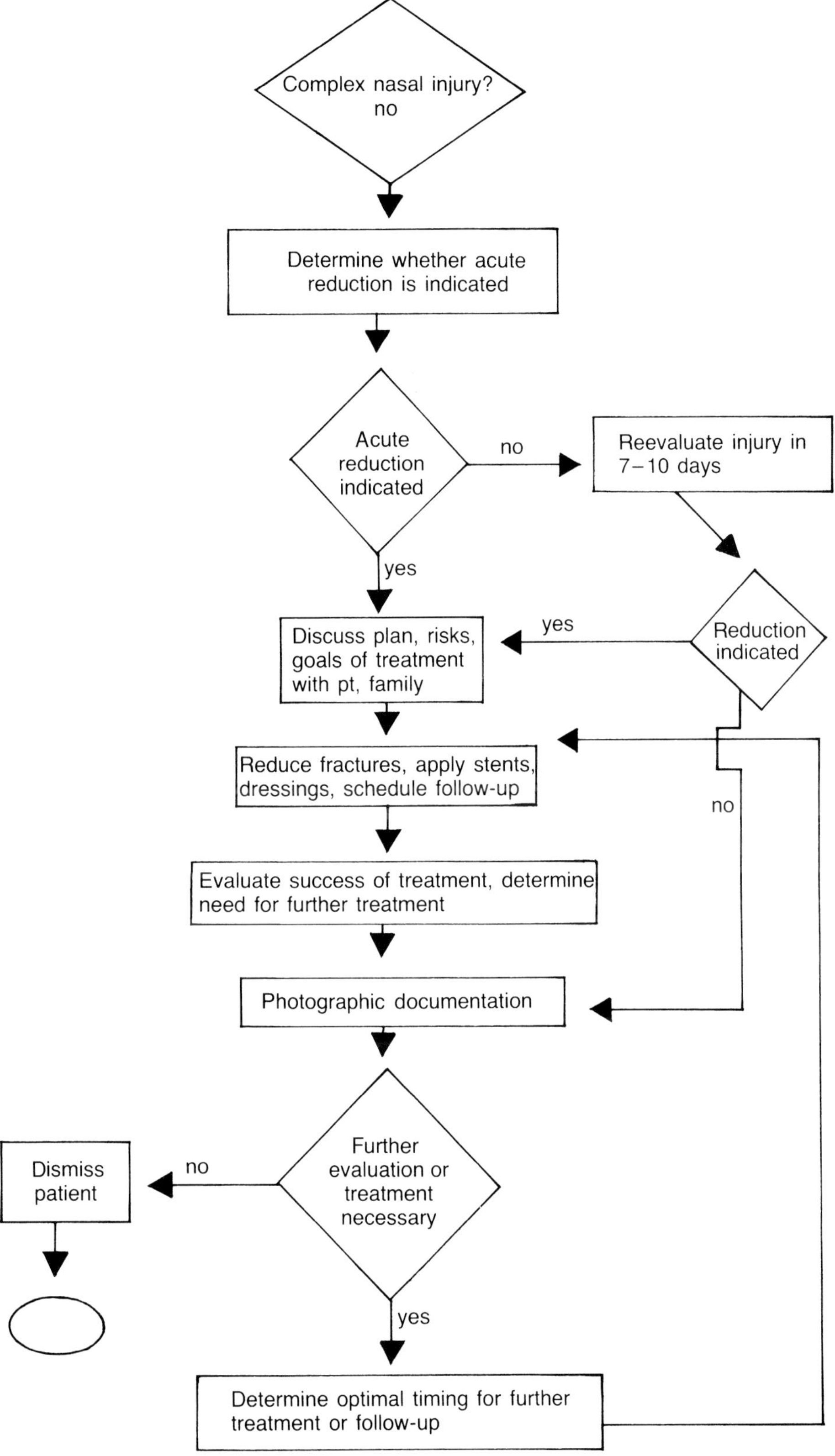

Figure 17–2. Management of simple nasal trauma.

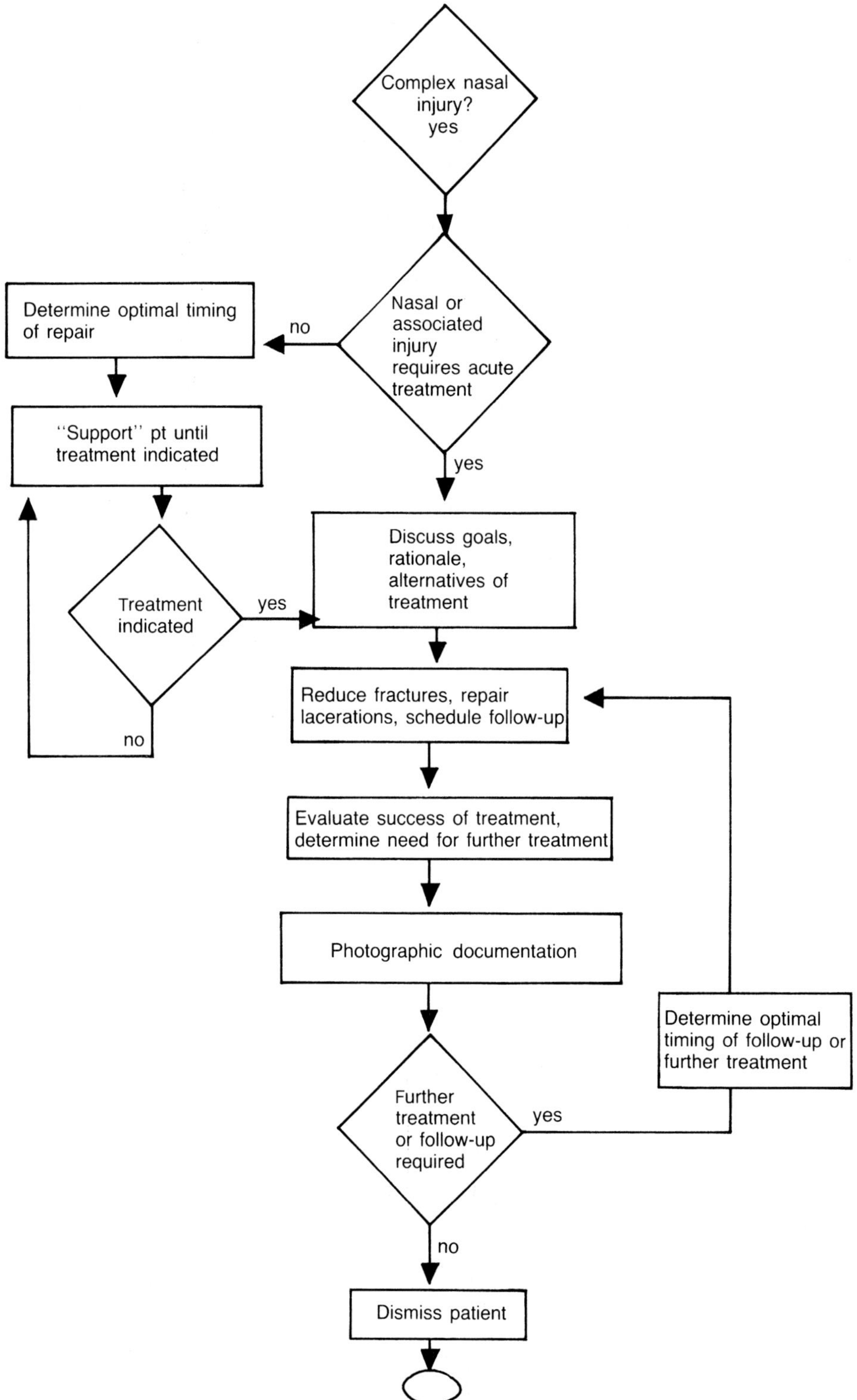

Figure 17–3.   Management of complex nasal trauma.

In simple nasal injuries, the focus of the treatment lies solely on addressing the nasal injury. In these cases, edema and availability of instrumentation typically determine the timing and setting of repair. In example 1, the patient presents with minimal edema several days after the injury and has no factors indicating a complex injury, and its acute reduction is possible. The patients in examples 2 and 3, however, both have factors that may prevent acute reduction and would qualify the nasal injuries as complex. The treating physician must be aware of the extent of injury, and this influences the timing of repair, the extent of surgical involvement, and the overall care of the patient. In example 2, factors that increase the complexity are primarily the significant epistaxis, potential hypovolemia, and the potential orbital fracture and injury. In example 3, the patient has a much more complex injury, and the physician must consider the stability of the cervical-spine, the urgency of repair as it relates to other life-threatening injuries, and the possibility of a cerebrospinal fluid leak. All these factors must be considered in the overall management that affect the timing and extent of repair.

Figure 17–2 depicts the decision-making steps and activity of the physician treating simple nasal fractures. At this point, the diagnosis should be well in hand, and the figure reinforces the need for continued evaluation of treatment in order to accurately diagnose any residual deformity associated with the initial trauma or reduction.

Figure 17–3 shows that the management of complex injuries is similar to that of simple nasal injuries with the exception of various supportive measures that may be needed and the decision-making process in the timing of reduction. Photographic documentation and follow-up need to be done to determine any residual external or intranasal deformities or other residual morbidity from the injury.

REFERENCES

1. Pollock RA: Nasal trauma. Pathomechanics and surgical management of acute injuries. *Clin Plast Surg* 1992; 19:133–147.
2. Renner GJ: Management of nasal fractures. *Otolarphgol Clin North Am* 1991; 24:195–213.
3. Logan M, O'Driscoll K, Masterson J: The utility of nasal bone radiographs in nasal trauma. *Clin Radio* 1994; 49:192–194.
4. Sharp JF, Denholm S: Routine x-rays in nasal trauma: the influence of audit on clinical practice. *J R Soc Med* 1994; 87:153–154.

18

Vasculitis and Granulomatous Disease

THOMAS J. McDONALD, M.D.

VASCULITIS

Vasculitis means inflammation of vessels, and within the context of this topic, it is useful for the otolaryngologist to be aware of various conditions whose sole or predominant histologic feature is inflammation of various vessels, including pulmonary vessels, even though the upper airway is not necessarily involved.

The vasculitides are essentially diseases of altered immunologic activity. In the assessment of inflammatory processes in the upper or lower airway, it is important to remember that infections can result in vasculitis (specifically in the lower airway) by extension of infectious pulmonary parenchymal disease into the vessel wall. Thus, in evaluation of "vasculitis," biopsy material from either the upper or the lower airway needs to be attained for culture.

Vasculitis Affecting the Lower Airway[1]

Polyarteritis nodosa (PAN) is characterized by necrotizing vasculitis that affects predominantly small or medium-sized muscular arteries of the systemic circulation. The predominant symptoms in PAN are related to the gastrointestinal tract, the kidneys, and the central nervous system. Hemoptysis, however, can occur, mostly due to complicating infections.

Takayasus's arteritis (pulseless disease) is a vasculitis whose main target seems to be the aorta and its major branches. Pulmonary artery involvement is also common. The clinical manifestations of this disease are mainly due to localized vascular insufficiency and include angina, headaches, syncope, impaired vision, and claudication.

Temporal (giant cell) arteritis is a relatively common systemic arteritis that affects older patients. Symptoms referable to the upper airway include sore throat,

370

hoarseness, a choking sensation, and tenderness of neck structures together with glossitis. These symptoms are most likely based on ischemic changes in arteries supplying the laryngeal and pharyngeal tissues.

Behçet's disease is usually considered to be characterized by multiple oropharyngeal ulcerations associated with anal-genital ulcerations. Behçet's disease, however, is a vasculitis, probably on the basis of immune complex deposition. Pulmonary manifestations usually appear 3 or 4 years after the onset of systemic disease and are characterized by hemoptysis, chest pain, dyspnea, and cough, usually due to pulmonary vasculitis.

Henoch-Schönlein purpura is characterized by purpura, abdominal pain, and gastrointestinal hemorrhage, together with arthralgias. The histologic picture is similar to that of a leukocytoplastic vasculitis that causes intra-alveolar hemorrhage and hemoptysis.

Leukocytolastic vasculitis is typified by a microangiitis, hypersensitivity vasculitis, and necrotizing alveolitis associated with alveolar hemorrhage and inflammation with necrosis of small parenchymal vessels. The abnormalities in this type of vasculitis are thought to represent an unusual histologic reaction rather than a specific disease entity such as Wegener's granulomatosis (WG).

The foregoing are important because at one time or another during the course of their disease, patients will have hemoptysis, shortness of breath, radiographic changes such as pulmonary cavitations, or laboratory values reflecting altered immunologic activity. Thus, there are significant overlaps among these diseases and two other types of vasculitis with both upper and lower airway manifestations, namely, Wegener's granulomatosis and allergic granulomatosis (Churg-Strauss syndrome).

WEGENER'S GRANULOMATOSIS

WG not only is classified as a vasculitis but also is a granulomatous as well as autoimmune disease.[2-4] It often behaves as a continuum. For example, when the disease first appears in the upper airway, if not treated it may proceed to the upper part of the trachea, lungs, and so on. As part of a continuum, it is therefore encountered in one of three roughly divided types: (1) a very limited form such as localized ulceration in the nose, (2) a more advanced type with multiple site involvement associated with systemic symptoms, and (3) a type characterized by systemic disease with major systemic symptoms and multiple organ involvement.

Etiology and Pathogenesis

In the more than 400 patients with WG who are currently being studied at the Mayo Clinic, the predominant involvement of the upper airway (nose, nasopharynx, and paranasal sinuses, as well as the upper trachea) strongly suggests an inhaled infectious agent as the etiologic catalyst. However, in this series of patients, cultures for all organisms have been negative (apart from the opportunistic gram-positive and gram-negative bacteria associated with localized mucosal ulceration). There is no doubt that it is an autoimmune process; one piece of evidence for this is the dramatic response to immunosuppressive treatment in a large majority of patients. The presence of granulomas in active lesions implies that there is a cell-mediated component in the pathogenesis. Furthermore, immunohistochemical studies show that most inflammatory cells in the parenchyma and vascular infiltrates are T-cells and monocytes, another indicator of a cell-mediated process.

Clinical Characteristics

Patients with a very limited form of WG usually present with bilateral nasal obstruction with serosanguineous drainage, often mimicking that of an upper respiratory tract infection that has become prolonged. The pathognomonic feature in this group of patients, and in fact in all patients with nasal involvement, is the significantly large crusts that are expelled from their nasal cavities. Apart from atrophic rhinitis, a disorder that is less and less common, WG is the only disease known to me that has these very long crusts as a feature. This group of patients may have a low-grade fever and vague mid-facial pain, but otherwise they feel well.

Removal of the crusts reveals a friable underlying mucosa, but in most cases the septum is intact. With the flexible telescope, erosion of the posterior part of the septum is noted, and there is crusty, dry scaliness in the nasopharynx. Computed tomography scanning of the paranasal sinuses shows pansinusitis, and there may or may not be unilateral or bilateral serous otitis.

The second group of patients, who have more advanced disease, may have nose and lung involvement with either solitary pulmonary nodules or multiple cavitating lesions seen on chest radiography. These patients are sicker and have more systemic symptoms.

The third group of patients, who have disseminated disease, often have fever, highly elevated erythrocyte sedimentation rate, hemoptysis, and progressive renal failure.

Laboratory Findings

In all three categories of WG, the sedimentation rate is almost universally increased. The sicker the patient, the higher the level. In patients with limited disease, the hemoglobin, creatinine, and urinalysis levels and chest radiography are usually negative. In more advanced disease, there may be anemia and also an abnormal urinary sediment with increased serum creatinine levels.

The antineutrophil cytoplasmic antibody (ANCA)[5] test is the most helpful test in the diagnosis and assessment of patients with WG. It correlates strongly with the presence of active disease and usually reflects response to treatment with the finding of normal results. The antibodies can be detected by indirect immunofluorescence or enzyme-linked immunosorbent assay (ELISA) techniques and appear to be related to several lysosomal enzymes. Positive ANCA results have been reported, but uncommonly so, in patients with idiopathic creascentic glomerulonephritis and allergic granulomatosis. ANCA testing is further useful when the biopsy is nonspecific or tissue is difficult to sample (for example, involvement of the upper trachea). In these instances, a positive ANCA result considered in combination with a constellation of typical symptoms and signs is diagnostic. The report of "nonspecific" histopathological findings is due sometimes to inadequately biopsied material or to pre-biopsy administration of corticosteroids. Corticosteroids tend to mask the vasculitis and interfere with the delineation of typical morphologic findings.

Histopathology

A frequent finding is inflammation of the mucosa and submucosa, with extensive necrosis and ulceration. Predominantly epithelioid necrotizing granulomas and vasculitis involving small arteries and veins are also evident. Some granulomas are nonnecrotizing, others have fibrinoid necrotic zones, and still others contain a central microabscess. Vasculitis can be identified as a variable degree of transmural infiltration of the vessel walls, often overshadowed by the inflammatory reaction of the necrotizing granuloma. Fibrinoid necrosis can be identified. Focal vascular lesions, healing vasculitis with vascular and intramural fibrosis, and focal loss of elastic tissue are also seen. In addition, granulation tissue containing cells of chronic inflammation, occasionally with abundant eosinophils, is evident.

Diagnosis

The history of serosanguineous nasal discharge in association with large nasal crusts overlying friable nasal mucosa diffusely and the appearance of an eroded vomer are strongly suggestive of WG involving the nose. In more advanced disease, abnormal blood test results such as an elevated sedimentation rate, a mild anemia, abnormal results of urinalysis, cavitating lesions on chest radiography (when there is pulmonary involvement), and a positive ANCA result are frequent findings.

The nasal biopsy, however, is a very vital part of the diagnostic process. Preferably, it should be done in the operating room with the patient under sedative intravenous anesthesia together with topically applied cocaine and adrenaline medication. The crusts must be removed, and up to 10 pieces of tissue are removed from turbinates, both abnormal and adjacently normal tissue. In addition to normal morphologic examination, tissue should be examined for fungal and acid-fast cultures (to rule out specific infections that cause a granulomatous reaction) and also for immunohistochemical studies.

Treatment

In patients with localized disease, treatment with corticosteroids is considered adequate, for example, 60 mg per day with a tapering dose schedule. In patients who have more advanced disease, corticosteroids given with cyclophosphamide are usually very successful. In a small select group of patients with very early disease, we have noted significant improvement with trimethoprim-sulfamethoxazole, double strength, 1 daily alone. It is also used with the other immunosuppressive treatment, and as the immunosuppressive treatment is discontinued, the use of trimethoprim-sulfamethoxazole is continued indefinitely.

Adjunctive therapy consists of daily nasal irrigation with water or saline followed by the application of aromatic oils such as rose of sesame with oil of geranium.

Prognosis

Review of the Mayo Clinic's current study of close to 500 patients shows that 85% are alive and well at 5 years.

Other Head and Neck Sites of Involvement in WG

WG can also cause episcleritis, unilateral or bilateral proptosis, unilateral or bilateral serous otitis media with or without suppurative otitis media and mastoiditis, cranial nerve neuropathies (especially cranial nerve VIII), and upper tracheal involvement.

Differential Diagnosis

Two clinical situations are commonly confused with WG. The first is due to previous or ongoing nasal substance abuse.[6] This problem classically presents in a young patient, either in the teenage years or early 20s or 30s, as an isolated, large septal perforation. The edges of the perforation are characteristically inflamed and crusty, and there is usually no history of external or intranasal trauma or previous surgical procedures involving the septum. With the exception of patients who present with similar types of perforation and who admit to a chronic factitial habit, isolated septal perforations with totally normal nasal mucosa and normal nasopharyngeal mucosa are often due to substance abuse. Careful questioning will usually elicit a history of cocaine abuse, and it should be considered the diagnosis, even if the abuse was "discontinued years ago." The differentiating signs are the presence of normal mucosa throughout the upper airway, nonspecific biopsy results, normal results of blood test, and, of course, a negative ANCA result.

The other disease very easily confused with WG is T-cell lymphoma of the nose.[7] In the last part of the past century and for most of this century, a clinical term applied to many patients with midline destructive lesions of the nose and face was "lethal midline granuloma." Most likely, many of these diseases were carcinomas involving the nose and face, diseases due to metabolic states (diabetic gangrenescens), fungal infections, and true malignant lymphomas. With modern morphologic and histochemical studies, these diseases can now be categorized correctly. The term "lethal midline granuloma" should be abandoned.

Until recently, other terms have been used to describe lymphoma-like lesions of the nose (T-cell), such as polymorphic reticulosis, lymphomatoid granulomatosis, and midline malignant reticulosis.

T-cell lymphoma of the nose is different from true malignant lymphoma of the nose because the "explosive" lesion is characterized by major ulceration, sometimes involving just one side of the nose with extension to the palate, adjacent sinuses, and often orbit and sometimes including soft tissues of the lip, nose, and so on. However, the lesion in WG is usually diffuse and, although it can involve bone, this is not common. The systemic symptoms of both, however, are very similar, including malaise, fevers, weakness, and arthralgias. In addition, cavitating lesions of the lungs are similar for both diseases but renal involvement is absent in patients with T-cell lymphoma of the nose.

The most helpful differentiating feature, however, is study of the biopsy specimen. WG is typified by necrotizing granulomas. T-cell lymphomas are characterized by a dense, lymphocytic pattern of large and small and usually benign lymphocytes (differentiating them from true malignant lymphoma, in which the lymphocytes are malignant). The explosive or infarctive nature of the lesion is caused by a typical angiocentric or angioinfiltrative pattern of behavior by these various types of lymphocytes.

Recently, immunohistochemical and molecular genetic techniques have allowed a clearer understanding of this disease. Immunohistochemical studies on biopsy specimens reveal a predominance of T cells with either a natural killer (CD2, CD56 positive) phenotype or T-cell phenotype. Analysis for the T-cell receptor gene is not usually of value.

WG responds well to chemotherapeutic agents, but limited forms of T-cell lymphoma respond well to radiation therapy. More disseminated forms of T-cell lymphoma are treated, however, with malignant lymphoma protocols and outcomes are poorer.

ALLERGIC GRANULOMATOSIS (CHURG-STRAUSS SYNDROME)[8]

For the diagnosis of allergic granulomatosis, several or more than one of the following criteria must be present: asthma, eosinophil value of more than 10% on differential leukocyte count, variable types of neuropathy, pulmonary infiltrates, paranasal sinus abnormalities, nasal polyps, and biopsy of nasal mucosa or nasal polyp containing a blood vessel showing vasculitis and extra-vascular eosinophils. Although it is sometimes considered a variant of WG, we believe it is a distinctly different syndrome.

Etiology and Pathogenesis

The cause is essentially unknown, but the association of asthma and rhinitis, the presence of increased levels of serum IgE, and a response to corticosteroids suggest a hypersensitivity reaction to an antigen.

Clinical Presentation

Usually, patients present with long-standing asthma and nasal polyps with pansinusitis. Some patients have abnormal chest radiographs, involvement of the skin, polyneuropathies, and lower urinary tract, spleen, gastrointestinal tract, and cardiac lesions.

Histopathology

Classically, vasculitis and necrotizing extravascular granuloma inflammation are present on morphologic examination. Inflammation occurs in small to medium-sized arteries and consists of a transmural infiltrate of histiocytes and multinucleated giant cells, as well as eosinophils. Chest radiography demonstrates nonsegmental air space consolidation and a peripheral distribution, very similar to eosinophilic pneumonia. In contrast to WG, there are usually no cavitating lesions. Asthma and peripheral blood and tissue eosinophilia are always present, as are allergic rhinitis and nasal polyps. There is a marked response to corticosteroid therapy.

GRANULOMATOUS DISEASE[9]

This portion of the chapter discusses granulomatous diseases caused by: (1) specific infectious agents such as mycobacterial tuberculous organisms, nontuberculous mycobacterial infections, fungal infections of the head and neck, and leprosy, and (2) granulomatous disease with unknown causes, such as sarcoidosis.

Mycobacteria

Mycobacteria are nonmotile, rod-shaped bacteria that are aerobic and differ from other bacteria in that they have an exceptionally high lipid content. This explains many of their properties, including resistance to drying, alcohol, alkali, and germicides. This acid-fast quality is helpful in their identification because when they are stained bright red with various dyes, the bacteria are able to resist discoloration by strong acid solutions. Both upper and lower airway infections can be caused by so-called classic mycobacterial tuberculosis but also by other nontuberculous bacteria, so-called atypical mycobacteria.

Mycobacterium tuberculosis

Nose and paranasal sinus involvement with traditional *M. tuberculosis* remains uncommon, and when it does occur it is almost always associated with pulmonary involvement. Typically there is ulceration of the nasal septum, both cartilaginous and bony, with sparing of the nasal floor.

The common systemic symptoms are fatigue, weakness, anorexia, and weight loss, and there is usually a history of contact with someone actively infected with tuberculosis. Sometimes there is hoarseness, usually a manifestation of concomitant laryngeal ulceration. The ulcers on the vocal cords are nonspecific.

Laboratory findings include positive results of tuberculous skin testing, and examination of stains of nasal or pulmonary secretions shows acid-fast bacilli. Nasal biopsy demonstrates caseating granulomas. Cultures usually grow *M. tuberculosis* or *M. bovis* organisms.

Nontuberculosis Mycobacterium (NTM)

NTM infections are becoming more and more common in the United States. They are being diagnosed in otherwise well children with normal socioeconomic backgrounds, sometimes with no evidence of other disease. Specifically (and in contrast to infections due to *M. tuberculosis*), NTM infections often occur without pulmonary involvement, and purified protein derivative test results may be normal. They present classically with either cervical or axillary node involvement. NTM infections of the nose and sinuses are uncommon. The most common NTM organism is *M. avium-intracellulare*. This is particularly common as an opportunistic infection in patients with human immunodeficiency virus infections. Other common NTM organisms are *M. kansasii* and *M. fortuitum*. The diagnosis of NTM infections is made with biopsy of infected tissue with subsequent staining and cultures. Treatment is directed at the removal of abscessed nodes, with or without conventional triple antituberculosis therapy of isoniazid, rifampin, and ethambutol.

Sarcoidosis

Sarcoidosis is a chronic systemic granulomatous disease capable of involving almost every organ in the body. It has a major predilection for involving many head and neck organs, especially the nose.

There are two types of nasal involvement. Externally, sarcoidosis may present as a raised papular lesion on the nose which can spread over the midline of the nose to adjacent malar regions bilaterally. Several of these lesions may collect to form bluish-red swelling. The lesions are firm and elastic when palpated. They may extend deeply to involve the entire thickness of the dermis. Intranasal sarcoidosis presents with atrophic, minimally ulcerated nasal mucosa with involvement of the paranasal sinuses. Another form of sarcoidosis intranasally is more common and is that of a "vasomotor rhinitis" presentation with large hyperplastic turbinates.

Diagnosis

Demonstration of noncaseous granulomas is essential in the diagnosis of sarcoidosis. The typical histopathologic picture is observed on nasal tissue or hilar nodes obtained by mediastinoscopy or by open lung biopsy. Biopsy specimens should also be cultured for acid-fast bacilli and fungal organisms. Newer studies suggest that sarcoidosis begins in the lung with alveolitis. It consists mainly of T-cells. These T-cells elaborate chemotactic factors that attract monocytic cells, which ultimately transform into epithelial cells. These cells form the granuloma that potentially leads to fibrosis. Serum angiotensin converting enzyme levels are an indicator of activity of sarcoidosis. Other findings include hypercalcemia and an increased erythrocyte sedimentation rate together with hypercalciuria and hypergammaglobulinemia.

Treatment

Treatment of sarcoidosis is controversial, with most of the controversy centering on pulmonary involvement. In patients with stage 1 pulmonary involvement, treatment is "watchful waiting" with periodic examinations. Seventy percent of patients with this type of sarcoidosis will have spontaneous remission. A patient with more advanced disease that is not improving or whose condition worsens should be treated with prednisone, 40 mg on alternate days. Almost always, nasal involvement is associated with pulmonary involvement. In my experience, nasal involvement responds well to topically applied steroid treatment.

Leprosy

Leprosy is a chronic granulomatous infection with major manifestations in three main organ systems: skin, peripheral nerves, and nasal mucosa. The organism is *Mycobacterium leprae* (Hansen's bacillus). Usually, patients present with some form of neuropathy associated with nonspecific nasal ulceration either on the turbinates or septum. The organism can be grown with routine culture methods and also has a characteristic reaction to the FITE stain. The disease responds to dapsone therapy.

Rhinoscleroma

This is a granulomatous disease caused by *Klebsiella rhinoscleromatis*. It presents with foul-smelling rhinorrhea followed by nasal atrophy. Ultimately, fibrosis and stenosis of the nose develop. The classic cell on morphologic examination is the Mikulicz cell containing typical "foamy"-looking histiocytes. Rhinoscleroma is treated primarily with tetracycline antibiotics, but patients may eventually have to have surgical treatment to remove the stenotic tissue, followed by relining of the nasal cavity with skin grafts.

FUNGAL DISEASES[10,11]

Aspergillosis

Aspergillus organisms are common saprophytes that grow as a mass of wide separate hyphae. Aspergillosis is contracted by inhaling airborne fungal spores found in decaying food, food grain, and plants. In the author's opinion, there are two forms of aspergillosis infection of the nose and paranasal sinuses (the most common organism being *Aspergillus fumigatus*). The first type is due to noninvasive aspergillosis, which can occur in normal persons. Patients present with a unilateral opacified maxillary or frontal sinus. The clinical examination is otherwise normal, and on removal, the appearance of the mass is that of a soft, yellow, cheesy appearance and is correctly described as a fungus ball. Fungal stains, particularly auramine-rhodamine, are useful. Eventually cultures "grow out" *Aspergillus fumigatus*. Removal is the treatment of choice for this type of problem.

The other type of aspergillosis infection is extremely dangerous. In the author's practice, it almost always occurs either in patients with HIV infections or in patients receiving chemotherapy for lymphoma or leukemia.

The hallmarks are distinct and twofold. First, there is deep, localized face pain followed by progressive neuropathies, particularly affecting cranial nerves III and VI. The association of deep, relentless facial pain with neuropathies in a patient receiving chemotherapy is highly suggestive of fungal infection, usually caused by *Aspergillus fumigatus*. The pursuit of the organism's precise identity must be relentless. Repeated computed tomography scans, both coronal and axial, must be obtained, followed by aggressive surgical intervention to obtain tissue and effect drainage and debridement. When the diagnosis is made, treatment with amphotericin B is essential.

Principals of Treatment With Amphotericin B

Amphotericin B is the most effective agent available for treating invasive fungal infections. It is used in patients with aspergillosis, candidiasis, histoplasmosis, coccidioidomycosis, and mucormycosis. It is administered intravenously over a period of several hours while the patient is carefully monitored to document the absence or presence of anaphylaxis. The usual dose is 0.3 mg/kg per day. This is increased to 0.5 or 0.6 mg/kg per day or as toxicity permits. Serum creatinine clearance levels are monitored to detect the development of nephrotoxicity. Once safe parameters have been determined, a double dose (1 mg/kg) is given on alternate days. Amphotericin B is not fungistatic, rather it is fungicidal so that long-term treatment, weeks to months, is necessary to achieve cure. Again, the adjunctive treatment of surgical intervention and debridement is important.

Mucormycosis

This major fungal infection of the nose and paranasal sinuses is also an opportunistic infection caused by certain members of the Mucorales family, which includes *Rhizopus*, *Mucor*, and *Absidia* species. In an otorhinolaryngologic practice, the most common presentation is a diabetic patient in ketoacidosis who presents with "rhinosinusitis" progressing to a rhino-orbital-cerebral infected state. These patients are sick with fever and have cranial nerve involvement, especially II, III, IV, and VI, associated with proptosis, facial swelling, mouth ulcers, and coma. Because the organism produces necrosis of nasal tissue, examination of the nose shows brick-red or black areas in both sides of the nose. A biopsy specimen should be taken and tissue stained (silver methenamine) to identify typical nonseptic hyphae. Tissue cultures should be performed on Sabouraud medium. Imaging studies shows opacification of all of the sinuses together with mucosal thickening and bone erosion. Computed tomographic imaging is essential to define soft tissue invasion and necrosis, early bone erosion, and cavernous sinus thrombosis. If involvement of major vessels is suspected, magnetic resonance imaging with or without gadolinium is most useful, particularly when carotid artery thrombosis is suspected. Magnetic resonance imaging is also the best way to evaluate intracranial extension. The treatment of rhinocerebral mucormyocosis is twofold. First, debridement of necrotic nasal tissue is done either through the nose, endoscopically, or by an open approach. If extensive necrosis has occurred, a more radical debridement has to be performed, proceeding as the extent of the disease dictates, even requiring the assistance of neurosurgical colleagues if skull base involvement has occurred. Rapid infusion of effective doses of amphotericin B is the second arm of treatment and is performed as described above.

Blastomycosis

Blastomycosis occurs in the nose as well-circumscribed, indurated, relatively painless lesions often confused with squamous cell carcinoma. The lesions are usually associated with ulcers involving the larynx oral cavity, pulmonary lesions, and skin lesions. Amphotericin B is the treatment of choice.

Candidiasis

Candidiasis (moniliasis) is a yeast-like fungus and its involvement of the paranasal sinuses and nose is unusual, but it does occur in some patients who are immunocompromised and have a deficiency of neutrophils. Treatment is directed at correcting the underlying cause together with the use of amphotericin B and fluconazole.

Coccidioidomycosis

The respiratory tract is the major portal of entry for the spores of coccidioidomycosis, and the nose and paranasal sinuses can be involved after establishment of the pulmonary infection. Major cutaneous involvement is also common, especially around the face and nose. The major lesion of the nose is that of diffuse ulceration, and the treatment is adequate local care and intravenous amphotericin B.

Histoplasmosis

This disorder is caused by *Histoplasma capsulatum*, a fungus with both mycelial and yeast phases. The patient usually has a nonspecific respiratory illness with hoarseness, cough, pleuritic pain, and shortness of breath. Infections are endemic in the valleys of the central United States (Missouri, Mississippi, and Ohio river valleys) and South America. It is transmitted through contact with soil contaminated with avian or bat feces. A disseminated form of histoplasmosis occurs in patients with HIV infections, and the nasal lesions are ulcerative and can be raised and confused with squamous cell carcinoma. A skin test known as a histoplasmin skin test provides a reliable diagnostic reaction, and the treatment is intravenous amphotericin B.

Rhinosporidiosis

This disease is caused by *Rhinosporidium seeberi*, which is a fungus-like organism not yet successfully grown in culture medium or transferred from a human to an animal host. The disease is contracted by immersion in contaminated waters in Asia and Africa. Initially, the nasal mucosal lesion in flat and sessile and enlarges to become a painless, polypoid growth that actually fills the nasal cavities.

Treatment consists of complete surgical excision. No medical treatment has been found to be effective. The classic histologic picture is that of pseudoepitheliomatous squamous cell metaplasia accompanying a granulomatous reaction.

REFERENCES

1. Fraser RS, Paré JAP, Fraser RG, Paré PD: *Synopsis of Diseases of the Chest*, ed 2. Philadelphia, WB Saunders, 1994, pp 392–443.
2. McDonald TJ, DeRemee RA, Kern EB, Harrison EG Jr: Nasal manifestations of Wegener's granulomatosis. *Laryngoscope* 1974; 84:2101–2112.
3. DeRemee RA, McDonald TJ, Harrison EG Jr, Coles DT: Wegener's granulomatosis: anatomic correlates, a proposed classification. *Mayo Clin Proc* 1976; 51:777–781.
4. DeRemee RA, McDonald TJ. Weiland LH: Wegener's Granulomatosis, Polymorphic Reticulosis, and Lymphomatoid Granulomatosis: A Comparative Analysis in Sarcoidosis and Other Granulomatous Diseases, in *Proceedings of the 8th International Conference on Sarcoidosis and Other Granulomatous Diseases*. United Kingdom, Alpha Omega Publishing, 1980, pp 738–742.
5. Specks U, Wheatley CL, McDonald TJ, et al: Anticytoplasmic antibodies in the diagnosis and follow-up of Wegener's granulomatosis. *Mayo Clin Proc* 1989; 64:28–36.
6. Becker GD, Hill S: Midline granuloma due to illicit cocaine use. *Arch Otolaryngol Head Neck Surg* 1988; 114:90–91.
7. Strickler JG, Meneses MF, Habermann TM, et al: Polymorphic reticulsois: a reappraisal. *Hum Pathol* 1994; 25:659–665.
8. Specks U, DeRemee RA: Granulomatous vasculitis: Wegener's granulomatosis and Churg-Strauss syndrome. *Rheum Dis Clin North Am* 1980; 16:377–397.
9. McDonald TJ: Granulomatous Diseases of the Nose, vol 2, in English GM (ed): *Otolaryngology*. Philadelphia, JB Lippincott Company, 1990, pp 1–14.
10. Blitzer A, Lawson W: Fungal infections of the nose and paranasal sinuses. Part I. *Otolaryngol Clin North Am* 1993; 26:1007–1035.
11. Sarosi GA, Davies SF: Therapy for fungal infections. *Mayo Clin Proc* 1994; 69:1111–1117.

19

Pediatric Sinusitis

ANIL GUNGOR, M.D.
JACQUELYNNE P. COREY, M.D., F.A.C.S.

DEFINITION OF TERMS

Acute sinusitis is defined as the persistence of upper respiratory infection beyond 7 to 10 days without improvement[1] or as disease of less than 30 days in duration[2] with more severe symptoms than the usual upper respiratory tract infection.[1] It is considered a possible diagnosis when the symptoms of upper respiratory tract virus last more than 10 days.[3] More severe symptoms than usual, such as a fever of more than 39°C, copious purulent nasal secretions, periorbital swelling, and facial discomfort are related to acute sinusitis.[1] According to criteria introduced by Shapiro and Rachelevsky,[4] acute sinusitis fulfills certain major and minor criteria (Table 19–1) and lasts longer than typical viral upper respiratory tract infections (more than 7 days). The presence of two major or one major and two or more minor criteria for more than 7 days is highly likely to signify acute sinusitis, which is usually bacterial. Acute onset of fever with purulent rhinorrhea is also considered highly likely to indicate acute bacterial sinusitis.

Chronic sinusitis has been defined as all of the following: signs and symptoms of sinusitis persisting longer than 3 months despite optimal medical therapy,[5] symptoms lasting more than 3 weeks after consideration is given to the possibility of inappropriate treatment of the initial episode,[1,6] more than four episodes of sinusitis occurring per year,[7] sinus disease lasting more than 3 months and manifesting as long-term symptoms with or without an ongoing need for antibiotic treatment,[4] or radiographic evidence of mucosal hyperplasia of the paranasal sinuses after adequate medical therapy for prolonged or recurrent symptoms of sinusitis.[4,8] Some authors define a patient who has three or more episodes of sinusitis within a year or requires three or more months of antibiotic therapy for sinusitis as sinusitis-prone.[9] Chronic sinusitis was defined by Shapiro and Rachelevsky[4] as the presence of two of three major clinical signs (rhinorrhea, postnasal drip, and cough) for 3 months or longer and confirmed by coronal computed tomography on the basis of mucosal thickening or opacification of the sinus or sinuses (Table 19–1).

Some authors prefer to differentiate acute from chronic disease based on evidence of mucosal hyperplasia on computed tomography after adequate medical treatment.[8]

**Table 19–1 Major and Minor Criteria
in the Clinical Diagnosis of Sinusitis**

Major criteria
  Purulent nasal discharge
  Purulent pharyngeal drainage
  Cough
Minor criteria
  Periorbital edema
  Headache
  Facial pain
  Tooth pain
  Earache
  Sore throat
  Foul breath
  Increased wheeze
  Fever

Modified from Shapiro GG, Rachelevsky GS: Introduction and definition of sinusitis. *J Allergy Clin Immunol* 1992; 90:417–418.

Acute sinusitis usually recurs when there are sufficient anatomical and structural changes in the infundibulum or when there is a defect of the mucociliary
system predisposing the patient to bouts of sinusitis.[5]

Subacute sinusitis is a term used by some to define disease lasting 30 to 120
days; the bacteriology is the same as that of acute sinusitis.[2,10]

PREDISPOSING FACTORS AND EPIDEMIOLOGY

Sinusitis is usually not an isolated process in children; many factors are involved
which should be looked for and treated in every child.[11] An important problem in
children is failure to recognize the disease before complications.[12]

Systemic disease associated with chronic sinusitis in children are viral upper
respiratory tract infections, allergic rhinitis, nonallergic rhinitis, asthma, cystic
fibrosis, immunodeficiency states, immotile cilia syndrome, Down's syndrome, aspirin sensitivity,[12] Young's syndrome,[13] and idiosyncratic reaction to drugs.[6] Cigarette
smoke,[5,14,15] chlorine, and air pollution[15] are local and environmental irritants predisposing to sinusitis.

Rhinitis medicamentosa, choanal atresia, cleft palate, nasal obstruction, septal
deviation, polyps, foreign bodies, tumors, trauma, barotrauma, chronic otitis media,
dental infection, adenotonsillar hypertrophy or infection, and swimming are local
factors associated with chronic sinusitis in children.[1,6,11,14]

The most common predisposing factors are viral upper respiratory tract infections and allergies.[5] The incidence of viral infections in acute and chronic sinusitis is
unknown.[16] Children have an average of six to eight such infections a year, and
adults have an average of 3 a year; sinusitis is more common in the pediatric
population.[1]

The initial mucosal changes are thought to arise from viral infection or allergic inflammation.[17] By age 16 years, 10% to 15% of children experience perennial allergic rhinitis or seasonal allergic rhinitis.[18] Allergic and nonallergic rhinitis have been thought to be risk factors for the development of chronic sinusitis.[6,19]

Rachelevsky[20] found that only 37% of children with chronic sinusitis have positive results of allergy skin tests. Van der Veken et al.[21] found no difference in the incidence of sinus disease between atopic and nonatopic patients. Orobello et al.[16] reported no observable correlation between the presence of positive results of allergy tests and positive results of sinus culture. In contrast, other authors have reported that 59% to 81% of skin tests are positive for allergens in pediatric patients who have chronic sinusitis[9,22] and 63% of allergic children have sinus abnormalities.[22] Respiratory allergy is generally recognized as a major factor that predisposes children to recurrent and chronic sinusitis.[3] In a study observing the response to allergen challenge in allergic patients and controls, radiographic changes of increased mucosal edema or opacification were noted in 78% of the patients with positive results of challenge tests and 16% of those with negative results of challenge tests. These radiographic changes resolved within 24 to 48 hours. The authors proposed a hypersensitivity mechanism initiated by antigen-antibody interaction that results in edema, obstruction, and accumulation of mucus and gas within the sinuses, with subsequent mucous membrane thickening, decreased aeration, increased fluid level and soft tissue mass.[23] In various studies, the minimum concordance of allergy and sinusitis is 25% and the maximum concordance is 70%.[15]

According to Wald et al.,[10] 5% to 10% of upper respiratory tract infections are complicated by sinusitis.

The association of chronic sinusitis with asthma has been reported by many authors.[24-26] Asthma is a highly significant variable in the natural history and response to medical therapy. Patients with asthma have higher recurrence rates of sinusitis.[8] Up to 80% of patients with asthma have symptoms of rhinitis, whereas 5% to 15% of patients with perennial allergic rhinitis have asthma.[3] Sinusitis has been shown to be an aggravating factor in both atopic and nonatopic children with asthma.[6] Sinusitis also has been found to be a more extensive disease in patients with asthma.[27] One study showed that 34.7% of patients who had chronic asthma had chronic sinusitis and 25.3% of pediatric patients who had chronic sinusitis had asthma.[22] The prevalence of sinus disease was 63% in atopic children with complaints of chronic respiratory disease.[19] There is suggestive evidence that sinusitis not only occurs in association with bronchial asthma but may also play a role in its pathogenesis. Proper treatment of sinusitis by medical and surgical means frequently results in significant improvement of asthma symptoms. Table 19-2 shows possible relationships between upper and lower airway disease. Nasal obstruction or a failure in the filtering function of the nose would increase the allergen/irritant burden to the lower airway, thus potentiating lower airway hyperresponsiveness.[3]

Chronic sinusitis is very common among children with respiratory complaints who seek a consultation with an allergist.[22] Allergic children with symptoms of rhinitis or asthma have a high frequency of sinusitis.[6] Patients presenting for evaluation of respiratory allergy have a high incidence of sinus disease.[3] Studies of the incidence of allergy among patients with sinusitis may be skewed upward by referral

Table 19–2   Association of Upper and Lower Airway Disease

Allergic rhinitis
  Fitter function failure; increases allergen/irritant burden on lower airway
  Heat and humidification failure; exercise-induced asthma
  Improvement in pulmonary symptoms by treatment of nasal symptoms
  Increased lower airway responsiveness: specific and nonspecific
Nasal polyps and asthma
Viral upper respiratory tract infection
Nasal-sinus-bronchial reflex

Modified from Slavin RG: Sinusitis and asthma. In Lusk RP (ed.), *Pediatric Sinusitis.* Raven, New York 1992, p 59.

preselection to the investigators' allergy/immunology practice. Slavin et al.[28] introduced the concept of "allergic sinusitis"; in three patients with ragweed allergic rhinitis who were evaluated with single photon emission computed tomography, hyperemia and increased metabolic activity were detected in the paranasal sinuses even though the radiographs were normal. Nasal antigen challenge in patients with chronic maxillary sinusitis caused changes on sinus radiographs, including increased mucosal edema or opacifications and pressure in the maxillary sinus area. Acute headache or otalgia often accompanied these changes. Acute nasal symptoms such as nasal blockage, hypersecretion, sneezing, and itching were present in all patients with positive results of challenge tests.[23] Major basic protein from eosinophils has toxic effects on the mucosal surface and on ciliary activity. The mucosa of allergic patients has been reported to be more vulnerable than the mucosa from normal persons; allergic patients may be at higher risk of sinus disease because of the known association of eosinophilia and allergy, that is, allergic persons are more likely to harbor nasal eosinophils, which have toxic potentials, and allergic mucosa may be more vulnerable than normal mucosa.[29] There is still no firm proof of a cause-and-effect relationship between allergy and sinusitis. No controlled study of the incidence of sinusitis among allergic and nonallergic patients has been done in children. However, respiratory allergy has been recognized as a major factor that predisposes children to recurrent and chronic sinusitis.[3]

Young children appear to be at even more risk of sinusitis because of small anatomical structures, more frequent viral infections, increased exposure to indoor allergens and irritants, child care, and perhaps an "immature" immune system.[2,15,30] In the first 3 years of life, 6% to 13% of children in day care centers experience sinusitis (defined as symptoms of upper respiratory tract infection lasting for 15 or more days).[1,10] Children in child care centers have protracted respiratory symptoms twice as often as children who are not in the centers. Smallness and the increased incidence of upper respiratory tract infections may increase the chance of obstruction and predispose these patients to recurrent sinus infections.[3]

Bacterial infections are associated with fewer ciliated cells, but they appear to grow back relatively quickly. There seems to be a longer lasting loss of ciliated cells with viral infections. Temporarily acquired ciliary defects have been observed in the nasal mucosa of children with acute viral upper respiratory tract infections.[31] Viral infection leads to abnormal cilia function, which recovers in 2 to 10 weeks.[12] Ciliary beat frequency is slower and mucociliary clearance with saccharin is prolonged due to toxins that are caused by the inflammatory response in patients with viral and bacterial infections.[32]

The younger the patient with chronic upper respiratory tract symptoms, the greater the risk of having chronic sinusitis.[22] Tonsils and adenoids may act as bacterial reservoirs. Partial obstruction due to adenotonsillar hypertrophy may lead to changes in the microenvironment and foster bacterial growth.[5] Also, young children have been noted to have immunoglobulin subclass deficiencies.[33,34] Some investigators believe that pediatric sinusitis is a self-limited disease and rarely occurs in children after 7 to 8 years of age, perhaps reflecting an immunologic immaturity of the young child.[30] The most common immunodeficiencies in children with refractory sinusitis are low levels of IgG3 and poor humoral antibody response to pneumococcal Ag 7. Some patients with refractory sinusitis may have normal immunoglobulin levels but fail to produce specific immunoglobulin when challenged (vaccine hyporesponsiveness).[35]

Immunodeficiencies can increase the incidence of infection with encapsulated organisms.[5] Immunodeficient children are sinusitis-prone. The most common immunodeficiencies in the sinusitis-prone child, in decreasing order of incidence, are common variable immunodeficiency, IgG subclass deficiency, selective antibody deficiency, IgA deficiency, C4 deficiency, X-linked agammaglobulinemia, ataxia-telangiectasia, and hyper-IgM syndrome.[3]

Bony anatomical abnormalities on computed tomography in children with sinusitis are similar to those in adults, except for a lower incidence of septal deformity.[27] Deformities disrupt laminar flow and cause anatomical obstruction at the ostiomeatal unit.[5] Although some reports indicate that chronic sinusitis in children is rarely associated with gross or obvious anatomical abnormalities,[22] various authors believe that chronic sinusitis usually occurs when there is an anatomical derangement.[14,27]

Viral upper respiratory tract infections, subtle anatomical abnormalities or variants, and possibly an immature local immune system or abnormal secretion of mucus may play a more significant role in the development of chronic sinusitis in children than previously suspected.[22] Proper movement of the mucous blanket is important in preventing infection and edema. The mucosa, the cilia, and the mucous blanket function as a unit. Chronic sinusitis is a result of disease in this functional unit.[3,5]

The mucous blanket is a double layer with a superficial viscid fluid layer and a serous layer underneath. The thick outer layer traps bacteria and debris. Cilia beat in the thin inner layer and just "touch" the outer layer; coordinated beating propels the thick layer. Cilia have two central microtubules surrounded by a ring of nine doublet microtubules connected by dynein arms. The cilia beat at a frequency of 1,000 cycles/minute.[3] Primary ciliary dyskinesia is a term used to describe diseases involving the cilia. One of these diseases is Kartagener's syndrome, which is an autosomal recessively transmitted disease involving the triad of situs inversus, bronchitis with bronchiectasis, and sinusitis. Male patients may be infertile as a result of sperm immotility. The cilia of these patients lack the ATPase-containing dynein arms necessary for ciliary movement. Kartagener's syndrome (immotile cilia syndrome) is the most common congenital cause of abnormal ciliary function.[12] Ciliary transport defects such as those that occur with viral infections or primary ciliary dyskinesias (viral short-term, primary ciliary dyskinesias long-term) and thick secretions such as those that occur in cystic fibrosis lead to an ineffective mucous blanket, which then causes stasis.[5]

Cystic fibrosis is an autosomal recessive disease with widespread involvement of the exocrine glands. Failure to clear mucous secretions, a paucity of water in mucous secretions, and an elevated salt content of sweat, and other serous secretions are characteristics of cystic fibrosis. Five percent of the white population are carriers of the recessive gene. One in 2,000 infants is affected; thus, cystic fibrosis is the most common life-threatening genetic trait in the white population and a major cause of severe, chronic lung disease in children. The head and neck manifestations of cystic fibrosis are chronic nasal obstruction, nasal polyposis, or sinusitis. Up to 10% of children with chronic sinusitis in a busy tertiary care otolaryngology practice may have cystic fibrosis.[3] Nasal polyposis is unusual in pediatric sinusitis, except in patients with cystic fibrosis, in whom the incidence may range from 5% to 86%.[5,36]

ANATOMY, DEVELOPMENT, AND PATHOLOGY

The size and shape of sinuses and the nasal structures in children are different from those in adults, a difference that is very important for the surgeon[37]; each age has specific anatomical features.[38]

Development of Paranasal Sinuses

The ethmoid and maxillary sinuses are present at birth and are developed at 3 years of age. The sphenoid sinus is present at 3 years of age and is fully developed at 12 years of age; the frontal sinus is generally present by 8 years of age and fully developed at 12 years of age.[17] With increasing age, the size of the maxillary sinus and the height of the lateral nasal wall increase.[27]

The newborn has very bulky turbinates; the bulla, uncinate process, and hiatus are present and their location is consistent, and the anterior and posterior ethmoid cells are almost completely developed in number but not in size. Most neonates have a superior turbinate. The maxillary sinus is spherical or pyramidal in shape; the sphenoid sinus is not developed in most cases, but the ostium is sometimes identifiable in neonates. The turbinates constrict all meatuses so that they are not a part of the respiratory cavity. The newborn breathes through a common nasal meatus. Because of this, moderate mucosal swelling causes severe nasal obstruction in the neonatal period.[37] Paired ethmoid cells are present at birth but are not easily visualized radiographically.[12] The surgical landmarks that are well developed and constant findings in the newborn are the uncinate process, ethmoid infundibulum, hiatus semilunaris, and the bulla ethmoidalis.[37]

Between the ages of 1 and 4 years, the ethmoid sinuses expand. The frontal sinus begins to pneumatize. The maxillary sinus expands rapidly, and the sphenoid pneumatization has begun. The superior turbinate is subject to involution.[37] The width of the anterior ethmoid doubles linearly from a mean of 0.39 cm between age 1 and 2 years to 0.79 cm at age 16 years. The width of the posterior ethmoid doubles linearly during this age range from 0.48 to 1.10 cm.[39]

Between the ages of 4 and 8 years, the frontal sinus expands laterally and medially. The maxillary sinus has expanded laterally past the infraorbital canal and inferiorly to the middle of the inferior meatus. Development is slow. Development of the ethmoid sinus is slower than that of the maxillary and frontal dinuses. During this period, injury to teeth from surgery is highly possible; interventions such as Caldwell-Luc, inferior meatal antrostomy, antral irrigation, fenestrations, and other inferior meatal procedures are hazardous and should be avoided because the only spongious bone lateral to the floor of the nose is here.[40] The lateral wall may also be easily injured because of the short medial-to-lateral distance. Fractures of the inferior turbinate may lead to chronic sinusitis.[38] Growth disturbances may occur after Caldwell-Luc procedures.[41] Also during this period, uncinate removal may lead to penetration of the lamina papyracea. Middle meatal antrostomies are dangerous also. The orbit may be penetrated accidentally as a result of the high attachment of the inferior turbinate.[37]

The infundibular length is linearly increased, but the width remains fairly constant at 0.2 cm throughout childhood into adolescence.[39]

From ages 8 to 12 years, there is almost complete development. The anatomy has reached adult proportions. The development of the choanae has finished. The maxillary sinus has reached the level of the floor of the nose, lateral to molar teeth, and medial to the nasolacrimal duct. The sphenoid sinus has reached its permanent size but not shape. Pneumatization accelerates again. The inferior meatus becomes part of the respiratory cavity. Connective tissue between ethmoid cells disappears, and the development is complete. Sinus proportions become similar to those of adults.

The development of the sinuses is directly linked to skull development and dentition. The size ratio between the ethmoid and maxillary sinuses is 2:1 in children, but 4:5 in adults.[42]

Developmental variants are most common with the frontal sinuses.[6] In a study assessing the effect of sinus disease on sinus development, no difference was found in the average size of the maxillary sinus between severe and mild disease groups. Growth of the maxillary sinus did not seem to be impaired by extensive or chronic disease, unlike the temporal bone; but, as the authors expressed, the children were not compared with normal controls.[27]

The most common pathophysiologic process leading to sinusitis is obstruction of the osteomeatal complex. This is the region of the middle meatus where the pathway of mucociliary flow converges from the maxillary, ethmoid, and frontal sinuses. It consists of the infundibulum, hiatus semilunaris, frontal recess, anterior ethmoid cells, ethmoid bulla, and the anterior wall of the middle turbinate. Conditions in the frontal and maxillary sinuses depend largely on the physiologic state of the anterior ethmoid sinuses. Therefore, improving drainage in this area often restores normal physiologic function to all three sinuses.[5,11,13] In the event of obstruction, a pathologic environment may develop as stagnant mucosa serves as a medium for bacterial overgrowth.[13] Tissue congestion worsens as the immune system responds to infection. The sinus cavity develops an acidic pH,[43] and anaerobic conditions evolve.[44] Anaerobes may thus emerge as important pathogens.[45–47] Eventually the mucosal surface, including cilia, is damaged, and ineffective mucociliary clearance further promotes chronic sinusitis. Obstruction of the sinus ostium leads to the development of negative intrasinus pressure due to resorbtion of air within the sinus cavity. If the patient blows the nose or sneezes, the obstruction is overcome, and an influx of bacteria from the nose into the sinus may occur.[12] When the ostia become obstructed, a vicious cycle of ciliary dysfunction, retention of secretions, obstruction of lymph drainage, edema, and mucosal hyperplasia develops and may at some point become irreversible disease.[3] Although it is clear that obstruction of the osteomeatal complex in children is *a* factor, it is not clear whether the obstruction is *the* primary cause of chronic or recurrent sinusitis in children.[3]

MICROBIOLOGY

Reported results regarding the bacteriology of sinusitis are variable and reflect the accuracy of the methods used to identify the pathogen. In acute and subacute sinusitis, anaerobes are uncommon,[7,48] whereas anaerobes should be suspected when protracted symptoms or symptoms requiring surgery are present.[2,45] Most studies imply that anaerobes do not play a significant role in acute sinusitis. Anaerobes are the most common bacteria in chronic sinusitis.[16,45,49,50]

Pathogens in acute sinusitis include *Streptococcus pneumoniae*, 30%; *Haemophilus influenzae*, 20%; and *Moraxella catarrhalis*, 20%.[2,17] In a study from Pittsburgh, 75% of *M. catarrhalis* organisms and 30% of *H. influenzae* organisms from cultures of sinus aspirates were β-lactamase-producing.[2] Another group reported β-lactamase-positive organisms in 25% of cultures of sinus aspirates in subacute maxillary sinusitis.[14] Studies indicating the emergence of resistant pneumococci are stressing the importance of taking appropriate cultures. There is some controversy over the use of nasal cultures, but many investigators believe that even cultures of the nasal discharge may be of value.[30]

H. influenzae organisms have a predilection for inhabiting virally damaged mucosa.[30] An experimental study showed that non-typeable *H. influenzae* organisms were associated only with mucous and structurally damaged cells; the bacteria were not associated with normal respiratory epithelium.[51]

Aerobic α-hemolytic *Streptococcus*, *Staphylococcus aureus*, *H. influenzae*, anaerobic *Bacteroides* species, and *Fusobacterium* species are reported in chronic sinusitis.[17] Muntz and Lusk[50] cultured the contents of 204 ethmoid bullae in chronic sinusitis and found mostly α-hemolytic *Streptococcus* and *S. aureus* organisms, which are the "normal" colonizing organisms of the nasal cavities.

Sinusitis in immunosuppressed patients may be associated with fungal infections such as *Aspergillus* species, *Rhizopus* species, and *Fusarium* species in cultures.[5,17] In one study, 90% of the cultures were positive; 50% contained more than one bacterial species, and 30% of the cultures contained anaerobes. These rates are all higher than those in nonimmunodeficient patients.[52]

Sinusitis in patients with cystic fibrosis was mostly associated with *Pseudomonas aeruginosa* and *S. aureus*.[5,17] Patients with cystic fibrosis have 100%

"sinus disease"; all patients with cystic fibrosis in a recent study had abnormal plain films.[53]

SIGNS, SYMPTOMS, AND PRESENTATION

Sinusitis is a dynamic disease with fluctuation in the severity of signs and symptoms.[54] Sinusitis rarely threatens life, but it causes considerable morbidity. In children, it frequently is not recognized or treated appropriately because many physicians believe or have been taught that the paranasal sinuses of the young child are not sufficiently developed.[6] Children with unrecognized chronic sinusitis are frequently referred for an allergy evaluation.[22,55,56]

Acute sinusitis presents in two ways. The less common presentation is a cold that is more severe than usual with a temperature of 39°C or higher, purulent rhinorrhea, and facial pain. The more frequent presentation is a prolonged cold with cough and nasal discharge persisting for more than 10 days; in this case, it is not the severity but the persistence of the symptoms that calls for attention.[1,7,57] Generalized malaise may be a symptom of sinusitis.[12] Periorbital swelling is an important finding and is most common in the morning; facial discomfort and a headache over and behind the eyes may be reported by the older child.[1] On the history obtained from parents, obstruction is frequently referred to as "congestion," "being stuffy," "mouth breathing," or "sinus."[3]

In general, symptoms and signs are not specific in pediatric sinusitis.[5] Especially in infants, irritability may be the only symptom. This may be due to the combined effect of a shallow sinus and a wider ostium in pediatric sinusitis, which prevents the occurrence of pressure symptoms in young children.[4,6,24] Older children have more defining symptoms such as purulent rhinorrhea, cough, nasal congestion, and chronic serous otitis media.[1,5,11,58] Headache and facial tenderness are uncommon in pediatric sinusitis.[4] Coughing is not diagnostic, but it is more common in chronic sinusitis.[3] Sinusitis is the second most common cause of chronic cough in children.[59] Purulent nasal discharge is almost universally present in children with acute and chronic sinusitis but is not characteristic in adults.[1,3] Viral upper respiratory tract infections also cause rhinorrhea, which may be purulent. A clinical diagnosis of sinusitis can be made when purulent drainage persists for more than 14 days.[17] In one study, the types of cough and nasal discharge were independent of the diagnosis; the nasal discharge was either thin and milky or thick and purulent, and the cough was either dry or associated with sputum production.[11] Van der Veken et al.[21] found that the prevalence of sinus disease was 64% in children with chronic rhinorrhea, nasal congestion, and cough.

Drainage or irritation of the upper lip due to purulent nasal discharge may be the presenting sign of chronic sinusitis.[3] Constant nasal discharge or drip that causes nasopharyngitis[1] and chronic persistent cough prompt parents to seek medical evaluation for their children.[3] Night cough is more common than day cough in chronic sinusitis, and sleep is frequently disrupted. Coughing in the morning just after awakening may be so severe that it results in emesis due to sinopulmonary reflex or thick postnasal drip.[3] Disease presenting with cough as the chief complaint (frequent viral upper respiratory tract infections, cough variant asthma, bronchitis, pneumonia, allergy) should be considered in the differential diagnosis of sinusitis.[59] Ocular "shiners" (suborbital venous congestion) and recurrent acute otitis media are found in 29% to 50% of patients with chronic sinusitis.[6] In one study, information on halitosis could be gained only by specifically asking.[3,9] Cervical lymphadenitis is not common in acute or chronic sinusitis.[3] Although rare, erythema of the tissue over the sinus is a sign of complicated sinusitis.[3] Complications of sinusitis are more common in infants than in older children.

Chronic sinusitis often is actually recurrent sinusitis. Recurrence is almost the norm in the otitis-sinusitis-prone child.[30] If the interval since the last sinusitis is less than 1 month, incompletely treated disease should be suspected. Three episodes in 6 months or four or five episodes in 12 months should lead to a thorough clinical evaluation.[1]

COMPLICATIONS

Patients with asthma or cystic fibrosis may have worsening of their disease during the course of sinusitis. Immunocompromised patients may have complicated sinusitis with unusual organisms, also resulting in dissemination of infection to other organ systems.[60]

Common sites of complications are the orbital and intracranial regions (Table 19–3). Infections that involve the orbit arise primarily in the ethmoid sinuses. Periorbital cellulitis is the most common complication of sinusitis in children.[17,60,61] Orbital infection results either from direct extension of a sinus infection through the

**Table 19–3   Complications of Sinusitis
in the Pediatric Age**

Complications	
Orbital	Stage 1: Periorbital cellulitis
	Stage 2: Orbital cellulitis
	Stage 3: Subperiosteal abscess
	Stage 4: Orbital abscess
	Stage 5: Cavernous sinus thrombosis
Intracranial	Meningitis
	Epidural abscess
	Subdural abscess
	Cavernous sinus thrombosis
	Cerebral abscess
Pulmonary	Bronchitis
	Asthma
	Cystic fibrosis
Other	Mucocele
	Osteomyelitis

Modified from Gurucharri MJ, Lazar RH, Younis RT: Current management and treatment of complications of sinusitis in children. *Ear Nose Throat* 1991; 70:107–112.

lamina papyracea or, less commonly, from local thrombophlebitis. Progression of orbital infection caused by sinusitis may include *periorbital cellulitis* (inflammation of the eyelid and conjunctiva), *periorbital abscess* (abscess formation in the subperiostal space), *orbital cellulitis* (spread of infection through the orbital septum), and *orbital abscess* (abscess formation within the orbital system: the globe becomes fixed and visual acuity diminishes).

Ophthalmologic examination is essential to assess visual status and to exclude concurrent problems in patients with signs and symptoms of orbital and periorbital inflammation. The cornerstone of diagnosis is high-resolution computed tomography with close-cuts to the orbit.[60] Any child with sinusitis and proptosis, ophthalmoplegia, or decreased visual acuity should have computed tomography of the sinuses with orbital detail to distinguish orbital cellulitis from periorbital (subperiosteal) abscess. Both cause proptosis and limited ocular movements. Evidence of abscess on computed tomography or progressive orbital findings after initial antibiotic treatment are indications for orbital exploration and drainage with external ethmoidectomy and orbital decompression.[17] Patients with orbital cellulitis or with orbital or periorbital abscess need to be hospitalized and treated with intravenously administered antibiotics. Initial antibiotic coverage should be broad-spectrum and effective against aerobic and anaerobic bacteria. Nafcillin, metronidazole, and ceftriaxone are common initial choices.[17] If management is inadequate, blindness may occur from occlusion of the central retinal artery, optic neuritis, corneal ulceration, or panophthalmitis. Further spread causes cavernous sinus thrombosis with sepsis and multiple cranial nerve involvement.[17] Most intracranial infections originate in the frontal sinus, and the spread is through direct extension along anatomical pathways, communicating veins, retrograde thrombophlebitis, or direct inoculation. Meningitis, epidural abscess, subdural empyema, cavernous sinus thrombosis, and cerebral abscess may occur.[17,60] Patients with central nervous system complications also have a high incidence of anaerobic organisms.[17] Because the frontal lobe is the most commonly affected area, subtle affective, personality, and behavioral changes may be the only findings. Altered neurologic function, altered consciousness, gait instability, and severe progressive headache may be the presenting symptoms.[17,60]

Long-standing sinus disease may cause a mucocele. Mucoceles may cause bony destruction as the result of local expansion, and the normal architecture of the bone in which expansion is taking place is destroyed. The treatment is surgical.[60] Another local complication is osteomyelitis, which requires long-term intravenous antibiotic therapy and occasionally concurrent surgical drainage of the infected sinus with debridement of the infected sinus.[60]

PHYSICAL DIAGNOSIS

The most commonly used basis for diagnosing sinusitis was clinical judgment in a recent mail survey conducted among pediatricians.[3] Peripheral smears and counts and erythrocyte sedimentation rate are usually not of clinical value. Transillumination is not reliable, and fiberoptic examination is not routinely recommended except for the highly skilled because of compliance problems in children.

Ultrasonography is specific but insensitive.[1,5,11,57] Magnetic resonance imaging is good in fungal sinusitis or sinus tumors.[5] A nasal smear with many neutrophils is considered confirmatory in sinusitis by some authors[4,22] but not by others.[62] Examination in the pediatric patient may be very difficult; endoscopes are frequently useless. The use of the otoscope to examine the anterior nasal cavity is helpful.[5] Examination shows boggy, edematous mucosa with significant obstruction that opens with vasoconstriction along with various amounts and type of nasal discharge.[3,11]

For cases in which the endoscope can be used, it aids in diagnosis, permitting objective evaluation of the nasal condition and its response to treatment. It enables the clinician to obtain representative cultures and tissue samples.[13,16] The histopathologic spectrum of chronic sinusitis is variable, and endoscopic examination enables the physician to detect and record the polypoid, fibrous, cystic, follicular, and papillary changes of the nasal and sinus mucosa and findings that are partially reversible with medical management despite intermittent remission of sinus symptoms.

Ethmoid culture and maxillary lavage are more effective for determining pathogens than nasal culture.[5] Middle meatal cultures correlate well with antral and ethmoid cultures, but nasopharyngeal cultures correlate poorly.[12,16] Intraoperative culture of antral mucosa seems to provide the most reliable findings of bacterial flora in chronic maxillary sinusitis.[47] In cases of persistent rhinorrhea, nasal cultures can be valuable in antibiotic selection,[30] although many believe that antibiotic selection directed by antral cultures alone is most efficient.[12]

IMAGING AND OTHER DIAGNOSTIC TESTING

It has been suggested that a high index of suspicion and screening sinus imaging (such as Waters view), especially between 2 and 10 years of age, are necessary for the diagnosis of pediatric sinusitis. The rationale is that the Waters view is easy to obtain and inexpensive, and if strict criteria are used (opacification, air-fluid level, mucosal thickness filling at least 50% of antrum), then the false-positive rate will decrease (but the high false-negative rate will remain). Many authors believe that clinical symptoms are not acceptably sensitive for differentiating sinusitis from allergic symptoms.[22] Others find the value of plain sinus radiography questionable because of the poor correlation with ethmoid disease and underestimation or overestimation of the sinus involvement. Correlations between total opacification and air-fluid levels in the maxillary sinuses are found on plain radiography, but the findings in the ethmoid sinuses are most frequently misinterpreted in chronic sinusitis. Caldwell views fail to localize ethmoid disease, and lateral films are of little use in children younger than 4 years because they frequently overread sphenoid sinus opacification.[5,54,63]

Clinical findings that correlate well with positive radiographs are rhinorrhea and copious purulent secretion along the nasal floor. Headache, nasal mucosal edema, and color of mucosa do not correlate.[12,64,65] Children younger than 1 year who cry during evaluation, irrespective of the condition of the sinus, may have abnormal sinus radiographs because of the pooling of tears within the sinus. Also, redundant maxillary sinus mucosa is present before 1 year of age and is an alternative reason for abnormal sinus radiographs.[66] After age 2 years, plain films of the maxillary sinuses are much more reliable.[66]

There has been a consensus among many physicians, however, that plain film imaging studies are not universally necessary for the diagnosis of sinus disease; instead, computed tomography (CT) is recommended to ascertain the extent of disease in patients who have chronic or recurrent disease, particularly before surgery.[4] CT detects sinusitis in 40% of cases in which sinus radiographs are normal.[67] It offers a more precise evaluation of the extent of the disease than nasal endoscopy,[8] shows areas of residual disease and anatomic abnormalities, and guides therapeutic intervention.[27] The correlation between plain radiographs and CT scans is poor; 40% to 46% of patients have a normal plain film and abnormal CT, and 36% have abnormal sinus films without a corresponding positive finding on CT.[21,63,67,68] Even CT may underestimate the extent of disease; CT should still be interpreted within the context of the history and clinical findings.[5] It should also be kept in mind that complete resolution of radiographic changes after an acute episode of sinusitis may take several months.[69] The degree of abnormality of radiographic findings is not well established.[22]

The type of CT performed should be high-resolution. Coronal cuts, 4-mm slices,[5,22] with both soft tissue and bone window images should be obtained to prevent false positive and false negative reading.[22] According to some authors, CT should include 3-mm axial cuts,[5] but this advice is not agreed on because the anatomical abnormalities are not easily recognized on axial scans and comparison with coronal scans is difficult.[27] The popular method of CT coronal scanning is as follows:[9] the patient is prone with the head hyperextended on the scanner bed. No intravenous contrast agent is used. A lateral computed radiograph is obtained, and the gantry is aligned perpendicular to the infraorbital line. Scanning is extended from the anterior frontal sinus to the posterior sphenoid sinus at 4-mm intervals. Scanner algorithms are chosen to best illustrate the soft tissue. Low-resolution CT scans, 5- to 10-mm slice width, and studies of soft tissue window alone[70] have many false positive readings and cannot classify the degree of abnormality of the radiographic findings. In children, sedation or anesthesia may be required to obtain adequate CT scans.

Many authors stress that a full medical regimen should be used in the workup before CT is performed[5] and CT *guides* therapeutic intervention only; surgery *must* be based on clinical judgment, and coronal CT alone should not serve as the basis for intervention. When obtained, CT should be used to guide the endoscopist to the site of disease to avoid complications.[71]

According to radiographic studies, the most commonly involved sinuses, in decreasing order of frequency, are the maxillary and anterior ethmoid, posterior ethmoid and frontal, and sphenoid sinus.[27] Because of the developmental characteristics, sphenoid and frontal sinuses may become infected between 8 and 18 years of age; maxillary and ethmoid sites are more commonly involved in children.[14] In a study of the incidence of sinus abnormality on CT scans in children,[5] children with allergy had a similar risk of having sinusitis as nonallergic children.

The most common anatomical abnormalities in pediatric sinusitis on coronal CT scans are the following: concha bullosa, Haller cells, septal deflection, paradoxical middle turbinate, atelectatic maxillary sinus, prominent ethmoid bulla, bilateral erosion of the uncinate process, and increased attenuation of soft tissue in the maxillary sinus.[27] The radiographic incidence of anatomical abnormalities varied from 4.2% to 19% for concha bullosa, 18% to 82% for Haller cells, and 13% for septal deformity.[22,27,39,72]

Patients with cystic fibrosis show the characteristic features of medial displacement of the lateral nasal wall in the middle meatus and demineralization of the uncinate process, creating the appearance of a maxillary sinus mucocele.[27]

In 10 of 260 patients who underwent surgical intervention on the basis of clinical findings without CT findings, mucosal disease was found in all.[37,73] Despite this, CT evaluation must be done with caution because the incidence of bony or mucosal disease in paranasal sinuses of asymptomatic children may be as high as 50%.[9,74] Also, given the amount of damage to the nasal mucosa and submucosa which often occurs with viral infections, it would be surprising if it were not so.[30] The asymptomatic child with an incidental paranasal sinus finding on CT scan need not have further workup unless clinical symptoms and signs are elicited.[68] In one study, 41% of scans showed some mucosal thickening or opacification in at least one of the sinuses. No difference was noted between groups in regard to age, presence or absence of otitis media, or respiratory tract disease (except clinical sinusitis).[68] Until the age of 12 years, the presence of mucosal thickening or sinus opacification is a common finding, and some authors believe that there is no better than a 50–50 chance that this represents sinus infection.[74] The incidence of abnormal radiographic findings is significantly lower in the age group 13 to 17 years than in the age group 1 to 2 years, but this difference does not seem to have any particular clinical significance.[74] Rates of ethmoid sinus opacification decrease steadily with age. In the age group 3 to 4 years, 58% had this finding, whereas the rate was 10% for ages 13 to 14 years.[21] The finding of sinus opacification or mucosal thickening in all asymptomatic children is incidental and without clinical correlation, nor is it predictive of clinically significant sinus disease.

Ultrasonography is a specific but insensitive method of diagnosing sinus disease. Its use has not gained widespread acceptance.

For cases in which severe-appearing radiographic sinus disease is found incidentally, the patient should be followed up clinically. An exhaustive history should be taken initially, and follow-up visits should be scheduled.[68] If a patient is classified as sinusitis-prone, serum immunoglobulin levels for G, A, M, and E and IgG subclass levels should be measured. If the history suggests respiratory allergy, appropriate allergy skin tests or in vitro tests should be performed, especially in chronic or recurrent sinusitis.[3,5,11] In vitro tests for allergy may be particularly useful as screens and in young children. The combination of these tests will detect approximately 75% of the immunodeficient patients and virtually all allergic patients.

If no immunologic abnormalities are found in these initial studies, a blood sample should be obtained for diphtheria or tetanus antibody titers, total hemolytic component, C4 level, and a preimmunization pneumococcal antibody level. If patients are older than 6 years, one should wait for the results of the pneumococcal antibody titers to ensure that a child is not already immune (antibody levels more than 300 ng/mL) before the vaccine is administered (to prevent painful Arthus reactions at the site of inoculation of pneumococcal polysaccharide vaccine in immune patients). Samples should be drawn 3 to 4 weeks after immunization. Antibodies to pneumococcal polysaccharide type 3, 7, 9, and 14 are generally measured, and postimmunization levels should exceed 300 mg/mL or the designated protective level for the laboratory used. If patients have low levels of all immunoglobulins, B- and T-lymphocyte populations should be measured in peripheral blood to discriminate between X-linked agammaglobulinemia, in which B cells are lacking, and common variable immunodeficiency, in which B cells are usually present. Patients with transient hypogammaglobulinemia of infancy, who may also be panhypogammaglobulinemic, should have normal T- and B-cell populations. The studies will also detect disorders with deficiencies of T cells or T-cell subpopulations. Vigorous medical management and surgical intervention often fail if the patient is not simultaneously receiving therapy for the immunodeficiency or allergy.[3]

TREATMENT

When medical or surgical treatment of pediatric sinusitis is considered, it should be kept in mind that acute sinusitis has a spontaneous cure rate of 40%.[2,75] Safety is important during treatment of a condition with a spontaneous cure rate of 40%. It is also important to know that most studies of antibiotic efficacy involve 25 to 30 patients (relatively small numbers) and so therapeutic regimens may appear to have similar success rates. Demonstration of a 10% difference between any two treatments requires many hundreds of patients in controlled trials.[2] It is also possible for chronic sinusitis to occur on a noninfectious basis,[4] although this issue is controversial.[30]

The goals of therapy in sinusitis are to eradicate the infection, to reverse sinus obstruction, and to return effective mucociliary clearance.[13]

Systemic decongestants and antihistamines are not routinely used to treat sinusitis in nonallergic children because these agents dry the normal sinus secretions and may decrease mucociliary clearance.[17] However, they should be considered in symptomatic allergic children.

Amoxicillin-clavulanate potassium, cefuroxime axetil, and erythromycin-sulfisoxazole have the most comprehensive antibacterial spectra (Table 19–4). Amoxicilin is appropriate for patients with uncomplicated sinusitis in geographic areas in which the prevalence of β-lactamase-producing pathogens is less than 20%. Gram-positive anaerobic *Streptococcus* and *Staphylococcus* respond to penicillin, and gram-negative *Bacteroides* with β-lactamase respond to amoxicillin-clavulanate potassium. If a patient does not respond to amoxicillin, or in areas in which there is a high prevalence of β-lactamase-producing bacterial species, alternative antimicrobials include amoxicillin-clavulanate potassium, erythromycin-sulfisoxazole, trimethoprim-sulfamethoxazole, cefaclor, cefuroxime axetil, cefixime, loracarbef, and cefpodoxime proxetil. For children who are allergic to penicillin/amoxicillin, the most suitable choices are erythromycin-sulfisoxazole in young children and cefuroxime axetil, which is newly available as a suspension. Cefixime has to be reserved for patients who do not respond to amoxicillin because it is less active against gram-positive cocci such as *Streptococcus pneumoniae*.[12,17] This schedule of the initial choice of antibiotics is not shared by all authors because these agents—

Table 19–4 Antibiotics for the Treatment of Pediatric Sinusitis

DRUG	FORM	DOSE	SPECTRUM	SPECIFICATIONS
Amoxicillin (Amoxil) (Trimox)	Caps* Chew Susp	40 mg/kg/24 h tid Food does not interfere with absorption	*S. pneumonia* *H. influenzae* *M. catarrhalis* β-lactamase unstable	Inexpensive Superinfection, anaphylaxis, urticaria
Amoxicillin- clavulanate (Augmentin)	Tabs Chew Susp	40 mg/kg/24 h tid Food does not interfere with absorption	*S. pneumoniae* *H. influenzae* *M. catarrhalis* Anaerobes *Staphylococcus* β-lactamase stable	Broad spectrum Diarrhea Superinfection, anaphylaxis, urticaria
Cefaclor (Ceclor)	Caps Susp	40 mg/kg/24 h tid Better peak concentration on empty stomach, total absorption same	*S. pneumoniae*	*H. influenzae* and *M. catarrhalis* are newly resistant *Staphylococcus* resistance Infants older than 1 month Gastrointestinal upset, diarrhea, rash Serum sickness-like reaction
Cefixime (Suprax)	Tabs Susp	8 mg/kg/24 h qd or bid Faster maximal absorption when taken on empty stomach	Gram-negative organisms β-lactamase stable	Broad spectrum Not active against *Staphyloccus* and *Pneumococcus* Children older than 6 months Diarrhea, gastrointestinal upset, rash, drug fever
Cefprozil (Cefzil)	Tabs Susp	30 mg/kg/24 h bid	*S. pneumoniae* *H. influenzae* *M. catarrhalis*	*H. influenzae* sensitivity *Staphylococcus* resistant Children older than 6 months Superinfection, gastrointestinal upset, dizziness Elevated liver enzyme values
Cefpodoxime proxetil (Vantin)	Tabs Susp	10 mg/kg/24 h bid Take with food	*Staphylococcus* *Streptococcus* *M. catarrhalis* *H. influenzae* β-lactamase stability not proven	Broad spectrum Diarrhea, nausea, vomiting, abdominal pain *C. difficile* Children older than 6 months

Table 19–4   *Continued*

DRUG	FORM	DOSE	SPECTRUM	SPECIFICATIONS
Cefuroxime axetil (Ceftin)	Tabs Susp	20–30 mg/kg/24 h bid Absorption is enhanced when given with food	*Staphylococcus* β-lactamase stable	Broad spectrum Children older than 3 months Diarrhea, nausea, vaginitis, hepatotoxicity
Clarithromycin (Biaxin)	Tabs Susp	15 mg/kg/24 h bid Food does not interfere with absorption	*H. influenzae* *M. catarrhalis* *S. pneumoniae* β-lactamase stable	Children older than 6 months Diarrhea, vomiting, abdominal pain
Clindamycin (Cleocin)	Caps Susp Vial	15–40 mg/kg/24 h tid Take with full glass of water	*Staphylococcus* Anaerobes	Broad spectrum Poor *H. influenzae* coverage Pseudomembranous colitis, diarrhea, Gastrointestinal upset, rash For persistent pneumococci
Erythromycin ethylsuccinate-sulfisoxazole (Pediazole)	Susp	50/150 mg/kg/24 h qid Food does not interfere with absorption	Staphylococcus	Broad spectrum Allergic reactions Increased theophylline and phenytoin levels Children older than 2 months Blood dyscrasias, hepatic or renal toxicity, crystalluria
Loracarbef (Lorabid)	Caps Susp	30 mg/kg/24 h bid Take on empty stomach	*Staphylococcus* Anaerobes β-lactamase stable	Children older than 6 months Gastrointestinal upset, rash, headache Weak against *H. influenzae*
Nafcillin (Unipen) (Nafcil)	Caps Soln Vial	25–50 mg/kg/24 h qid Poor oral absorption	Penicillinase-producing *Staphylococcus*	Superinfection, anaphylaxis, urticaria, gastrointestinal upset
Trimethoprim-sulphamethoxazole (Bactrim, Septra)	Tabs Susp Vial	8/40 TMP/SMX mg/kg/24 h bid Take on empty stomach	*S. pneumoniae* *H. influenzae* *M. catarrhalis* β-lactamase unstable	Inexpensive Group A streptococci not covered Sulfa hypersensitivity, blood dyscrasias Megaloblastic anemias, hepatic or renal toxicity Infants older than 2 months

Generic names followed by brand names in parentheses.

amoxicillin-clavulanate potassium, erythromycin-sulfisoxazole, and cefaclor—are *not* the drugs of choice for any of the above-mentioned organisms. *Haemophilus influenzae*, in particular, can persist despite these agents, possibly because of new bacteria at play.[30]

Amoxicillin has replaced ampicillin because it is twice as well absorbed, has a longer half-life, can be administered three times a day, is relatively inexpensive, and is safe. Its susceptibility to the action of β-lactamases is overcome by the introduction of amoxicillin-clavulanate combinations. Erythromycin cannot be used alone because of its ineffectiveness against *H. influenzae*.[2] Trimethoprim-sulfamethoxazole is inexpensive, but sulfa hypersensitivity is a potentially serious problem and group A streptococci are also not covered by sulfa combinations.[2,76]

First-generation cephalosporins lack activity against *H. influenzae* and should be avoided; cefaclor (second generation) is susceptible to β-lactamases from *Moraxella catarrhalis* and *H. influenzae*. Moreover, it is associated with a 1% incidence of serum sickness-like reaction in children who are given multiple courses of the drug.[2,77]

Cefuroxime axetil, a second-generation cephalosporin, has a more expanded spectrum than amoxicillin, and is resistant to β-lactamases. It is available in suspension form; gastrointestinal toxicity is similar to that with amoxicillin-clavulanate.[2]

Cefixime is a third-generation cephalosporin, can be used once daily, and is effective against β-lactamase-producing bacteria such as *H. influenzae* and *M. catarrhalis*,[2,78] but it is not effective against gram-positive cocci.[30]

Cefpodoxime proxetil is a newly introduced cephalosporin that has no proven effect on β-lactamase-producing strains of *H. influenzae*.

Loracarbef[17] has significant anaerobic coverage but, like cefprozil, is not as effective against *H. influenzae*.[30]

Clarithromycin is a macrolide that has β-lactamase stability and is also available in liquid form.

The empiric therapy of previously treated pediatric rhinosinusitis poses a more difficult problem but can be overcome by using a schedule based on knowledge of the antimicrobial effectiveness of various drugs.[30]

There is substantial variation among authors in regard to the duration of treatment, an issue that has not been studied systematically. Some use antibiotic treatment for acute sinusitis for at least 14 days,[17] whereas others, stressing the fact that sinusitis is a mucosal disease, advise a 7- to 10-day course of the correct antibiotic,[30] indicating that if the antibiotic is not effective in 1 week, it will not be effective if used longer. Another approach is to treat acute sinusitis for 10 to 14 days and assess the response to treatment in 72 hours. If no response is seen in 72 hours, an alternative agent is selected.[2] If a slow improvement is found on the 10th day of therapy and the patient is still symptomatic, the course is extended for 1 more week.[2] One clinical approach can be applied as the rule of thumb: antibiotic therapy is extended 1 week beyond the time when symptoms have completely resolved. This approach can lead to complete eradication of all bacteria.[2,17] But, because of the natural course of the disease, one can expect reinfection with *new* organisms.[30] Fixed schedules such as a 3-week course of β-lactamase-resistant antibiotic plus topical steroids are used by some authors. Sometimes a short course of systemic steroids and a topical vasoconstrictor is added for 3 to 5 days in acute cases.[5]

Prophylactic antibiotics[24] have not gained uniform acceptance. Saline nasal douches and continued use of nasal steroids to prevent ostial occlusion from swelling are also controversial.

For the treatment of chronic sinusitis, the duration of medical therapy is generally longer, continued for 3 to 6 weeks,[17] with extensive medical treatment consisting of a course of at least 4 weeks with a β-lactamase-resistant antibiotic and intranasal steroids.[27] Persistent pneumococci can be treated with clindamycin, vancomycin, and even rifampin.[30]

Limited evidence suggests that daily ingestion of yogurt with active cultures of *acidophilus* may help preclude some of the diarrheal effects that occur with certain antibiotics and may decrease the incidence and severity of yeast infections related to prolonged use of antibiotics.[79,80]

The rationale of functional endoscopic sinus surgery, as advocated by Stammberger,[81] can be summarized as follows: "most paranasal sinus infections spread from the nose to the sinuses, recurring sinusitis probably results from a focus of infection within the sinuses which is secondary to insufficient outflow or obstruction of natural sinal ostia into the nose, the sites of obstruction or partial stenosis are the ethmoid infundibulum, at the entrance of the maxillary sinus or the frontal recess at the entrance to the frontal sinus."

Functional endoscopic sinus surgery is essentially surgery of the ostiomeatal complex with or without other added features. The technique frequently includes opening the complex and removing sinus disease with minimal manipulation of surrounding normal tissue; the pediatric form is a two-stage operation requiring follow-up nasal cleaning with the patient under general anesthesia.[11]

The surgical treatment of pediatric sinusitis is a very controversial issue and has many advocates as well as opponents. The opponents argue that an enlightened medical therapy is substantially more effective than surgery and is more rational. According to this approach, pediatric sinusitis is analogous to recurrent acute otitis media and is actually part of the same disease process. The picture is usually one of multiple respiratory tract infections, viral and bacterial, in children with exposure to other children (such as in day care centers). The surgical intervention with tubes in otitis media has no equivalent in sinusitis and some physicians believe that recommending surgery is the equivalent of suggesting a mastoidectomy for recurrent acute otitis media. Pediatric ethmoid surgery may also interfere with facial growth. The most common organism, *H. influenzae*, has a predilection for inhabiting virally damaged mucosa. Surgical drainage of the ethmoids does not seem likely to change that. Even gross radiologic disease, or extensive mucosal disease, has repeatedly been shown to be potentially reversible.[30,82] It seems to be a very dangerous approach that some pediatricians have been led to believe that an abnormal CT scan (one showing disease of the ostiomeatal complex) essentially translates into surgical disease, which may cause many unnecessary interventions.[30] The indications for surgery consist of persistent or recurrent symptoms; often, unabated rhinorrhea, failure of "maximal medical therapy, and an abnormal CT scan are not considered to bear scientific scrutiny.[30] Polyposis, complications of sinus disease, mucoceles, mucopyoceles, and retention cysts are not considered in the concept of the medical treatment range.[30,82]

Advocates of surgical treatment have a careful approach, which can vary between institutions. Young patients with a history of disease of less than 1 year are treated conservatively with minimal sinus surgery. Older patients with a history of disease of more than 1 year are candidates for functional endoscopic sinus surgery rather than minimal surgical intervention.[5] Minimal sinus surgery is described as inferior meatal antrostomy and antral lavage. Antral lavage does not seem to offer significant advantage over antibiotics alone but can be used to obtain a specimen for culture if medical treatment fails. Inferior meatal antrostomy also is ineffective, although patients with ciliary dyskinesia may benefit from nasal antral windows.[5,54] In patients younger than 4 yrs who have a significant adenotonsillar component, minimal sinus surgery can be used in combination with tonsillectomy or adenoidectomy,[5] although some find that tonsillectomy or adenoidectomy does not cause any improvement in sinusitis symptoms and should not be used simultaneously with functional endoscopic sinus an surgery.[9] A conservative approach dictates that surgery should be done in infants only in emergency orbital or cerebral disease, and acutely ill children should not have an operation.[9] According to this approach, the patient qualifies for surgery when medical therapy has failed, as determined by the pediatrician and the surgeon. Medical treatment is defined as multiple prolonged courses of broad-spectrum antibiotics, with consideration given to allergies, asthma, and immunodeficiencies.[9] Whenever possible, allergic patients should not have an operation during the season of their symptoms or when there is evidence that their disease is not under good control.[83] Localized mucosal disease seems to benefit from surgical intervention, whereas patients with mucosal disease originating from systemic causes are poor candidates for surgical intervention because the diseased mucosa must reline the surgical defect.[35] The success rate of intranasal ethmoidectomy in asthma patients was reported to be 50%, whereas in nonasthmatic patients the success rate was 88%.[43]

At surgery, care must be taken to preserve the natural anatomy of the middle turbinate.[84] Some authors recommend the use of special pediatric instruments,[3,9] whereas some do not encounter any difficulty with the use of adult instruments.[5] The overall success rate for functional endoscopic sinus surgery in children has been reported to be 80%,[11,58,73] which is similar to that in adults.[85,86] The rate of symptom relief with surgery was 85% for nasal obstruction, 86% for cough, 83% for nasal discharge, and 84% for headache in 260 children and 513 adults, as reported by Lazar et al.[73] In another study of children whose chief complaint was nasal obstruction, 81% were better after surgery. Nasal discharge improved in 88%, postnasal drip in 61%, chronic cough in 84%, halitosis in 75%, headaches in 96%, and behavioral and social problems in 94% of children.[9] Nineteen percent of the allergic patients did not require allergy treatment postoperatively. In patients with asthma, the average number of attacks decreased from 6.7 to 2.5 per month after surgery. Ninety-six percent had fewer or no attacks. Fifty-eight percent were asymptomatic, and 79% had a decrease in the number of emergency visits per year. Eighty-eight percent of the patients who remained symptomatic had less severe symptoms.[9] After surgery, missed school days, asthmatic symptoms, and antibiotic use diminished.[5]

Functional endoscopic sinus surgery is generally accepted to be a safe technique. The complication rate is the same as that with nonendoscopic techniques. In one study, synechiae, persistent or recurrent polyposis, and bleeding were the most frequent complications, and no major complications were encountered.[5] The most common findings during the second-stage endoscopy were adhesions and granulation formation.[11] Complications of the procedure are orbital ecchymosis, dacryocystorhinitis, severe ear pain, blindness, cerebrospinal fluid rhinorrhea, extraocular muscle injury, meningitis, and revision.[11]

Revision operation is done in 1 year, mostly because of synechiae between the middle turbinate and lateral nasal wall, which cause occlusion of the ostiomeatal unit. Persistent polyps of the frontal recess, adhesions, granulation tissue, and significant crusting are other indications for revision surgery.[5,11]

SUMMARY

The variations in the presentation of sinusitis and its signs and symptoms in the pediatric age group are poorly understood. Physicians vary in their understanding of sinus disease, and this difference leads to variations in the diagnosis of sinusitis. There is also considerable inconsistency in the recommendations concerning the method, duration, and timing of therapeutic intervention. Although the etiologic factors leading to the disease are widely discussed, assessment of these factors in clinical practice may fail to take advantage of the full range of possible causes. This in turn leads to excessive use of some therapeutic methods (such as surgery or prolonged courses of antibiotics) and underscores the importance of therapeutic interventions directed at the cause or simple watchful waiting. The natural course of pediatric sinusitis in association with related respiratory tract diseases also poses an important aspect of the disease process, which is another point of disagreement. Allergies and viral upper respiratory tract infections are among the most common predisposing factors of sinus disease.

REFERENCES

1. Fireman P: Diagnosis of sinusitis in children. *J Allergy Clin Immunol* 1992; 90:433–436.
2. Wald ER: Antimicrobial therapy of pediatric patients with sinusitis. *J Allergy Clin Immunol* 1992; 90:469–473.
3. Lusk RP (ed): *Pediatric Sinusitis*. New York, Raven Press, 1992.
4. Shapiro GG, Rachelevsky GS: Introduction and definition of sinusitis. *J Allergy Clin Immunol* 1992; 90:417–418.
5. Willner A, Lazar RH, Younis RT, Beckford NS: Sinusitis in children: current management. *Ear Nose Throat J* 1994; 73:485–491.
6. Rachelevsky GS, Katz RM, Siegel SC: Chronic sinusitis in the allergic child. *Pediatr Clin North Am* 1988; 35:1091–1101.
7. Wald ER, Reilly JS, Casselbrant M, et al: Treatment of acute maxillary sinusitis in childhood: a comparative study of amoxicillin and cefaclor. *J Pediatr* 1984; 104:297–302.
8. Friedmann W, Katsantonis GP: Staging systems for chronic sinus disease. *Ear Nose Throat J* 1994; 73:480–484.
9. Parsons DS, Phillips SE: Functional endoscopic surgery in children: a retrospective analysis of results. *Laryngoscope* 1994; 103:899–903.
10. Wald ER, Guerra N, Byers C: Upper respiratory tract infections in young children: duration of and frequency of complications. *Pediatrics* 1991; 87:129–133.
11. Lazar RH, Younis RT, Gross CW, et al: Pediatric functional endonasal sinus surgery: review of 210 patients. *Head Neck* 1992; 14:92–98.
12. Duplechain JK, Miller RH: Pediatric sinusitis: diagnosis and treatment with endoscopic techniques. *J La State Med Soc* 1994; 143:7–13.

13. Lanza DC, Kennedy DW: Nose and sinus mucosal inflammation and infection, including medical therapy. *Curr Opin Otolaryngol Head Neck Surg* 1994; 2:27–32.
14. Reilly JS: The sinusitis cycle. *Otolaryngol Head Neck Surg* 1990; 103:856–862.
15. Furukawa CT: The role of allergy in sinusitis in children. *J Allergy Clin Immunol* 1992; 90:515–517.
16. Orobello PW Jr, Park RI, Belcher LJ, et al: Microbiology of chronic sinusitis in children. *Arch Otolaryngol Head Neck Surg* 1991; 117:980–983.
17. Dunham ME: New light on sinusitis. *Contemp Pediatr* 1994; 11:102–117.
18. Fireman P: Allergic Rhinitis, in Bluestone CD, Stool SE, Scheetz MD (eds.): *Pediatric Otolaryngology*, ed. 2. Philadelphia, WB Saunders, 1990, pp 793–804.
19. Rachelevsky GS, Goldberg M, Katz RM, et al: Sinus disease in children with repiratory allergy. *J Allergy Clin Immunol* 1978; 61:310–314.
20. Rachelevsky GS: Chronic sinusitis: the disease of all ages (editorial). *Am J Dis Child* 1989; 143:886–888.
21. Van der Veken PJW, Clement PAR, Buisseret TH, et al: CT-scan study of the incidence of sinus involvement and nasal anatomic variations in 196 children. *Rhinology* 1990; 28:177–184.
22. Nguyen KL, Corbett ML, Garcia DP, et al: Chronic sinusitis among pediatric patients with chronic respiratory complaints. *J Allergy Clin Immunol* 1993; 92:824–830.
23. Pelikan Z, Pelikan-Filipek M: Role of nasal allergy in chronic maxillary sinusitis—diagnostic value of nasal challenge with allergen. *J Allergy Clin Immunol* 1990; 86:484–491.
24. Manning SC: Surgical management of sinus disease in children. *Ann Otol Rhinol Laryngol* 1992; 101 Suppl 155:42–45.
25. Phipatankul CS, Slavin RG: Bronchial asthma produced by paranasal sinusitis. *Arch Otolaryngol* 1974; 100:109–112.
26. Slavin RG, Cannon RE, Freidman WH, et al: Sinusitis and bronchial asthma. *J Allergy Clin Immunol* 1980; 66:250–257.
27. April MM, Zinreich SJ, Baroody FM, Naclerio RM: Coronal CT scan abnormalities in children with chronic sinusitis. *Laryngoscope* 1993; 103:985–990.
28. Slavin RG, Zilliox AP, Samuels LD: Is there such an entity as allergic sinusitis (abstract)? *J Allergy Clin Immunol* 1988; 81:284.
29. Hisamatsu K, Ganbo T, Nakazawa T, et al: Cytotoxicity of human eosinophil granule major basic protein to human nasal sinus mucosa in vitro. *J Allergy Clin Immunol* 1990; 86:52–63.
30. Poole MD: Pediatric sinusitis is not a surgical disease. *Ear Nose Throat J* 1992; 71:622–623.
31. Mygind N, Pedersen M, Nielsen MH: Primary and secondary ciliary dyskinesia. *Acta Otolaryngol (Stockh)* 1983; 95:688–694.
32. Wilson R, Sykes DA, Currie D, Cole PJ: Beat frequency of cilia from sites of purulent infection. *Thorax* 1986; 41:453–458.
33. Morell A, Skvaril F, Hitzig WH, Barandun S: IgG subclasses: development of the serum concentrations in "normal" infants and children. *J Pediatr* 1972; 80:960–964.
34. Schur PH, Rosen F, Norman ME: Immunoglobulin subclasses in normal children. *Pediatr Res* 1979; 13:181–183.
35. Shapiro GG, Virant FS, Furukawa CT, et al: Immunologic defects in patients with refractory sinusitis. *Pediatrics* 1991; 87:311–316.
36. Duplechain JK, White JA, Miller RH: Pediatric sinusitis: the role of endoscopic sinus surgery in cystic fibrosis and other forms of sinonasal disease. *Arch Otolaryngol Head Neck Surg* 1991; 117:422–426.
37. Wolf G, Anderhuber W, Kuhn F: Development of the paranasal sinuses in children: implications for paranasal sinus surgery. *Ann Otol Rhino Laryngol* 1993; 102:705–711.
38. Stammberger H, Zinreich SJ, Kopp W, et al: Surgical treatment of chronic recurrent sinusitis—the Caldwell-Luc versus a functional endoscopic technique. *HNO* 1987; 35:93–105.
39. Munat S, Riding M, Kirkpatrick D: Development of the osteomeatal unit in childhood. A radiological study. *J Otolaryngol* 1992; 21:307–314.
40. Peter K: Vergleichende Anatomie und Entwicklungsgeschichte der Nase, in Denker A, Kahler O (eds.): *Handbuch der Hals-Nasen-Ohrenheilkunde*. Berlin, Springer-Verlag, 1925, pp 184–221.
41. Mühler G: Sinusitis maxillaris bei Sauglingen und Kleinkindern. *Z Laryngol Rhinol Otol* 1971; 50:255–260.
42. Plenk H, Tschabitscher M: Entwicklung, Makro und Mikromorphologie der Kieferhohle. New York, Springer-Verlag, 1986.
43. Lawson W: The intranasal ethmoidectomy: an experience with 1,077 procedures. *Laryngoscope* 1991; 101:367–371.
44. Aust R, Drettner B: Oxygen tension in the human maxillary sinus under normal and pathological conditions. *Acta Otolaryngol (Stockh)* 1974; 78:264–269.
45. Brook I: Bacteriologic features of chronic sinusitis in children. *JAMA* 1981; 246:967–969.

46. Westrin KM, Norlander T, Stierna P, et al: Experimental maxillary sinusitis induced by *Bacteroides fragilis*. A bacteriological and histological study in rabbits. *Acta Otolaryngol (Stockh)* 1992; 112:107–114.
47. Su W-Y, Liu C, Hung S-Y, Tsai WF: Bacteriological study in chronic maxillary sinusitis. *Laryngoscope* 1983; 93:931–934.
48. Wald ER, Byers C, Guerra N, et al: Subacute sinusitis in children. *J Pediatr* 1989; 115:28–32.
49. Frederick J, Braude AI: Anaerobic infection of the paranasal sinuses. *N Engl J Med* 1974; 290:135–137.
50. Muntz HR, Lusk RP: Bacteriology of the ethmoid bullae in children with chronic sinusitis. *Arch Otol Head Neck Surg* 1991; 117:179–181.
51. Wilson R, Read R, Cole P: Interaction of *Haemophilus influenzae* with mucus, cilia, and respiratory epithelum. *J Infect Dis* 1992; 165 Suppl 1:S100–S102.
52. Lusk RP, Polmar SH, Muntz HR: Endoscopic ethmoidectomy and maxillary antrostomy in immunodeficient patients. *Arch Otolaryngol Head Neck Surg* 1991; 117:60–63.
53. Amodio JB, Berdon WE, Abramson S, Baker D: Cystic fibrosis in childhood: pulmonary, paranasal sinus, and skeletal manifestations. *Semin Roentgenol* 1987; 22:125–135.
54. Lusk RP, Lazar RH, Muntz HR: The diagnosis and treatment of recurrent and acute sinusitis in children. *Pediatr Clin North Am* 1989; 36:1411–1421.
55. Shapiro GG: The role of allergy in sinusitis. *Pediatr Infect Dis* 1985; 4 Suppl 6:S55–S59.
56. Richards W, Roth RM, Church JA: Underdiagnosis and undertreatment of chronic sinusitis in children. *Clin Pediatr* 1991; 30:88–92.
57. Wald ER, Milmoe GJ, Bowen A, et al: Acute maxillary sinusitis in children. *N Engl J Med* 1981; 304:749–754.
58. Lusk RP, Muntz HR: Endoscopic sinus surgery in children with chronic sinusitis: a pilot study. *Laryngoscope* 1990; 100:654–658.
59. Holinger LD: Chronic cough in infants and children. *Laryngoscope* 1986; 96:316–322.
60. Gurucharri MJ, Lazar RH, Younis RT: Current management and treatment of complications of sinusitis in children. *Ear Nose Throat J* 1991; 70:107–112.
61. Harrington PC: Complications of sinusitis. *Ear Nose Throat J* 1984; 63:163–171.
62. Zimmermann B, Stringer D, Feanny S, et al: Prevalence of abnormalities found by sinus x-rays in childhood asthma: lack of relation to severity of asthma. *J Allergy Clin Immunol* 1987; 80:268–273.
63. McAlister WH, Lusk R, Muntz HR: Comparison of plain radiographs and coronal CT scans in infants and children with sinusitis. *AJR* 1989; 153:1259–1264.
64. Shapiro GG: Sinusitis in children. *J Allergy Clin Immunol* 1988; 81:1025–1027.
65. Shapiro GG, Furukawa CT, Pierson WE, et al: Blinded comparison of maxillary sinus radiography and ultrasound for diagnosis of sinusitis. *J Allergy Clin Immunol* 1984; 77:59–64.
66. Caffey J: *Pediatric X-Ray Diagnosis*. Chicago, Year Book, 1972; pp 104–111.
67. Lazar RH, Younis RT, Parvey LS: Comparison of plain radiographs, coronal CT, and intraoperative findings in children with chronic sinusitis. *Otolaryngol Head Neck Surg* 1992; 107:29–34.
68. Lesserson JA, Kieserman SP, Finn DG: The radiographic incidence of chronic sinus disease in the pediatric population. *Laryngoscope* 1994; 104:159–166.
69. Leopold D: Pollution: the nose and sinuses. *Otolaryngol Head Neck Surg* 1992; 106:713–719.
70. Glasier CM, Ascher DP, Williams KD: Incidental paranasal sinus abnormalities on CT of children: clinical correlation. *AJNR* 1986; 7:861–864.
71. Zinreich SJ, Kennedy DW, Rosenbaum AE, et al: Paranasal sinuses; CT imaging requirements for endoscopic surgery. *Radiology* 1987; 163:769–775.
72. Bolger WE, Butzin CA, Parsons DS: Paranasal sinus bony anatomic variations and mucosal abnormalities: CT analysis for endoscopic sinus surgery. *Laryngoscope* 1991; 101:56–64.
73. Lazar RH, Younis RT, Long TE: Functional endonasal sinus surgery in adults and children. *Laryngoscope* 1993; 103:1–5.
74. Diament MJ, Senac MO Jr, Gilsanz V, et al: Prevalence of incidental paranasal sinus opacification in pediatric patients: a CT study. *J Comput Assist Tomogr* 1987; 11:426–431.
75. Wald ER, Chiponis D, Ledesma-Medina J: Comparative effectiveness of amoxicillin and amoxicillin-clavulanate potassium in acute paranasal sinus infections in children: a double-blind, placebo-controlled trial. *Pediatrics* 1986; 77:795–800.
76. Henderson FW, Gilligan PH, Wait K, Goff DA: Nasopharyngeal carriage of antibiotic-resistant pneumococci by children in group day care. *J Infect Dis* 1988; 157:256–263.
77. Levine LR: Quantitative comparison of adverse reactions to cefaclor vs. amoxicillin in a surveillance study. *Pediatr Infect Dis* 1985; 4:358–361.
78. Marchant CD, Shurin PA, Turcyzk VA, et al: A randomized controlled trial of cefaclor compared with trimethoprim-sulfamethoxazole for treatment of acute otitis medis. *J Pediatr* 1984; 105;633–638.

79. Black F, Einarsson K, Lidbeck A, et al: Effect of lactic acid producing bacteria on the human intestinal microflora during ampicillin treatment. *Scand J Infect Dis* 1991; 23:247–254.
80. Hilton E, Isenberg HD, Alperstein P, et al: Ingestion of yogurt containing *Lactobacillus acidophilus* as prophylaxis for candidal vaginitis. *Ann Intern Med* 1992; 116:353–357.
81. Stammberger H: Endoscopic endonasal surgery—concepts in treatment of recurring rhinosinusitis. Parts I and II. *Otolaryngol Head Neck Surg* 1986; 94:143–156.
82. Wigand ME: *Endoscopic Surgery of the Paranasal Sinuses and Anterior Skull Base.* New York, Thieme Medical Publishers, 1990.
83. Davis WE, Templer JW, Lamear WR, et al: Middle meatus antrostomy: patency rates and risk factors. *Otolaryngol Head Neck Surg* 1991; 104:467–472.
84. Messerklinger W: On the drainage of the normal frontal sinus of man. *Acta Otolaryngol* 1967; 63:176–181.
85. Schaefer SD, Manning S, Close LG: Endoscopic paranasal sinus surgery: indications and considerations. *Laryngoscope* 1989; 99:1–5.
86. Kennedy DW, Zinreich JS: Functional endoscopic surgery. *Adv Otolaryngol Head Neck Surg* 1989; 3:1–20.

Index

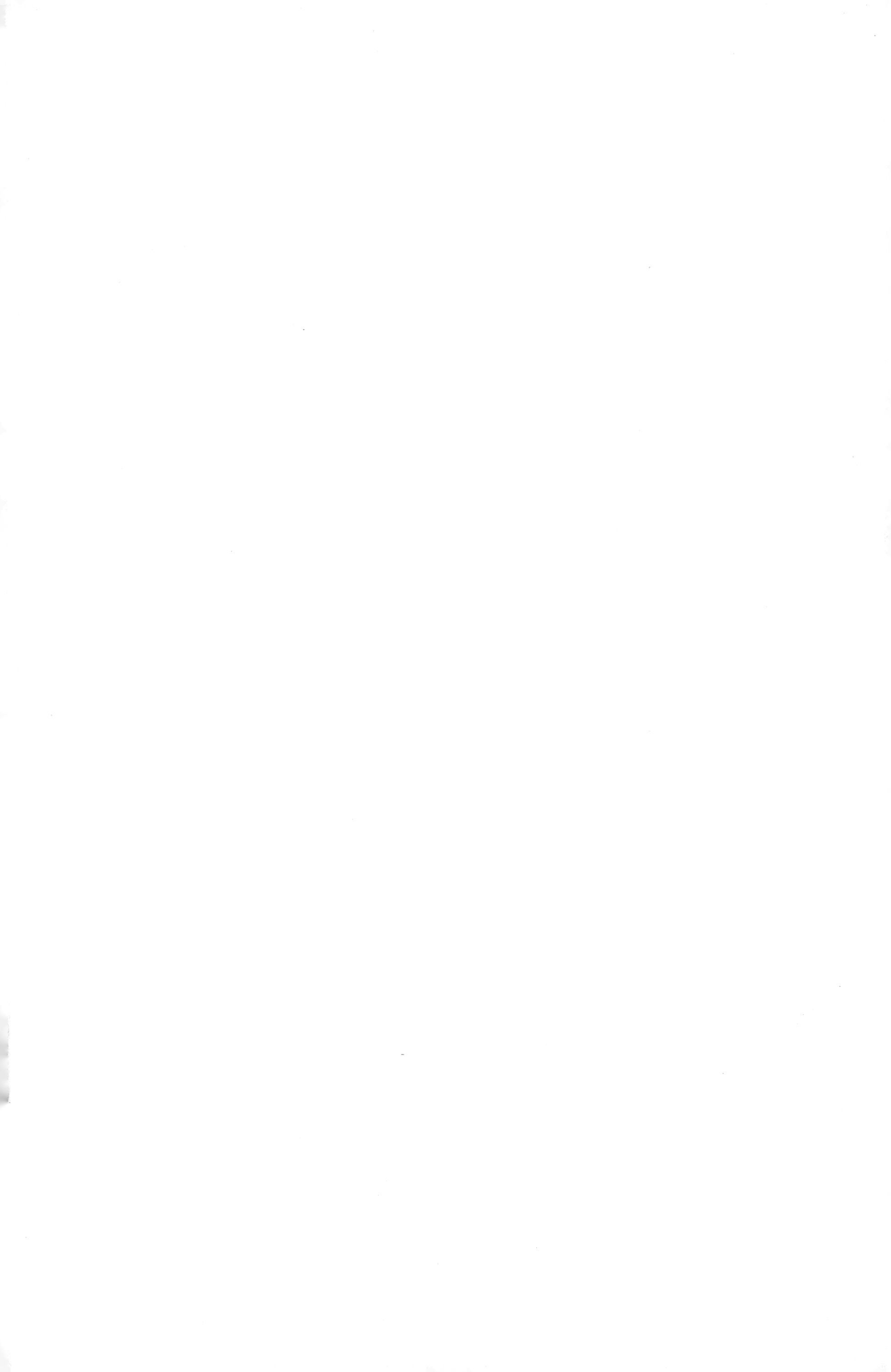